DIAGNOSIS AND RISK PREDICTION

OF PERIODONTAL DISEASES, VOL 3

THE AXELSSON SERIES
ON PREVENTIVE DENTISTRY

The world-renowned authority on preventive and community dentistry presents his life's work in this five-volume series of clinical atlases focusing on risk prediction of dental caries and periodontal disease and on needs-related preventive and maintenance programs.

Volume 1 An Introduction to Risk Prediction and Preventive Dentistry

Provides a general overview of current and future trends in risk prediction, control, and nonaggressive management of caries and periodontal disease; preventive dentistry methods and programs; and quality control.

Volume 2 Diagnosis and Risk Prediction of Dental Caries

Includes a comprehensive discussion of the etiology, pathogenesis, diagnosis, risk indicators and factors, individual risk profiles, and epidemiology of caries.

Volume 3 Diagnosis and Risk Prediction of Periodontal Diseases

Presents a comprehensive discussion of the etiology, pathogenesis, diagnosis, risk indicators and factors, individual risk profiles, and epidemiology of periodontal diseases. Considers periodontal diseases as a possible risk factor for systemic diseases and presents current and future trends in the management of periodontal diseases, including nonaggressive debridement and preservation of the root cementum.

Volume 4 Preventive Materials, Methods, and Programs

Discusses self-care and professional methods of mechanical and chemical plaque control, use of fluorides and fissure sealants, and integrated caries prevention. Addresses needs-related preventive programs based on risk prediction and computer-aided epidemiology analysis for quality control and outcome.

Volume 5 Nonaggressive Treatment, Arrest, and Control of Periodontal Diseases and Dental Caries

Details current and future trends in nonaggressive treatment methods that seek to preserve the root cementum; surgical versus nonsurgical periodontal therapy; repair and regeneration of periodontal support; management of furcation-involved teeth; restricted use of antibiotics; arrest of noncavitated enamel, dentin, and root caries lesions; nonaggressive mini-preparations; esthetic and hygienic aspects of restorations; and management of erosions. Focuses on needs-related maintenance programs to ensure the long-term success of treatment and to prevent recurrence of periodontal disease and dental caries.

DIAGNOSIS AND RISK PREDICTION
OF PERIODONTAL DISEASES, VOL 3

Per Axelsson, DDS, Odont Dr

Professor and Chairman
Department of Preventive Dentistry
Public Dental Health Service

Karlstad, Sweden

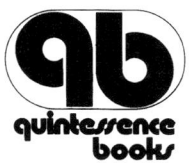

Quintessence Publishing Co, Inc
Chicago, Berlin, Tokyo, Copenhagen, London, Paris, Milan, Barcelona,
Istanbul, São Paulo, New Delhi, Moscow, Prague, and Warsaw

To my wife Ingrid, my daughter Eva, and my son Torbjörn

Library of Congress Cataloging-in-Publication Data

Axelsson, Per, D.D.S.
  Diagnosis and risk prediction of periodontal diseases / Per Axelsson.
    p. ; cm. — (Axelsson series on preventive dentistry ; v. 3)
Includes bibliographical references and index.
  ISBN 0-86715-363-6
  1. Periodontal disease—Diagnosis. 2. Periodontal disease—Risk
factors.
  [DNLM: 1. Periodontal Diseases. 2. Periodontal Diseases—etiology.
3. Risk Factors. WU 240 A969d 2002] I. Title.
  RK361 .A95 2002
  617.6'32—dc21

                                     2002001978

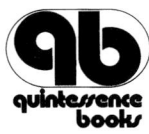

quintessence
books

© 2002 Quintessence Publishing Co, Inc

Quintessence Publishing Co, Inc
551 Kimberly Drive
Carol Stream, IL 60188
www.quintpub.com

Editor: Kathryn O'Malley
Production: Thomas Pricker

Printed in Slovakia

CONTENTS

PREFACE

The etiology of periodontal diseases is well understood, and we have now developed efficient methods for prevention, treatment, arrest, and control of these diseases. For example, over the last 10 years in County of Värmland, Sweden, large-scale implementation of our preventive programs has led to an increased number of remaining teeth in 65-year-old patients by more than 15% and a reduced loss of periodontal support by more than 20%, at the same time reducing the percentage who are edentulous from 17% to 7%. In addition, in a 15-year longitudinal adult study, we maintained the periodontal attachment level unaltered irrespective of age.

According to the principles of *lege artis*, all members of our profession are obliged to offer treatment based on the most current scientific and clinical knowledge available. As we now have entered the new millenium, we must therefore continue to concentrate our efforts on preventing, controlling, and arresting the development of dental caries and periodontal diseases. However, needs-related preventive and maintenance programs must be cost effective and should be based on information derived from comprehensive diagnoses, histories, and risk predictions at group, individual, and tooth-surface levels. For quality control and evaluation of such programs, computer-aided analytic epidemiology, using relevant variables, should be introduced.

The aim of this book, the third volume of a five-volume series of textbooks and atlases, is to give the reader updated knowledge about the etiology, modifying factors, risk evaluation, pathogenesis, diagnosis, and epidemiology of periodontal diseases, as well as the relationship between periodontal diseases and other diseases.

Sufficient knowledge about the above topics is the first prerequisite for efficient and needs-related prevention, treatment, arrest, and control of periodontal diseases. New materials and methods for prevention, nonaggressive treatment, arrest, and control of periodontal diseases are comprehensively discussed and illustrated in volumes 4 and 5.

In this book, detailed scientific backgrounds, well-illustrated guides to implementing the "state of art," and conclusions and future recommendations are provided for each topic addressed. Thus, the book is useful not only for dentists and dental hygienists, but also for undergraduate and postgraduate students.

In the chapter on etiology of periodontal diseases, the updated evidence-based role of nonspecific plaque formation rate, the specific periopathogenic microflora, and ecologic conditions, as well as new microbiologic tests such as the "checkerboard" DNA-DNA hybridization technology, are discussed.

New developments in the relationship between external (environmental) and internal (endogenous) risk indicators, risk factors, and prognostic risk factors, as well as principles for risk prediction and establishment of risk profiles as a tool for communication with the patient, are comprehensively discussed and illustrated. In particular, some genetic factors, in combination with smoking, are discussed in detail as the most important modifying risk factors.

New research on periodontal diseases as a possible risk indicator, risk factor, or prognostic risk factor for coronary heart diseases, stroke, infective endocarditis, pneumonia, preterm low birth weight, and poorly controlled diabetes is discussed. The new system for classification of periodontal diseases, which is used throughout this volume, is presented, and recent research on the pathogenesis of periodontal diseases is described step by step and is well-illustrated from clinical and cellular levels down to the molecular level.

In the chapter on diagnosis of periodontal diseases, techniques and validity of clinical probing of attachment loss versus radiographs are discussed and illustrated. New tools for computerized digital subtraction radiography, controlled-force probing, measurement of periodontal pocket temperature (fever) and gingivae fluid amount, and content of molecules related to active periodontal destruction are also discussed and illustrated.

Finally, the great importance of analytic epidemiology at population, group, individual, and tooth-surface levels for quality control, outcome of therapy, design, and evaluation of prevention and maintenance are discussed.

This project could not have been completed without the assistance and support of my family, friends, and colleagues. I offer my deepest thanks to my wife Ingrid, my daughter Eva, and my son Torbjörn and their families, as well as to all my other relatives and friends, for their patience and understanding throughout the last 5 years in which I have spent almost every night, weekend, and vacation preparing the material for these five volumes. I also wish to thank my wonderful staff at the Department of Preventive Dentistry, Public Dental Health Service, county of Värmland, for all their services, and particularly my assistant, Pia Hird, who typed most of my manuscript. I owe special thanks to Art Director Fredrik Persson, Dr Jörgen Paulander, and the Dumex Company for their excellent support with computer-aided illustrations and to Associate Professor Joan Bevenius for her work in checking my English manuscript.

I am very grateful to all my colleagues and friends around the world and to several publishers (Munksgaard International, The American Academy of Periodontology, S. Karger Medical and Scientific Publisher, FDI World Dental Press, and WHO Oral Health Unit) who have generously permitted me to use their illustrations (about 30% of the total). Last but not least, the excellent cooperation of the publisher is gratefully acknowledged.

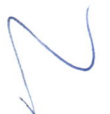

CHAPTER 1

ETIOLOGY OF PERIODONTAL DISEASES

Gingivitis and periodontitis are unquestionably caused by microorganisms; ie, both are infectious diseases. These microorganisms colonize the gingival region of the tooth surfaces, supragingivally as well as subgingivally, forming dentogingival plaque, a so-called biofilm. In diseased pockets, microorganisms also grow subgingivally, without attaching to the tooth surfaces, and may invade the periodontal tissues (Frank and Voegel, 1978; Listgarten, 1976; Saglie et al, 1982a, 1982b).

In 1965, Löe and coworkers conducted a pioneering study of experimental gingivitis in humans: When dental plaque was allowed to accumulate undisturbed, students with healthy gingiva developed clinical signs of gingivitis within 2 or 3 weeks; on resumption of oral hygiene, the inflammation subsided within a week. An initial gingival lesion develops within about 4 days of free plaque accumulation (Page and Schroeder, 1976), and subclinical signs of gingival inflammation appear, in the form of an exudate from the gingival sulcus (Egelberg, 1964). In a 6-week study in students, Lang and coworkers (1973) showed that if plaque was thoroughly removed at least every second day, no clinical signs of gingival inflammation appeared; with less frequent plaque removal, only every third or fourth day, gingivitis developed. Bosman and Powell (1977) induced experimental gingivitis in a group of students: With plaque removal only every third or fifth day, gingival inflammation persisted, whereas healing occurred within 7 to 10 days in the two groups who cleaned their teeth at least every second day.

These studies provided evidence that prevention of gingivitis should be based on plaque control: Thorough mechanical cleaning of all tooth surfaces every second day is more effective than daily cosmetic brushing of the buccal and lingual surfaces that are not at risk. Experimental animal studies have shown that untreated, plaque-induced gingivitis can eventually progress to periodontitis (Lindhe et al, 1975; Saxe et al, 1967). In humans, although gingivitis is very common, progressive periodontitis develops in only a minority of individuals and sites. At the First European Workshop on Periodontology (Lang and Karring, 1994), consensus was reached that periodontitis is always preceded by gingivitis. Prevention of gingivitis should also, therefore, prevent periodontitis (for details on the pathogenesis of gingivitis and periodontal diseases, see chapter 4).

Although there are more than 400 species of bacteria in the oral cavity, only a few have the ability to colonize a newly cleaned tooth surface. It is estimated that 1 mL of saliva contains about 200 million bacteria but that only 1 mm³ of dental plaque contains the same number of bacteria; ie, the density of bacteria is about 1,000 times higher in dental plaque than it is in saliva.

Current laboratory techniques allow culture of about 70% of the bacteria disclosed by microscopy in a sample from the gingival margin. There are several reasons why not all bacteria are detected (Moore, 1987). Laboratory conditions are not conducive to growth of some bacteria, particularly the gram-negative anaerobic motile subgingival microflora. Others may be killed by the methods used to disperse the bacterial samples. However, the new DNA probe technique allows detection of species that have not to date been successfully cultured.

Three different theories have been proposed for the etiology of periodontal diseases: the nonspecific plaque hypothesis, the ecological plaque hypothesis and the specific plaque hypothesis.

Since the aforementioned experimental gingivitis and periodontitis studies were conducted, the nonspecific plaque hypothesis has been most frequently and successfully applied for the prevention and control of gingivitis and periodontitis. It asserts that many of the microorganisms in the heterogenous mixture in the plaque (biofilm) could play a role in the development of gingivitis and periodontal diseases and that these diseases are a result of the overall interaction of the microflora with the host (Theilade, 1986). It also explains why, in longitudinal clinical studies, frequent mechanical removal or disruption of the biofilm by self-care, supplemented by needs-related professional mechanical toothcleaning (PMTC) and subgingival debridement, has been so successful in the prevention and control of gingivitis and periodontitis (Axelsson and Lindhe, 1977, 1981a, 1981b; Axelsson et al, 1991; Badersten et al, 1981, 1984a, 1984b, 1985a, 1985b, 1985c, 1985d, 1987a, 1987b; Lövdal et al, 1961; Söderholm, 1979; Suomi et al, 1971).

The recently introduced ecological plaque hypothesis (Marsh, 1994) proposes that a change in a key environmental factor (or factors) will trigger a shift in the balance of the resident plaque microflora and that this change might predispose a site to disease. The occurrence of potentially path-ogenic species as minor members of the resident plaque microflora would be consistent with this proposal. Under the conditions that prevail in health, these organisms would be only weakly competitive and might also be suppressed by intermicrobial antagonism, so that they would constitute only a small, clinically insignificant percentage of the plaque microflora. Microbial specificity in disease would be attributed to the fact that only certain species are competitive under the altered environmental conditions.

It is a basic tenet of microbial ecology that a major change to an ecosystem produces a corresponding disturbance in the stability of the resident microbial community. With respect to the etiology of periodontal diseases, this may be exemplified by the following sequence. Undisturbed gingival plaque gradually results in gingivitis: edema of the gingival margin (pseudopocket formation) and secretion of gingival crevicular fluid (GCF). The resultant improved nutritional conditions and lowered redox potential in the gingival sulcus favor subgingival growth of the gram-negative anaerobic microorganisms, including the most important periopathogens. The ecological plaque hypothesis explains why a successful method for treatment of periodontal diseases is surgical elimination of pockets, supported by excellent control of gingival plaque in the subsequent maintenance program (Axelsson and Lindhe, 1981b; Lindhe and Nyman, 1984; Nyman et al, 1975; Rosling et al, 1976a, 1976b; Westfelt et al, 1983).

The specific plaque hypothesis (Loesche, 1976) proposes that, of the diverse collection of microorganisms constituting the resident plaque microflora, only a very limited number are actively involved in causing disease. This hypothesis, however, does not explain cases in which disease is diagnosed in the apparent absence of the putative pathogens or those in which pathogens are present at sites with no evidence of disease.

At the 1996 American Academy of Periodontology Workshop, there was consensus that particularly *Porphyromonas gingivalis, Actinobacillus actinomycetemcomitans,* and *Bacteroides forsythus,* as well as *Prevotella intermedia* and *Treponema denticola,* should be considered true periopathogens, strongly correlated with the etiology of periodontal diseases (American Academy of Periodontology, 1996c). Both *P gingivalis* and *A actinomycetemcomitans* are regarded as exogenous, transmissible periopathogens and *B forsythus, P intermedia,* and *T denticola* as opportunistic. Several studies have shown a relationship between *A actinomycetemcomitans* and aggressive periodontitis in children and young adults. In a recent prospective study, periodontal pockets containing *B forsythus* exhibited seven times higher risk for further loss of periodontal attachment than did *B forsythus*–negative sites (Machtei et al, 1997). It has also been shown that *A actinomycetemcomitans* and *P gingivalis,* particularly, may invade the periodontal soft tissues. This may partly explain why diseased periodontal pockets treated by nonsurgical subgingival debridement sometimes fail to heal but may respond to a combination of mechanical removal of the subgingival biofilm and use of antibiotics (van Winkelhoff et al, 1992). The etiology of periodontal diseases is explained not by any one of these hypotheses alone, but by a combination of all three theories.

ORAL ENVIRONMENT

The oral cavity as macroenvironment

In some aspects, the oral cavity may be regarded as a single microbial ecosystem, or macroenvironment. The oral environment is dominated by the flow of saliva, at the rate of approximately 0.4 mL/min under resting conditions and 2.0 mL/min under stimulated conditions; the average flow rate during waking periods is 0.6 mL/min. Around 15% of the adult population has a stimulated flow rate of less than 0.7 mL/min, which may be related to medication with anticholinergic drugs, irradiation, or disease. The total daily secretion has been estimated to be 600 to 700 mL. The resting volume of saliva is approximately 7 mL and is replenished about 10 times per minute during waking hours. Salivary flow almost ceases during sleep. During sleep, the salivary flow rate may be as low as 0.25 mL per minute.

In addition to saliva, the oral fluid contains tissue fluid, originating predominantly from the gingival sulci or crevices. The volume of crevicular fluid is dependent on the health of the periodontal soft tissues.

The oral fluid is very complex in composition. It contains organic and inorganic components. The organic components consist of a variety of proteins, carbohydrates, enzymes, and so on. Each component plays an important role in controlling the oral environment. For example, secretion of immunoglobulin (sIgA), agglutinins, antimicrobial enzymes (lysozymes, lactoperoxidase, and lactoferrins), glycosyltransferase, and others will significantly influence the number and variety of oral microflora as well as the plaque formation rate (Axelsson, 1987, 1991).

Although saliva is not a good medium for supporting the growth of many bacteria, as stated earlier, 1 mL of whole saliva may contain more than 200 million microorganisms, representing more than 400 different species. Several periodontal pathogens can be cultured from saliva (Asikainen et al, 1991a; Petit et al, 1993; van Winkelhoff et al, 1988a). It is likely that organisms shed from intraoral reservoirs find transient residence in saliva. Investigation of untreated subjects with suppurating periodontitis revealed that *P gingivalis* and *P intermedia* could be detected in saliva at levels exceeding 106 cells/mL (van Winkelhoff et al, 1988a), implying that saliva facilitates intraoral spread of these organisms. This is supported by the observation that trypsin-like activity, a characteristic of *P gingivalis,* can be detected before treatment in the saliva of patients with periodontitis (Zambon et al, 1985).

It is also likely that microbes attached to desquamated epithelial cells spread via saliva to different tooth surfaces and typically colonize sheltered regions: interproximal spaces, gingival margins, and occlusal fissures (Saxton, 1975).

In addition, it is important to recognize that there are several major and minor compartments in the oral cavity, each constituting a separate microenvironment not easily affected by major events in the oral cavity. These environmental factors significantly influence the access and release of antimicrobial agents from different delivery systems. For example, suspensions of charcoal in water placed in the vestibule of one side of the mouth of an individual who is not talking or chewing will spread within about 5 minutes to the dorsum of the tongue and the hard palate on the same side of the mouth. However, no spread to the other side of the mouth occurs, even after prolonged conversation. If placed initially under the tongue, the charcoal moves so that the entire dorsum of the tongue will be covered within 1.5 minutes, but the hard palate on both sides will not be covered for at least 4 minutes (Jenkins and Krebsbach, 1985).

Thus, even the major subcompartments within the oral cavity, for example, the sublingual space and the vestibule, are not in immediate communication. There are also many discrete compartments within the oral cavity, such as the interproximal spaces, gingival crevices, gingival pockets, occlusal fissures, the papillae of the dorsum of the tongue, and the crypts and fissures of the tonsils, each of which creates a special microenviroment within the open system of the oral cavity as a whole.

All the surfaces of the oral cavity are colonized by microorganisms. Facultatively anaerobic streptococci constitute an essential part of the microflora that constantly colonize the mucous membranes and the teeth. Microorganisms are regularly swallowed with saliva and the amount within the oral cavity fluctuates, simply because the microbial deposits building up on mucous membranes and in particular on tooth surfaces grow and multiply, and thus provide a reservoir for the oral environment. Fluctuations occur during sleeping and waking hours and as a result of such activities as eating, drinking, and oral hygiene procedures.

The microflora in mixed saliva comprises mainly microorganisms shed from the oral surfaces and to some extent reflects the gross composition of the microbial deposits on the various oral surfaces.

Specific environments for microbial deposits

A specific area that supports a bacterial flora is termed a *habitat.* The flora of a habitat develop through a series of stages, collectively called *colonization.* Colonization is a complex process, because it involves not only interaction between bacteria and their environment but also interaction among bacteria.

The first important aspect of colonization of a habitat by bacteria is one of access. Because the organisms must be able to enter the habitat, there must be a means of transmission from one habitat to another. For example, mothers can serve as reservoirs for oral bacteria that colonize their children's mouths, and, within a single host, bacterial reservoirs can aid the survival of the organism. In the human mouth, the tongue and tonsils as well as the oral mucosa may serve as reservoirs for bacteria that, given the right conditions, may colonize periodontal pockets; several investigators have observed that black-pigmented species, including *P gingivalis* and *P intermedia,* can be cultured from the dorsum of the tongue (van Winkelhoff et al, 1988a), the tonsils (van Winkelhoff et al, 1988a), and the oral mucosa (Van Winkelhoff et al, 1986). It has also been demonstrated that *A actinomycetemcomitans* may attach to the teeth, tongue, and buccal mucosa (Asikainen et al, 1995; Slots et al, 1980).

Comparison of the microbiota on the tongue and tonsillar area in subjects with and without periodontitis indicates a correlation between disease and the presence of *P intermedia* and motile bacteria in these areas (Van Winkelhoff et al, 1986). Similarly, in a group of untreated subjects with *A actinomycetemcomitans*–associated periodontitis, the subgingival load of *A actinomycetemcomitans* has been associated with the number of *A actinomycetemcomitans* on cheek mucosa. It is well-known that the dorsum of the tongue is the main reservoir for *Streptococcus salivarius,* a very potent cariogenic (acidogenic) bacteria. In one study, however, higher numbers of *Streptococcus mutans* were repeatedly found on the dorsum of the tongue after five thorough scrapings with a tongue scraper than prior to scraping, indicating that this is an important reservoir for *S mutans* (Axelsson et al, 1987). Lindquist et al (1989) found a significant correlation between the prevalence of *S mutans* in saliva and that of *S mutans* on the dorsum of the tongue.

These data support the inclusion of the dorsum of the tongue in oral hygiene procedures, at least for patients highly infected by periopathogens and/or cariogenic bacteria such as *S mutans,* using the so-called complete-mouth disinfection principle (Axelsson et al, 1987; Mongardini et al, 1999; Quirynen et al, 1995). The tongue-cleaning procedure should include initial thorough mechanical removal of deposits from the dorsum of the tongue, followed by rinsing with an efficient antimicrobial agent (chlorhexidine), because the dorsum of the tongue is normally covered by thick deposits that prevent penetration of the antimicrobial solution. Studies using DNA fingerprints have shown that there are reservoirs, or fugitive habitats, where, for example, *S mutans* and periopathogens can survive chlorhexidine treatment (Kozai et al, 1991).

The oral cavity presents two types of surfaces for colonization by bacteria: the soft tissues and the hard tooth surfaces, both modified to some extent by a coating of saliva or, in the case of the hard surfaces, by a pellicle, formed by adsorption of salivary components. A distinct and important difference between the two types of surface is that the soft tissue surfaces desquamate, while the hard tissues do not. Bacteria colonizing the soft tissue surfaces are lost when the cells are shed: For survival in this habitat, readherence is essential. Unlike the hard surfaces, which will support heavy deposits of bacteria in dental plaque, the soft tissue surfaces do not develop complex layers of bacteria (biofilms).

In defining different habits in the oral cavity, it is important to recognize that the physical dimensions of a habitat do not fall within specific limits. The whole oral cavity, an occlusal tooth surface, or even a defined area on the occlusal surface may be considered a habitat. These habitats, together with their physiologic characteristics, are referred to as *microenvironments.*

In oral microbiology, changes in the flora of a habitat such as the mouth may indicate, for example, patients at risk of caries, while changes in tooth surface microenvironments can identify a surface at risk of disease. Thus, although general definitions of habitats can be made, studies of the oral microflora should always include careful definition of the habitats being examined. Generally, the oral cavity includes local habitats, such as the mucosa, tongue, saliva, and tooth surfaces. Included in the microenviroments are local areas, where hard surfaces and soft tissues are juxtaposed, such as the gingival sulcus and periodontal pockets.

FORMATION OF PLAQUE BIOFILMS

Role of saliva in pellicle and plaque formation

The saliva contains many different proteins and some other small organic molecules that, together, protect the oral cavity (the soft tissues and the teeth) from frictional wear, dryness, erosion, pathogenic bacteria, and so on. Almost all salivary proteins are glycoproteins; ie, they contain variable amounts of carbohydrates linked to the protein core. Glycoproteins are often classified according to their cellular origin and subclassified on the basis of their biochemical properties. A characteristic feature is that many occur in multiple forms, constituting families, which may, however, exhibit remarkable functional differences.

Mucous glycoproteins, the mucins, are of acinar cell origin, have a high molecular weight, and

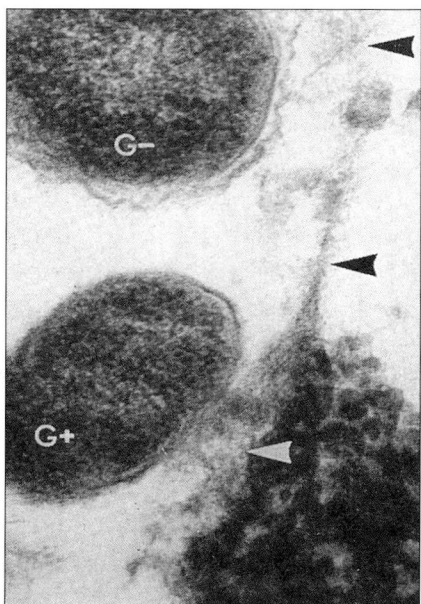

Fig 1 Attachment of a gram-positive (G+) pioneer coloniz-er to the pellicle-covered tooth surface *(white arrow)* in con-trast to the relationship between a gram-negative bacterium (G-) and the pellicle *(black arrows)* (original magnification ×90,000). (From Lie, 1978. Reprinted with permission.)

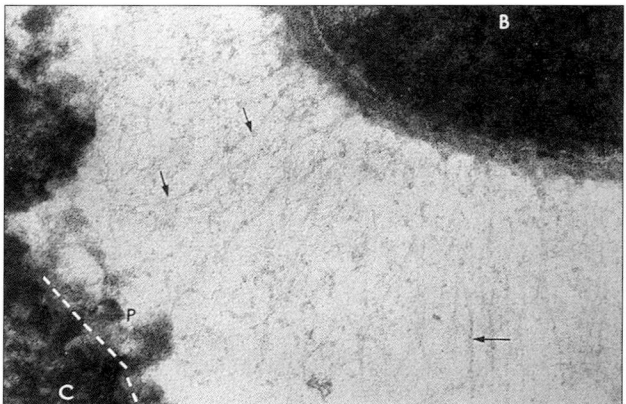

Fig 2 Closeup of the attachment *(arrows)* between a gram-positive bacterium (B) and the pellicle (P). C = Hydroxya-patite crystals (original magnification ×150,000). (From Lie, 1978. Reprinted with permission.)

contain more than 40% carbohydrate. The mucins are produced by the minor salivary glands in the palate and provide a nonfrictional, lubricant layer, protecting the soft tissues from wear and tear and facilitating swallowing of food. Because the mucins have a strongly negative charge, other negatively charged molecules, such as those con-tained in the cell walls of many oral bacteria, are repelled from the mucin-coated oral mucosa. Among other properties, the mucins also bind water and thereby protect the oral mucosa from drying out.

Serous glycoproteins have a much lower mol-ecular weight than mucins and contain less than 50% carbohydrate. Many belong to a group called *proline-rich glycoproteins* (PRPs), of which sever-al are phosphorylated. These proteins are secret-ed from the parotid and submandibular glands.

The collective name *glycoprotein* for all car-bohydrate-linked proteins encompasses a large, heterogenous group. Most salivary proteins, such as secretory IgA, lactoferrin, peroxidases, and ag-glutinins, belong to this group. Because human saliva is supersaturated with respect to most cal-cium phosphate salts, some proteins are neces-sary to inhibit their spontaneous precipitation in the salivary glands and their secretions. Such pro-teins include statherin and PRPs. Statherin is pres-ent in both submandibular and parotid salivas. Proline-rich proteins form a complex group of proteins with large numbers of genetic variants, some of which also have the ability to inhibit spon-taneous precipitation of calcium phosphate salts.

A newly proposed biologic function for these proteins is the ability of adsorbed acidic PRPs to selectively mediate bacterial adhesion on tooth surfaces. Recently, it was shown that the negative charge of these acidic PRPs binds electrostatical-ly to calcium on the tooth surfaces; the outer ends, consisting of proline and glutamine amino acids, attract and bind very strongly to the harmless and protective normal microflora of the teeth *(Strep-tococcus oralis, Streptococcus sanguis,* and *Strep-tococcus mitis).* This may explain early electron micrographs by Lie (1978), which show how a gram-positive "pioneer colonizer," unlike gram-negative bacteria, attaches to the pellicle-covered tooth surface (Figs 1 and 2).

This primary colonization of the protective normal microflora occurs during the first 24 hours after cleaning. However, recent research has shown that so-called secondary colonization by other, more pathogenic microorganisms (gram-positive as well as gram-negative) is strongly related to the binding between galactose amine structures on the surfaces of the normal microflora as well as the "secondary colonizers." The production and the individual structures of acidic PRPs and galactose amines are genetically related and may partly explain individual variations in plaque formation rates. This is a field of ongoing research (Strömberg, 1996).

As described earlier, saliva plays a significant role in maintaining an appropriate balance within the ecosystem associated with tooth surfaces. This is of great importance in the control of the oral microflora, because saliva enhances the ability of some bacteria to survive and reduces the competitiveness of others. This control over the oral flora is achieved by salivary components, which may be present constantly or activated by a specific host response.

The major antimicrobial proteins are listed in Box 1. Many studies have shown that most of these proteins can inhibit the metabolism, adherence, or even the viability of pathogenic microorganisms in vitro, but their role in vivo is largely unknown. It seems that they are important for the control of microbial overgrowth in the mouth, but their selectivity against pathogens has not been determined.

The lysozyme (LZ) in whole saliva is derived from the major and minor salivary glands, gingival crevicular fluid, and salivary leukocytes (polymorphonuclear neutrophil leukocytes [PMNLs]). Salivary LZ is present in newborn babies at levels equal to those of adults, suggesting a pre-eruptive antimicrobial function. The classic concept of the antimicrobial action of LZ is based on its muramidase activity, ie, the ability to hydrolyze the

bond between N-acetylmuramic acid and N-acetylglucosamine in the peptidoglycan layer of the bacterial cell wall. Gram-negative bacteria are more resistant to LZ because of the protective function of the outer lipopolysaccharide layer. In addition to its muramidase activity, LZ is strongly cationic, and can activate bacterial "autolysins" that can destroy components of the cell wall.

Lactoferrin (LF) is an iron-binding glycoprotein secreted by the serous cells of the major and minor salivary glands. Polymorphonuclear leukocytes are also rich in LF and release it into gingival fluid and whole saliva. The biologic function of LF is attributed to its high affinity for iron and its consequent expropriation of this essential metal from pathogenic microorganisms. This bacteriostatic effect is lost if the LF molecule is saturated with iron, a factor that should be taken into account in areas where the drinking water is rich in iron. In its iron-free state, LF (apo LF) has also a bactericidal, irreversible effect on a variety of microorganisms.

Salivary peroxidase is produced in the acinar cells of the parotid and submandibular glands but not in the minor salivary glands. Salivary peroxidase systems have two major biologic functions:

Box 1 Major antimicrobial proteins of human whole saliva*

Nonimmunoglobulin proteins
- Lysozyme
- Lactoferrin
- Salivary peroxidase system (enzyme-SCN^--H_2O_2)
- Myeloperoxidase system (enzyme-SCN^-/halide-H_2O_2)
- Agglutinins
  - Parotid saliva glycoproteins
  - Mucins
  - Secretory immunoglobulin A
  - 2-Microglobulin
  - Fibronectin
- Histidine-rich proteins (histatins)
- Proline-rich proteins

Immunoglobulins
- Secretory immunoglobulin A
- Immunoglobulin G
- Immunoglobulin M

*From Tenovuo and Lagerlöf (1994).

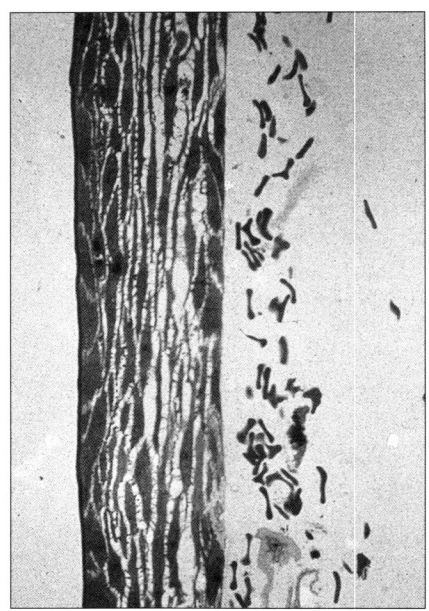

Fig 3 Undisturbed pellicle in cross section *(left)*. It is formed in different layers. Many nonattaching bacteria *(right)* are close to the outer surface of the pellicle.

(1) antimicrobial activity and *(2)* protection of host proteins and cells from hydrogen peroxide toxicity.

Salivary agglutinins are glycoproteins that have the capacity to interact with unattached bacteria, resulting in clumping of bacteria into large aggregates that are more easily flushed away by saliva and swallowed; the term *aggregation is* therefore often used synonymously with *agglutination.* Listed in Box 1 are salivary proteins with agglutinating capacity. The most potent agglutinin is a high-molecular-weight glycoprotein that has been isolated from human parotid saliva. Despite a concentration in parotid saliva of only 0.001%, it is very effective. Mucins are also able to agglutinate bacteria. In high-molecular-weight glycoproteins, sugar residues and sialic acid are important for the interaction with bacteria.

The secretory immunoglobulins, most notably secretory sIgA, act by aggregating bacteria. They target specific bacterial molecules, such as adhesions, or enzymes, such as glucosyl transferase. Saliva also contains immunoglobulin G (IgG) and immunoglobulin M (IgM), derived from serum and produced locally in the gingival tissues.

Formation and functions of pellicle

Saliva is seldom in direct contact with the tooth surface but rather is separated from it by the acquired *pellicle,* defined as an acellular layer of salivary proteins and other macromolecules, approximately 2 to 10 μm thick, adsorbed onto the enamel surface. It forms a base for subsequent adhesion of microorganisms, which, under certain conditions, may develop into dental plaque biofilms. The pellicle layer, although thin, has an important role in protecting the enamel from abrasion and attrition, but it also serves as a diffusion barrier.

The undisturbed pellicle is formed in different layers (Fig 3). There are many nonattaching bacteria close to the outer surface of the pellicle. Because of abrasion, for example from toothbrushing, the thickness will vary between 2 and 10 μm, depending on the intervals between brushing. Saxton (1976) showed that complete removal of the pellicle requires about 5 minutes' application of pumice in a rotating rubber cup.

Figure 4 shows a groove in the pellicle down to the enamel surface, made by a knife. Such grooves were earlier thought to be abrasive defects in the enamel surface, caused by use of abrasive toothpaste. Figure 5 shows the thickness of new pellicle several hours after intensive cleaning.

In the pellicle, movement of molecules by forces other than diffusion is low compared to that in most other parts of the salivary film. The relatively undisturbed layer of liquid in the pellicle will certainly influence the solubility of the enamel surface. Adsorption to the enamel of macromolecules, usually originating from the saliva, is selective; ie, certain macromolecules show a higher affinity for the mineral surface than do others.

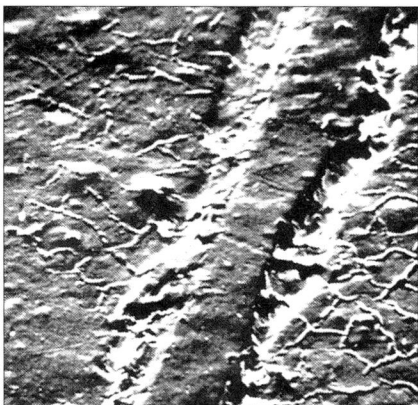

Fig 4 Groove in the pellicle, down to the enamel surface. The groove was made with a knife. (From Saxton, 1976. Reprinted with permission.)

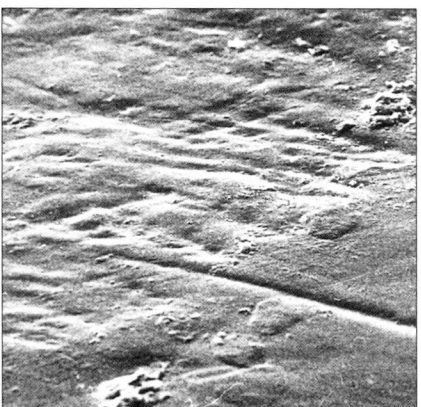

Fig 5 The groove shown in Fig 4 was removed by 5 minutes' intensive cleaning. The pellicle-free enamel surface was partly covered with nail varnish *(left)*, while the other part *(right)* was exposed to saliva for several hours. The surface is shown after removal of the nail varnish. (From Saxton, 1976. Reprinted with permission.)

In the normal oral pH range, the enamel surface has a negative net charge because of the structure of hydroxyapatite, in which phosphate groups are arranged close to the surface. Counterions (of opposite charge) eg, calcium, are attracted to the surface, forming a hydration layer of unevenly distributed charges. The exact composition of this layer will be determined by several factors (eg, pH, ionic strength, and the type of ions present in the saliva). Normally the hydration layer close to the enamel surface contains mainly calcium and phosphate ions in the proportion of 10:1, but other ions, such as sodium, potassium, fluoride, and chloride, must also be present. Because calcium predominates, the resulting net charge of the enamel surface with its hydration layer is positive, implying that the hydration layer will attract negatively charged macromolecules (Figs 6 and 7).

Negative charges on macromolecules are found in acidic side chains with end groups of phosphate or sulfate. These side chains have a high affinity to the tooth surface. Recent research has shown that the bulk of the pellicle consists of salivary micelle-like structures of great importance for reducing diffusion through the pellicle and reducing friction between the teeth and other oral tissues.

Not all of the proteins contributing to the pellicle are well defined. However, salivary proteins such as amylase, lysozyme, peroxidase, IgA, IgG, and glucosyl transferase participate in pellicle matrix formation, together with mucins and breakdown products from macromolecules of both salivary and bacterial origin. Of special interest are the acidic PRPs mentioned earlier, which bind via their amino-terminal segments to the tooth surface, leaving their carboxy-terminal regions directed toward the oral cavity, where they may interact with oral microorganisms.

Pellicle formation is rapid during the first hour and then decreases. It seems likely that adsorption of the first layer of molecules on a clean surface is instantaneous. The formation rate varies among

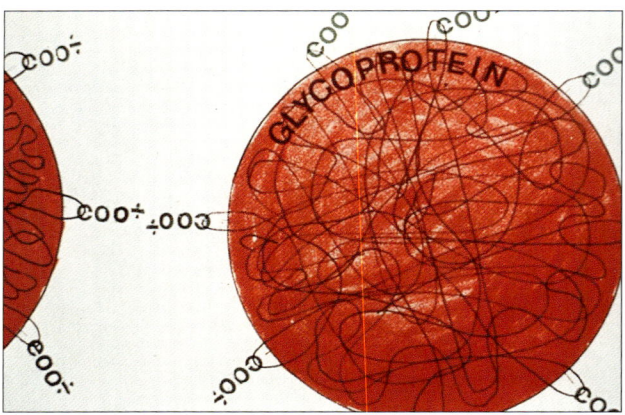

Fig 6 Illustration representing the glucoprotein macromolecule. (Illustrated by J. Waerhaug. Courtesy of Department of Periodontics, University of Oslo.)

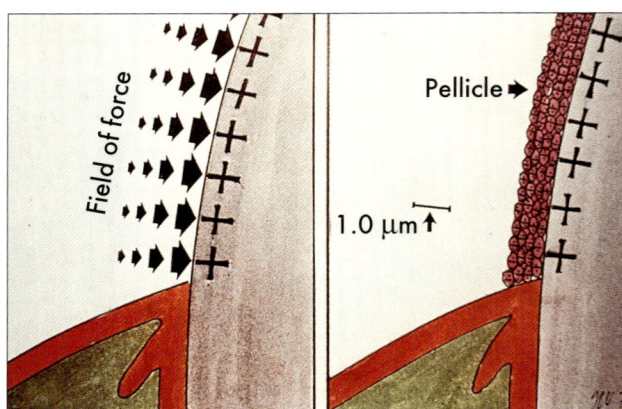

Fig 7 Illustration of the mechanism for attachment of the glucoprotein macromolecules on the enamel surface during formation of the pellicle. (Illustrated by J. Waerhaug. Courtesy of Department of Periodontics, University of Oslo.)

individuals, probably because of differences in salivary composition.

Formation and composition of supragingival plaque biofilms

Dawes et al (1963) described dental plaque as "the soft tenacious material found on tooth surfaces which is not readily removed by rinsing with water." Nolte (1973) defined dental plaque as: "the non-mineralized microbial accumulation that adheres tenaciously to tooth surfaces, restorations, and prosthetic appliances, shows structural organization with predominance of filamentous forms, is composed of an organic matrix derived from salivary glycoproteins and extracellular microbial products, and cannot be removed by rinsing or water spray."

The most readily discernible plaque on the smooth surfaces of the teeth along the gingival margin is termed *dentogingival plaque*. Dentogingival plaque on the approximal surfaces, apical to the contact points, is termed *approximal dental plaque*. Plaque occurring below the gingival margin, in the gingival sulcus or in the periodontal pocket, is termed *subgingival plaque* (Theilade and Theilade, 1976).

It is estimated that only 1 mm³ of dental plaque, weighing about 1 mg, contains more than 200 million bacteria. Other microorganisms, such as mycoplasma, "yeasts," and protozoa also occur in mature plaque; sticky polysaccharides and other products form the so-called plaque matrix, which constitutes 10% to 40% by volume of the supragingival plaque. The composition and structure of dental plaque indicate how the elements of dental plaque, predominantly bacteria, are organized and interrelated. Mature dental plaque is a well-organized "society." The dentogingival plaque is therefore regarded as a *biofilm,* defined as "matrix-enclosed bacterial populations adherent to each other and/or to surfaces or interfaces" (Costerton et al, 1994).

The first condition for plaque formation is a solid surface. In the oral cavity, only the pellicle-covered tooth surfaces offer such conditions. On the soft tissues of the oral cavity, the microorganisms may attach to the outer surface of the epithelial cells. However, no plaque can form because the outermost layers of epithelial cells are continuously desquamated. At best, the microorganisms on desquamated epithelial cells may be transported by the oral fluid, eventually attaching to a solid tooth surface; only then can formation of colonies and plaque begin.

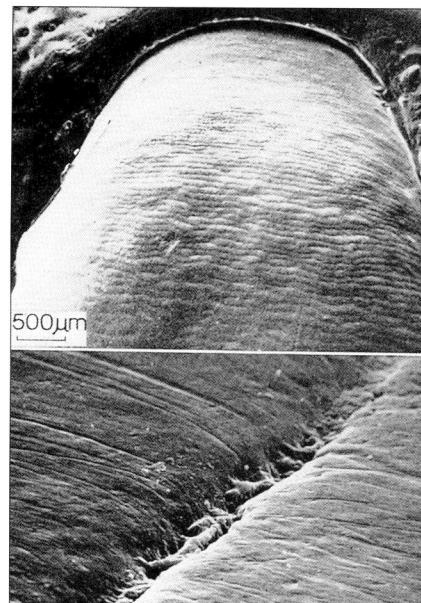

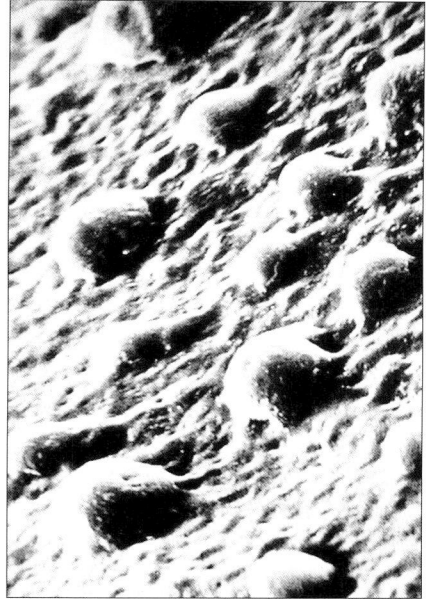

Fig 8 *(top)* Facial enamel surface of a newly erupted and cleaned permanent central incisor. The perikymata are still discernible. *(bottom)* Increased magnification of the view. (From Saxton, 1975. Reprinted with permission.)

Fig 9 Formation of bacterial colonies (original magnification ×4,000). (From Saxton, 1975. Reprinted with permission.)

Figure 8 is a scanning electron micrograph (SEM) of the facial enamel surface of a newly erupted and cleaned permanent central incisor. The perikymata are still discernible. The first cells to adhere to pellicle on tooth surfaces or other solid surfaces are coccoid bacteria, epithelial cells, and polymorphonuclear leukocytes; the bacteria occur singly or as aggregates, either on or within the pellicle. Larger numbers of microorganisms may be carried to the tooth surface by epithelial cells, as described earlier. During the first few hours, bacteria that resist detachment from the pellicle may start to proliferate, forming small colonies of morphologically similar organisms (Fig 9).

Plaque growth also may be initiated by microorganisms harbored in minute irregularities, such as grooves in tooth surfaces, the margins of restorations, the cementoenamel junction, and the gingival sulcus, where they are protected from natural cleaning of the tooth surface (Figs 10a and 10b). As early as 1975, Saxton showed that gingival crevicular fluid (GCF) released from inflamed gingiva results in increased reaccumulation of bacterial colonies and plaque immediately after toothcleaning because GCF is rich in nutrients not readily available in the saliva. Figure 11 shows seepage of GCF from the gingival sulcus and bacterial colonies in the same area. The largest colonies are located close to the GCF (Fig 12).

Four hours after cleaning, there are 103 to 104 bacteria per 1 mm² of tooth surface (Nyvad and Kilian, 1987), predominantly streptococci and actinomycetes. Within a day, the number of bacteria increases 100- to 1,000-fold, mainly because of the growth of streptococci.

The initial bacteria are called *pioneer colonizers* because they are hardy and successfully compete with the other members of the oral flora for a place on the tooth surface (Gibbons and van Houte, 1980). The deposition of these pioneer species is not a chance happening but the result of an exquisitely sensitive interaction between

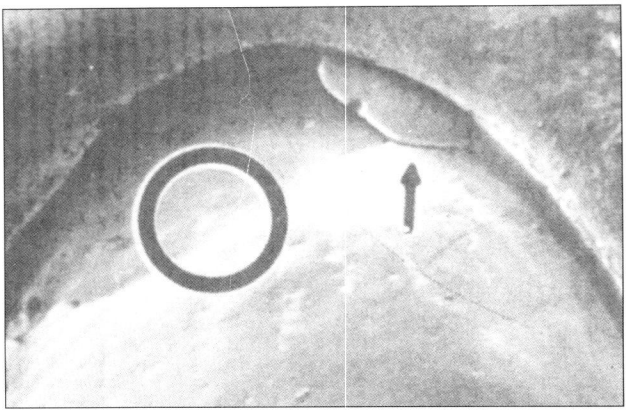

Fig 10a SEM of exposed cementoenamel junction, a potential area of plaque retention. Some gingival exudate *(arrow)* was present during the taking of the impression (original magnification ×50). (From Bevenius et al, 1994. Reprinted with permission.)

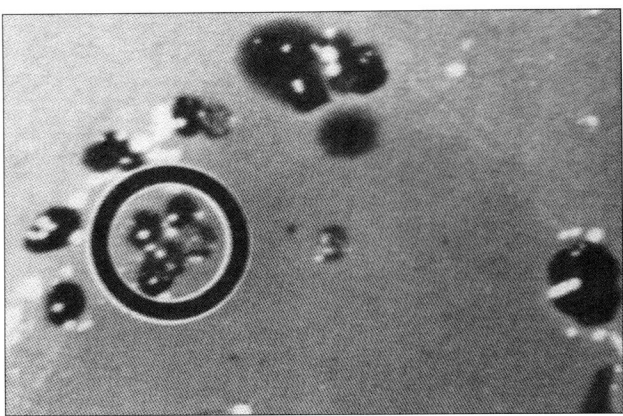

Fig 10b Plaque growth in inset area of Fig 10a (original magnification ×2000). (From Bevenius et al, 1994. Reprinted with permission.)

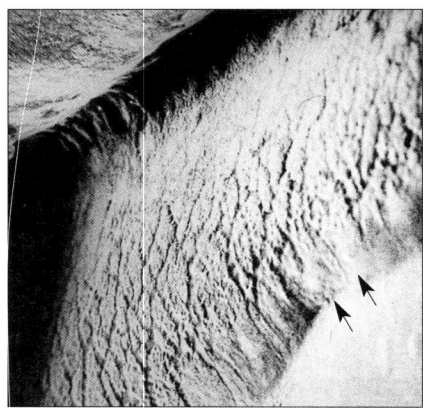

Fig 11 Relationship between bacterial colonies *(arrows)* and seepage of gingival crevicular fluid from the sulcus (original magnification ×200). (From Saxton, 1975. Reprinted with permission.)

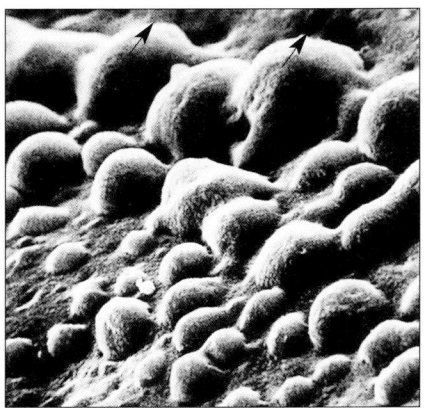

Fig 12 The largest bacterial colonies *(arrows)* are located close to the gingival crevicular fluid (original magnification ×4,000). (From Saxton, 1975. Reprinted with permission.)

protein adhesions on the surface of the colonizing bacteria and carbohydrate receptors on the salivary components adsorbed to the tooth surface, as previously described.

After deposition, clones of pioneer colonizing bacteria, *S sanguis,* begin to expand away from the tooth surface to form columns that move outward in long chains of palisading bacteria. These parallel columns are separated by uniformly narrow spaces (Fig 13). Plaque growth proceeds by deposition of new species into these open spaces (Listgarten et al, 1975).

These newly deposited species attach to pioneer species in a specific molecular lock-and-key manner. Expansion of existing species in a lateral direction causes the interbacterial spaces to merge. It is hypothesized that, once the spaces are close enough, a starter substance is secreted by

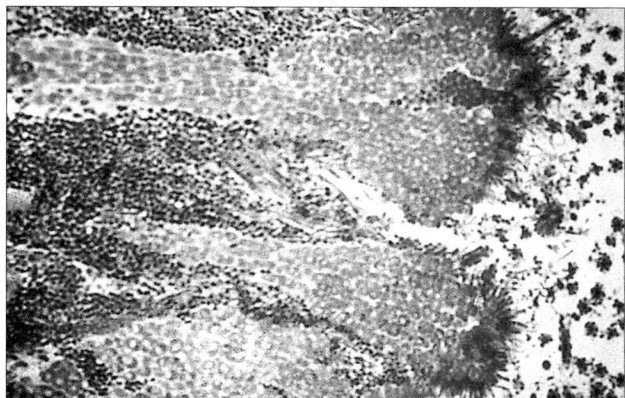

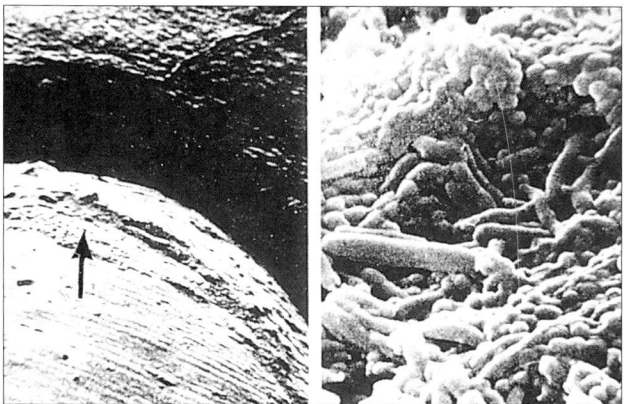

Fig 13 Cross section of columns of colonizing bacteria, separated by open spaces. (From Listgarten et al, 1975. Reprinted with permission.)

Fig 14 *(left)* Plaque formation along the gingival margin after 24 to 48 hours *(arrow)* (original magnification ×100). *(right)* Increased magnification revealing that the plaque is dominated by streptococci and a few rods (original magnification ×4,000). (From Saxton, 1973. Reprinted with permission.)

bacteria within the plaque matrix, stimulating a growth spurt in the surrounding bacteria. The tooth surface adjacent to the gingiva is rapidly covered by intermeshed bacteria. New bacteria, derived from saliva or surrounding mucous membranes, now sense only the bacteria-laden landscape of the tooth surface and attach by a bonding interaction to bacteria already attached to the plaque. These associations, called *intergeneric coaggregations,* are mediated by specific attachment proteins that occur between two partner cells. All this activity occurs within the first 2 days of plaque development and for descriptive purposes is called *phase I* of plaque formation (Theilade et al, 1976).

Continuous plaque has formed along the gingival margin after 24 to 48 hours (Fig 14). The plaque is dominated by streptococci and a few rods. Figures 15 to 17 show 2 days' free plaque accumulation in a caries-free young adult without gingivitis. Even in such a healthy mouth, there has been continuous plaque accumulation at so-called stagnant zones (interproximally and along the gingival margins), ie, sites at which plaque can accumulate undisturbed by friction from chewing and tongue movements. Figure

18 shows gingivitis at mandibular lingual and interproximal sites in another young adult, in whom much more plaque reaccumulated in less than 2 days.

During the first 2 days, the dentogingival plaque is dominated by the relatively "harmless" normal microflora of the tooth surface, consisting of facultatively anaerobic gram-positive streptococci (*S sanguis* and *S mitis)* and a minority of gram-positive rods *(Actinomyces* species), which may impede infiltration of more pathogenic microorganisms.

In phase II, from around day 3, filamentous bacteria can be found on the surface of the predominantly coccoid plaque (Figs 19 and 20). Figure 21 illustrates the thickness of freely accumulated gingival plaque after 2, 3, and 4 days. Note the dramatic increase of plaque thickness after 3 and 4 days compared to the first 2 days.

In phase III, competitive growth among the predominantly coccoid microbial colonies continues for about 1 week. Filamentous bacteria then begin to penetrate the coccoid plaque from the surface, and it gradually becomes predominantly filamentous. The process may continue for about 2 weeks more; the columnar microbial

Figs 15 to 17 Two days' free plaque accumulation in a caries-free young adult without gingivitis. Plaque has accumulated in stagnant zones.

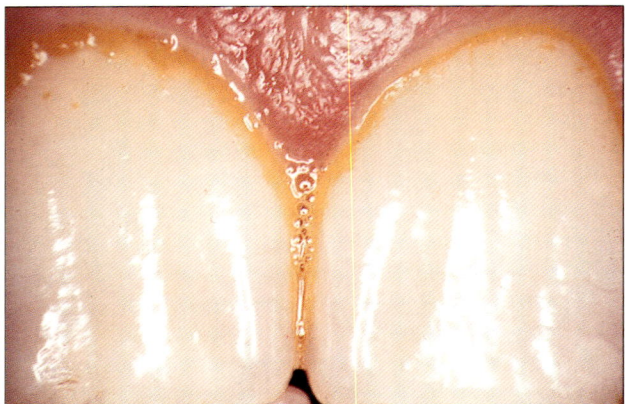

Fig 15

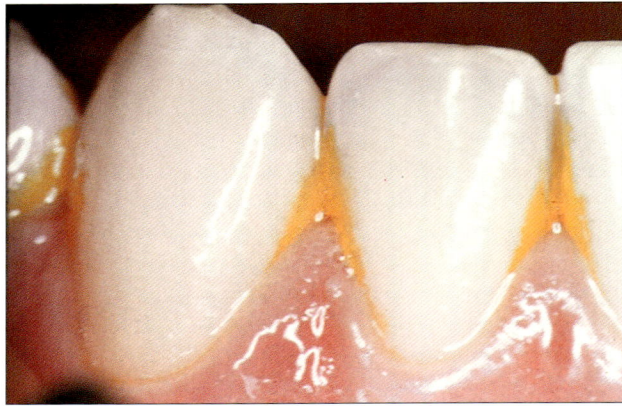

Fig 16

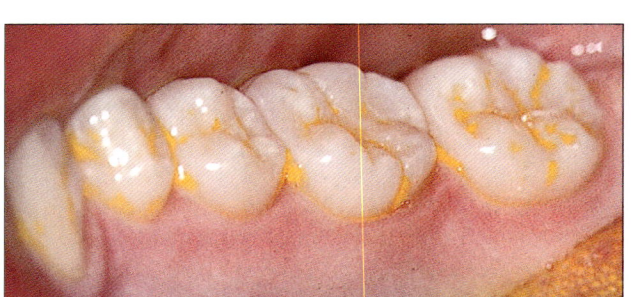

Fig 17

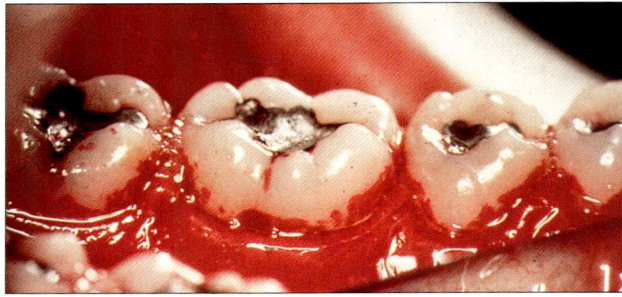

Fig 18 Gingivitis at mandibular lingual and interproximal sites in another young adult. Much more plaque has accumulated in less than 2 days in this individual than in the patient shown in Figs 15 to 17.

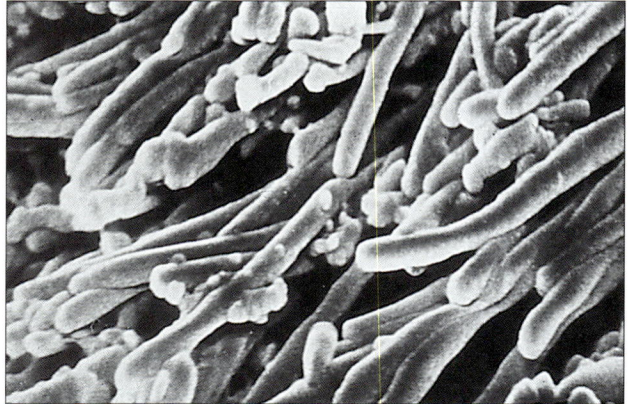

Fig 19 Outer surface of plaque in phase II of plaque development, covered by gram-positive tall rods (original magnification ×8,000). (From Saxton, 1973. Reprinted with permission.)

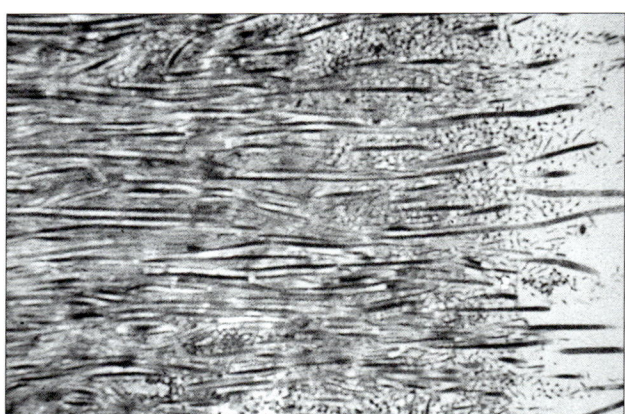

Fig 20 Filamentous bacteria on the surface of predominantly coccoid plaque during phase II of plaque development (original magnification ×1,500). (From Listgarten et al, 1975. Reprinted with permission.)

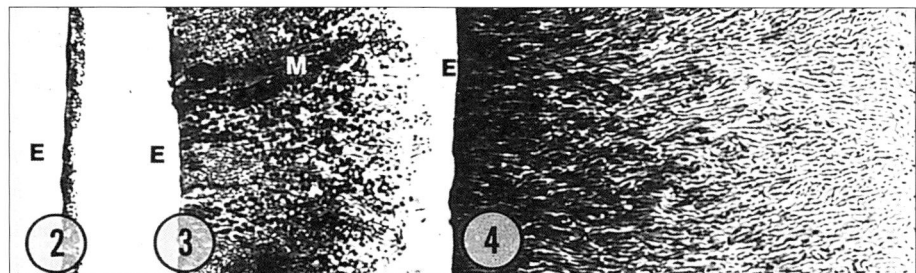

Fig 21 Thickness of freely accumulated gingival plaque after 2, 3, and 4 days. E = Enamel; M = Columnar microcolony (original magnification ×1,000–1,500). (From Listgarten, 1976. Reprinted with permission.)

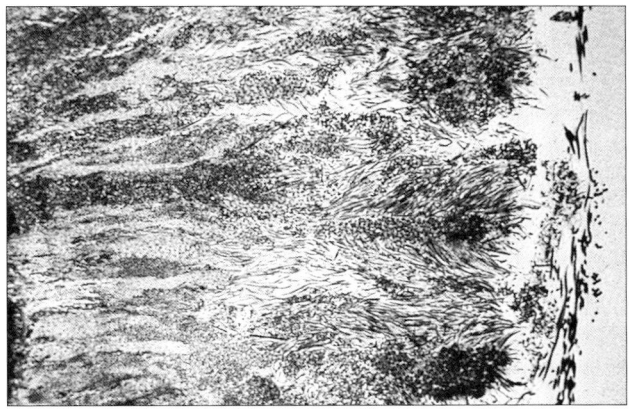

Fig 22 Dense mat of filamentous bacteria, oriented roughly perpendicular to the colonized surface, in phase III of plaque formation. (From Listgarten et al, 1975. Reprinted with permission.)

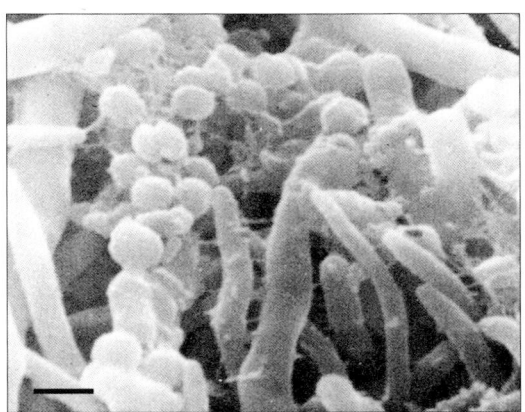

Fig 23 Surface of phase III plaque (bar = 5μm). (From Adriaens et al, 1988b. Reprinted with permission.)

colonies are replaced by a dense mat of filamentous bacteria, oriented roughly perpendicular to the colonized surface (Figs 22 and 23).

It has also been observed that several species of coccoid bacteria are able to aggregate with some of the filamentous bacteria to produce "corncob" formations that are detectable on the plaque surface in this phase, particularly along the gingival margin (Figs 24 to 27). Corncob formations may persist on the plaque surface along the gingival margin. This new structural organization is relatively consistent over time and can be identified in supragingival plaque samples known to be 3 weeks old.

In phase IV, 1 to 2 weeks after initiation, the diversity of the flora has increased to include motile bacteria, spirochetes, and vibrios as well as fusiforms. Attached gingival plaque fills the gingival sulcus, while spirochetes and vibrios move around in the outer and more apical regions of the sulcus (Fig 28). Gradually the gingival margin becomes inflamed, resulting in an increase in vol-

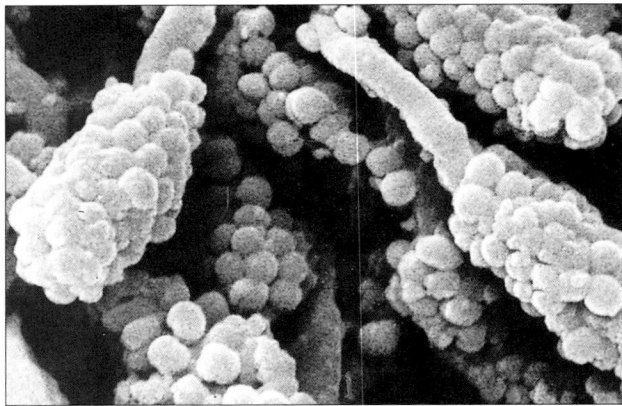

Fig 24 Corncob formation of coccoid and filamentous bacteria in phase III of plaque formation (original magnification ×8,000). (From Saxton, 1973. Reprinted with permission.)

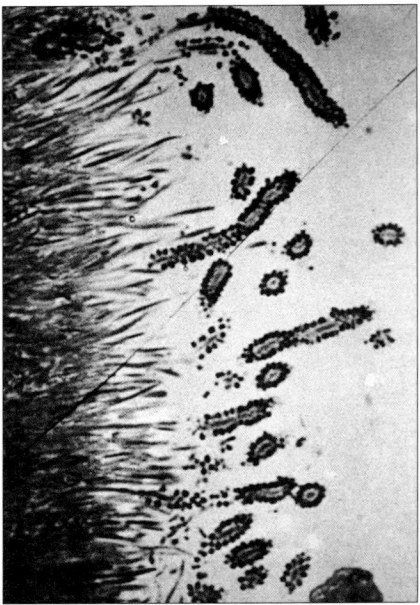

Fig 25 Cross section of the outer surface of gingival plaque, containing several corncob formations (original magnification ×1,000). (From Listgarten, 1976. Reprinted with permission.)

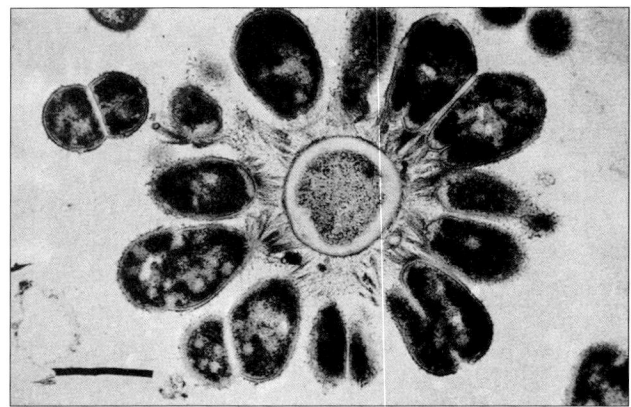

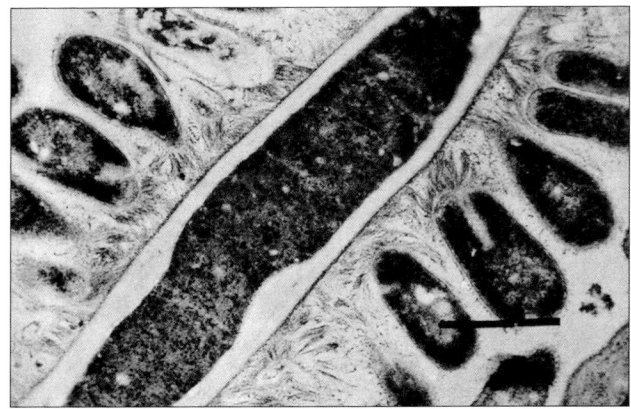

Figs 26 and 27 Close-ups of formations in Fig 25 reveal strong organic connections between the coccoid and filamentous bacteria (original magnification ×30,000). (From Listgarten, 1976. Reprinted with permission.)

ume of GCF. In the depths of the plaque that fills the sulcus, minerals from the GCF accumulate, forming black calculus (Fig 29). In addition, the anaerobic environment in the depths of such thick, mature plaque leads to a shift toward gram-negative anaerobic microflora; ie, growth conditions favorable to most periopathogens are created.

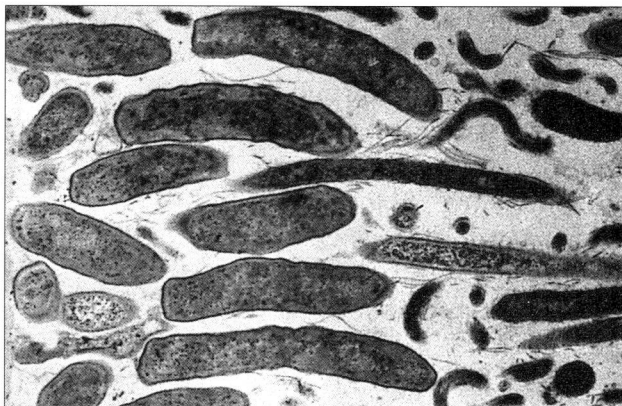

Fig 28 Cross section of gingival plaque filling the gingival sulcus while spirochetes and vibrios move around in the outer and more apical regions of the sulcus during phase IV of plaque development (original magnification ×12,000). (From Listgarten,1976. Reprinted with permission.)

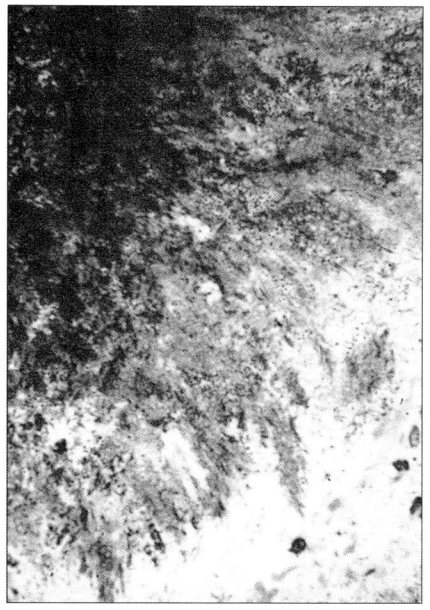

Fig 29 Accumulation of minerals in the deeper part of the plaque, resulting in calculus formation (original magnification ×400). (From Listgarten, 1976. Reprinted with permission.)

Formation and composition of subgingival biofilms and nonattached microflora

Periodontitis is always preceded by gingivitis. If undisturbed, the supragingival biofilm elicits in the gingival margin a typical inflammatory response (gingivitis), ie, edema, deepening the gingival sulcus by formation of a pseudopocket in which the relatively anaerobic conditions favor the establishment of an anaerobic microbiota.

Colonization of the gingival sulcus and the subsequently developing periodontal pocket originates in the already established supragingival plaque. Thus, the bacterial composition of subgingival plaque at specific sites is partly influenced by the composition of the preexisting supragingival plaque.

However, growth conditions are determined by the subgingival environment, and the difference in bacterial composition between subgingival and adjacent supragingival plaque may be attributable to several factors:

- Access to the oral cavity is limited, favoring anaerobic development.
- Nutrients are readily available from the gingival exudate, the volume of which increases as a result of gingival inflammation.
- Detachment of already established microorganisms is limited by the protecting gingival tissues, allowing organisms without special adhesive mechanisms to survive.
- Access for bacteria transported by saliva is limited or impossible.

Anaerobic bacteria that colonize the subgingival region include motile rods and spirochetes. They are able to increase their mass by contributing to the deepening of the sulcus, thereby increasing the volume of their ecological niche. Because many of the subgingival microorganisms are motile, the structural organization of this microbial population is quite different from that of supragingival plaque.

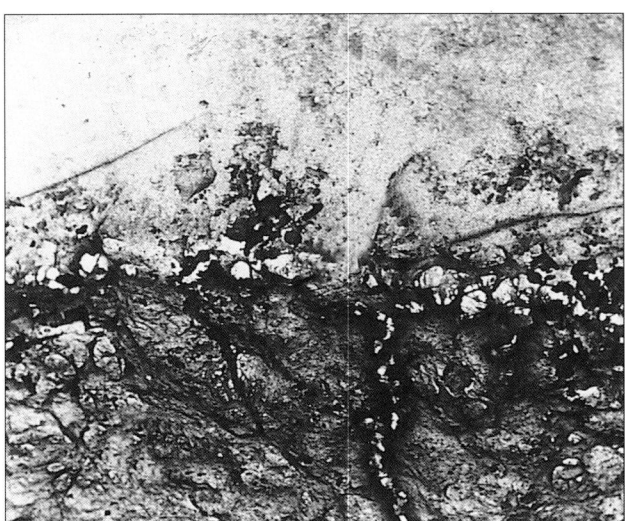

Fig 30 SEM showing the relatively smooth enamel surface *(top)* compared with the rough intact root cementum *(bottom)* from a newly erupted premolar (original magnification ×210).

Formation of subgingival plaque

As soon as tissue breakdown results in loss of periodontal support, the rough root surface becomes accessible to bacterial colonization. The morphology of the rough, plaque-retentive surfaces of intact root cementum and the cementoenamel junction is in stark contrast to that of the enamel surface (Fig 30). Cross-sectional views illustrate how well the microorganisms of the subgingival biofilm attach to the root cementum (Figs 31 and 32).

Evidence suggests that bacteria move subgingivally by at least two mechanisms, which probably share biologic messages: First, the nonmotile bacteria piggyback into the subgingival space on motile bacteria, and second, the tooth-attached bacteria progress by direct, amoeba-like, creeping migration from the supragingival to the subgingival space. Migration may occur at random, but it is more likely to be directed by a chemical gradient. A relatively thin layer of adherent bacteria covers the root surface. Rods and filaments tend to be arranged in a palisading pattern in which the long axis of the cells is perpendicular to the tooth surface (see Figs 31 and 32).

Unique bacterial aggregates, resembling bottlebrushes, can be found attached to the adherent plaque and extending into the space between the bacterial layer and the adjacent soft tissue wall (Fig 33). The "bristles" of these brush formations are gram-negative filamentous bacteria, some of which may be flagellated, and the axial portion of the brush comprises single or several long filaments, held together by an amorphous extracellular matrix.

The tendency for bacteria to colonize tooth surfaces freshly exposed by disruption of the junctional epithelium leads to a gradual deepening of the sulcus, or pocket, and, 3 to 12 weeks after the beginning of supragingival plaque formation, to the establishment of a distinctive subgingival microbiota, predominantly gram-negative anaerobic bacteria, including a number of motile species. The process is dependent on a series of interrelated events: the successive colonization of the tooth surface by different bacterial populations, each of which appears to facilitate colonization by the next wave of bacterial settlers. As discussed earlier, most putative periodontal pathogens are anaerobic gram-negative species whose main ecological niche is in the subgingival region. In this protected environment, they maintain and expand their habitat by destruction of the periodontal tissues.

The bulk of the subgingival microbiota consists of a complex mixture of predominantly anaerobic bacteria that surround and cover the bottlebrush formations. The lack of well-defined microbial colonies in this environment may be due to the high degree of motility of the resident microbiota. The peripheral region of the subgingival microbiota is composed of a high concentration of spirochetes that are in direct contact with the gingival tissue wall as well as with the apical lining of the sulcus or pocket (Fig 34). Sometimes a layer of leukocytes, mostly neutrophils that have migrated out of the junctional epithelium, separates the bacterial mass from the sulcus or pocket epithelium.

The base of the sulcus, or pocket, consists of the coronal, desquamative surface of the junc-

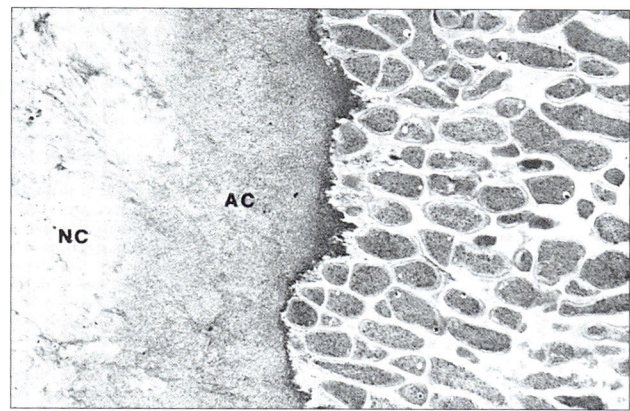

Fig 31 Cross section demonstrating attachment of subgingival microorganisms to the root cementum. AC = Altered afibrillar cementum; NC = Normal cementum (original magnification ×7,000). (From Listgarten, 1976. Reprinted with permission.)

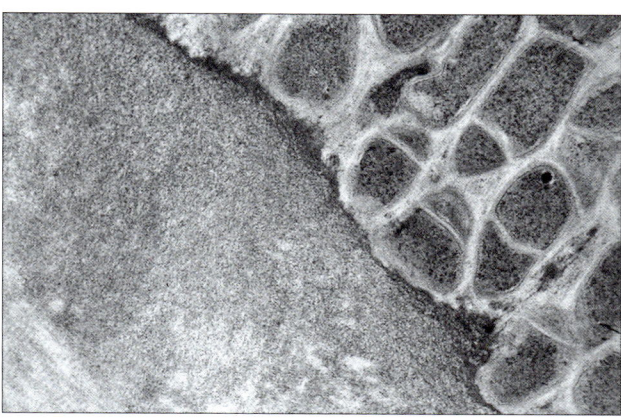

Fig 32 Increased magnification of Fig 31 (original magnification ×20,000). (From Listgarten, 1976. Reprinted with permission.)

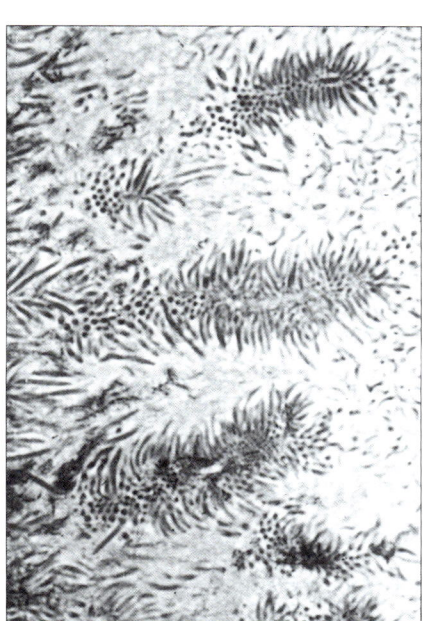

Fig 33 Bottlebrush formation of aggregated bacteria in adherent plaque surrounded by nonattaching spriochetes (original magnification ×1,500). (From Listgarten,1976. Reprinted with permission.)

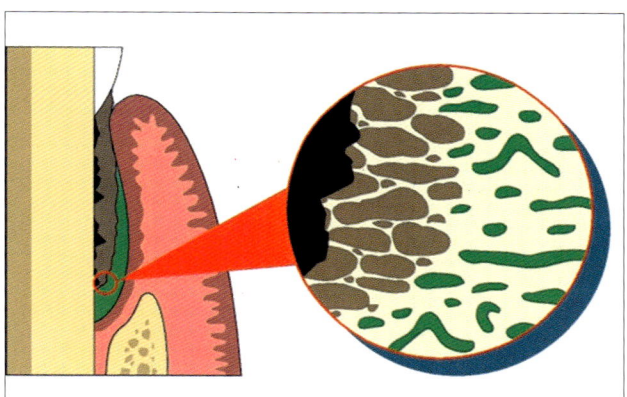

Fig 34 Diseased periodontal pocket containing attached subgingival plaque and nonattaching, motile subgingival microflora (spirochetes, vibrios, and straight rods with flagella). Note the calculus (black) covered by the subgingival plaque biofilm (brown).

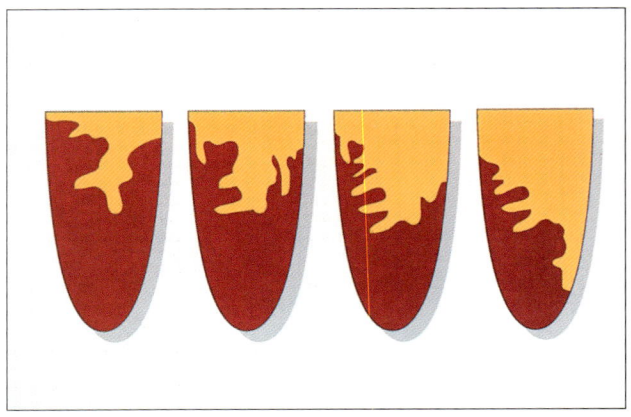

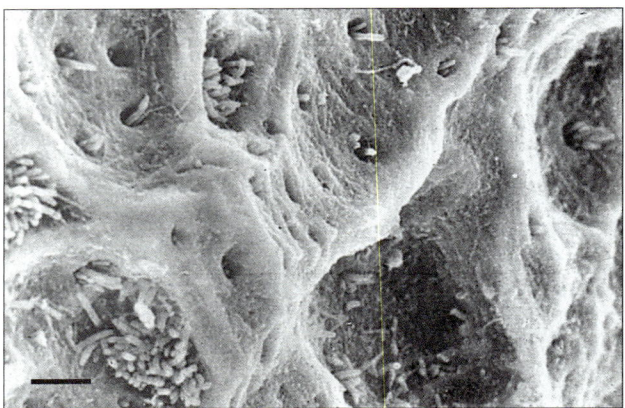

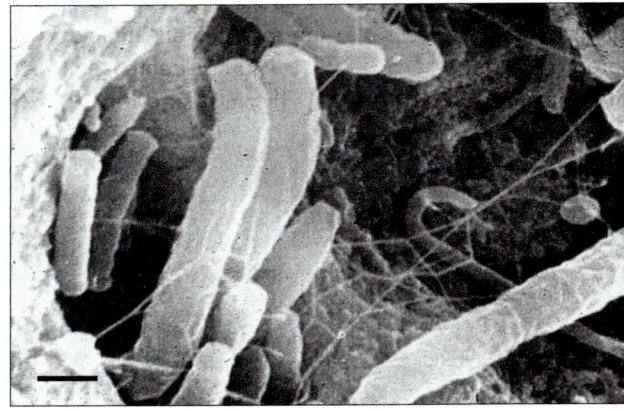

Fig 35 Iatrogenic grooves, cementum hypoplasia, etc may result in irregular lateral as well as apical migration of subgingival bacteria.

Figs 36a and 36b Invasion of bacteria in dentinal tubules via apertures denuded of cementum during aggressive scaling and root planing ([Fig 36a] bar = 10 μm; [Fig 36b] bar = 1 μm). (From Adriaens et al, 1988b. Reprinted with permission.)

tional epithelium, which is attached to the tooth surface on one side and to the gingival connective tissue on the other. This portion of the junctional epithelium is subject to both bacterial and mechanical injuries, which may result in enlarged intercellular spaces and vertical tears. These disruptions to the integrity of the junctional epithelium allow gradual apical colonization of the tooth surface by coccoid cells and rods. Irregularities in the root surface, such as those caused by localized root resorption, may shelter plaque microorganisms and contribute to their retention at such sites.

Even iatrogenic grooves left by aggressive scaling with rough instruments may result in lateral and apical migration of subgingival microbiota, with corresponding loss of periodontal support (Fig 35). Subgingival bacteria may also be

able to invade dentinal tubules via apertures denuded of cementum by aggressive scaling and root planing or by cementum hypoplasia (Figs 36a and 36b). This is a potential source of reinfection of the subgingival space following periodontal treatment. The role of exposed radicular dentin in periodontal infection has also been highlighted in studies by Ehnevid et al (1995) demonstrating that, in the absence of root cementum, bacteria or their products may migrate from infected root canals to the root surface, initiating or maintaining local periodontitis.

Figure 37 clearly shows the close correlation between the remaining periodontal membranes and junctional epithelia and the pattern of subgingival plaque deposits. Figure 38 shows that subgingival calculus, derived from minerals in the

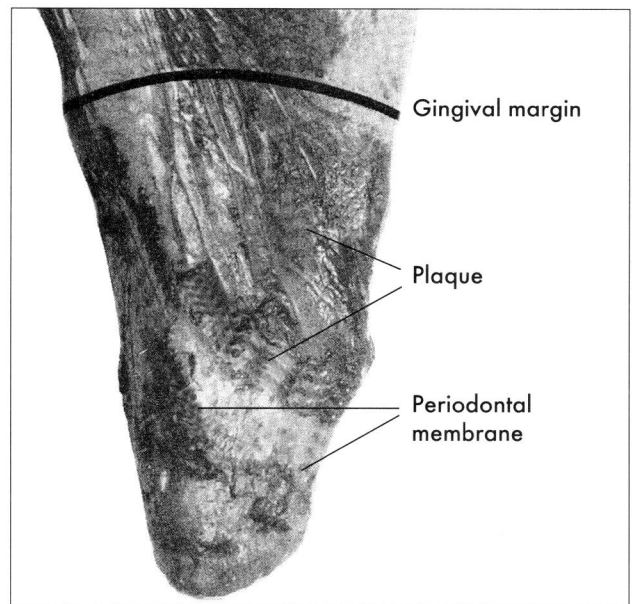

Fig 37 Close correlation between the remaining periodontal membrane and junctional epithelia and the pattern of subgingival plaque. (From Waerhaug, 1977. Reprinted with permission.)

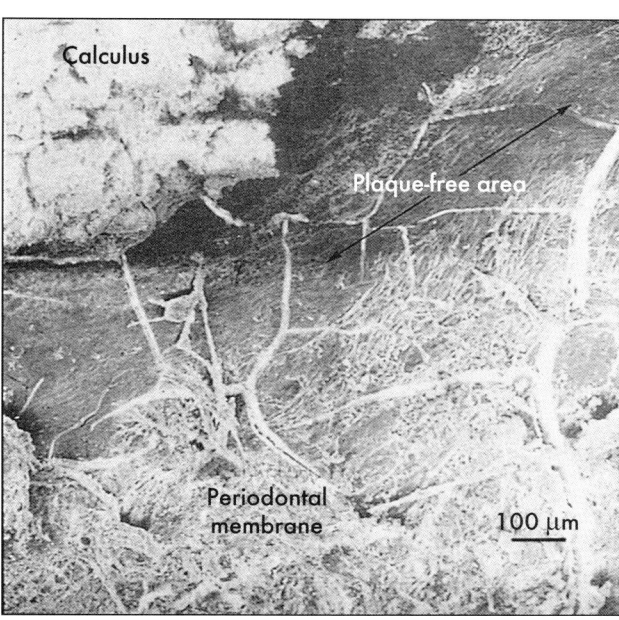

Fig 38 Subgingival calculus restricted to the base of the attached subgingival plaque biofilm. (From Waerhaug, 1977. Reprinted with permission.)

GCF, is restricted to the base of the attached subgingival plaque biofilm. The so-called "plaque-free zone" (0.2 to 1.0 mm) between subgingival plaque and calculus and the remaining periodontal membrane represents the sum of the area occupied by nonattaching motile microorganisms and the junctional epithelium. Recent studies by Noiri and Ebisu (2000) showed that *P gingivalis, Campylobacter rectus, T denticola, Prevotella nigrescens,* and *Actinomyces viscosus* were present in the "plaque-free zone."

The biofilm concept

Dental plaque is a microbial biofilm. *Biofilms* are defined as "matrix-enclosed bacterial populations adherent to each other and/or to surfaces or interfaces" (Costerton et al, 1994). More recent research into their molecular organization, physiochemical properties, and growth characteristics has led to the concept of biofilms as ecological communities that evolved to permit survival of the community as a whole (Costerton et al, 1995). Evidence from a variety of sources is consistent with the concept of coevolution of a mixed microbial community to live in proximity to the tooth surface, above and below the gingival margin. This is supported by the presence of a primitive circulatory system and metabolic cooperation (Darveau et al, 1997), but there is as yet no published documentation of mutational analysis and structure-function analysis, in vitro or in vivo (Fig 39).

Although the capacity to attach plays a key role in the variety of different microbial species

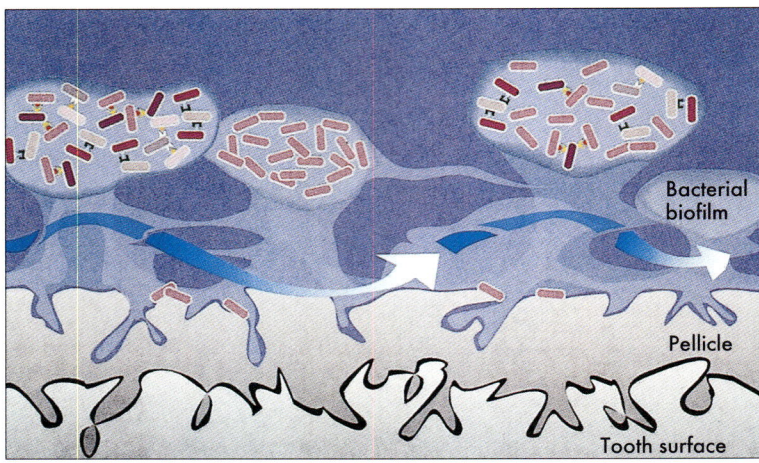

Fig 39 Schematic illustration of a plaque biofilm. The pellicle and biofilm extracellular matrix are depicted as firmly embedded in each other, contributing to the well-known recalcitrance of dental plaque. The unique shape of biofilms are believed to facilitate growth and symbiosis among the microbiota. The large arrows depict solvent flow that occurs through both large and small aqueous channels that are believed to carry nutrients and metabolic products to different members of the community. (From Darveau et al, 1997. Reprinted with permission.)

that constitute the dental plaque biofilm, bacterial growth is the primary determinant of the relative proportions of the bacteria. Plaque-doubling times are rapid in early development and slower in more mature films because of the structure of the biofilms, which contain areas of high and low bacterial biomass interlaced with aqueous channels of different sizes. It is believed that these channels transport nutrients and metabolic waste products within the colony. For example, dissolved oxygen in living biofilms was measured to be at nearly anoxic values within microcolonies but at significant concentrations at all levels in cell-free aqueous channels (Costerton et al, 1994). This structure provides a means by which the different bacterial species can benefit from their juxtaposition, facilitating a type of physiologic cooperation not seen in mixed populations of planktonic organisms. The unique conditions of physiologic cooperation in biofilms may influence the occurrence of bacterial blooms (periods of rapidly accelerated growth of specific species or groups of species) described in periodontal plaque (Sissons et al, 1995). Further investigation is needed to define the factors that influence

growth of selected microcolonies in dental plaque biofilms.

An excellent discussion of the factors that may influence growth of the subgingival plaque has recently been published (Shah and Gharbia, 1995). The main nutritional component is gingival crevicular fluid, which accounts for the predominance of asaccharolytic species. In addition, interspecies cooperation in the metabolism of α-gingipain in digested proteins was suggested. Although this cysteine protease is considered to be an important virulence factor for *P gingivalis,* it may have evolved simply to provide nutrition in this environment.

In contrast to the supragingival biofilm, the subgingival biofilm is protected from intraoral abrasion or salivary host defense components. As long as it is not disrupted by mechanical debridement, the microorganisms are inaccessible to antimicrobial agents and host factors. The main determinants limiting growth are physical space and the innate host defense system.

Because gingival crevicular fluid is rich in nutrients, growth is unlikely to be limited by poor nutrition. In periodontal health, the subgingival

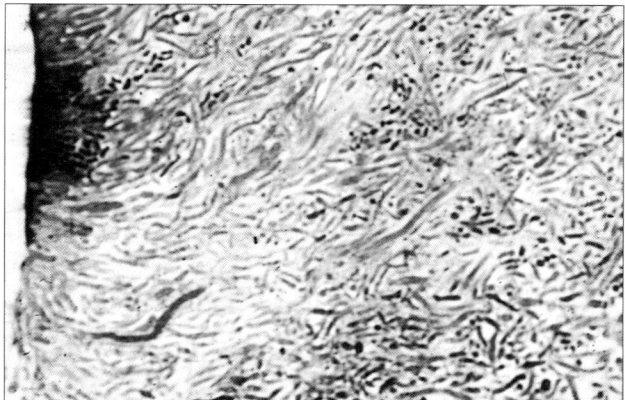

Fig 40 Attached biofilm with calculus in the interior *(left)* surrounded by an assortment of nonattached motile microorganisms (original magnification ×1,500). (From Listgarten, 1976. Reprinted with permission.)

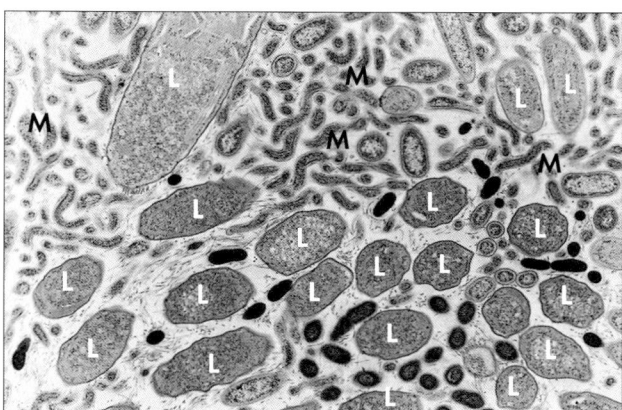

Fig 41 Increased magnification of Fig 40 revealing many motile microorganisms (M) as well as leukocytes (L) (original magnification ×15,000). (From Listgarten, 1976. Reprinted with permission.)

space available for bacterial growth is limited, but one effect of subgingival plaque accumulation is a continual increase in this space, resulting from a reduction of epithelial cell attachment levels and an increase in pocket depth.

The innate host defense system limits this spread by maintaining an intact epithelial cell barrier. Gingival crevicular fluid contains a potent array of antimicrobial agents. It is similar in composition to serum and contains the innate and adaptive components of host defense, which prevent bacteremia and systemic infection. Innate components include lysozyme, complement, and a variety of vascular permeability enhancers, such as bradykinin, thrombin, and fibrinogen. Adaptive components include antibodies and lymphocytes. Of major importance is the role of the phagocytozing neutrophils (PMNLs), representing the first line of nonspecific defense in walling off further apical migration of the subgingival biofilm as well as motile spirochetes.

Nonattached subgingival microflora

On the periphery of the subgingival plaque biofilm are high concentrations of spirochetes and other nonattaching microorganisms in direct contact with the gingival tissue wall and the apical lining of the sulcus or pocket. Figure 40, which shows the apical region of a deep periodontal pocket, reveals attached biofilm, with calculus in the interior surrounded by a great assortment of nonattached motile microorganisms. Figure 41 shows not only many motile microorganisms but also leukocytes (PMNLs and monocytes) in this "community." The predominant motile microflora are shown in Figs 42 and 43. Long spirochetes on the periphery of the subgingival biofilm are shown in Fig 44.

The major role of the phagocytozing PMNLs in preventing bacterial invasion of the tissues is discussed in chapters 4 and 5. Many "aggressive" competent PMNL cells that migrate into the pocket, guided by chemotactic forces, are very beneficial, as shown by Saglie et al (1982b). An aggressive, competent PMNL cell can engulf many bacteria, even long rods or spirochetes. By form-

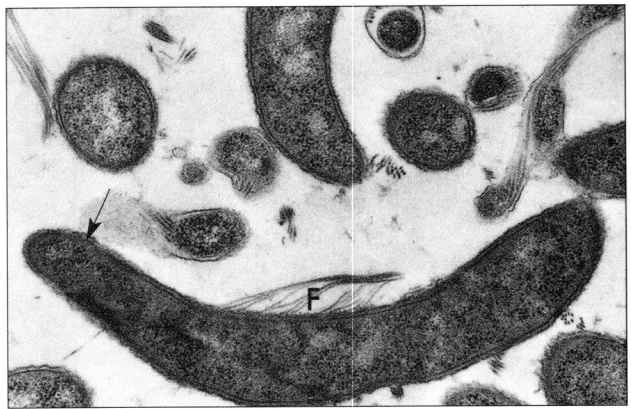

Fig 42 Predominant motile microflora: vibrio (arrow) with flagella (F) in longitudinal section (original magnification ×28,000). (From Listgarten, 1976. Reprinted with permission.)

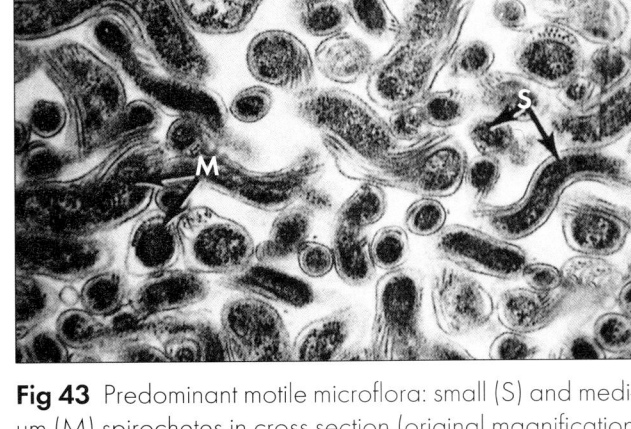

Fig 43 Predominant motile microflora: small (S) and medium (M) spirochetes in cross section (original magnification ×15,000). (From Listgarten, 1976. Reprinted with permission.)

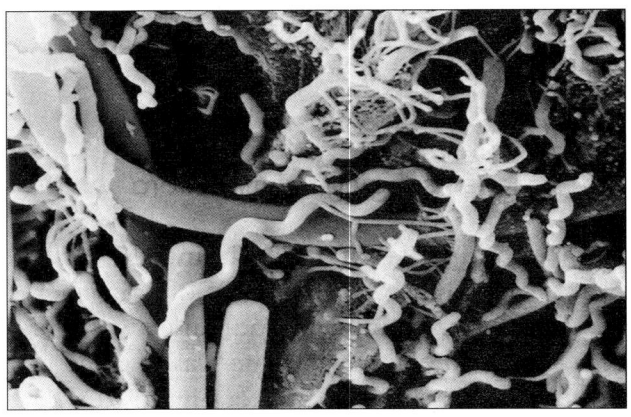

Fig 44 Long spirochetes on the periphery of the subgingival biofilm (original magnification ×8,000). (Courtesy of L. Nilsson.)

ing a barrier of viable phagocytic cells between the subgingival plaque and the gingival tissue, PMNLs prevent apical and lateral extension of the subgingival plaque.

If the gingival crevice or periodontal pocket lacks adequate numbers of vital, aggressive, phagocytosing PMNLs of sufficient versatility (lysosymal enzymes, etc), periopathogenic bacteria may invade the periodontal tissues during acute (active) phases of periodontitis (bursts or exacerbation) (Figs 45 to 48), sometimes resulting in formation of microabscesses or macroabscesses (Frank and Voegel, 1978; Saglie et al, 1982a, 1982b, 1987, 1988a, 1988b; Saglie, 1991).

It has also been shown that bacteria invade the pocket epithelial cells (Saglie et al, 1982b). Experimentally, Madianos et al (1996) have shown that the well-known periopathogen *P gingivalis* may not only invade the epithelial cells, but also multiply in the cells. Other studies have shown that in cases of aggressive periodontitis, *A actinomycetemcomitans* and even *Mycoplasma* invade the pocket epithelium and connective tissue. Figure 49 shows several mycoplasmas attacking a lymphocyte. In other recent studies, periopathogens were found in 80% of atheromas removed from the carotid arteries of patients receiving endarterectomy because of carotid stenosis. These observations may to some extent explain the relationship between periodontal diseases and cardiovascular diseases (Haraszthy et al, 2000).

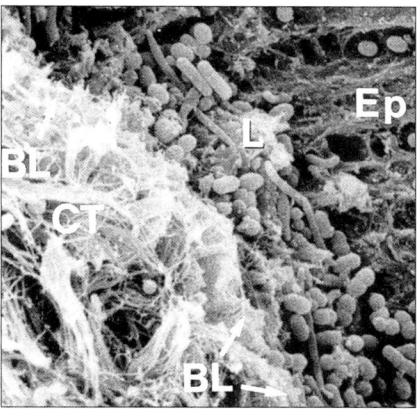

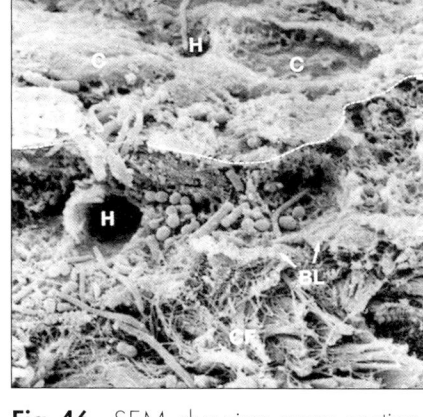

Fig 45 SEM showing cross section of pocket epithelium–connective tissue interface. Large accumulation of cocci, rods, and filaments can be seen on the epithelium side. BL = Basement lamina; Ep = Epithelium; CT = Connective tissue; L = Leukocyte (PMN) (original magnification ×6,000). (From Saglie et al, 1982a. Reprinted with permission.)

Fig 46 SEM showing cross section of the epithelium–connective tissue interface. The inner surface of the pocket epithelium is on top. Observe how cocci and tall rods enter into the epithelium via opened intercellular holes (H). Arrows show that the bacteria also penetrate basement lamina (BL) into the connective tissue. C = Epithelial cells; CF = Connective tissue fibers (original magnification ×8,000). (From Saglie et al, 1982a. Reprinted with permission.)

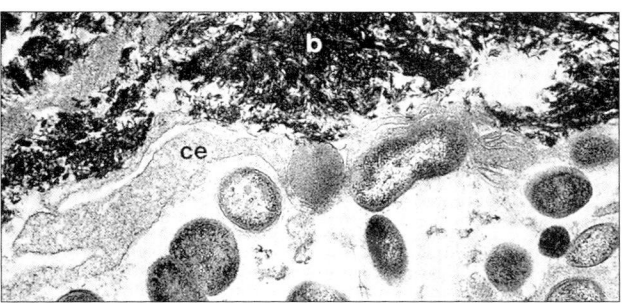

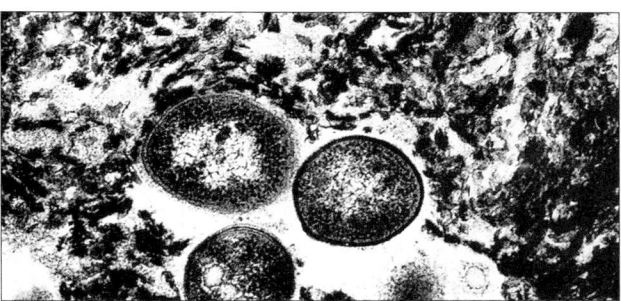

Fig 47 Advancing bacteria separated from the alveolar bone (b) by osteoclastic cells (ce) in advanced periodontitis (original magnification ×27,000). (From Frank and Voegel, 1978. Reprinted with permission.)

Fig 48 Gram-negative bacteria in direct contact with an actively resorbing bone surface in an advanced periodontitis site (original magnification ×42,000). (From Frank and Voegel, 1978. Reprinted with permission.)

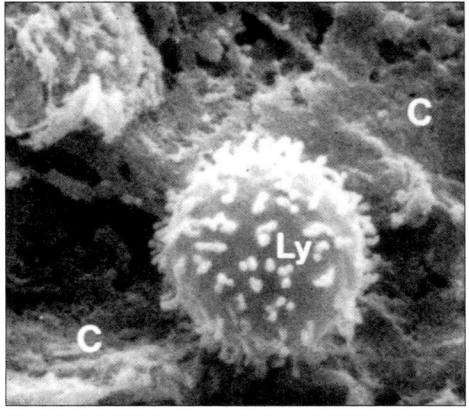

Fig 49 Several mycoplasmas attacking a lymphocyte (Ly). C = Epithelial cells (original magnification ×8,000). (From Saglie et al, 1982c. Reprinted with permission.)

AMOUNT OF PLAQUE
Plaque indices

The presence and/or the amount of supragingival plaque is usually measured by one of the established plaque indices, which have been used for many years to record oral hygiene standards in epidemiologic studies, clinical trials, and clinical practice. Assessment may be based on the presence or absence of plaque at certain sites, the area or thickness of plaque, or gravimetric measurement. Recordings are usually made from the exposed buccal and/or lingual surfaces of the teeth, although interproximal determinations can be attempted by supplementary probing. Disclosing agents may be applied to highlight the colorless plaque for the examiner and particularly for the patient (see Figs 15 to 18). Although simplified indices are often used in epidemiologic studies, complete-mouth recordings are strongly recommended in clinical trials and clinical practice.

Oral Hygiene Index

The original Oral Hygiene Index (OHI) was based on measurement of 12 tooth surfaces (Greene and Vermillion, 1960). Subsequently, the Simplified Oral Hygiene Index (OHI-S) was introduced (Greene and Vermillion, 1964), based on recordings from only six tooth surfaces: the labial surfaces of teeth 11, 16, 26, and 31 and the lingual surfaces of teeth 36 and 46. The index has two components, one for soft deposits and one for calcified deposits. The Simplified Calculus Index (CI-S) is not used extensively. Most clinicians use only one component of the OHI-S, the Simplified Debris Index (DI-S), which has the following criteria for assigning scores of 0 to 3:

- 0 = no debris or stain
- 1 = soft debris covering not more than one third of the exposed tooth surfaces or the presence of extrinsic stains without debris, regardless of surface area covered
- 2 = soft debris covering more than one third,

but no more than two thirds, of the exposed tooth surfaces
- 3 = soft debris covering more than two thirds of the exposed tooth surfaces

The DI-S score is calculated by dividing the sum of the debris score for all teeth by the number of surfaces scored. At least two of the six surfaces must have been included to calculate the score, and adjacent teeth may be substituted if the usual index teeth are missing. This relatively simple assessment is reproducible. To give the DI-S index clinical relevance, oral cleanliness is also rated:

- Good = 0.3 to 0.6
- Fair = 0.7 to 1.8
- Poor = 1.9 to 3.0

Ramfjord Plaque Index

The prototype for contemporary plaque indices was introduced by Ramfjord (1959, 1967), as part of his periodontal disease index. A modified version of this system has been applied extensively. The modified system comprises examination of the facial and lingual surfaces of six selected teeth (teeth 16, 21, 26, 36, 41, and 44), and restricts the scoring of plaque to the gingival half of the interproximal surfaces. The following scoring system is used:

- 0 = absence of dental plaque
- 1 = dental plaque in the interproximal area or at the gingival margin, covering less than one third of the gingival half of the facial or lingual surface
- 2 = dental plaque covering more than one third but less than two thirds of the gingival half of the facial or lingual surface
- 3 = dental plaque covering two thirds or more of the gingival half of the facial or gingival surface of the tooth

To derive a mean score, the total score is divided by the number of teeth examined.

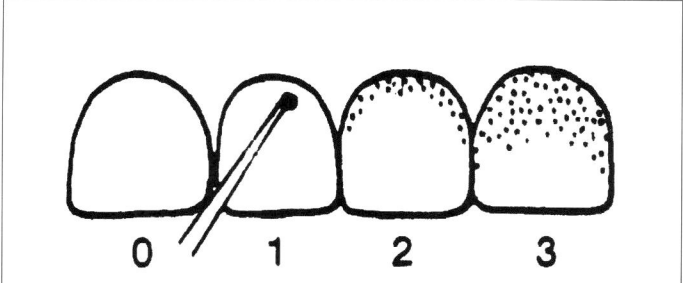

Fig 50 Silness and Löe Plaque Index (1964): 0 = The tooth surface is clean; 1 = The tooth surface appears clean, but dental plaque can be removed from the gingival third with a sharp explorer; 2 = Visible plaque is present along the gingival margin; 3 = The tooth surface is covered with abundant plaque.

Quigley and Hein Plaque Index

The plaque index developed by Quigley and Hein (1962) and modified by Turesky et al (1970) is acknowledged as reliable, using an estimate of the area of the tooth covered by plaque. By scoring plaque on the buccal and lingual surfaces, it offers comprehensive assessment, suitable for evaluating antiplaque procedures such as toothbrushing and flossing as well as chemical antiplaque agents. This index highlights the difference in plaque accumulation in the gingival third of the tooth. The scoring system is as follows:

- 0 = no plaque
- 1 = separate flecks of plaque at the cervical margin of the tooth
- 2 = a thin continuous band of plaque (up to 1 mm) at the cervical margin
- 3 = a band of plaque wider than 1 mm but covering less than one third of the crown
- 4 = plaque covering at least one third but less than two thirds of the crown
- 5 = plaque covering two thirds or more of the crown

Silness and Löe Plaque Index

The plaque index most extensively applied in clinical trials during the last few decades is that originally described by Silness and Löe (1964). The method is based on estimated measurements of plaque by examination of the whole or parts of the dentition. It has been applied to studies in children as well as adults and is reliable for evaluating both mechanical and chemical plaque control. Each of the four gingival areas of the tooth is given a score from 0 to 3; this is the Plaque Index (PI) for the area. The scores from the four areas of the tooth may be added and then divided by four to give the PI for the tooth. The scores for individual teeth (incisors, premolars, and molars) may be grouped to designate the PI for groups of teeth. By adding the area scores for each tooth and dividing by the number of teeth examined, the plaque index for the individual is obtained.

Each gingival area is scored as follows (Fig 50):

- 0 = The gingival area of the tooth surface is literally free of plaque. The surface is tested by running a pointed probe across the tooth surface at the entrance to the gingival crevice after the tooth has been properly dried. If no soft matter adheres to the point of the probe, the area is considered clean.
- 1 = No plaque can be observed in situ by the

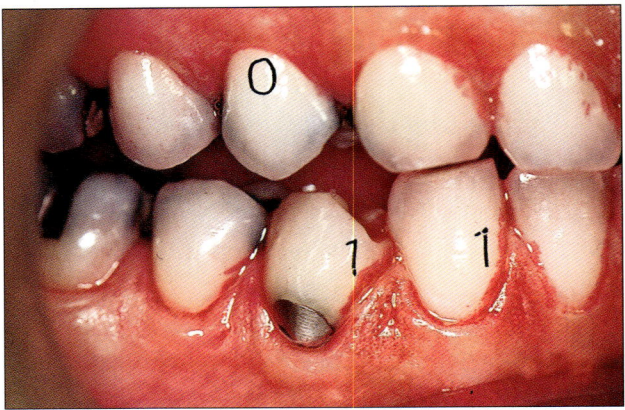 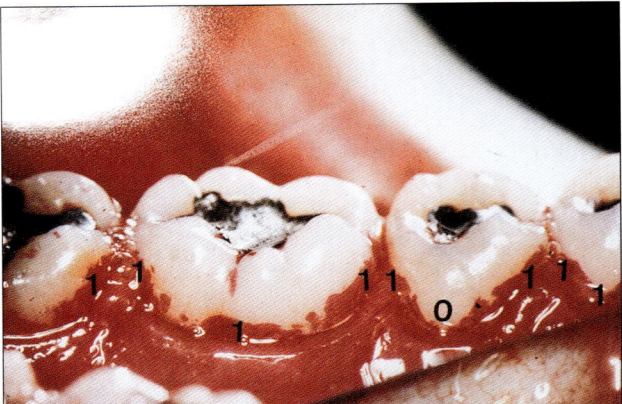

Figs 51 and 52 Examples of scoring with the Plaque Control Record (O'Leary et al, 1972). Plaque is scored as present (1) or absent (O) on four or six surfaces per tooth. The number of positively scored surfaces is divided by the total number of surfaces evaluated, and the result is multiplied by 100 to obtain a percentage.

naked eye, but plaque is visible on the point of a probe drawn across the tooth surface at the entrance of the gingival crevice. Disclosing solution was not used in the original investigation but may be useful for recognizing this film of plaque.

- 2 = The gingival area is covered by a thin to moderately thick layer of plaque, visible to the naked eye.
- 3 = There is heavy accumulation of soft matter, filling the niche produced by the gingival margin and the tooth surface. The interdental area is full of soft debris.

The plaque index scores record only differences in the thickness of the soft deposits on the gingival area of the tooth surfaces and not the coronal extent of the plaque. Plaque deposited on calculus deposits, restorations, and crowns is assessed. A major criticism of the Silness and Löe index is the subjectivity involved in estimating plaque, which becomes apparent when several examiners are participating in a study. It is therefore recommended that a single examiner be trained and used with each group of patients throughout a clinical trial.

The Silness and Löe Plaque Index is not linear, and nonparametric methods are therefore necessary for analysis of the data. It is essential not only

to note the actual plaque scores recorded but also to monitor the fate of the scores through the course of the study. For example, a record should be kept of the scores that change from 0 to 1 or to some other score.

The Silness and Löe Plaque Index has frequently been used in longitudinal plaque control studies to evaluate the correlation between PI and scores found using the Löe and Silness Gingival Index (GI) (1963). Strong correlations have been found at group, individual, and tooth-surface levels (Ainamo, 1970; Axelsson and Lindhe, 1974, 1977).

Plaque Control Record

A very simple and therefore reliable method for evaluating oral hygiene procedures was proposed by O'Leary and coworkers (1972). On a dichotomous basis, the disclosed plaque accumulations on all teeth are scored. Four (mesial, buccal, distal, and lingual) or six (mesiobuccal, buccal, distobuccal, mesiolingual, lingual, and distolingual) surfaces per tooth are recorded. The number of positively scored units is divided by the total number of tooth surfaces evaluated, and the result is multiplied by 100 to express the index as a percentage. With this method, the topographic distribution of plaque throughout the dentition can be readily assessed. Repeated scorings of that nature facilitate evaluation of the efficacy of oral hygiene programs in daily practice.

Figures 51 and 52 exemplify some positive and negative scores according to O'Leary et al (1972). This index is particularly useful in clinical practice for monitoring a patient's standard of oral hygiene and as a basis for individual education in self-care. However, it reveals only areas that the patient has failed to clean effectively, despite a special effort on the day of the dental appointment; it does not indicate the rate at which plaque forms in the individual, or the oral hygiene status 1 week before or after the dental appointment (for reviews on plaque indices, see Barnes et al, 1986; Fischman, 1986; Lang, 1998).

Pattern of plaque in toothbrushing populations

The pattern and quantity of plaque remaining after people "clean their teeth" will vary widely among populations and individuals, depending on factors such as the oral hygiene aids being used, differences in instruction in self-care, socioeconomic conditions, and so on. The habit of brushing daily is generally well established, whereas interproximal cleaning is not (Kuusela et al, 1997).

Specific individual patterns of plaque accumulation have been recognized in young individuals who have had no special instruction in home care (Cumming and Löe, 1973) and have been attributed to patterns in the quality of local plaque control. Although the pattern was unique to each of the subjects in the study, a general pattern for the whole group emerged. While some regions of the dentition were sometimes plaque free and sometimes covered by plaque, other areas in the mouths of all subjects were either consistently clean or consistently covered by plaque.

The pattern of remaining plaque, based on the Silness and Löe Plaque Index (1964), is shown in

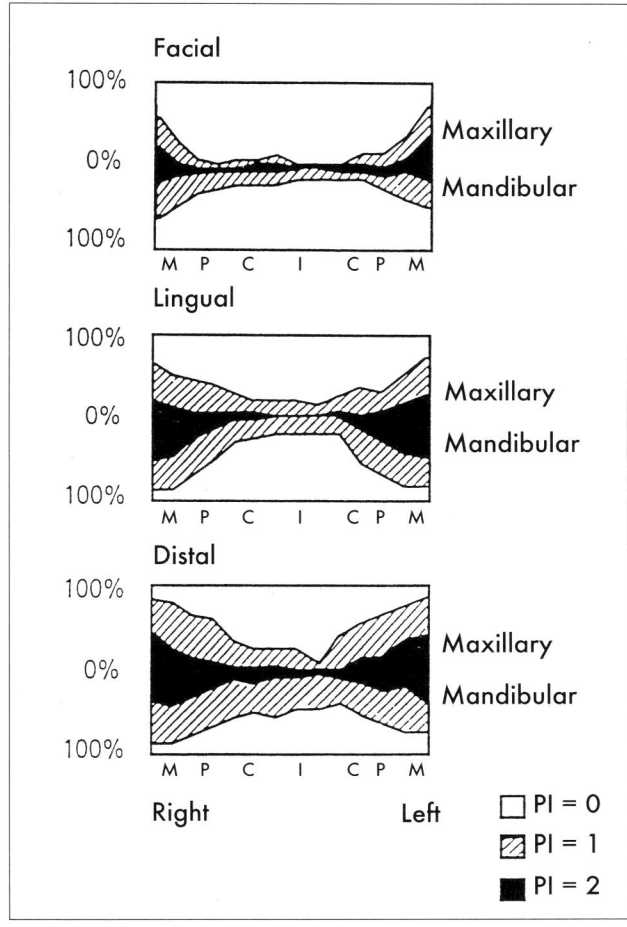

Fig 53 Pattern of remaining plaque, based on the Silness and Löe Plaque Index (PI). The frequency of plaque deposits is lowest on the facial surfaces and greatest at interproximal sites. M = Molar; P = Premolar; C = Canine; I = Incisor. (Modified from Cumming and Löe, 1973.)

Fig 53. The lowest frequency of plaque deposits was recorded for the facial surfaces. Plaque was slightly more common on mandibular teeth than on maxillary teeth, and far more frequent on molars than on incisors and premolars. The pattern was repeated for mandibular surfaces: Remaining plaque was observed more frequently on lingual than on facial aspects. Interproximal surfaces harbored the highest amount of plaque, and the distribution was similar to that on the other surfaces.

Similar findings were made in a study of the patterns of plaque removal in students and faculty members of a dental school (Lang et al, 1977):

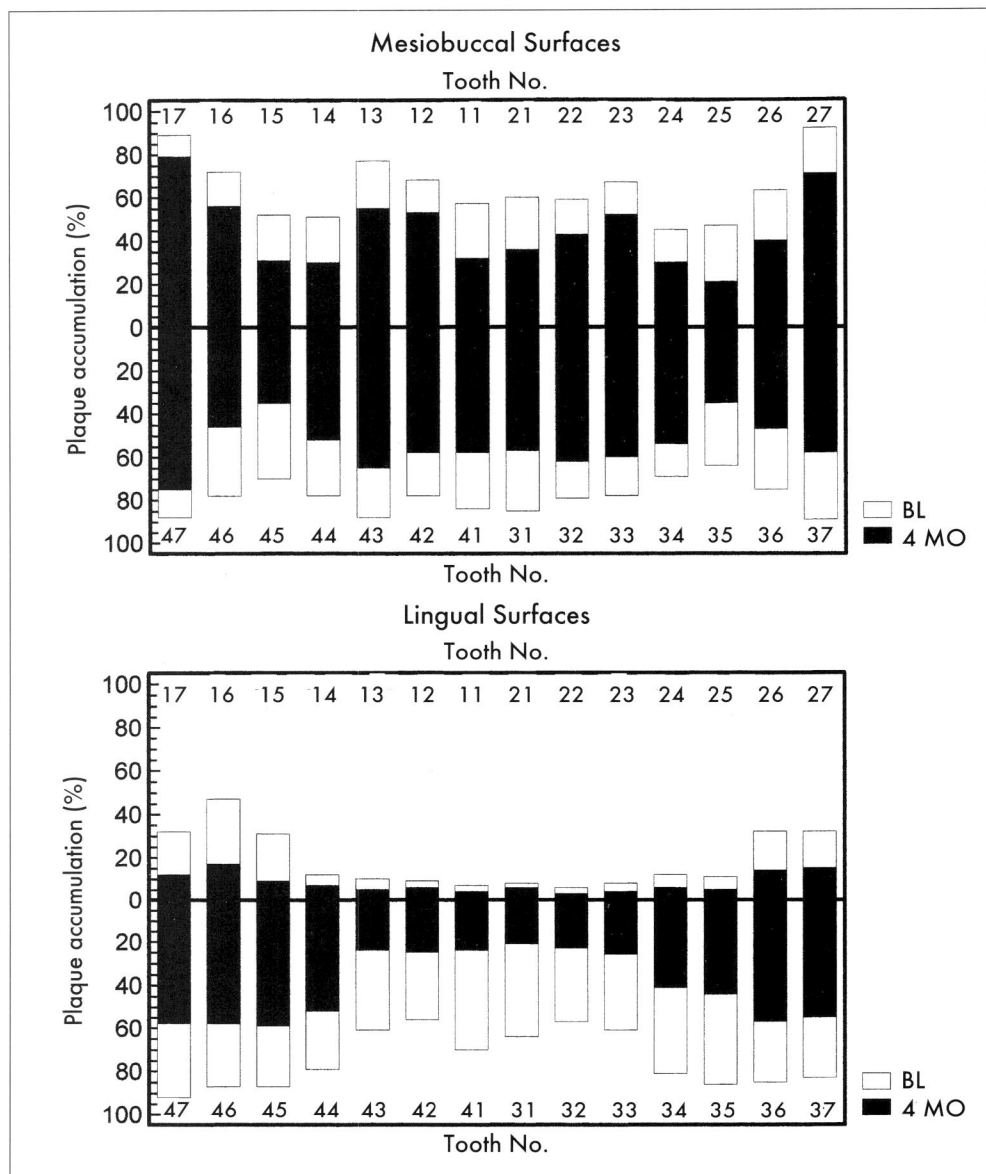

Fig 54 Effect of 4 months' Meridol (amine fluoride + stannous fluoride) therapy on plaque accumulation on mesiobuccal and lingual surfaces. Observe the pattern of existing plaque on the mesiobuccal surface vs the lingual surfaces at baseline (BL). 4 MO = 4 Months. (From Axelsson et al, 1994. Reprinted with permission.)

Oral cleanliness (PI) and gingival health (GI) were assessed in 150 dental students and 101 faculty members. Analysis of plaque distribution showed that posterior teeth consistently had more plaque than anterior teeth and that the heaviest deposits were interproximal. Furthermore, a positive relationship was found between oral hygiene habits and the subjects' academic status and involvement in clinical dentistry.

Axelsson et al (1994) studied a selected group of 100 subjects, aged 18 to 19 years, with established daily toothbrushing habits but relatively high gingivitis scores. Disclosed plaque was recorded at baseline and after 4 months' mouthrinsing twice a day with Meridol (amine fluoride + stannous fluoride). The mean patterns of disclosed plaque on the mesiobuccal and lingual surfaces are shown in Fig 54. Plaque was almost negligible on the lingual surfaces of the maxillary teeth. Because of poor accessibility, the antiplaque mouthrinse was less effective on the mesiobuccal surfaces than on the lingual surfaces.

Although mean plaque scores observed by examining a number of representative tooth surfaces might identify the need for improved oral hygiene in general, they would fail to identify specific potential problem regions in subjects with better-than-average oral hygiene standards. Because each individual appears to perform plaque control in specific patterns, the clinician has to identify inadequacies in personal oral hygiene programs by serial registrations of plaque deposits on single surfaces. Generally, in undisturbed plaque accumulation, the heaviest deposits seem to form interproximally and on the lingual mandibular posterior surfaces. Because this is also the case in the average patient without special home-care instruction (Cumming and Löe, 1973), it is obvious that special attention has to be paid to interdental cleansing when clinicians motivate patients.

RATE OF PLAQUE FORMATION

The amount and location of plaque recorded at clinical examination discloses only where the patient has been unsuccessful in cleaning, despite extra effort on the day of the dental appointment. It does not reveal the age of the plaque, the rate of accumulation, or the patient's usual standard of oral hygiene. It is therefore important to appreciate the difference between plaque indices, which are static, and the plaque reaccumulation rate, which is dynamic. An understanding of plaque formation rates and patterns is an essential foundation for successful strategies for primary and secondary prevention of periodontal diseases. According to the nonspecific plaque hypothesis, mechanical removal of dental plaque, being causally directed, is a rational method for prevention and control of periodontal diseases. However, for cost effectiveness, it should be related to the pattern and rate of plaque reaccumulation and otherwise-predicted risk. In the past three decades, questions regarding the rate of plaque growth and its

pattern of development on the dentition have been addressed by several investigators.

After mechanical removal, plaque slowly reaccumulates along the gingival margins of the teeth over the following 2 days. After the second day, the thickness increases dramatically, reaching a maximum after 7 days (Lang et al, 1973; Listgarten et al, 1975; Löe et al, 1965; Saxton, 1973). Forty-eight hours after toothcleaning, plaque has reaccumulated on 70% to 100% of the approximal surfaces and 90% to 100% of the lingual surfaces of the mandibular molars and premolars, to a visible plaque score of 2 on the Silness and Löe (1964) scale (Lang et al, 1973).

The aim of a clinical study by Lang et al (1973) was to assess the rate and pattern of plaque development in 32 dental students with excellent oral hygiene and clinically healthy gingival conditions. Four groups of volunteers performed complete plaque removal every 12, 48, 72, or 96 hours. For a period of 6 weeks, PI (Silness and Löe, 1964) was recorded immediately before cleaning. Figure 55 illustrates the different levels of plaque accumulation in the four groups: The mean level of undisturbed plaque accumulation after 12 hours was significantly lower than that after 48, 72, or 96 hours.

Plaque Formation Rate Index

The quantity of plaque that forms on clean tooth surfaces during a given time represents the net result of interactions among etiologic factors and many internal and external risk indicators and risk factors, as well as protective factors:

- The total oral bacterial population
- The quality of the oral bacterial flora
- The anatomy and surface morphology of the dentition
- The wettability and surface tension of the tooth surfaces
- The salivary secretion rate and other properties of saliva

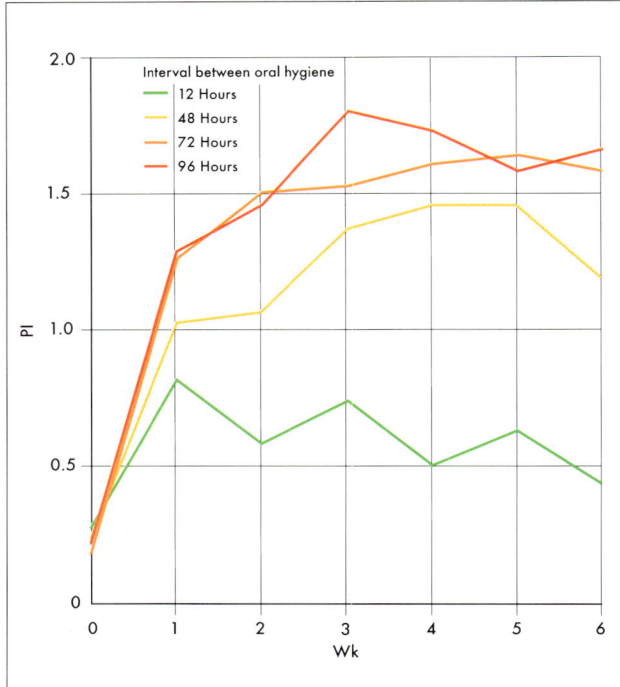

Fig 55 Levels of plaque accumulation in dental students performing oral hygiene measures at differing intervals. The Silness and Löe Plaque Index (1964) was significantly lower after 12 hours than it was after any of the other time intervals. (From Lang et al, 1973. Reprinted with permission.)

- The intake of fermentable carbohydrates
- The mobility of the tongue and lips
- The exposure to chewing forces and abrasion by foods
- The eruption stage of the teeth
- The degree of gingival inflammation and volume of gingival exudate
- The individual oral hygiene habits
- The use of fluorides and other preventive products, such as chemical plaque-control agents

This observation has been the rationale for the construction of the Plaque Formation Rate Index (PFRI) by Axelsson (1987, 1991). It includes all but the occlusal tooth surfaces and is based on the amount of plaque freely accumulated (de novo) in the 24 hours following PMTC, during which period subjects refrain from all oral hygiene. In a pilot study on 50 adult subjects, adherent plaque

was disclosed on 5% to 65% of the total number of tooth surfaces. On the basis of this study, the following five-point scale was constructed for the PFRI:

- Score 1 = 1% to 10% of surfaces affected: very low
- Score 2 = 11% to 20% of surfaces affected: low
- Score 3 = 21% to 30% of surfaces affected: moderate
- Score 4 = 31% to 40% of surfaces affected: high
- Score 5 = > 40% of surfaces affected: very high

In 1984, the PFRI was evaluated in a cross-sectional study of 667 schoolchildren aged 14 years in the city of Karlstad, Sweden. The subjects were followed over a 5-year period, up to the age of 19 years (Axelsson, 1987, 1991). Many indicators and factors possibly related to PFRI were also evaluated, including the following:

- Caries prevalence and caries incidence
- Gingival inflammation
- Plaque Index
- Dietary intake during the 24 hours of free plaque accumulation
- Salivary levels of *S mutans* and glucosyl transferase
- Agglutinin levels in resting saliva
- Oral hygiene, dietary and fluoride habits, etc

Figure 56 shows the frequency distribution of the 14-year-old schoolchildren according to PFRI scores. Most were low (Score 2 = 48%) or moderate (Score 3 = 27%) plaque formers, but the standard of oral hygiene is very high among schoolchildren in Karlstad, and as a consequence the gingival index and caries prevalence are low.

Among other observations from the study were:

- Individuals with a PFRI score of 4 or 5 had considerably higher scores for gingival bleeding than did those with a score of 1 or 2.
- An initially high Plaque Index usually correlated with PFRI scores 3 to 5.

- There was no significant correlation between different salivary *S mutans* levels and PFRI scores.
- The level of salivary glucosyl transferase was lower in individuals with a PFRI score of 4 or 5 than in those with a score of 1 or 2, probably because glucosyl transferase had already accumulated in the matrix of the plaque in the fast and very fast plaque formers.
- The scores tended to remain constant over the 5-year period for individuals with very low and low PFRI (scores 1 and 2) but tended to vary in some individuals with scores of 3 to 5, increasing or decreasing by 1 unit.

This final observation indicates that in subjects with a score of 4 or 5, plaque formation rates can be reduced. Thorough evaluation of such subjects should identify the factors contributing to the rapid plaque formation. Needs-related preventive measures could then be introduced. For example, there is a strong correlation among plaque formation rate, the severity of gingival inflammation, and the volume of gingival exudate (Axelsson, 1987; Quirynen et al, 1991; Ramberg et al, 1994, 1995; Saxton, 1973, 1975). Initially intensive and frequent mechanical and chemical plaque control, both self-care and professional, is indicated in individuals with a PFRI score of 4 or 5 and high Gingival Index scores in order to heal all inflamed sites as quickly as possible and thereby reduce the plaque formation rate.

If the high plaque formation rate is associated with inadequate salivary secretion, frequent plaque control (before every meal) should be supplemented with salivary stimulation through the use of fluoride chewing gum immediately after every meal.

A high intake of fermentable carbohydrates, particularly sucrose, will result in sticky plaque, rich in polysaccharides, and an increased plaque formation rate (Carlsson and Egelberg, 1965). Needs-related prevention for individuals with a PFRI score of 4 or 5 and a frequent intake of sugar-containing products should therefore emphasize not only frequent plaque control but

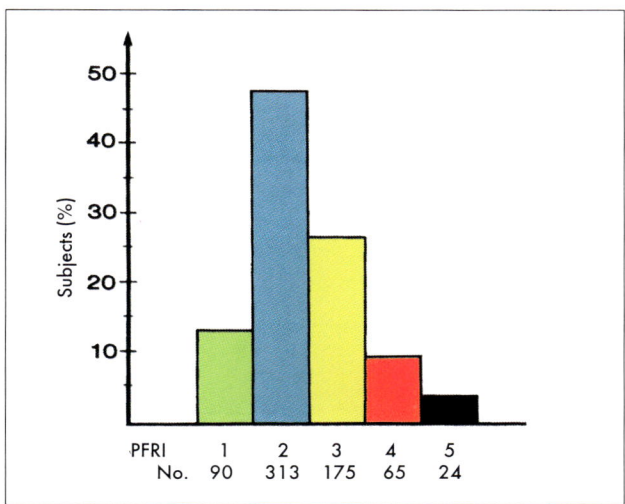

Fig 56 Stratification of Plaque Formation Rate Index (PFRI) in 14 year olds in Karlstad, Sweden. (From Axelsson, 1987, 1991. Reprinted with permission.)

also a reduction in frequency of sugar intake. In this study, a high consumption of bananas during the 24-hour period of free plaque accumulation was noted in some individuals with a PFRI score of 5.

The PFRI has recently been applied in studies on different populations and age groups. From more than 1,000 individuals aged 17 to 19 years in the city of Karlstad, 30% with the highest GI were selected to participate in a 4-month double-blind mouthrinse study. At baseline, most of the subjects had a PFRI score of 3 (more than 40%) or 4 (about 25%) (Axelsson et al, 1994). Subjects with the highest GIs also had the highest PFRI scores. In addition, sites with gingival inflammation had significantly higher plaque formation rates than did healthy gingival sites (Ramberg et al, 1995).

Brazil has the highest caries prevalence in the world. In São Paulo, a 3-year caries-preventive study based on self-diagnosis and self-care was conducted in 12- to 15-year-old schoolchildren. The PFRI was used as a tool for self-diagnosis and establishment of needs-related oral hygiene habits. At baseline, almost 100% of the 12-year-old schoolchildren had a PFRI score of 5. The mean percentage of surfaces with reaccumulated plaque was more than 70%, probably because of

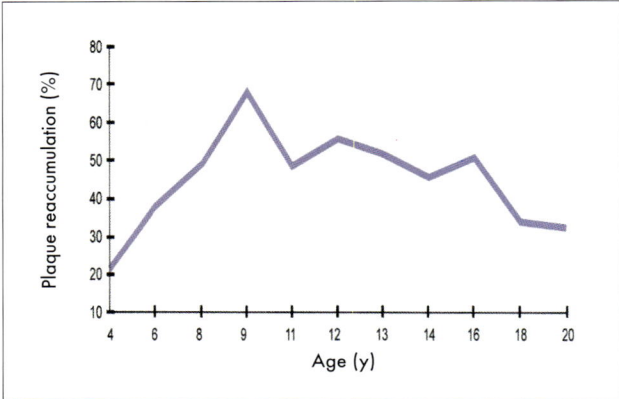

Fig 57 Plaque reaccumulation by age (percentage of surfaces with plaque). (From Cunea and Axelsson, 1997. Reprinted with permission.)

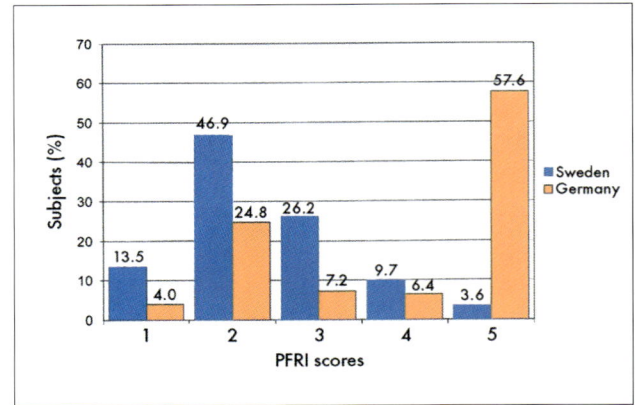

Fig 58 Comparison of Plaque Formation Rate Index (PFRI) scores of German and Swedish children. (From Cunea and Axelsson, 1997. Reprinted with permission.)

the extremely high caries prevalence, a high Gingival Index, and the presence of erupting permanent teeth. At reexamination 3 years later, the PFRI had dropped significantly: Most of the 15 year olds had a score of 3 or 4. The main contributing factors were improvement in oral hygiene habits and gingival health and the fact that all teeth were now fully erupted (Albandar et al, 1994; Axelsson et al, 1994; Buischi et al, 1994).

In Duisburg, Germany, the PFRI was evaluated in different age groups of children: preschool children, children with mixed dentitions and erupting permanent teeth, and children with fully erupted teeth. Children with erupting teeth had the highest PFRI scores (Fig 57). According to the World Health Organization's Data Bank (1993), caries prevalence in German 12-year-old children is high, and the German children generally had higher PFRI scores than did Swedish children of comparable age with very low caries prevalence, excellent gingival conditions, and good oral hygiene habits (Fig 58) (Axelsson, 1991; Cunea and Axelsson, 1997).

Pattern of plaque reaccumulation

As discussed earlier, the plaque formation rate is influenced by such factors as:

- The anatomy and surface morphology of the teeth
- The stage of eruption and functional status of the teeth
- The wettability and surface tension of the tooth surfaces (both intact and restored surfaces)
- The gingival health and volume of gingival exudate

The pattern of plaque reaccumulation will also be influenced by these factors, but may differ somewhat on tooth surfaces exposed to chewing forces, abrasion from foods, and friction from the dorsum of the tongue, lips, and cheeks and on less accessible areas, such as approximal sites, along the gingival margin, and in irregularities such as occlusal fissures. These areas are often designated "stagnation areas" for plaque.

In the 6-week study by Lang et al (1973) described earlier, plaque reaccumulation was registered in four groups of dental students with different frequencies of oral hygiene procedures: mechanical toothcleaning by self-care twice daily or every second, third, or fourth day. Figure 59

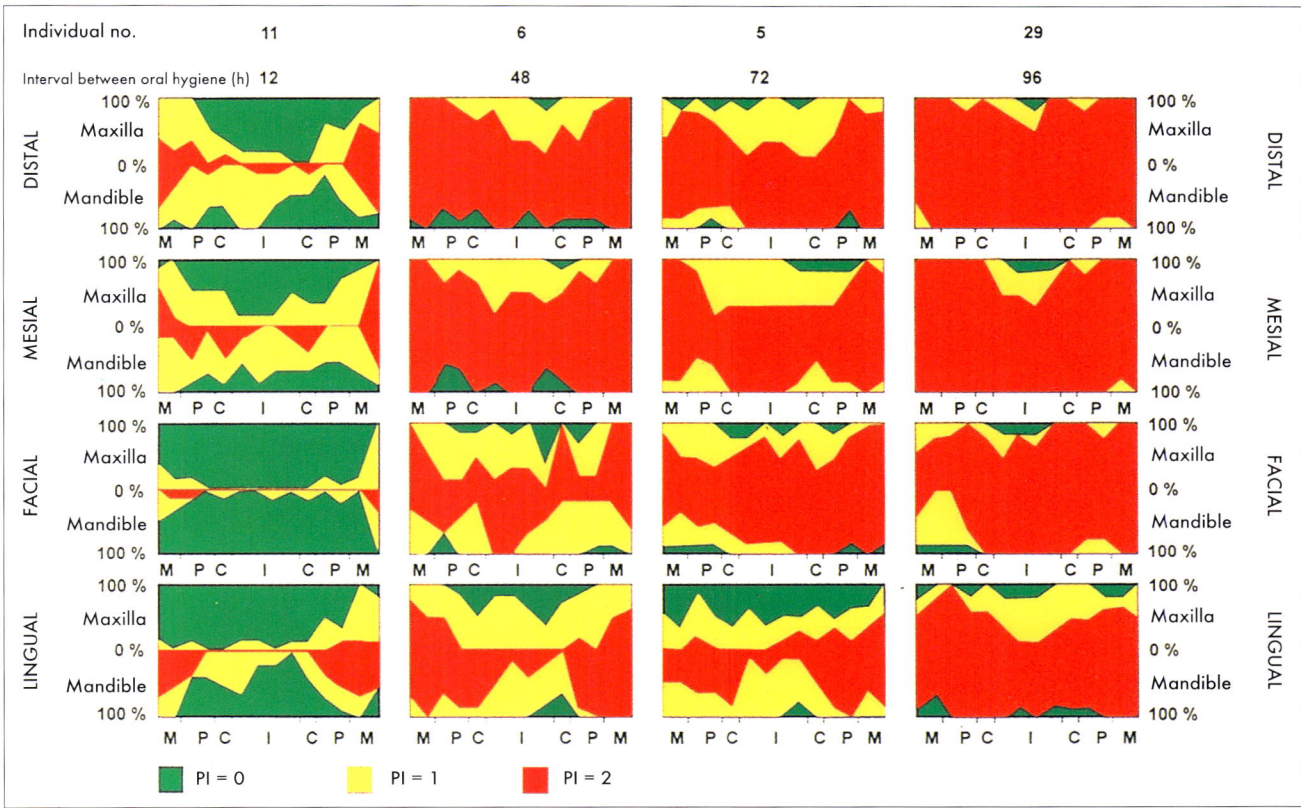

Fig 59 Patterns of plaque reaccumulation in subjects with various frequencies of plaque removal. Plaque was measured with the Silness and Löe (1964) Plaque Index (PI). (Modified from Lang et al, 1973. Reprinted with permission.)

shows the pattern of reaccumulated plaque, measured with the Silness and Löe (1964) Plaque Index (scores 0 to 3) on the surfaces of the maxillary and mandibular teeth. After only 24 hours of free plaque reaccumulation, there was visible plaque on some of the approximal surfaces of the molars and the lingual surfaces of the mandibular molars (score 2). After 48 hours, almost 100% of these surfaces and most of the remaining approximal surfaces had a score of 2 or 3. The pattern of visible plaque after 2 and 3 days seemed to be similar, except for the facial surfaces.

According to Listgarten (1976), freely accumulated plaque is about 5 times thicker after 3 days than after 2 (see Fig 21). This explains why gingivitis developed in the group of students cleaning only every third or fourth day, but not in those who cleaned their teeth at least every second day.

Figure 60 presents the percentage of freely accumulated (de novo) plaque, 24 hours after PMTC, from the large-scale study on 667 children aged 14 years in the city of Karlstad (Axelsson, 1987, 1991). Plaque reaccumulation was greatest on the mandibular mesiolingual and distolingual surfaces (33%), particularly on the molars, followed by the mesiobuccal and distobuccal surfaces of both maxillary and mandibular teeth, particularly the molars. There was almost no plaque reaccumulation (3%) on the lingual surfaces of the maxillary teeth, mainly because of friction from the rough dorsum of the tongue.

Figure 61 illustrates the percentage of de novo plaque, 24 hours after PMTC, in 3- to 5-, 6- to 7-, 8- to 12-, 13- to 16-, and 16- to 21-year-old German subjects (Cunea and Axelsson, 1997). The highest percentages are found in 6 to 14 year olds, who

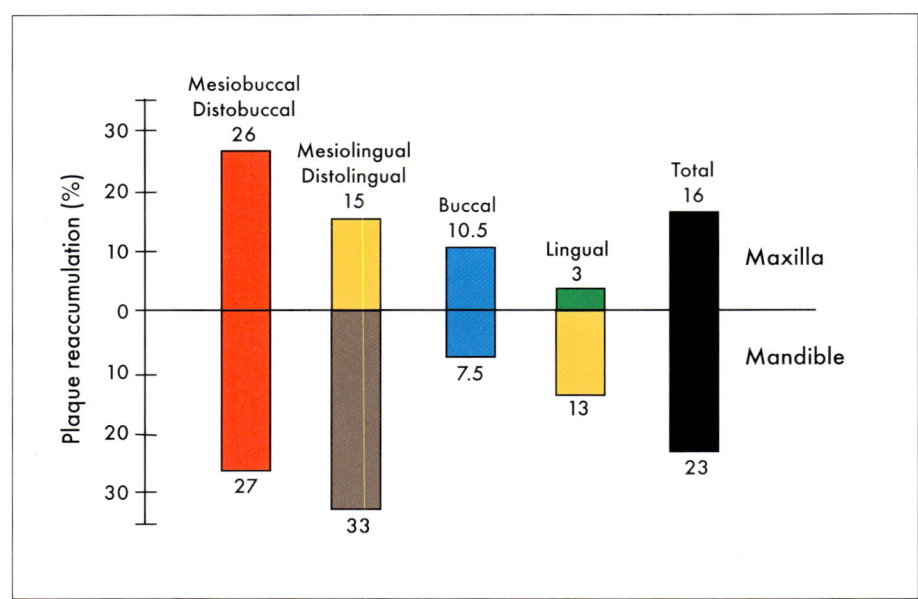

Fig 60 The pattern of plaque formation rate in 14-year-old subjects 24 hours after PMTC. (From Axelsson, 1987, 1991. Reprinted with permission.)

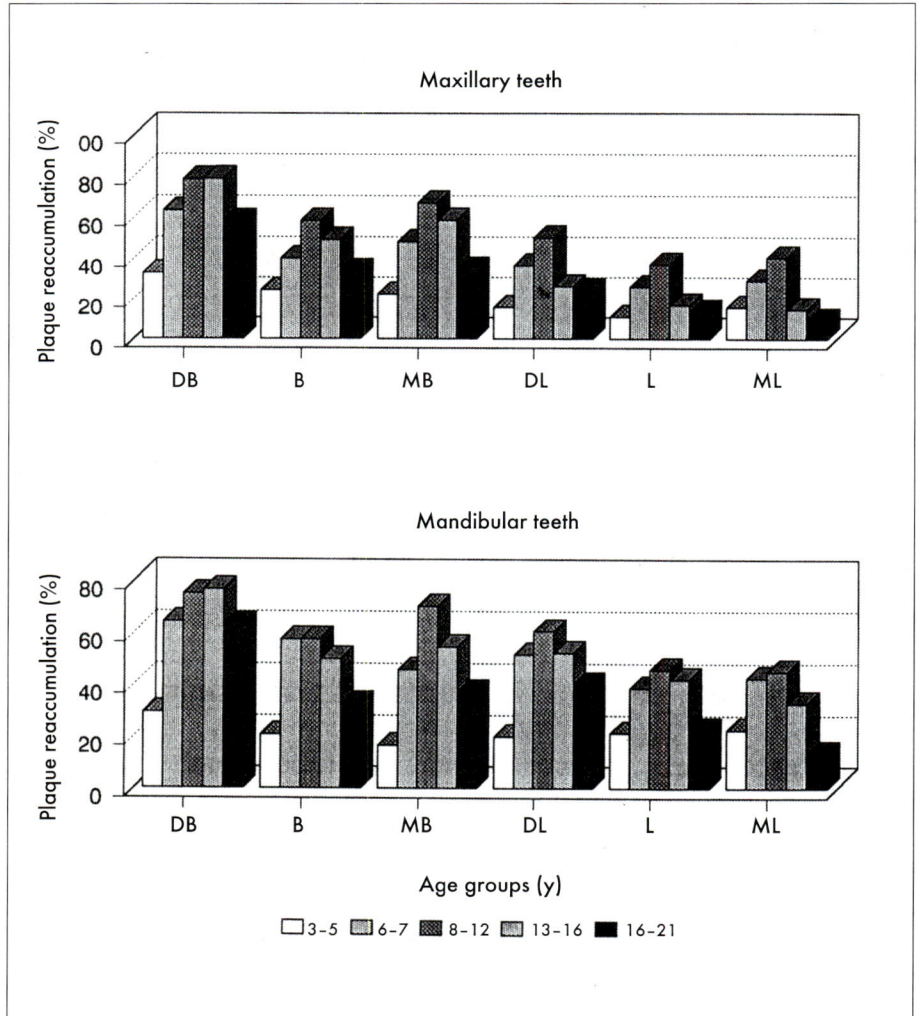

Fig 61 Percentage of new plaque accumulation related to age on distobuccal (DB), buccal (B), mesiobuccal (MB), distolingual (DL), lingual (L), and mesiolingual (ML) surfaces of teeth 24 hours after PMTC. (From Cunea and Axelsson, 1997. Reprinted with permission.)

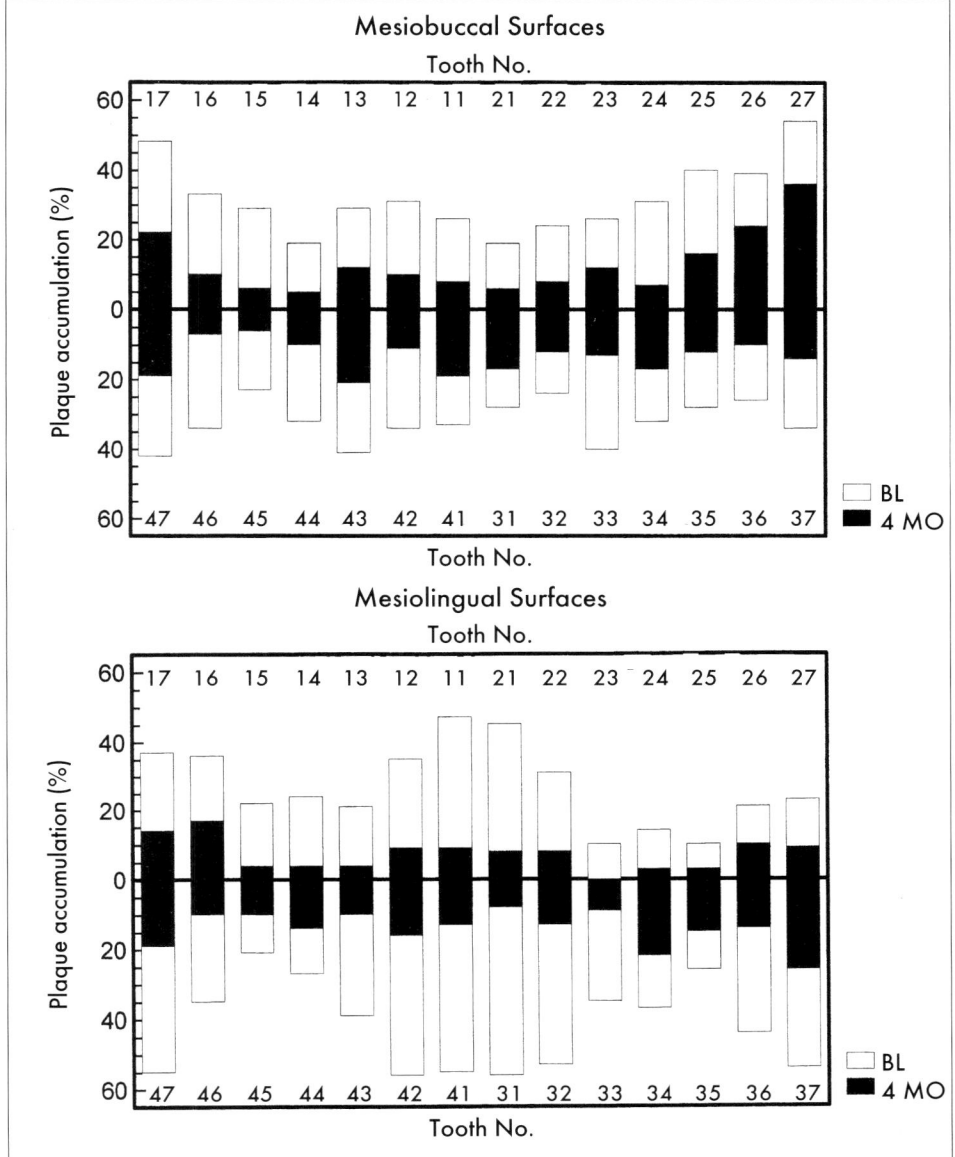

Fig 62 Effect of chlorhexidine on plaque reaccumulation on mesiobuccal and mesiolingual surfaces. BL = Baseline score; 4 MO = Score after 4 months' use of 0.1% chlorhexidine twice daily. (From Axelsson et al, 1994. Reprinted with permission.)

have many teeth under eruption; on distobuccal and mesiobuccal surfaces of molars; and on distolingual and mesiolingual surfaces of mandibular molars.

Figure 62 illustrates the pattern of de novo plaque reaccumulation, 24 hours after PMTC and after 4 months of rinsing twice a day with 0.1% chlorhexidine, in 100 subjects aged 17 to 19 years selected because of high gingival index scores. At both the baseline examination and the end of the trial, the mesiobuccal and mesiolingual surfaces

of both maxillary and mandibular teeth had the highest percentage of reaccumulated plaque. The lingual surfaces of the maxillary teeth exhibited by far the lowest percentage (close to 0%) of reaccumulated plaque. The most significant reduction in plaque formation achieved by the chemical plaque control agent was on the mandibular lingual surfaces, indicating that the rinsing solution had inadequate access to the approximal surfaces, where the plaque formation rate was greatest (Axelsson et al, 1994).

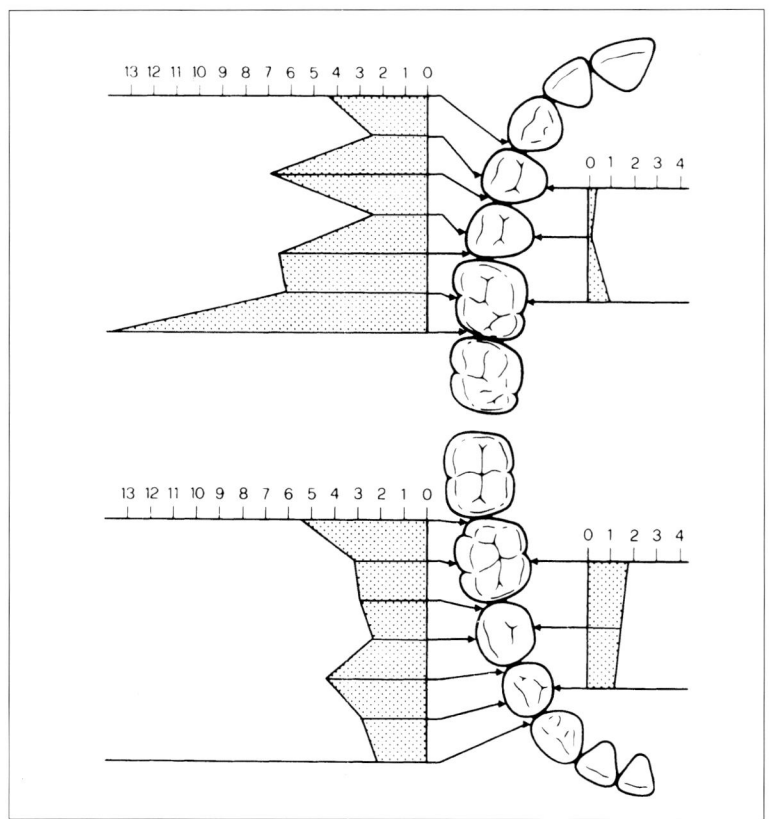

Fig 63 Bacterial counts in subgingival plaque from various intraoral sites. Numbers represent × 10⁶ organisms/mL. (From Mombelli et al, 1990a. Reprinted with permission.)

In another study (Furuichi et al, 1992), the pattern of de novo plaque formation after 1, 4, 7, and 14 days of undisturbed plaque accumulation was studied in 10 subjects aged 24 to 29 years. At the beginning of the study, the subjects received a thorough dental prophylaxis and oral hygiene instruction. At the end of a 2-week preparatory phase, the subjects were examined to ensure that the gingivae were healthy at baseline. Mechanical toothcleaning was discontinued, and plaque accumulation was recorded as PI (Silness and Löe, 1964). During a 2-week period without oral hygiene, most plaque formed during the first 4 days and was greater on mandibular than on maxillary teeth. Deposits were greatest on the approximal surfaces and least on the palatal surfaces. These differences, observed on day 4, persisted throughout the 2-week monitoring period. These findings verified the patterns of plaque formation described by Lang et al (1973) and Axelsson (1987, 1991).

In a microbiologic study, Mombelli et al (1990) analyzed subgingival plaque samples from maxillary and mandibular right canines, premolars, and first molars (distal, midbuccal, and lingual) in 10 healthy subjects who had refrained from oral hygiene procedures for 4 days. The samples were examined by darkfield microscopy. Distobuccal samples contained more bacteria than did buccal samples, and buccal samples contained more than lingual samples. Bacterial counts were higher in samples from posterior sites than from anterior sites and significantly higher in maxillary samples than in mandibular samples (Fig 63). This microscopic study also appeared to confirm the distinct pattern of plaque development on clean tooth surfaces.

In conclusion, on plaque-free tooth surfaces, a pattern of plaque growth starting with plaque accumulation on the interproximal areas of the premolars and molars is evident. Furthermore, gingival health may be maintained by complete removal of plaque at least once every 48 hours (for reviews on plaque formation rate and pattern of plaque reaccumulation, see Axelsson, 1991, 1998; Furuichi, 1998; Ramberg et al, 1995; Straub et al, 1998).

NONSPECIFIC PLAQUE HYPOTHESIS

It is now generally accepted that gingivitis and most periodontal diseases are caused by bacteria in dental plaque biofilms. The evidence for the infectious nature of periodontal disease comes from several sources including (1) studies that correlate most forms of gingivitis and periodontitis with accumulated dental plaque; (2) treatment studies that demonstrate that elimination of plaque microorganisms can be correlated with clinical improvement; and (3) in vivo and in vitro studies demonstrating the relative virulence of different plaque bacteria.

Although the infectious etiology of periodontal diseases is generally accepted, the relative importance of individual bacterial species within dental plaque is still unresolved, and this is reflected in the distinction between the nonspecific and the specific plaque hypotheses. The so-called ecological plaque hypothesis also considers the role of the environment on the composition of the microflora. The nonspecific plaque hypothesis proposes that the bacterial dental plaque that accumulates around teeth is a relatively homogenous mass that causes periodontal disease when it accumulates to the point of overwhelming the host's defense mechanisms.

Some debate about these hypotheses may be in part semantic (eg, the definitions of *specific* and *nonspecific),* because plaque-mediated diseases, while not necessarily having a totally specific etiology, do show evidence of specificity.

Experimental gingivitis

Evidence for the nonspecific plaque hypothesis has most frequently been tested in experimental gingivitis studies. In their classic "experimental gingivitis study," Löe and associates (1965) demonstrated that, in students with clinically healthy gingiva, clinical symptoms of gingivitis developed within 2 to 3 weeks if dental plaque was allowed to accumulate freely. Once adequate oral hygiene was resumed, the gingival inflammation subsided within a week.

The thickness of the gingival plaque gradually increased during the 3-week experimental period (Löe et al, 1965). For the first few days, plaque is composed of gram-positive cocci and rods, representing the indigenous microflora of the tooth surface. After 4 to 5 days, filamentous organisms and gram-negative cocci and rods "infect" the gingival plaque, nonattaching spirochetes gradually appear in the gingival sulcus, and the assortment of microorganisms in the gingival biofilm increases continuously. The first clinical signs of gingivitis develop within 2 to 3 weeks. When accumulated plaque is mechanically removed and daily oral hygiene is reestablished, the gingivae heal within about a week.

These findings have since been confirmed in many human and animal studies (Egelberg, 1964; Lindhe and Rylander, 1975; Lindhe et al, 1975; Saxe et al, 1967; see chapter 5). Figure 64, from the study by Lang et al (1973), illustrates the mean GI (Löe and Silness, 1963) for all gingival units in subjects cleaning every 12, 48, 72, or 96 hours over an observation period of 6 weeks. Clinical signs of gingivitis developed only in the groups, with 72 and 96 hours of plaque accumulation, and not in subjects cleaning every 12 or 48 hours, despite an almost identical mean PI among all groups. Plaque accumulation of more than 48 hours may have greater pathogenic potential than less mature plaque. This might be attributable to the dramatic change that occurs between 2 days and 3 to 4 days of de novo plaque accumulation (Listgarten, 1976): a massive increase in the thickness of the plaque and thereby the total number of plaque

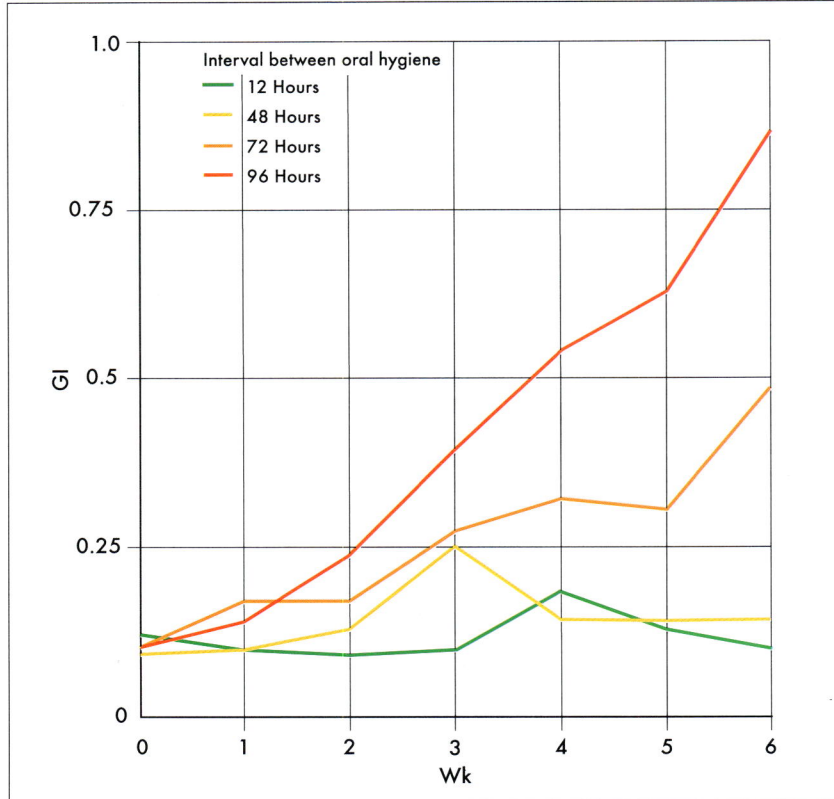

Fig 64 Mean Löe and Silness (1963) GI for all gingival units in subjects cleaning at various intervals during a 6-week study. (From Lang et al, 1973. Reprinted with permission.)

microorganisms. This study by Lang et al (1973) clearly demonstrated that effective and complete plaque control at intervals of 48 hours was compatible with the absence of clinical signs of gingival inflammation; at greater intervals, gingivitis developed.

In another study, Bosman and Powell (1977) induced gingivitis experimentally and then randomly allotted the subjects to one of four test groups, using a chemical plaque-control program by rinsing with 0.2% chlorhexidine solution twice a day or every second, third, or fourth day. Gingivitis was eliminated within 7 to 10 days in all subjects who rinsed twice a day and every second day but persisted among the subjects who rinsed only every third or fourth day. This study confirmed the findings by Lang et al (1973) that plaque control at least every second day eliminates or prevents the development of gingivitis.

Effect of mechanical removal of plaque

More than 30 years ago, in a 5-year-study, Lövdal et al (1961) showed that a maintenance program based on oral hygiene training and scaling two to four times per year reduces gingivitis and tooth loss. In 1973, Ramfjord et al reported the results of a 7-year study showing that periodontal attachment could be maintained in patients with advanced periodontal disease. After initial nonsurgical or surgical periodontal treatment, the patients had been recalled every third month for oral hygiene training, PMTC, and subgingival scaling or debridement. Nonsurgical and surgical treatment were shown to be equally effective. Similar results were reported by Wennström et al (1986) in a 6-year longitudinal study of a selected group of patients with a history of aggressive periodontitis.

Frequent PMTC has also been successfully used in maintenance programs after initial nonsurgical or surgical treatment of marginal periodontitis. In a 2-year study by Rosling et al (1976a), patients with a high prevalence of infrabony pockets were randomly allotted to a test or a control group. After initial open-flap surgery, scaling, and root planing, the test group received PMTC every second week. On reexamination, about 95% of the infrabony pockets had healed, and the gingival condition was excellent. In the matched control group without intensive mechanical plaque control, there was advanced recurrence of periodontal attachment loss.

Axelsson and Lindhe (1981b) also demonstrated the value of a carefully designed maintenance program following treatment of advanced periodontal disease. Seventy-seven patients were examined before treatment, 2 months after the last surgical procedure, and 3 and 6 years postsurgery. Two of every three patients (52) were enrolled in a supervised maintenance program that included oral hygiene instruction, PMTC, and needs-related debridement every 2 months for the first 2 years and every 3 months for the last 4 years of the observation period. The remaining 25 patients resumed care with the referring dentist, who was informed of the importance of checking their oral hygiene, calculus formation, gingival conditions, and periodontal conditions (nonrecall group). The recall patients were able to maintain proper oral hygiene and unaltered attachment levels. In the nonrecall group, plaque scores increased markedly from the baseline values, as did the number of inflamed gingival units. Concomitantly, there were obvious signs of recurrent periodontitis.

According to Lindhe and Nyman (1975), well-motivated patients who maintain high levels of oral hygiene can be managed with extended recall intervals, even if they have advanced loss of attachment at the time of treatment. Seventy-five such patients, with initial loss of alveolar bone amounting to half the length of the roots or more, were treated and subsequently received PMTC, scaling, and oral hygiene instruction every 3 to 6 months. After 5 years, there was no radiographic evidence of further loss of alveolar bone. In 1984, Badersten et al demonstrated that, for single-rooted teeth, a single

session of meticulous subgingival scaling and root planing is at least as effective as three sessions, even in patients with advanced periodontitis, provided that the patients are recalled for special oral hygiene training and PMTC at needs-related intervals (Badersten et al, 1984b).

Although so-called supragingival plaque control is considered to have little effect on the subgingival microflora of deep periodontal pockets, this may not apply to PMTC in moderately deep pockets (4 to 6 mm). A series of studies have shown that both probing depth and the total number of subgingival microflora gradually decrease in such pockets as a result of frequent PMTC without prior subgingival scaling. In addition, there is a shift from a periopathogenic to a less pathogenic microflora (for reviews, see Axelsson, 1994; Kieser, 1994). This may be attributable to the repeated removal of 2 to 3 mm subgingival plaque by PMTC, rather than the supragingival plaque control.

The most cost-effective means of treatment and control of periodontal diseases is initial, comprehensive, subgingival, "nonaggressive" scaling, root planing, and debridement, followed by a maintenance program based on meticulous gingival plaque control: self-care, supplemented by PMTC at needs-related intervals.

These principles have been tested in a 15-year longitudinal study in adults (Axelsson et al, 1991). Two groups of subjects from one geographic area were recruited. Of 555 individuals, 375 were assigned to a test group and 180 to a control group, stratified into three age groups: 20 to 35 years, 36 to 50 years, and 51 to 70 years. During the first 6-year period, the control patients were seen regularly once a year and given traditional dental care. The subjects in the test group underwent initial "nonaggressive" scaling, root planing, and debridement and were then recalled every 2 months for the first 2 years, and once every third month for the following 4 years. They were individually educated in proper oral hygiene techniques, based on self-diagnosis. Professional mechanical toothcleaning, supplemented by debridement when necessary, was provided by a dental hygienist. Reexaminations were carried out toward the end of the third and sixth years of the study.

On average, the control group lost 1.2 mm of periodontal attachment per individual, while the test group lost none. Although there was no attachment loss in most of the subjects in the control group, there was serious deterioration in a few, with continued attachment loss (Axelsson and Lindhe, 1978, 1981a). For ethical reasons, after the 6-year period, the control subjects were also offered needs-related prevention, and many accepted.

For the following 9-year period, up to the 15-year reexamination, all test subjects received an individualized secondary preventive program, supervised by the same dental hygienist. To maximize cost effectiveness, both the preventive measures and the recall intervals were based strictly on individual needs: About 65% of patients visited the dental hygienist only once a year, 30% twice a year, and 5% (the high-risk individuals) three to six times a year.

Over the 15-year period, only 0.23 teeth were lost per individual (Axelsson et al, 1991). These results could be extrapolated to imply that a 50-year-old subject involved in such a program would be more than 100 years old before losing another single tooth. During the same 15-year period, it is estimated that the Swedish adult population lost, on average, two to three teeth per individual (Håkansson, 1991).

The mean gain in probing periodontal attachment per individual, regardless of age, was 0.3 mm. This gain was roughly the same in the 66 to 85 year olds as it was in the 36 to 50 year olds. It was estimated that the annual costs for dental care in the test group were only about 50% of the average annual costs for Swedish adult patients.

ECOLOGICAL PLAQUE HYPOTHESIS

This hypothesis is based on the theory that the unique local microenvironment influences the composition of the oral microflora. From an ecological point of view, the oral cavity is an open growth system; ie, nutrients and microbes are repeatedly introduced to and removed from the system. The flow rate of saliva is so high that, in order to colonize the surfaces of the oral cavity, the organisms must be able to adhere or be retained in some other way. Not only the flow of saliva but also the flow of the gingival fluid, friction from chewing, oral hygiene procedures, and desquamation of epithelial cells from the mucous membranes remove bacteria from the oral surfaces. Some bacteria may simply obtain a refuge in pits and fissures or in the protected areas between the teeth. Other microorganisms have to rely on specific mechanisms of adherence to overcome the strong removal forces on the oral surfaces.

The characteristics of the oral surfaces are unique, and only specific bacteria have the ability to adhere. This means that the oral cavity harbors a unique microbiota, and most species are unable to colonize any other site in the human body. The oral cavity consists of several distinct sites, each of which will support the growth of a characteristic microbial community, and there are therefore pronounced differences in the composition of the microbiota on the mucous membranes, the tongue, and the teeth and in the gingival sulcus. It has even been demonstrated that the composition of the microbiota may vary from site to site on a single tooth surface. For example, facultative anaerobes able to attach to the solid tooth surfaces predominate in thin supragingival plaque on buccal and lingual surfaces, while obligate anaerobic spirochetes predominate at the base of deep periodontal pockets.

Similarly, low pH and access to fermentable carbohydrates such as sucrose provide a favorable environment for aciduric and acidogenic bacteria (eg, *S mutans* and lactobacilli). Dental practitioners spend most of their clinical time dealing with problems caused by the oral microflora and emphasize improved methods of removing or inhibiting this source of inflammation and disease. However, the normal oral microflora is an important defense factor acting in concert with other host defenses to help prevent colonization by exogenous, and often pathogenic, microorganisms. Nevertheless, imbalances in the stability of the resident oral microflora do occasionally occur and predispose a site to disease. This may result from changes in diet or hormonal balance, the use of antimicrobial agents, deficiencies in the host defenses, or inadequate plaque control. Therefore, during the treatment of patients, the aims of the dentist should be to identify any predisposing factors and to select strategies to control, rather than eliminate, the oral microflora, so as to preserve the beneficial properties of the harmless normal oral microflora.

Bacterial homeostasis

Once established, the microflora at a site remain relatively stable over time, despite regular minor disturbances in the oral environment (Marsh, 1989). This stability (termed *microbial homeostasis)* stems not from any metabolic indifference among the components of the microflora but rather from a dynamic balance of microbial interactions, including both synergism and antagonism.

It has been proposed that the ability to maintain homeostasis within a microbial community increases with its species diversity. In dental plaque, diversity is enhanced by the development of food chains among bacterial species and their use of complementary metabolic strategies for the catabolism of endogenous nutrients, such as glycoproteins and proteins. Individual species possess different but overlapping patterns of enzyme activity, so that certain mixed cultures of oral bacteria can synergistically degrade complex host molecules (van der Hoeven and Camp, 1991). Several food chains have been recognized among

plaque bacteria, such as the utilization of lactic acid by *Veillonella* species and succinate by spirochetes.

Antagonism is also a major mechanism in maintaining microbial homeostasis in plaque. Bacteriocins and bacteriocin-like substances are produced by many genera of oral bacteria (Marsh, 1989). Although the specific benefit of bacteriocins is unclear, their production can confer an ecological advantage on an organism during colonization. Other inhibitory factors produced by plaque bacteria include organic acids, hydrogen peroxide, and enzymes.

The production of such inhibitory substances might also be a major factor in determining the composition of the plaque microflora. It was found that subgingival plaque samples from healthy subjects contained organisms that could inhibit the growth of several periopathogens (Hillman and Socransky, 1989). In contrast, plaque from sites with localized aggressive periodontitis or with refractory periodontitis invariably lacked organisms that produce inhibitors. Subsequent studies identified some of the antagonistic bacteria as *S sanguis* and the inhibitor as hydrogen peroxide (Hillman and Socransky, 1989). Such interactions can also contribute to colonization resistance.

Supragingival plaque accumulates preferentially at stagnant or retentive sites, unless removed by diligent oral hygiene, as described earlier. As plaque mass increases, saliva is less able to penetrate plaque and protect enamel. Microbial homeostasis can break down, and major shifts in the composition of the microflora can occur.

Relationship to gingivitis and periodontitis

Gingivitis is associated with the accumulation of plaque around the gingival margin. The host mounts an inflammatory response to this microbial challenge, and the flow of gingival crevicular fluid is increased. The composition of subgingival plaque shifts from a streptococci-dominated microflora to one with higher levels of *Actinomyces* species and an increase in capnophilic and obligately anaerobic bacteria such as *Capnocytophaga, Fusobacterium,* and *Prevotella* species (Moore et al, 1987a; Savitt and Socransky, 1984).

Gingivitis may lead to more advanced forms of periodontal disease in which the microflora can become even more diverse. Depending on the type of disease, bacteria belonging to the genera *Actinobacillus, Campylobacter, Selenomonas, Treponema,* and *Wolinella* may be isolated. Tissue damage can result directly from the activity of the subgingival microflora and indirectly from the release of lysosomal enzymes during phagocytosis or from the production of cytokines that stimulate resident connective tissue cells to release metalloproteinases (for details on the pathogenesis of periodontal diseases, see chapter 5).

In patients with periodontal disease, the redox potential is lower in pockets than it is at healthy sites. The inflammatory host response also leads to increased secretion of GCF and a small rise in local pH, from just below neutrality in health to approximately pH 7.5 during disease (Eggert et al, 1991). The GCF not only delivers components of the host defense, but also provides a continuous supply of proteins, glycoproteins, and cofactors that can act as novel nutrients for bacteria, especially asaccharolytic and obligately anaerobic species (Box 2).

In an early longitudinal clinical study, black-pigmented anaerobes increased from 0.01% to 0.20% of the subgingival flora when gingivitis progressed to a bleeding stage (Loesche and Syed, 1978). This is noteworthy, because these organisms require hemin for growth, and this cofactor can be derived from the degradation of host molecules in GCF. Similarly, it was reported that some species that predominate in periodontitis but are undetectable in the healthy gingiva can be found as a small proportion of the microflora in gingivitis (Moore et al, 1987b). This also suggests that environmental conditions that develop during gingivitis (eg, bleeding, increased GCF flow) may favor the growth of species implicated in periodontitis.

The possible effect of GCF on the stability of the subgingival microflora has been studied in the laboratory by repeated passing of plaque through human serum (used as a substitute for GCF) (ter Steeg et al, 1987) or by the prolonged, continuous culture of plaque on serum (ter Steeg et al, 1988). Both experimental approaches resulted in the enrichment of species implicated in periodontal disease (eg, anaerobic streptococci, *P intermedia, Fusobacterium nucleatum,* and *T denticola),* which were present in the inoculum at levels too low to be detected.

Likewise, the effect of the clinically observed rise in pH during inflammation on the proportions of three black-pigmented anaerobes has been studied in mixed continuous culture. At or below pH 7.00, the culture was dominated by *Prevotella melaninogenica.* As the pH was increased to 7.25, *P intermedia* became predominant. At pH 7.50 and higher, the culture comprised more than 99% *P gingivalis* (McDermid et al, 1990). These studies have demonstrated the significant influ-

---

Box 2 Components of gingival crevicular fluid that might affect the composition of the subgingival microflora*

Host defenses
- Immunoglobulin G
- Immunoglobulin A
- Immunoglobulin M
- Complement
- B lymphocytes
- T lymphocytes
- Neutrophils (polymorphonuclear leukocytes)
- Macrophages

Novel nutrients
- Hemin, iron
- Albumin
- α-2-Globulin
- Transferrin
- Hemopexin
- Hormones
- Haptoglobin
- Hemoglobin
- Proteins, glycoproteins

*From Marsh (1994). Reprinted with permission.

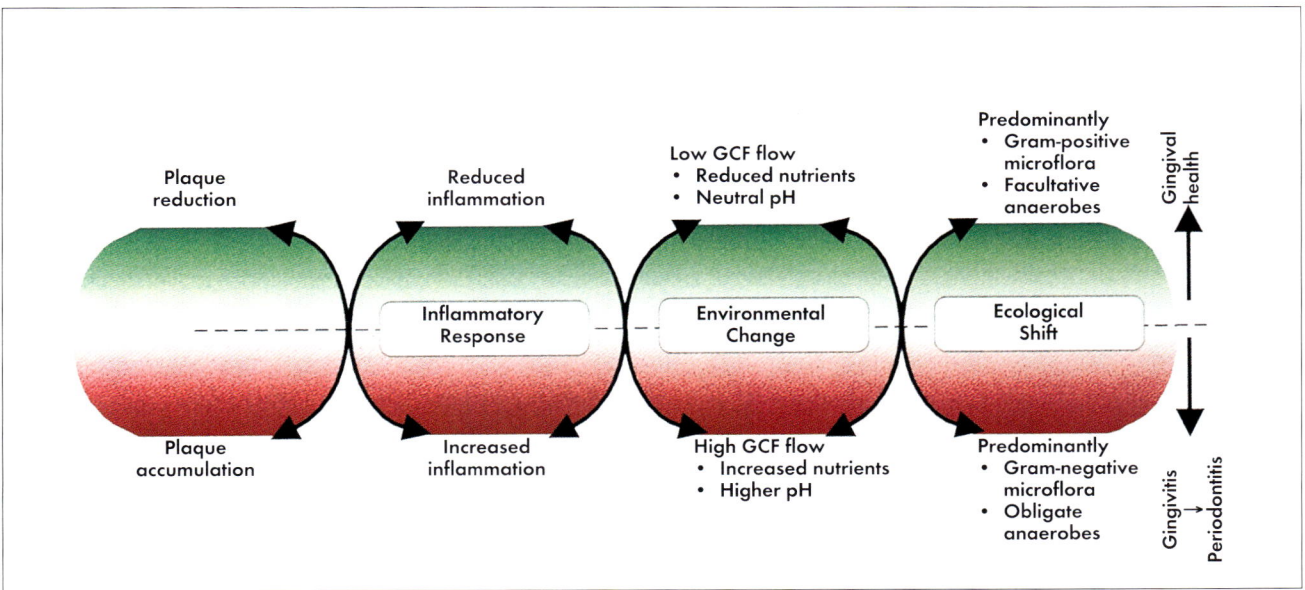

Fig 65 Ecological plaque hypothesis and the prevention of periodontal disease. (Modified from Marsh, 1994.)

ence an altered supply of nutrients and even a small change in local pH can have in determining the balance of the microflora.

In an attempt to unify some of these clinical and laboratory observations, Marsh (1991) proposed the ecological plaque hypothesis: A change in a key environmental factor (or factors) will trigger a shift in the balance of the resident plaque microflora, and this might predispose a site to disease. The occurrence of potentially pathogenic species as minor members of the resident plaque microflora would be consistent with this proposal. In health, these organisms would be only weakly competitive and might also be suppressed by intermicrobial antagonism and therefore would constitute only a small, clinically unimportant proportion of the plaque microflora. Microbial specificity in disease would be due to the fact that only certain species are competitive under the new (changed) environmental conditions. It is a basic tenet of microbial ecology that a major change in an ecosystem produces a corresponding disturbance in the stability of the resident microbial community.

In periodontal diseases, the changes in nutrient profile of the gingival crevice resulting from GCF secretion will lead to increased plaque biomass, the metabolism of which will lower the redox potential of the site and raise the pH. These changes will tend to enrich the previously low levels of obligately anaerobic and often asaccharolytic gram-negative bacteria and so fuel the inflammatory response (Fig 65). Other predisposing factors might include the state of the host defenses, so that leukotoxin-producing strains of *A actinomycetemcomitans* might exploit the pocket environment in individuals with neutrophil deficiencies and gain a competitive advantage (Genco and Slots, 1984). These sequences of events can in part explain the lack of total specificity in the microbial etiology of periodontal diseases and account for the pattern of bacterial succession often seen during disease progression in clinical studies.

Within the pocket, the major nutritional sources of bacterial metabolism are the periodontal tissues, the GCF, and blood. Therefore, many bacteria found in periodontal pockets produce hydrolytic enzymes that break down complex macromolecules from the host into simple peptides and amino acids. These enzymes are thought to be a major factor in the destructive processes of periodontal tissues.

Because differences in the composition of the subgingival microbiota have been attributed in part to the local availability of blood products, redox potential, and po2, an unresolved question is whether the presence of specific microorganisms in patients or distinct sites is the cause or the consequence of disease. Many organisms considered to be periodontal pathogens are fastidious, strict anaerobes and, as such, may contribute little to initiation of disease in sites that are still shallow and exposed to oxygen. If their preferred habitat is the deep pocket, they would be linked to disease progression in preexisting sites rather than to initial bursts of disease in shallow sites.

Prevention and control of periodontal diseases based on the ecological plaque hypothesis

One inference of the ecological plaque hypothesis is that disease might be prevented not only by inhibiting the putative pathogens but also by interfering with the factors responsible for the transition of the plaque microflora from a commensal to a pathogenic relationship with the host (Marsh, 1991). A consideration of the principles behind the ecological plaque hypothesis can lead to the identification of new strategies to prevent disease and offer new perspectives on existing approaches (Box 3). These strategies will be discussed in terms of their ecological implications.

Reduction in probing depths

Reduction in probing depths, surgical or nonsurgical, has long been successful in treatment of periodontal disease, achieving an immediate, dra-

matic ecological change that favors a facultative anaerobic gingival microflora and depriving the subgingival anaerobic microflora of its anaerobic environment at the base of deep pockets. However, without a maintenance program based on excellent gingival plaque control, there is frequently recurrence of deep, diseased pockets.

Mechanical removal or disruption of the subgingival biofilms

As discussed earlier, the subgingival biofilm represents a well-organized community of microorganisms, matrix material, "nutrition channels," and so on, in which most of the microorganisms are inaccessible to host defense factors (PMNLs, antibodies, complement, etc) and antimicrobial agents. Mechanical removal or disruption of this homeostatic biofilm changes the ecology and the remaining microorganisms become accessible to both host factors and antimicrobial agents.

Use of anti-inflammatory and antimicrobial agents

Anti-inflammatory agents might break the cycle of tissue destruction caused by both bacterial and

---

Box 3 Prevention strategies and the ecological plaque hypothesis*

Altered subgingival environment
- Reduction in probing depth
- Mechanical removal or disruption of the subgingival plaque biofilm
- Use of anti-inflammatory agents
- Use of antimicrobial agents (subminimum inhibitory concentration)
- Application of oxygenating or redox agents

Replacement theory
- Preemptive colonization
- Competitive displacement

*Modified from Marsh (1994).

---

host-derived proteases (Johnson and Curtis, 1994). This would also reduce the supply of GCF and thereby restrict the availability of nutrients essential for the growth of some periodontal pathogens. Some of the antimicrobial agents being used in dental health products are broad spectrum and can reduce plaque, especially at sites that are difficult to clean. Care has to be taken with the regular, unsupervised use of such agents, so that the natural ecology of dental plaque will not be disrupted (Page, 1989).

Studies have suggested that, at their concentrations in the mouth, the activity of some of these agents may be more selective than hitherto suspected. In analogy with the use of chlorhexidine for selective suppression of mutans streptococci in plaque (Köhler et al, 1984), preparations containing triclosan and zinc citrate in combination with other agents have been found to be highly effective against periodontal pathogens in vitro (Bradshaw et al, 1993) and in vivo (Jones et al, 1990), leaving streptococci associated with sound enamel and a health periodontium relatively unaffected. In a recent 3-year longitudinal study, daily use of a toothpaste containing triclosan and copolymer resulted in significant reduction in probing depths, gain in clinical attachment, and reduction in subgingival periopathogens compared to a placebo paste (Rosling et al, 1997a, 1997b), probably attributable to the documented antiplaque and anti-inflammatory effects of triclosan. At subminimum inhibitory concentrations, several antimicrobial agents inhibit bacterial proteases implicated in tissue destruction, another potentially valuable property (Cummins, 1991; Marsh, 1992; Scheie, 1989).

Application of oxygenating and redox agents

Another approach has been to try to raise the redox potential of the pocket (which is lowered during disease) to create an environment incompatible with the growth of obligate anaerobes. This has been tried, with varying success, with molecular oxygen or an oxygenating agent. The use of redox dyes has been proposed: Although they do not release oxygen, the dyes can raise the redox potential of an ecosystem. In a study by Wilson et al (1992), methylene blue dye was applied subgingivally on a daily basis for 7 days at 25 test sites; in the same patients, water was applied to control sites. The treatment resulted in a significant reduction in flow of GCF and a reduction in the proportions of obligate anaerobes and motile organisms in the subgingival microflora, with a concomitant increase in facultative anaerobes and cocci (Wilson et al, 1992). These early studies confirm the theoretical basis of the ecological plaque hypothesis by showing that a preventive strategy that interferes with a critical event in the breakdown of microbial homeostasis in plaque can shift the ecological balance of plaque back toward one that is compatible with dental health.

Replacement therapy

The phenomenon by which one member of an ecosystem can inhibit the growth of another is termed *bacterial interference.* The idea that antagonistic organisms could be used to control pathogens and prevent disease has been proposed for more than 100 years and is termed *replacement therapy.* This approach has the potential advantage of providing lifelong protection with minimal cost or compliance on behalf of the recipient, once colonization by the "effector" strain has been achieved (Hillman and Socransky, 1989).

There are two main approaches to the use of replacement therapy to prevent periodontal diseases: preeruptive colonization and competitive displacement. In preeruptive colonization, ecological niches (functions) within plaque are filled by a harmless or potentially beneficial organism before the undesirable strain has had an opportunity to colonize or become established. The initial colonizer becomes integrated in the ecosystem and subsequently excludes the pathogen. This principle is more useful in prevention of dental caries than periodontal diseases because the cariogenic microflora may be established as soon as the primary teeth erupt.

In the alternative approach, competitive displacement, a more competitive strain is derived that would displace a preexisting organism from plaque (Donoghue, 1990). This is of potentially greater clinical value, because it is not dependent on treatment with the effector strain at or before colonization by the undesired organism (Hillman and Socransky, 1989).

Competitive displacement has been considered in the treatment of localized aggressive periodontitis. Hillman and Socransky (1982), as stated earlier, showed that plaque from periodontally healthy sites contains organisms such as hydrogen peroxide–producing strains of S sanguis, which inhibit the growth of A actinomycetemcomitans, whereas the converse is true for plaque from sites with localized aggressive periodontitis. In gnotobiotic rats, levels of A actinomycetemcomitans are markedly reduced by superinfection with wild-type S sanguis, but attempts to implant S sanguis in humans have had variable results (Hillman and Socransky, 1989). However, at present, conventional approaches involving debridement and selective use of antibiotics remain the optimal form of treatment.

Before replacement therapy can be considered as a practical alternative to existing treatment, the problems of implanting effective effector strains will have to be overcome, and assurances of the safety of these strains will be required. Molecular biology is being explored to develop suitable effector strains with the desired properties. Nevertheless, the use of bacterial interference to produce plaque with either a lower disease potential or an increased level of colonization resistance would be consistent with the principles of the ecological plaque hypothesis.

SPECIFIC PLAQUE HYPOTHESIS

In recent years, the specific plaque hypothesis has dominated discussions of the etiology of periodontal diseases. To determine the etiologic agents of destructive periodontitis, researchers have focused on the classic approach of verifying Koch's postulates (1884): (1) a causative organism must be isolated from every case of disease; (2) the agent must not be recovered from other forms of disease or in the absence of pathosis, except in a carrier state; and (3) after isolation, the pathogen should be able to induce disease in animals.

In periodontics, classic postulates have, however, been extended to include the criteria of: (1) association with disease, ie, the need to detect higher levels of pathogens in affected patients than in control subjects; (2) treatment elimination, ie, the influence of successful therapy on both clinical parameters and the associated microbiota; (3) induction of a host response by bacteria or bacterial components gaining access to the underlying periodontal tissues; (4) pathogenicity in animal models, ie, the ability to cause disease in experimental animals; (5) formation of virulence factors and maintenance of a pathogenic environment, ie, production of pathogenicity factors that give bacteria a selective advantage in destruction of host tissue or evasion of host defenses (Socransky, 1977; Socransky and Haffajee, 1990, 1992, 1997).

Composition of the microflora

In health, the periodontal microflora consists of a highly complex association of bacterial species (Listgarten and Helldén, 1978; Newman and Socransky, 1977; Slots, 1977). In their landmark studies examining the predominant cultivable microbiota in different periodontal conditions, Moore and coworkers described the presence of more than 300 bacterial species or groups in subgingival plaque (Moore, 1987; Moore and Moore,

1994; Moore et al, 1982, 1983, 1985, 1991, 1993). Among this highly heterogenous microflora, some species are considered to be present occasionally, while others are part of a "resident" colonizing flora.

The microflora associated with destructive periodontitis has been carefully scrutinized to identify specific periodontal pathogens associated with breakdown of the attachment apparatus in aggressive periodontitis, chronic periodontitis, and refractory periodontitis. The general approach has consisted of an initial association of potential pathogens in predominant cultivable studies and verification of their role in larger study groups by the use of selective media. These association studies implicated *P gingivalis, P intermedia, Eikenella corrodens, C rectus, Eubacterium* species, *Selenomonas* species, *B forsythus,* and largely noncultivable spirochetes (Listgarten and Levin, 1981; Listgarten et al, 1978; Loesche et al, 1985) in adult disease forms. *A actinomycetemcomitans, Capnocytophaga ochraceus, P intermedia,* and *E corrodens,* on the other hand, seem to predominate in the early-onset forms of breakdown.

Evidence for a specific role of some bacteria in periodontal diseases includes the following:

- The existence of different bacterial profiles in health, experimental gingivitis, chronic gingivitis, and different forms of periodontal disease (Listgarten, 1994)
- The presence of increased proportions of some species in sites with evidence of recent attachment loss (Dzink et al, 1985, 1988; Tanner et al, 1984).
- The characterization of specific virulence factors and animal pathogenicity (for review, see Socransky and Haffajee, 1991)
- The correlation between specific periopathogens and attachment loss in prospective longitudinal studies (Machtei et al, 1997; Papapanou et al, 1997a)
- The link between suppression of specific microorganisms and clinical improvement and the link between high levels of those species

and increased risk for further breakdown (Bragd et al, 1987; Carlos et al, 1988; Dahlén et al, 1996; Grossi et al, 1994; Haffajee and Socransky, 1994; Haffajee et al, 1991b, 1991c; Renvert et al, 1998)

The theory that some bacteria have a specific role in periodontal diseases is challenged by the following arguments:

- Most of the available data are derived from retrospective analysis: The disease develops before the microbiota are identified.
- Demonstration of association is not proof of cause: Microbial changes may be the consequence, rather than the cause, of the disease. (Is the presence of specific microorganisms a risk factor or a risk indicator for periodontal disease?)

Table 1 identifies the most prominent microbial species associated with various clinical forms of periodontitis. Box 4 lists representative species related to periodontal health and diseases.

Figures 66 to 71 attempt to illustrate the relative proportions of different facultatively anaerobic and anaerobic gram-positive and gram-negative bacteria associated with clinically healthy gingiva (Fig 66), established gingivitis (Fig 67), acute necrotizing ulcerative gingivitis (Fig 68), aggressive periodontitis (Fig 69), acute necrotizing ulcerative periodontitis (Fig 70), and chronic periodontitis (Fig 71). Bacteria implicated in the etiology are underlined.

Table 1 Microbial species associated with various forms of periodontitis*

Species	Localized aggressive periodontitis	Aggressive periodontitis	Chronic periodontitis	Refractory periodontitis	Failing guided tissue regeneration
Fusobacterium species	+	++	+++	++	+++
Actinobacillus actinomycetemcomitans	+++	++	++	++	++
Porphyromonas gingivalis	±	+++	+++	++	++
Prevotella intermedia/Prevotella nigrescens	++	+++	+++	+++	+++
Bacteroides forsythus	±	++	+++	++	++
Campylobacter rectus	+	++	++	+	+++
Peptostreptococcus micros	±	++	+++	++	+++
Eubacterium species	–	+	++	+	+
Treponema species	++	+++	+++	++	++
Enteric rods and pseudomonads	–	–	±	+	±
β-Hemolytic streptococci	?	++	++	++	+
Candida species	–	–	–	±	–

*From Mombelli (1998) (data from Dougherty and Slots, 1993; Loesche et al, 1985; Nowzari and Slots, 1994; Nowzari et al, 1995; Slots and Rams, 1990). Reprinted with permission.
– = Not elevated in comparison to health; ± = Occasionally isolated; + = Less than 10% of the patients positive; ++ = Less than 50% of the patients positive; +++ = More than 50% of the patients positive; ? = Unknown

Box 4 Microbial species associated with periodontal health and diseases*

Health
- Streptococcus sanguis
- Streptococcus mitis
- Veillonella parvula
- Actinomyces naeslundii
- Actinomyces viscosus
- Rothia dentocariosus

Gingivitis
- Actinomyces species
- Streptococcus species
- Veillonella species
- Fusobacterium species
- Treponema species
- Prevotella intermedia

Chronic periodontitis
- Treponema species
- Prevotella intermedia
- Porphyromonas gingivalis
- Bacteroides forsythus
- Peptostreptococcus micros
- Campylobacter rectus
- Actinobacillus actinomycetemcomitans

- Eikenella corrodens
- Fusobacterium species
- Selenomonas species
- Eubacterium species

Aggressive periodontitis in children
- Actinobacillus actinomycetemcomitans
- Other bacterial species (?)

Aggressive periodontitis in adults
- Actinobacillus actinomycetemcomitans
- Porphyromonas gingivalis
- Bacteroides forsythus
- Campylobacter rectus
- Eikenella corrodens

Refractory periodontitis
- Actinobacillus actinomycetemcomitans
- Porphyromonas gingivalis
- Prevotella intermedia
- Bacteroides forsythus
- Campylobacter rectus
- Peptostreptococcus micros
- Enteric rods
- Candida species

*From Listgarten (1994). Reprinted with permission.

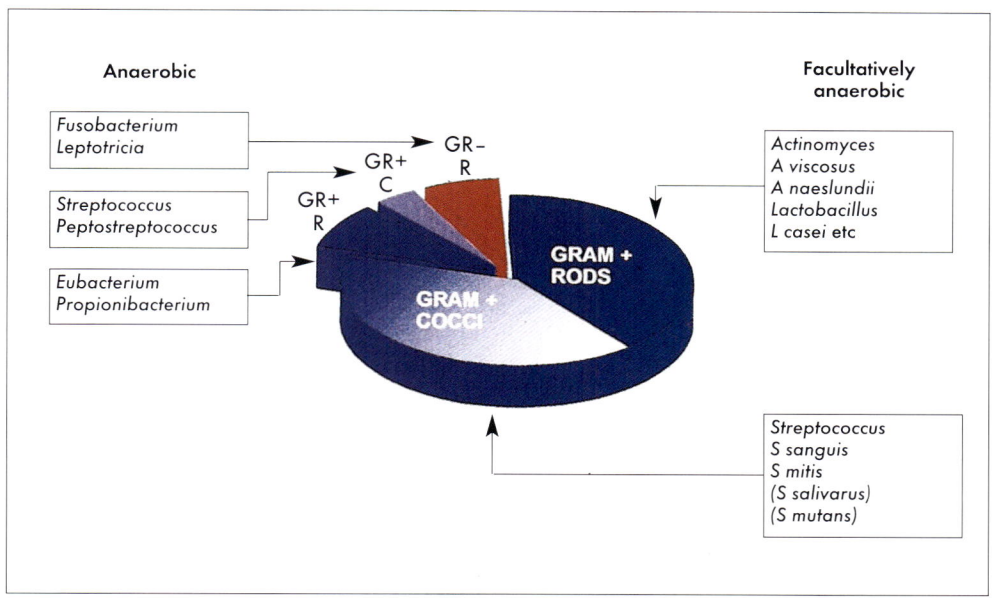

Fig 66 Composition of the gingival microflora associated with clinically healthy gingiva. GR+ = Gram-positive *(blue)*; GR– = Gram-negative *(red)*; C = Cocci; R = Rods.

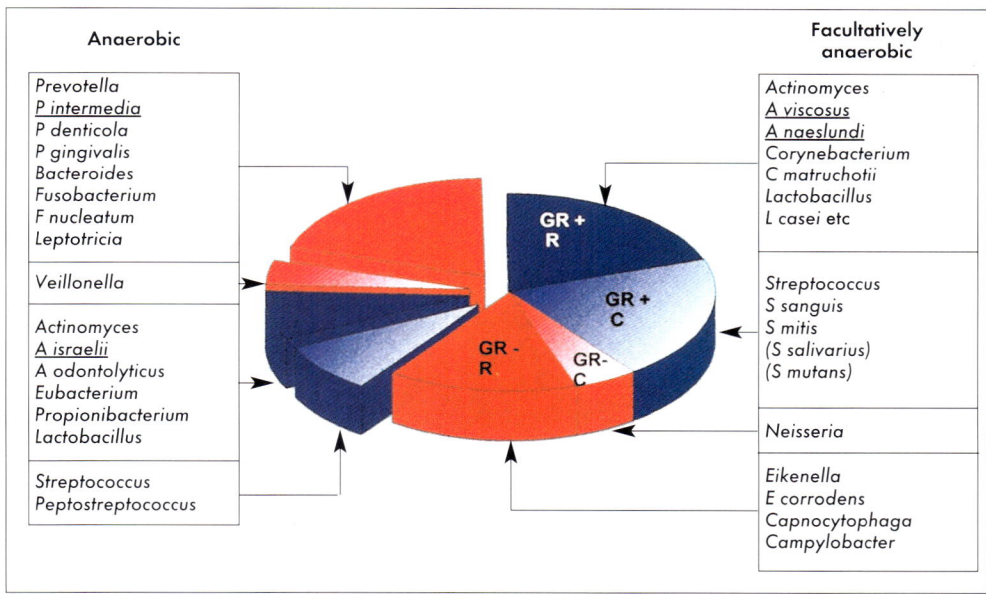

Fig 67 Composition of the subgingival microflora associated with gingivitis. GR+ = Gram-positive *(blue)*; GR– = Gram-negative *(red)*; C = Cocci; R = Rods. The most important pathogens are underlined.

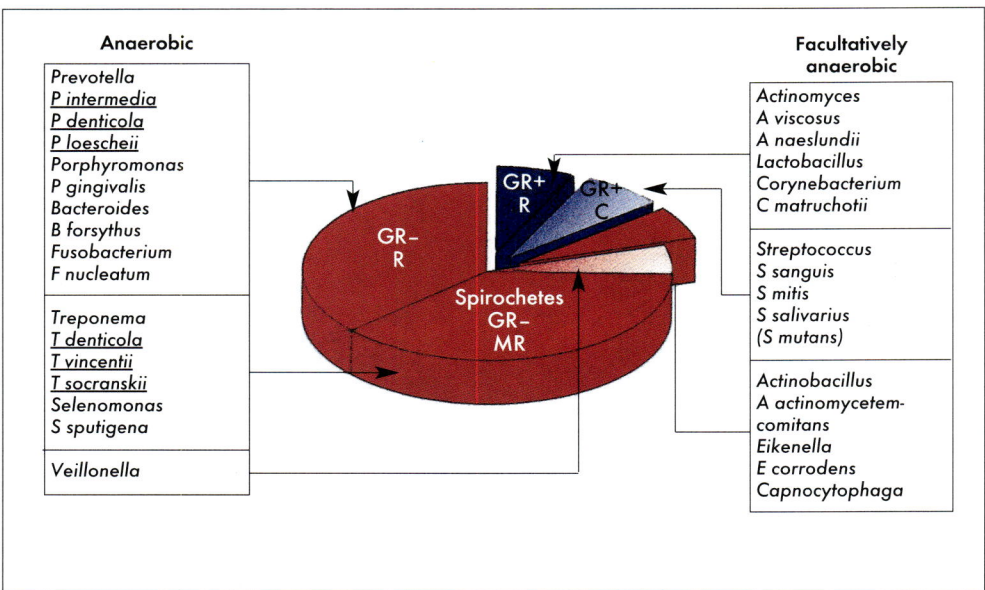

Fig 68 Composition of the subgingival microflora associated with acute necrotizing ulcerative gingivitis. GR+ = Gram-positive *(blue)*; GR– = Gram-negative *(red)*; C = Cocci; R = Rods; MR = Motile rods. The most important periopathogens are underlined.

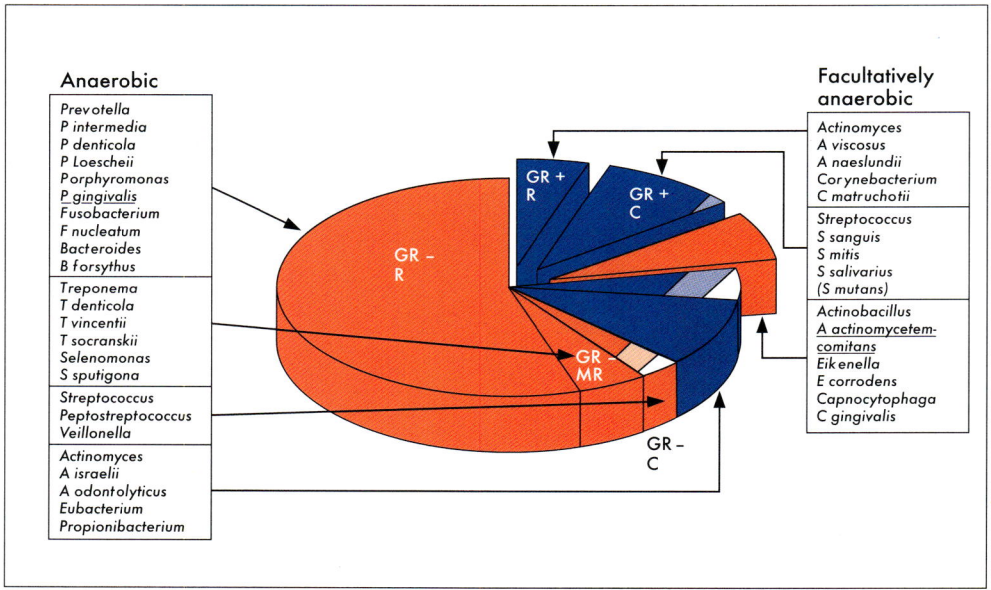

Fig 69 Composition of the subgingival microflora associated with aggressive periodontitis. GR+ = Gram-positive *(blue)*; GR– = Gram-negative *(red)*; C = Cocci; R = Rods; MR = Motile rods. The most important periopathogens are underlined.

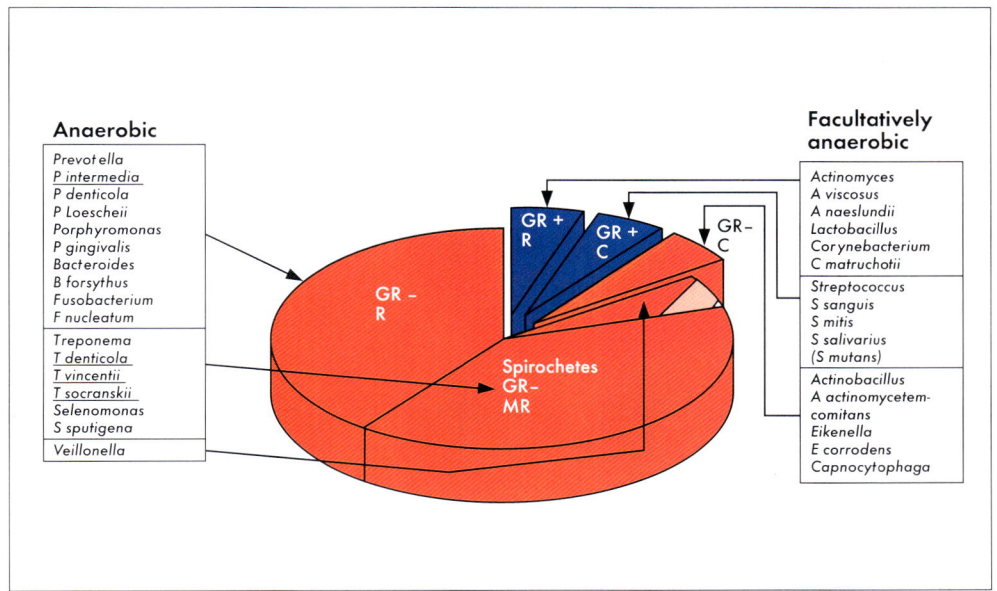

Fig 70 Composition of the subgingival microflora associated with acute necrotizing ulcerative periodontitis. GR+ = Gram-positive *(blue)*; GR– = Gram-negative *(red)*; C = Cocci; R = Rods; MR = Motile rods. The most important periopathogens are underlined.

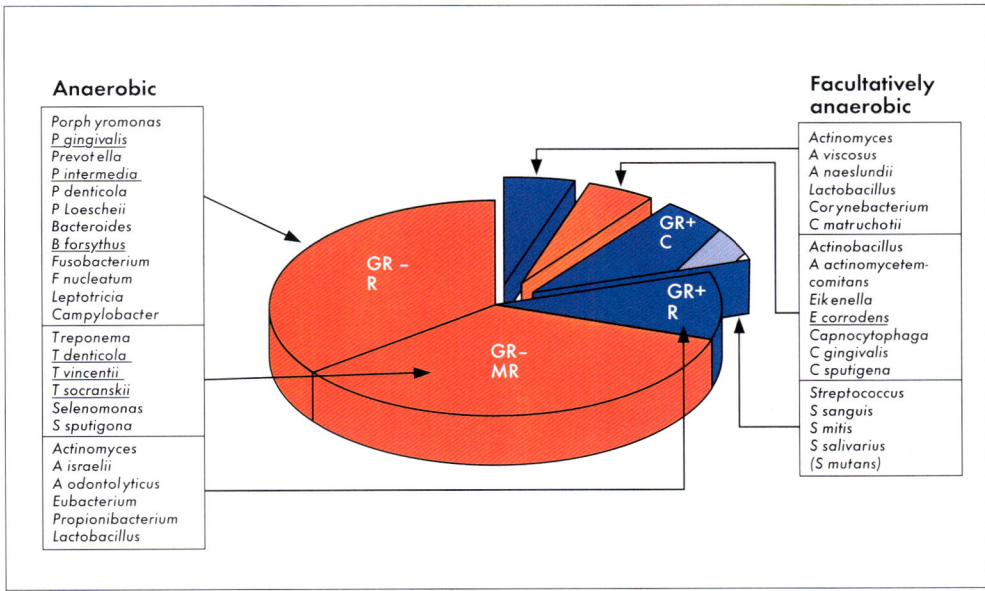

Fig 71 Composition of the subgingival microflora associated with chronic periodontitis. GR+ = Gram-positive *(blue)*; GR– = Gram-negative *(red)*; C = Cocci; R = Rods; MR = Motile rods. The most important periopathogens are underlined.

53

Major microorganisms implicated in periodontal diseases

At the latest American Workshop on Periodontology (American Academy of Periodontology, 1996c), there was consensus that particularly *A actinomycetemcomitans, P gingivalis,* and *B forsythus,* but also *P intermedia* and *T denticola,* should be considered as causative periopathogens. Of these, *A actinomycetemcomitans* and *P gingivalis* are regarded as exogenous and transmissible, while *B forsythus, P intermedia,* and *T denticola* are endogenous and opportunistic; ie, when pocket depth increases, they increase in number and participate directly and indirectly in destruction of periodontal tissue. Both *A actinomycetemcomitans* and *P gingivalis* are regarded as true exogenous periopathogens for the following reasons:

- There is low prevalence of *A actinomycetemcomitans* and *P gingivalis* in the presence of periodontal health or gingivitis (Europe and North America) (Ashimoto et al, 1996).
- There is evidence for transmission, eg, from parent to child or between spouses (Di Rienzo, 1991; Loos et al, 1990, 1992; Ménard and Mouton, 1995; Poulsen et al, 1994; Von Troil-Lindén et al, 1995).
- There is low genetic variability of target organisms within patients (patients are infected by only one strain (Ali et al, 1997; Loos et al, 1990; Saarela et al, 1993; van Steenbergen et al, 1993).
- Immune responses to *A actinomycetemcomitans* and *P gingivalis* markedly exceed those expected for endogenous infections (Slots and Listgarten, 1988).
- Clinical studies show that *A actinomycetemcomitans* and *P gingivalis* can be eliminated by appropriate mechanical treatment and adjunctive antibiotic therapy (Pavicic et al, 1994; Rams et al, 1992).

If *A actinomycetemcomitans* and *P gingivalis* are true exogenous pathogens, avoidance of exposure to these organisms is relevant to the prevention of periodontal disease: Their mere presence would be an indication for intervention and thus highly sensitive qualitative tests would be valuable diagnostic tools. The prevention of opportunistic infections, however, implies the continuous control of ecological conditions regulating growth of the resident flora. In this case, quantitative tests would be required and sensitivity would not be a critical issue. This question has assumed practical importance as DNA probes and other diagnostic tools for the detection of several putative pathogens have been developed and made available to dentists.

Actinobacillus actinomycetemcomitans

One of the strongest associations between a suspected pathogen and destructive periodontal disease (at least in terms of number of publications) is provided by *A actinomycetemcomitans. A actinomycetemcomitans* is a small, facultatively anaerobic, nonmotile, gram-negative, saccharolytic, capnophilic, round-ended rod that forms small, convex colonies with a star-shaped center when grown on blood agar plates.

This species was first recognized as a possible periodontal pathogen because it was found more frequently and in higher numbers in lesions of localized forms of aggressive periodontitis (Chung et al, 1989; Mandell and Socransky, 1981; Newman et al, 1976; Newman and Socransky, 1977; Slots, 1976; Slots et al, 1980; Zambon et al, 1983a, 1983b) than it was in plaque samples from other clinical conditions, including periodontitis, gingivitis, and health. Soon thereafter, it was demonstrated that the majority of subjects with a localized form of aggressive periodontitis had an enormously elevated serum antibody response to this species and that there was local synthesis of antibody to this species. When subjects with this form of disease were treated successfully, the species was eliminated or its numbers were decreased; treatment failures were associated with failure to reduce the numbers of the species in treated sites (Christersson et al, 1985a, 1985b; Christersson and

Zambon, 1993; Haffajee et al, 1984; Kornman and Robertson, 1985; Mandell et al, 1986; Pavicic et al, 1994; Preus, 1988; Saxén and Asikainen, 1993; Slots and Rosling, 1983).

In experimental animals, the species produced a number of potentially damaging metabolites, including a leukotoxin, and induced disease (Irving et al, 1978). *A actinomycetemcomitans* also has been shown to have the ability to invade human gingival epithelial cells cultured in vitro (Blix et al, 1992; Sreenivasan et al, 1993). Perhaps the strongest association data come from studies of "active lesions," in which the numbers of *A actinomycetemcomitans* were greater in active sites than in inactive sites (Haffajee et al, 1984; Mandell 1984, Mandell et al, 1987) and prospective studies of unaffected siblings of subjects with localized aggressive periodontitis (Di Rienzo et al, 1994). Collectively, the data suggest that *A actinomycetemcomitans* is a probable pathogen of localized aggressive periodontitis. However, this should not be interpreted to mean that *A actinomycetemcomitans* is the sole cause of this clinical condition.

The species can also be an important organism in the subgingival flora of patients with refractory chronic periodontitis (Rodenburg et al, 1990). In a recent study of patients with refractory periodontitis, Colombo et al (1998) found that *A actinomycetemcomitans, P gingivalis, B forsythus;* and *T denticola* were equally prevalent. In addition, Renvert et al (1998) recently found greater numbers of *A actinomycetemcomitans* in smokers than in nonsmokers, after nonsurgical treatment.

Van Winkelhoff et al (1992) treated 50 adult subjects with "severe generalized periodontitis" and 40 subjects with refractory periodontitis who were culture positive for *A actinomycetemcomitans*. Therapy included mechanical debridement and systemically administered amoxicillin and metronidazole for 7 days. Only 1 of 90 subjects was culture positive for *A actinomycetemcomitans* 3 to 9 months posttherapy (Van Winkelhoff et al, 1992) and one of 48 subjects was culture positive 2 years posttherapy (Pavicic et al, 1994).

There was a significant gain in attachment level and decrease in probing depth in virtually all patients after therapy. Data such as these suggest that *A actinomycetemcomitans* also plays a role in periodontal disease in some, but certainly not all, adult subjects.

Serotype-dependent variance in virulence has been suggested for *A actinomycetemcomitans*. Differences in serotype distribution have been noted between patients with periodontal disease and apparently unaffected carriers of *A actinomycetemcomitans*. Serotype b has been found particularly often in subjects with aggressive periodontitis (Asikainen et al, 1991b, 1995; Zambon et al, 1983b, 1996b). Several properties of *A actinomycetemcomitans* are regarded as important determinants of virulence and pathogenic potential, ie, leukotoxin production, which is considered highly significant for its possible role in evasion of local host defense by *A actinomycetemcomitans*. A substantially higher prevalence (10- to 100-fold) of highly leukotoxic strains has been reported in patients with localized aggressive periodontitits than from chronic periodontitis patients or from healthy subjects (Zambon et al, 1996b).

Table 2 lists some of the evidence implicating *A actinomycetemcomitans* in the etiology of destructive periodontal diseases.

Porphyromonas gingivalis

Porphyromonas gingivalis is the second most intensively studied periopathogen after *A actinomycetemcomitans*. In contrast to the facultatively anaerobic *A actinomycetemcomitans*, it is fastidious, strictly anaerobic, and gram negative. It is nonmotile and asaccharolytic and usually coccoid or short rod–shaped, and belongs to the black-pigmented anaerobes (formerly, black-pigmented *Bacteroides),* of which it is considered the most virulent. Black-pigmented anaerobes produce several potent enzymes, in particular collagenases and proteases; endotoxin; fatty acids; and other possibly toxic agents (Shah, 1993).

Table 2 Evidence implicating *A actinomycetemcomitans* in the etiology of destructive periodontal diseases[*]

Criterion	Findings
Association	Elevated in lesions of LAP, prepubertal, or adolescent periodontal disease.
	Lower in healthy sites, sites with gingivitis, and edentulous subjects.
	Elevated in some lesions of chronic periodontitis.
	Elevated in active lesions of LAP.
	Detected in apical area of pockets or in tissues from lesions of LAP.
Elimination	Elimination or suppression resulted in successful therapy.
	Recurrent lesions harbored species.
Host response	Elevated antibody in serum or saliva of patients with LAP.
	Elevated antibody in serum or saliva of patients with chronic periodontitis.
	Elevated local antibody in patients with LAP.
Virulence factor	Leukotoxin, collagenase, endotoxin, epitheliotoxin, fibroblast inhibitory factor, bone resorption–inducing factor, induction to cytokine production from macrophages, modification of neutrophil function, degradation of immunoglobulins.
	Invaded epithelial cells in vitro.
Animal studies	Induced disease in gnotobiotic rats and subcutaneous abscesses in mice.

[*] Modified from Socransky and Haffajee (1997). Reprinted with permission.
LAP = Localized aggressive periodontitis.

Studies initiated in the late 1970s and continuing today have reinforced the association of *P gingivalis* with disease and have demonstrated that the species occurs only rarely and in low numbers in health or gingivitis but more frequently in destructive forms of disease. It has been shown to be reduced in successfully treated sites but common in sites with recurrence of disease (Bragd et al, 1987; Haffajee et al, 1988a; van Winkelhoff et al, 1988b). Refractory lesions often contain elevated numbers of *P gingivalis.*

In subjects with various forms of periodontitis, *P gingivalis* has been shown to induce elevated systemic and local immune responses (Mahanonda et al, 1991). In recent years, investigators have not only compared antibody responses in subjects with and without disease, but also examined the relative avidities of antibody (Lopatin and Blackburn, 1992; Mooney et al, 1993; Whitney et al, 1992), the subclass of antibody (Lopatin and Blackburn, 1992; Wilton et al, 1992), the effect of treatment (Chen et al, 1991; Johnson et al, 1993), and the nature of the antigens that elicit the elevated responses (Curtis et al, 1991; Duncan et al, 1992; Ogawa et al, 1989).

The consensus of the antibody studies is that many, but not all, subjects who have experienced periodontal attachment loss exhibit elevated levels of antibody to antigens of *P gingivalis*, suggesting that this species gained access to the underlying tissues and may have initiated or contributed to the observed pathosis.

P gingivalis–like organisms are also strongly related to destructive periodontal disease in naturally occurring or ligature-induced disease in dogs, sheep, or monkeys. The species or closely related organisms were greater in number in lesion sites than in nonlesion sites in naturally occurring disease. When disease was induced by ligature in dogs or monkeys, the level of the species rose at the diseased sites concomitant with the detection of disease. Of great interest were the observations of Holt et al (1988) that a microbiota suppressed by systemic administration of rifampin (without detectable *P gingivalis*) would not cause ligature-induced disease but that the reintroduction of *P gingivalis* to the microbiota resulted in initiation and progression of the lesions.

As stated above, *P gingivalis* is noted particularly for its abundance of extracellular proteases, including an arginine-specific cysteine proteinase that increases vascular permeability, resulting in an increase in gingival crevicular fluid, thereby providing a rich source of nutrients for the subgingival plaque community. In addition, bacterial invasion of gingival epithelial cells has been demonstrated not only for *A actinomycetemcomitans* but also for *P gingivalis* (Duncan et al, 1993; Lamont et al, 1995; Leonhardt et al, 1992; Sandros et al, 1994). Recent studies have shown that *P gingivalis* multiplies and persists within human epithelial cells in vitro (Madianos et al, 1996), inhibits transepithelial migration of PMNLs (Madianos et al, 1997) and induces interleukin-lβ (messenger) RNA expression in oral epithelium (Madianos et al, 1997; Madianos, 1997).

The ability of bacteria to invade host cells probably reflects a long adaptive process between the host and these bacteria. Like the plaque biofilm, host cells are another "safe haven" from innate host defense. Although the importance of this process in periodontal disease remains to be determined, host epithelial cells harboring *A actinomycetemcomitans* and *P gingivalis* may be a source of reinfection after mechanical debridement. Invasion of epithelial cells by *A actinomycetemcomitans* was recently shown to facilitate cell-to-cell spread and may represent a mechanism by which the organism is able to rapidly colonize a host and mediate extensive tissue destruction (Leonhardt et al, 1995).

Invasion by *A actinomycetemcomitans* and *P gingivalis* required bacterial protein synthesis, which may reflect the fact that epithelial cell contact triggers de novo bacterial protein synthesis. This is an exciting possibility, because host cell contact by other pathogenic bacteria was recently shown to activate regions of the bacterial chromosome termed *pathogenicity islands* (Galan, 1996). These regions of DNA are believed to be transmitted in blocks and may represent a major

evolutionary step in the transition to a pathogen. The presence of pathogenicity islands in periodontal pathogens would be strong evidence for the true evolutionary and adaptive processes that occur in the periodontal environment.

A key component of the biofilm paradigm for dental plaque and the development of periodontitis is that different organisms play different roles in the disease process. Darveau et al (1995) have found that *P gingivalis* differs from other gram-negative bacteria in that it does not have the capacity to directly stimulate the production of E-selectin by human endothelial cells (Fig 72). In addition, it has recently been shown that a co-infection of *P gingivalis* and human cytomegalovirus (HCMV) appears to be particularly deleterious in subjects with aggressive periodontitis (Michalowicz et al, 2000). This co-infection may be one of the reasons why *P gingivalis* occurs and multiplies intracellularly. As a consequence, leukocytes cannot bind to endothelial cells and migrate into the extravascular compartment. Through this mechanism, *P gingivalis* blocks a key step in the inflammatory response. Animal studies have confirmed that the lipopolysaccharide from *P gingivalis* does not elicit an immediate innate host inflammatory response (Reife et al, 1995).

Further examination revealed that *P gingivalis* is able to inhibit the ability of other bacteria to stimulate E-selectin expression on human endothelial cells. Additional studies extended these observations and showed that *P gingivalis* or its lipopolysaccharide is able to inhibit monocyte chemotaxis protein 1, interleukin-8, and intracellular adhesion molecule expression in human endothelial cells, gingival fibroblasts, and gingival epithelial cells (Cunningham et al, 1996). These observations may not be applicable to all cell types, but are consistent with a role of *P gingivalis* in suppressing the innate host inflammatory response to bacteria. Theoretically, this could facilitate colonization and growth of the members of the subgingival plaque biofilm community that are able to take advantage of the ecological niche established by *P gingivalis*. The absence of an ef-

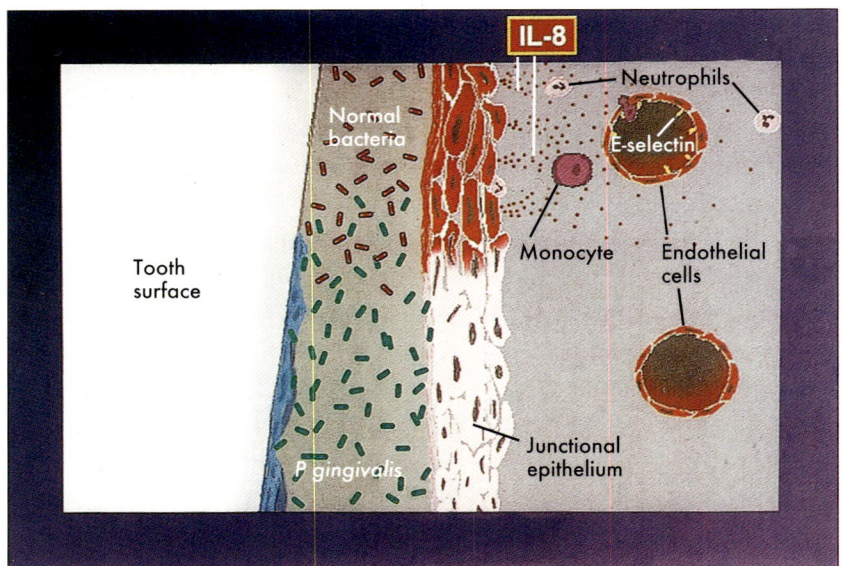

Fig 72 Early stage of *P gingivalis*–associated periodontitis. *P gingivalis* in the deeper part of the gingival sulcus results in a lack of chemoattractive interleukin-8 (IL-8) and E-selectin in the same area. The local inhibition of these inflammatory mediators results in a lack of sufficient phagocytozing leukocytes (PMNLs) to properly control formation of plaque biofilms in the same area. (From Darveau et al, 1997. Reprinted with permission.)

Table 3 Evidence implicating *P gingivalis* in the etiology of destructive periodontal diseases*

Criterion	Findings
Association	Elevated in lesions of periodontitis.
	Lower in healthy sites, sites with gingivitis, and edentulous subjects.
	Elevated in actively progressing lesions.
	Detected in tissues or cells from lesions.
Elimination	Elimination resulted in successful therapy.
	Recurrent lesions harbored species.
	Therapy altered level and/or avidity of antibody to *P gingivalis*
Host response	Elevated antibody in serum or saliva of subjects with various forms of periodontitis.
	Altered local antibody in patients with periodontitis.
Virulence factors	Collagenase, endotoxin, trypsinlike activity, fibrinolysin, other proteases, phospholipase A, degradation of immunoglobulin, fibroblast inhibitory factor, H_2S, NH_3, fatty acids, factors that adversely affect polymorphonuclear lymphocytes, bone resorption–inducing factor, induction of cytokine production from various host cells, generation of chemotactic activity.
	Reduced leukocyte migration of inhibiting E-selectin and interleukin-8.
	Invaded epithelial cells and multiplies in vitro.
	Induced interleukin-1β messenger RNA expression in human epithelial cells.
	Inhibited transepithelium migration of polymorphonuclear leukocytes.
Animal studies	Important in experimental pure or mixed subcutaneous infections.
	Induced disease in gnotobiotic rats.
	Studies in monkeys, sheep, and dogs.
	Immunization diminished disease in experimental animals.

*Modified from Socransky and Haffajee (1997). Reprinted with permission.

fective innate host response is proposed as a major factor in the development of periodontal disease (Darveau et al, 1997). These bacteria could attain the large numbers characteristic of periodontitis. As mentioned earlier, a pathogenic biofilm contains several periodontal pathogens that release antigens more prone to misdirect the inflammatory response and induce bone loss.

Table 3 lists findings implicating *P gingivalis* in the etiology of destructive periodontal diseases.

Bacteroides forsythus

Bacteroides forsythus was first described in 1979 as a "fusiform" *Bacteroides* species (Tanner et al, 1979). The organism is a gram-negative, anaerobic, spindle-shaped, highly pleomorphic rod. Growth is enhanced by cocultivation with *F nucleatum,* with which it commonly occurs in subgingival sites (Socransky et al, 1988a). *B forsythus* is found in higher numbers in sites of destructive periodontal disease than in sites with gingivitis or healthy sites (Lai et al, 1987) and is detected more frequently and in higher numbers in active than in inactive periodontal lesions (Dzink et al, 1988).

Initially, *B forsythus* was thought to be a relatively uncommon subgingival species. However, Lai et al (1987), using fluorescent-labeled polyclonal antiserums, demonstrated that levels of *B forsythus* are much higher in subgingival than in supragingival plaque samples and are higher in sites that show breakdown after periodontal therapy than in sites that remain stable or gain attachment. Studies by Gmür et al (1989), who used monoclonal antibodies to enumerate the species directly in plaque samples, suggested that it is more common than previously found by culture, its levels being strongly related to increasing probing depth.

These findings are confirmed in current studies using checkerboard DNA-DNA hybridization techniques to examine subgingival plaque samples. Using this technique, Forsyth Dental Center demonstrated that *B forsythus* is the most com-

mon species detected on or in epithelial cells recovered from periodontal pockets. It is infrequently detected in epithelial cell samples from healthy subjects. Double-labeling experiments demonstrated the presence of *B forsythus* both on and in periodontal pocket epithelial cells, indicating its invasive ability. Listgarten et al (1993) reported *B forsythus* to be the species most frequently detected in subjects with refractory disease. Serum antibody to *B forsythus* has been found to be elevated in a number of patients with periodontitis (Taubman et al, 1992) and often extremely elevated in a subset of subjects with refractory periodontal disease.

The role of this species in periodontal diseases is being clarified by ongoing studies in numerous laboratories, using noncultural methods of enumeration such as DNA probes or immunologic methods. For example, Grossi et al (1994, 1995) considered *B forsythus* to be the most significant microbial risk indicator distinguishing subjects with periodontitis from those who are periodontally healthy. In the subsequent prospective, longitudinal part of this study, it was shown that, compared to *B forsythus*–negative sites, sites infected by *B forsythus* carried a sevenfold greater risk for future attachment loss (odds ratio, 7.8); the odds ratios for sites with pocket depths more than 3.2 mm, sites infected by *P gingivalis,* and smokers versus nonsmokers were 3.0, 6.1, and 5.4, respectively (Machtei et al, 1997). These findings confirmed *B forsythus,* particularly, and *P gingivalis* to be very powerful microbial prognostic risk factors for further attachment loss in diseased periodontal pockets.

Prevotella intermedia

Prevotella intermedia is the second black-pigmented *Bacteroides* species to attract considerable interest. The levels of this gram-negative, short, round-ended anaerobic rod have been shown to be particularly elevated in acute necrotizing ulcerative gingivitis (Loesche et al, 1982) and certain forms of periodontitis (Dzink et al,

1983; Moore et al, 1985; Tanner et al, 1979). *P intermedia* appears to have a number of the virulence properties exhibited by *P gingivalis*, and injection into laboratory animals has been shown to induce mixed infections. Elevated serum antibodies to this species have been observed in some but not all subjects with refractory periodontitis (Haffajee et al, 1988b).

Recently, strains of *P intermedia* that show identical phenotypic traits have been separated into two species, *P intermedia* and *P nigrescens* (Shah and Gharbia, 1992). This distinction makes earlier studies difficult to interpret, because data from the two species may inadvertently have been pooled. However, new studies that discriminate the species in subgingival plaque samples should clarify the role of both in the pathogenesis of periodontal disease.

In the prospective longitudinal human study by Machtei et al (1997) described earlier, it was also shown that sites infected with *P intermedia* lost more attachment than did *P intermedia*–negative sites.

Fusobacterium nucleatum

Fusobacterium nucleatum is a gram-negative, anaerobic, spindle-shaped rod that has been recognized as part of the subgingival microbiota for about 100 years (Plaut, 1894; Vincent, 1899). It is the most common isolate in cultures of subgingival plaque samples, constituting approximately 7% to 10% of total isolates from different clinical conditions (Dzink et al, 1985, 1988; Moore et al, 1985).

Although a difference in levels of this species in active and inactive periodontal lesions has been detected (Dzink et al, 1988), inadvertent pooling of subspecies may have masked an even more pronounced difference. This is supported by antibody responses in subjects with different forms of periodontal disease to different hormology groups of *F nucleatum*. The role of *F nucleatum* may be clarified by individual evaluation of subspecies with respect to their association with disease status and progression.

Campylobacter rectus

Campylobacter rectus is a gram-negative, anaerobic, short, motile vibrio (see Fig 42). It is unusual in that it utilizes H_2 or formate as its energy source. It is a member of the "vibrio corrodens," a group of short, nondescript rods that formed small, convex, "dry spreading" or "corroding" (pitting) colonies on blood agar plates. These organisms were eventually shown to include members of a new genus *Wolinella* (some species have been redefined as *Campylobacter*), *E corrodens*, and *Campylobacter (Bacteroides) gracilis*.

C rectus has been shown to be present in higher numbers in diseased sites than in healthy sites (Lai et al, 1992; Lippke et al, 1991; Moore et al, 1983, 1985) and was found in higher numbers and more frequently at sites of active periodontal destruction (Dzink et al, 1985, 1988; Rams et al, 1993; Tanner and Bouldin, 1989). Like *A actinomycetemcomitans*, *C rectus* has been shown to produce a leukotoxin (Gillespie et al, 1992).

Eikenella corrodens

Eikenella corrodens is a gram-negative, capnophilic, asaccharolytic, regular, small rod with blunt ends. It is found more frequently in sites of periodontal destruction than in healthy sites (Savitt and Socransky, 1984) and is found more frequently and at higher levels in active sites (Dzink et al, 1985; Tanner et al, 1987) and in sites of subjects who respond poorly to periodontal therapy (Haffajee et al, 1988b). Successfully treated sites harbor lower proportions (Tanner et al, 1987). *E corrodens* has also been found in association with *A actinomycetemcomitans* in some lesions of localized aggressive periodontitis (Mandell, 1984; Mandell et al, 1987). While there is some association of this species with periodontal disease, to date this association has not been particularly strong (Chen et al, 1989).

Spirochetes

Spirochetes are gram-negative, anaerobic, helical, highly motile microorganisms that are common in many periodontal pockets (see Figs 28, 34, 43, and 44). Their role in the pathogenesis of destructive periodontal diseases deserves extended comment. A spirochete has been clearly implicated as the probable etiologic agent of acute necrotizing ulcerative gingivitis, on the basis of its presence in large numbers in tissue biopsies from affected sites (Listgarten and Socransky, 1964; Listgarten, 1965). The role of spirochetes in other forms of periodontal disease is less clear.

The organisms have been considered as possible periodontal pathogens since long ago. In the 1970s and 1980s they were used as possible diagnostic indicators of disease activity and/or therapeutic efficacy (Keyes and Rams, 1983; Listgarten and Helldén, 1978; Rams and Keyes, 1983), mainly because of their increased numbers in sites with increased probing depth. Healthy sites exhibit few, if any, spirochetes; sites of gingivitis but no attachment loss exhibit low to moderate levels, while many deep pockets harbor large numbers.

The major difficulty encountered in defining the role of spirochetes has been the difficulty in distinguishing individual species. At least 15 species of subgingival spirochetes have been described, but in most studies of plaque samples spirochetes are combined either in a single group or in groups based on cell size, ie, small, medium, or large. Thus, while there may be pathogens among the spirochetes, their role may have been obscured by unintentional pooling with non-pathogenic spirochetes.

The role of individual spirochete species may soon be clarified by the use of immunologic or DNA probe techniques to detect their presence in plaque samples. Enumeration of even uncultivable spirochete taxa is possible with oligonucleotide probes (Tanner et al, 1994) or specific antibody. Studies based on these techniques allow better distinction of species of spirochetes and a clearer understanding of their possible role in disease.

Treponema denticola. In recent years, specific species of spirochetes have been correlated to periodontal breakdown. *T denticola* has been found to be more common in periodontally diseased than healthy sites and more common in subgingival than supragingival plaque (Riviere et al, 1992; Simonson et al, 1988). Levels of *T denticola* were shown to decrease in successfully treated periodontal sites but did not change or increased in unresponsive sites (Simonson et al, 1992b). Cultural studies have suggested that *T denticola* is found more frequently in patients with severe periodontitis than in healthy or gingivitis sites (Moore et al, 1982).

Treponema pallidum. Riviere et al (1991a, 1991b, 1991c, 1992) employed a monoclonal antibody directed against *Treponema pallidum,* the etiologic agent of syphilis, to examine supragingival and subgingival plaque samples and/or tissues from healthy subjects and subjects with periodontitis or acute necrotizing ulcerative periodontitis. This antibody cross-reacted with antigens of uncultivated spirochetes in many of the plaque samples. These pathogen-related oral spirochetes (PROS) were the most frequently detected spirochetes in supragingival and subgingival plaque of patients with periodontitis and were the most numerous spirochetes found at periodontitis lesion. The PROS were also detected by using immunohistochemical techniques on plaque samples (Riviere et al, 1991c) and tissue biopsies from patients with acute necrotizing ulcerative gingivitis (Riviere et al, 1991a). The PROS were also shown to have the ability to penetrate a tissue barrier in vitro (Riviere et al, 1991b). These studies and others suggest that certain species of spirochetes are important in the pathogenesis of acute necrotizing ulcerative gingivitis and certain forms of periodontitis.

Relative importance of pathogenic bacteria

In a recent investigation, Haffajee et al (1998) compared the site prevalence of subgingival species in 203 subjects: 30 periodontally healthy subjects

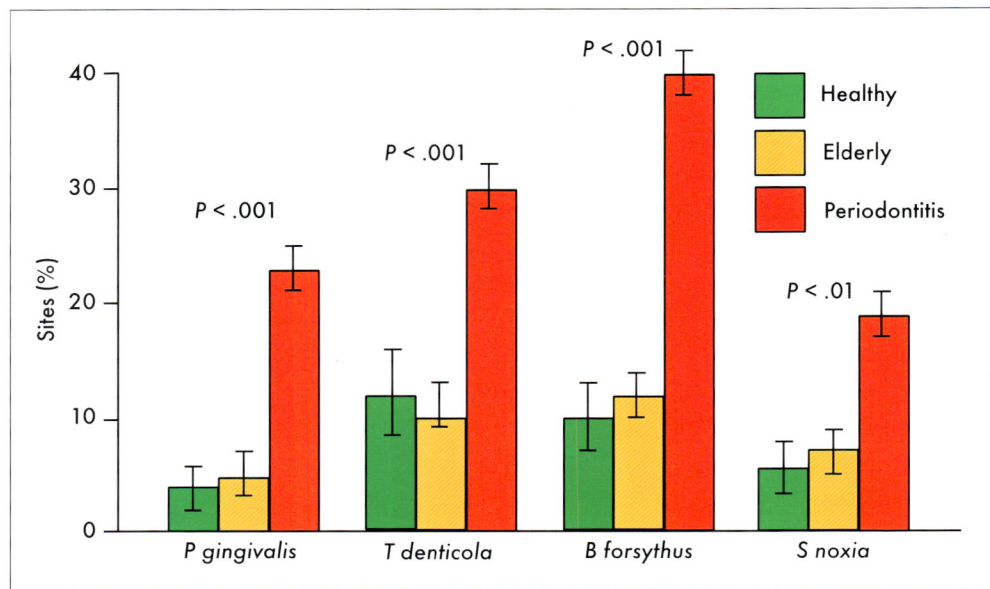

Fig 73 The mean prevalence of *P gingivalis*, *T denticola*, *B forsythus*, and *S noxia* in periodontally healthy subjects, elderly subjects with a well-maintained periodontium, and subjects with chronic periodontitis. (From Haffajee et al, 1998. Reprinted with permission.)

(mean age, 36 ± 9 years), 35 elderly subjects with a well-maintained periodontium (mean age, 77 ± 5) and 138 subjects with chronic periodontitis (mean age, 46 ± 11). At baseline, subgingival plaque samples were taken from the mesial aspect of each tooth (up to 28 samples) in the 203 subjects. The presence and levels of 40 subgingival taxa were determined in 5,003 plaque samples, using whole genomic DNA probes and checkerboard DNA-DNA hybridization. Clinical assessments, including dichotomous measures of gingival redness, bleeding on probing, plaque accumulation, and suppuration, as well as duplicate measures of probing depth and attachment level, were made at six sites per tooth. The percentage of sites colonized by each species (prevalence) was computed for each subject.

Commonly detected species, such as *Actinomyces naeslundii* genospecies 2, *S sanguis*, and *S oralis* did not differ significantly among subject groups. After results were adjusted for multiple comparisons, four species were found in significantly greater numbers and at greater prevalence in the periodontitis group. The mean percentage of sites (± SEM) colonized by *B forsythus* was 10% ± 3%, 12% ± 2%, and 40% ± 2% ($P < .001$) for the healthy, elderly, and periodontitis groups, re-

spectively. When *B forsythus* was detected at more than 5% of sampled sites, the odds ratio that a subject had periodontitis was 14.4:1. The mean prevalence of *P gingivalis* was 4% ± 2%, 5% ± 2%, and 23% ± 2% ($P < .001$); the prevalence of *T denticola* was 12% ± 4%, 10% ± 3%, and 30% ± 2% ($P < .001$); and that of *Selenomonas noxia* was 6% ± 2%, 7% ± 2%, and 19% ± 2% ($P < .01$) among the healthy, elderly, and periodontitis groups, respectively (Fig 73). When only sites with probing depths of 0 to 4 mm were analyzed, similar differences were observed among the subject groups. The data suggest an etiologic role for *B forsythus*, *P gingivalis*, *T denticola*, and *S noxia* in chronic periodontitis.

Table 4 is an attempt to rank putative periodontal pathogens according to the strength of their relationship to periodontal diseases.

Table 5 summarizes some of the data implicating subgingival species other than the exogenous, transmissible periopathogens *A actinomycetemcomitans* and *P gingivalis* in the pathogenesis of destructive periodontal diseases.

As discussed earlier, the identification of bacteria as causative risk factors, rather than risk indicators, requires prospective longitudinal clinical trials. Because such trials are time-consuming

Table 4 Strength of relationships between periodontal pathogens and periodontal disease

Very strong	Strong	Moderate	Early stage of investigation
A actinomycetemcomitans	B forsythus	Streptococcus intermedius	Selenomonas
Spirochete of acute necrotizing ulcerative gingivitis	P intermedia	P nigrescens	Gram-negative enteric rods
P gingivalis	C rectus	Peptostreptococcus micros	Staphylococcus species
	Eubacterium nodatum	F nucleatum	Bacteroides gracilis
	Treponema species	Eubacterium species	
		E corrodens	

*From Haffajee and Socransky (1994). Reprinted with permission.

Table 5 Evidence implicating subgingival bacterial species in the etiology of destructive periodontal diseases*

	Association	Elimination	Host response	Virulence factors	Animal studies
P intermedia	+++	+++	++	+++	++
F nucleatum	+++	+	++	++	+
B forsythus	+++	++	+	+	+
C rectus	+++	+	+	+	
E corrodens	+++	+	+	+	+
P micros	++	+	+	+	
Selenomas species	++				
Eubacterium species	++		++	+	
S intermedius	+				

*From Socransky and Haffajee (1997). Reprinted with permission.
+ = 1–3 References; ++ = 4–10 References; +++ = > 10 References

and very costly, bacterial risk indicators are generally identified by analysis of cross-sectional data. However, cross-sectional studies cannot determine whether a disease marker occurred before the onset of disease.

It is also important that a clear distinction be made between prospective and retrospective studies and specially why it is important to base identification of etiologic (risk) factors on prospective studies. Retrospective bacterial studies may monitor clinical sites over time but characterize specific bacteria only after attachment loss has occurred. The disadvantage is that only an association can be determined. In a prospective study, sites are monitored longitudinally, both clinically and microbiologically, and plaque is characterized for specific bacteria both before

and after periodontal destruction has occurred. A disadvantage is that, if disease progression is slow and can be measured only in a limited number of subjects, a large number of patients and/or sites must be followed over a long period of time to detect change.

The introduction of immunologic and DNA probe techniques to identify specific bacteria in plaque as an alternative to culture methods has helped reduce the prohibitive cost of such studies, and the application of these techniques could determine a possible association between a bacterial pathogen and future periodontal destruction. Identification of such a microorganism in plaque could then serve as a screening test for predicting future periodontal deterioration.

Longitudinal studies of the specific plaque hypothesis

Recently, a few longitudinal retrospective and prospective studies have been conducted to correlate specific periopathogens to periodontal tissue breakdown and the outcome of periodontal therapy.

In a prospective study by Dahlén et al (1996), the aim was to eliminate *A actinomycetemcomitans* and *P gingivalis* and reduce *P intermedia* to less than 5% of the total viable count in patients with advanced periodontitis. After baseline examination of probing depth, clinical attachment level, bleeding on probing, plaque recording, and microbial sampling, all the patients underwent comprehensive subgingival scaling, root planing, and debridement and received oral hygiene education. This was followed after 3 months by supplementary PMTC and oral hygiene training.

After 6 months, the results were evaluated by duplicate microbiologic samplings and clinical measurements made 1 week apart. If the indicator bacteria, *A actinomycetemcomitans* or *P gingivalis,* were revealed, or if *P intermedia* was detected in more than 5% in one of the duplicate samples, according to Bragd et al (1987), the sampled areas were subjected to treatment phase II, which consisted of either redebridement or periodontal surgery in a split-mouth design. Surgical measures included a reverse bevel incision, elevation of a full-thickness flap, removal of inflamed tissue, debridement, and root planing of the teeth. At this point, sites that did not fulfill the microbiologic criteria for treatment were left without intervention.

At 18 months, a reevaluation was performed, including duplicate microbiologic samplings and clinical measurements made 1 week apart. Again, if the sites fulfillled the treatment criteria, they were subjected to treatment phase III, which included surgery combined with systemic administration of tetracycline (250 mg, four times a day, for 3 weeks). All sites were then reevaluated by duplicate microbiologic sampling and clinical measurements after 27, 33, 39, 51, and 63 months.

In one patient, in whom treatment stages I, II, and III had failed to eradicate the indicator bacteria, further destruction was noted after 33 months. Destruction was even more pronounced after 39 months. For ethical reasons, this patient underwent redebridement and was given a combination of systemic metronidazole (250 mg) and amoxicillin (375 mg) three times a day for 28 days.

The patients were recalled for maintenance every third month during the first 3 years, and every 6 months thereafter. At each visit, plaque was disclosed, oral hygiene instruction was reinforced, and PMTC was carried out. No subgingival scaling or cleaning was performed in the experimental areas at any time. None of the patients received any other antibiotic regimen during the 5-year study period. The patients showed highly individual patterns with respect to the presence of indicator bacteria, type of treatment needed to accomplish treatment goals, clinical response, and bacterial and disease recurrences. The results suggested that the presence of the indicator bacteria in microbial samples taken after treatment may identify patients at risk for recurrent periodontitis.

In another prospective study by Renvert et al (1998), 28 patients (13 smokers and 15 nonsmokers) with untreated advanced periodontal disease received sessions of oral hygiene instruction and nonsurgical treatment. The baseline values for clinical data did not differ significantly between the groups. Six months after therapy, the complete-mouth bleeding score was 36.5% for the smokers and 22.7% for the nonsmokers ($P < .05$). Probing depth was reduced by 1.9 mm for smokers and by 2.5 mm for nonsmokers, a statistically significant difference ($P < .05$). Compared to baseline, the levels of *P gingivalis* and *P intermedia/P nigrescens* were reduced in both groups, but *A actinomycetemcomitans* demonstrated a slight increase in mean values at 6 months. This was especially notable for smokers, in whom *A actinomycetemcomitans* was more difficult to eradicate. In this study, the microbiologic response seemed to be in conformity with the clinical response.

An investigation by Colombo et al (1998) compared clinical variables and the sites, prevalence, and levels of 40 subgingival species in 94 patients with successfully treated or refractory periodontitis. Patients were treated with scaling and root planing and, if needed, periodontal surgery and systemic tetracycline. Twenty-eight subjects with refractory disease showed mean full-mouth attachment loss greater than 2.5 mm and/or more than three sites with attachment loss greater than 2.5 mm within 1 year posttherapy; 66 successfully treated subjects showed mean attachment level gain and no sites with attachment loss greater than 2.5 mm. Baseline subgingival plaque samples were taken from the mesial aspect of each tooth, and the presence and levels of 40 subgingival taxa were determined with whole genomic DNA probes and checkerboard DNA-DNA hybridization. The mean levels and percentage of sites colonized by each species (prevalence) were computed for each subject, and differences between groups were calculated.

Most of the species tested, including *A actinomycetemcomitans, P gingivalis, T denticola,* and *B forsythus,* were equally or less prevalent in the group with refractory disease. *P nigrescens* was significantly more prevalent in successfully treated subjects, while subjects with refractory disease harbored a larger proportion of *Streptococcus* species, particularly *Streptococcus constellatus.* The odds that a subject would have refractory disease were 8.6 (*P* < .001) if *S constellatus* constituted more than 3.5% of the total DNA probe count.

Because there were few microbiologic differences in treatment outcome using DNA probes to known species, the predominant cultivable microbiota of 33 subgingival samples from 14 subjects with refractory periodontitis was examined, and 85% of the 1,649 isolates were identified by probes for 69 recognized subgingival species. Many sequenced isolates were of taxa considered uncommon in the oral microbiota, such as *Acinetobacter baumanni, Gemella haemolysans, Enterococcus faecalis, Staphylococcus warneri, Pseudomonas aeruginosa,* and novel species in the genera *Bartonella, Ralstonia, Neisseria, Eubacterium, Rothia, Gordona, Gemella, Corynebacterium, Leptotrichia,* and *Actinomyces.* Based

on their subgingival microbiota, subjects with refractory disease constituted a heterogenous group: They did not harbor more of the "classic" periopathogens, although elevated proportions of *S constellatus* were found.

In a prospective treatment study by Shiloah et al (1997), the overall goal was to determine the short-term anti-infective effects of four randomized treatment modalities on *A actinomycetemcomitans, P gingivalis,* and *B forsythus* and determine the effects of bacterial survival on treatment outcomes in patients with chronic periodontitis. The subjects were 12 adults with moderate periodontitis: All had at least one tooth in each quadrant that had an inflamed pocket with a probing depth greater than 5 mm and probing attachment loss and that harbored at least one of the following three periodontal pathogens: *A actinomycetemcomitans, P gingivalis,* or *B forsythus.* The number of target organisms per site was determined preoperatively and at 1 week, 1 month, and 3 months postoperatively with DNA probes. One quadrant in each patient was randomly assigned to the following four treatment groups: *(1)* scaling and root planing; *(2)* pocket reduction through osseous surgery and epically positioned flap; *(3)* modified Widman flap; *(4)* modified Widman flap and topical application of saturated citric acid at pH 1 for 3 minutes. All four treatments were carried out at the one appointment. No postoperative antibiotics were used. The patients were instructed to supplement their daily oral hygiene with chlorhexidine oral rinse during the study.

The study produced the following results:

- None of the treatment modalities was effective in eliminating the target species.
- The incidence of infected sites for all groups was 100.0% preoperatively and 62.5%, 33.3%, and 31.3% at 1 week, 1 month, and 3 months postoperatively, respectively.
- These infected sites lost 1.1 ± 0.4 mm of probing attachment while uninfected sites gained 0.0 ± 0.3 mm. The infected sites had higher mean Plaque Index and bleeding on probing

values (0.9 ± 0.3 and 73% ± 12%, respectively) than did the uninfected sites (0.3 ± 0.1 and 30% ± 8%, respectively).

Shiloah et al (1997) drew the following conclusions: Although the number of samples does not allow for statistical consideration of sites within patient interactions, the data from this report strongly suggest that mechanical therapy alone, or in conjunction with topical application of citric acid, is not a predictable approach for elimination of the target species evaluated in this study. All four treatment modalities significantly reduced the bacterial load, but failed to predictably eliminate the target species. The survival of these species was associated with a higher incidence of bleeding on probing postoperatively and a deleterious effect on probing attachment level. These results indicate that survival of highly pathogenic bacterial species negatively affects the short-term clinical outcomes of nonsurgical and surgical periodontal therapy in a patient population with chronic periodontitis.

Haffajee et al (1997) evaluated the effect of complete-mouth scaling and root planing on the subgingival microbiota in 57 subjects with chronic periodontitis. The subjects were monitored clinically prior to therapy and at 3, 6, and 9 months posttherapy. Subgingival plaque samples were taken from the mesial aspect of each tooth in each subject at each of these appointments. Counts of 40 subgingival species in each plaque sample were determined by using modifications of the checkerboard DNA-DNA hybridization technique.

The clinical findings were in accordance with those of other studies. There was an overall small but statistically significant decrease in probing depth and probing attachment level measurements, most marked at pockets deeper than 6 mm and less measuring at pockets 4 to 6 mm; there was virtually no change at sites with an initial probing depth of less than 4 mm. In general, scaling and root planing did not have a major effect on the subgingival microbiota, although three species, *B forsythus*, *T denticola*, and *P gingivalis*,

were significantly decreased in mean levels and percentage of sites colonized posttherapy; this reduction was maintained at 6 and 9 months posttherapy. Other species increased in prevalence and levels posttherapy: Most notable was the significant increase in mean levels of *A viscosus* posttherapy. Other putative beneficial species, such as *S mitis* and *Streptococcus gordonii*, also showed modest increases posttherapy. Nonetheless, the majority of species were not significantly changed by scaling and root planing.

Of 57 subjects, 18 lost attachment as a result of scaling and root planing. These subjects did not differ significantly in any clinical, demographic, or environmental parameter examined but had lower levels of *T denticola*, *P gingivalis*, and *B forsythus* (the species primarily affected by scaling and root planing) pretherapy and/or low levels of the putative beneficial species, *A viscosus*. At a biologic level, it is probably preferable that scaling and root planing does not alter the majority of the subgingival microbiota, which has co-evolved with, and in most instances is in quiet harmony with, the host. On occasion, pathogens of one or more species disturb this equilibrium and lead to tissue damage. If the most common periodontal therapy dramatically and randomly altered the subgingival equilibrium in large proportions of patients, then superinfection by an undesirable microbial complex would be very likely. Thus, it is rather reassuring that scaling and root planing induce small but useful alterations, which in virtually all instances benefit the host.

In a 10-year retrospective longitudinal study (Papapanou et al, 1997a), checkerboard DNA-DNA hybridization technology was used to study the epidemiology of 18 microbial species associated with various states of periodontal health and disease. The researchers examined a sample of 148 Chinese subjects, aged 30 to 39 and 50 to 59 years, who had never been exposed to systematic dental therapeutic intervention. The aims were to (1) describe the prevalence of these microorganisms; (2) correlate the microbiologic and clinical profiles of the subjects; and (3) examine the association between the microbiologic variables and the longitudinal changes of periodontal status that occurred over a preceding 10-year period.

A maximum of 14 subgingival samples was obtained from each subject: 1,864 in all. The frequency of occurrence of the 18 species examined was high at both subject and tooth-site levels. However, not all species were equally capable of reaching high numbers in the subgingival samples and, as a rule, the species colonized heavily only limited proportions of tooth sites within each mouth. In deep pockets or progressing sites, there was a profound increase in certain species, such as *P gingivalis, T denticola,* and *B forsythus.*

Multivariate statistical analyses of the subgingival profile could effectively discriminate between deep and shallow pockets and progressing and stable tooth sites. The microbiologic variables showed an enhanced discriminating potential when classifications were performed at an individual subject level. Colonization by *P gingivalis, B forsythus, C rectus,* and *T denticola* at levels exceeding a certain threshold was associated with a significantly increased probability (odds ratio, > 4) that an individual subject would harbor deep pockets or progressing tooth sites. Figure 74 shows the levels of various species of bacteria in subjects with no deep pockets and subjects with three or more deep pockets.

In the prospective longitudinal study by Machtei et al (1997), discussed previously, 79 patients with established periodontitis were monitored longitudinally for 1 year. Complete-mouth clinical measurements, plaque, gingival, and calculus indices, and probing depth and attachment level measurements were repeated every 3 months. Complete-mouth radiographs were taken at baseline and 12 months, to determine changes in crestal bone height, using an image enhancement technique. Subgingival plaque samples were taken at baseline and every 3 months. Immunofluorescence assays were performed for the battery of target microorganisms.

The overall mean attachment loss and bone loss were almost identical (0.159 mm and 0.164 mm, respectively). Individual patient variation was large (-0.733 to +1.004 mm). An overall 6.89%

of sites were active. Mean probing depth showed minimal change over the study period, suggesting that most, if not all, of the attachment loss was accompanied by concomitant gingival recession. Smokers exhibited greater attachment loss and radiographic bone loss than did nonsmokers. *B forsythus, P intermedia,* and *P gingivalis* were common in these patients; their presence at baseline was associated with further disease progression. Subjects with a mean baseline probing depth of 3.2 mm or greater were at greater risk for future bone loss 1 year later (odds ratio, 2.97). Smokers were at significantly greater risk for further attachment loss than were nonsmokers (odds ratio, 5.41). Subjects harboring *B forsythus* at baseline were at seven times greater risk for increased probing depth (odds ratio, 7.84). The presence of *P gingivalis* resulted in six times increased risk (odds ratio, 6.15). Thus, past periodontal destruction, smoking habits, and the organisms *B forsythus, P gingivalis,* and *P intermedia* are prognostic risk factors for further periodontal breakdown. In this context, Zambon et al (1996a) reported that counts of *B forsythus* in diseased sites were significantly greater in smokers than in nonsmokers and former smokers.

When clinical trials are designed, or when epidemiologic data are evaluated, it is most important to make allowance for these factors, and treatment strategies should attempt to eliminate or modify them. In another prospective longitudinal study, Tanner et al (1998) compared the subgingival microbiota in the presence of periodontal health, gingivitis, and initial periodontitis using predominant culture and a DNA-probe, checkerboard-hybridization method. Fifty-six healthy adult subjects with minimal periodontal attachment loss were clinically monitored at 3-month intervals for 12 months. More sites demonstrated small increments of attachment loss than attachment gain over the monitoring period.

Sites showing more than 1.5 mm periodontal attachment loss during monitoring were sampled as active lesions for microbial analysis. Twelve subjects had interproximal lesions, and five had attachment loss at buccal sites (recession). Cul-

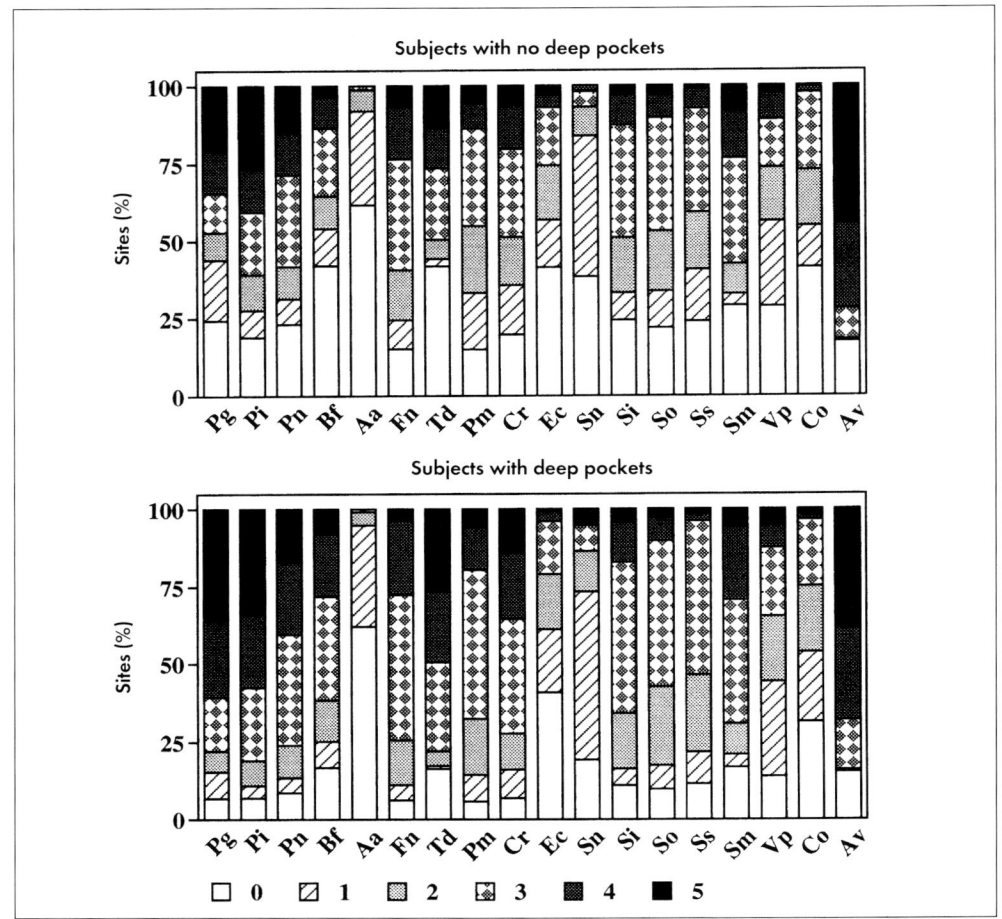

Fig 74 Percentage of sites found to harbor various levels of bacterial species in subjects with no deep pockets and subjects with 3 or more deep pockets. Sites were examined for 18 species: *P gingivalis (Pg), P intermedia (Pi), P nigrescens (Pn), B forsythus (Bf), A actinomycetemcomitans (Aa), F nucleatum (Fn), T denticola (Td), P micros (Pm), C rectus (Cr), E corrodens (Ec), S noxia (Sn), S intermedius (Si), S oralis (So), S sanguis (Ss), S mutans (Sm), Veillonella parvula (Vp), C ochraceus (Co),* and *A viscosus (Av).* Scores were assigned using the following scale: O = No bacteria; 1 = < 10^5 Bacteria; 2 = 10^5 Bacteria; 3 = > 10^5 but < 10^6 Bacteria; 4 = 10^6 Bacteria; 5 = > 10^6 Bacteria. (From Papapanou et al, 1997a. Reprinted with permission.)

tural studies identified *B forsythus, C rectus,* and *S noxia* as the predominant species associated with active interproximal lesions (9 subjects), whereas *A naeslundii* and *S oralis* were the dominant species colonizing active buccal sites. *A naeslundii, C gracilis,* and *B forsythus* (at lower levels than were found at active sites) were the predominant species cultured from sites with gin-

givitis (10 subjects). Health-associated species (10 subjects) included *S oralis, A naeslundii,* and *Actinomyces gerencseriae.* The DNA probe data identified higher mean levels of *B forsythus* and *C rectus* at sites with active periodontitis (7 subjects) than at sites with inactive periodontitis.

P gingivalis and *A actinomycetemcomitans* were detected infrequently. Cluster analysis of the cultural microbiota grouped eight of nine active interproximal lesions in one subcluster, characterized by a mostly gram-negative microbiota, including *B forsythus* and *C rectus*. The data suggest that *B forsythus*, *C rectus*, and *S noxia* were major species characterizing sites in transition from periodontal health to disease. The differences in location and microbiota of active interproximal and buccal sites suggested that different mechanisms may be involved in increased attachment loss. While interproximal attachment loss was associated with deeper pockets and caused by periopathogens, buccal attachment loss was probably associated with shallow pockets and caused mainly by iatrogenic recession resulting from toothbrushing.

Role of mixed infections

During the last few decades, attention has focused on the possible role of individual species as risk factors for destructive periodontal diseases. However, microbial complexes colonizing the subgingival area can have a spectrum of relationships with the host, ranging from beneficial (the organisms prevent disease) to harmful (the organisms cause disease). The presence of two pathogens at a site could have no effect, or it could diminish the potential pathogenicity of one or the other of the species. Alternatively, pathogenicity could be enhanced in either an additive or a synergistic manner (see the earlier discussions on the role of *P gingivalis*). Studies on the relative risk for further attachment loss showed that the risk was two to three times greater at sites with a count of more than 10^5 of both *P gingivalis* and *A actinomycetemcomitans* than it was for the two separate species (Gunaratnam et al, 1992). It seems likely that mixed infections occur in subgingival sites because so many diverse species inhabit this niche.

Based on evidence from examination of plaque samples by culture, certain combinations of species have been suggested as important in human periodontal diseases. These combinations include *F nucleatum*, *B forsythus*, and *C rectus*; *S intermedius*, *P gingivalis*, and *P micros*; and *S intermedius* and *F nucleatum*, with and without *P gingivalis* (Haffajee et al, 1988b; Socransky et al, 1988b). *P gingivalis* was also found in combinations with *A actinomycetemcomitans* (Tanner et al, 1979), *B forsythus* (Gmür et al, 1989), and *T denticola* (Simonson et al, 1992a). Recently Michalowicz et al (2000) found that a co-infection of *P gingivalis* and HCMV resulted in significantly more loss of periodontal attachment in patients with aggressive periodontitis than did infections of *P gingivalis* or *A actinomycetemcomitans* in the absence of HCMV. The pathogenic role of these mixtures in human periodontal diseases awaits confirmation by further testing.

A comprehensive examination of the relationship among multiple species in plaque has become possible with the advent of techniques such as checkerboard DNA-DNA hybridization (Socransky et al, 1994), which permits concurrent identification of large numbers of bacterial species in large numbers of plaque samples. The technique was employed to examine the associations of species in subgingival plaque samples and demonstrated the relationship among certain groups of bacterial species, including *P gingivalis*, *B forsythus*, and *T denticola*. Another closely related group of species included *F nucleatum* subspecies, *P intermedia*, *P nigrescens*, *P micros*, and *C rectus* (Socransky et al, 1994).

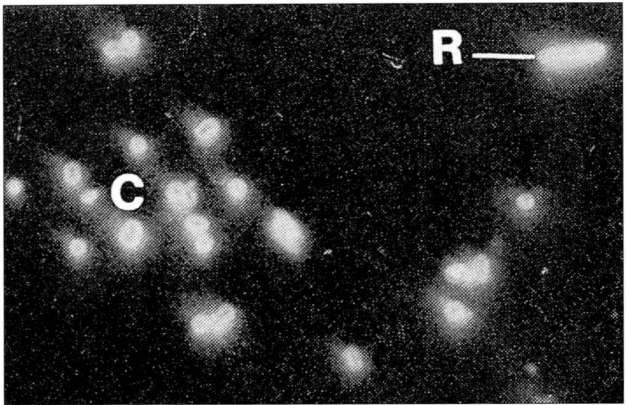

Fig 75 Microscopy revealing cocci (C) and short rods (R) in healthy gingival pockets. (From Listgarten and Helldén, 1978. Reprinted with permission.)

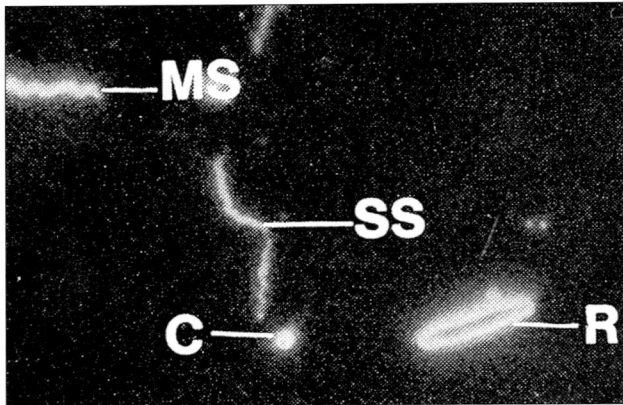

Fig 76 Microscopy revealing small (SS) and medium spirochetes (MS), rods (R), and cocci (C) in diseased pockets. (From Listgarten and Helldén, 1978. Reprinted with permission.)

ORAL MICROBIOLOGY TESTS

Direct microscopy

Microscopy, particularly darkfield and phase-contrast microscopy, has been used as a microbiologic assay of dental plaque for several decades. It has been promoted as the monitoring component of the nonsurgical periodontal therapy known as the *Keyes approach*. Microscopy can provide useful information. The phase-contrast or darkfield microscopic technique can be used to make a chairside evaluation of the relative proportions of the subgingival microflora related to shape and motility. In studies by Listgarten and Helldén (1978), samples from healthy pockets were characterized by cocci and short rods (Fig 75). Small, medium, and large spirochetes and long rods predominated in samples from diseased pockets (Fig 76). However, this technique often underestimates the numbers of small cells and cocci. Because the method is rapid and can be used at the chairside, it is useful for screening and patient motivation.

When plaque samples are compared over time, microscopy can detect shifts in the morphology and motility of the plaque flora in patients with periodontitis. The ability to detect such shifts has clinical relevance. There are, for example, positive correlations between the microscopic determination of motile rods and clinical levels of gingival inflammation as well as between microscopic counts of spirochetes and clinical probing depth (Listgarten and Helldén, 1978). Therefore, clinical efficacy can be demonstrated by shifts from a disease-associated to a health-associated flora. Further, darkfield microscopy has been used to demonstrate differences in the distribution of bacterial morphotypes that occur in subgingival plaque in a coronal to apical direction. These assays show good reproducibility, as reported in studies of repeated plaque samples from patients with periodontitis and edentulous patients with implants (Listgarten and Helldén, 1978).

The major shortcoming of both darkfield or phase-contrast microscopy for detecting periodontal pathogens is that the methods cannot discriminate individual bacterial species: These techniques cannot determine whether the small rod microscopically visible in a plaque sample is *A actinomycetemcomitans, P gingivalis,* or any of the other rod-shaped bacteria in dental plaque. Therefore, although they are useful in demonstrating gross shifts in plaque bacteria that occur following periodontal therapy and in motivating patients to perform better oral hygiene, they fall short as microbiologic methods for identifying particular species of periodontal pathogens.

Microbial culture

Bacterial culture is regarded as the "gold standard" microbiologic assay against which other tests are compared and validated.

Laboratories that base their work on selective media deliberately exclude other portions of the flora. Good selective media or serologic reagents detect very low concentrations of a species. However, the importance of a species is usually directly proportional to its concentration, and this relationship may be overlooked. With selective media, not all the colonies belong to the species being studied. The care with which the resulting colonies are identified can make an important difference in the final data.

When selective media are used, nonselective media or microscopic counts may be used to determine the relative concentrations of species, but quantitative errors are associated with both methods.

No single medium or method grows all of the bacterial types that are present. Therefore, laboratories use different parts of the flora, even though there may be some overlap.

In addition to analytical differences, there is a highly significant difference in the composition of the periodontal flora of different people, and a smaller (but sometimes statistically significant) difference in flora composition from site to site or from time to time within subjects. For this reason, several laboratories have reported different results after they have examined additional subjects or different conclusions after they have compared the flora of healthy control subjects (for reviews see Socransky and Haffajee, 1997).

Finally, interpretation of the same data may vary among authors. In view of these differences, it is surprising how much agreement there is among reports on periodontal bacteriology.

Samples of the subgingival microflora are usually collected with paper points or curettes. In bacterial culture, patient plaque samples are dispersed by sonication or by vortex mixing, distributed onto various types of agar media, and cultured under aerobic as well as anaerobic conditions. However, most of the subgingival microflora are anaerobic.

The plates are examined after a suitable incubation period, and individual colonies are subcultured. These bacterial strains are identified with multiple tests, including colony and cellular morphology, Gram stain, patterns of sugar fermentation, biochemical tests, and chromatographic analysis of metabolic acid end products. The clinical laboratory report details both the types of bacterial species present in the patient plaque sample and their relative proportions or absolute numbers.

The paper point technique by Slots is especially useful in diseased pockets, where insertion of a curette will cause bleeding (Figs 77 to 80). Dental plaque is removed from the gingival sulcus by PMTC (Fig 77). A sterile plane instrument is used to open the gingival pocket, and two sterile paper points are inserted to the base (Fig 78).

A flask containing Viable Medium Gothenburg (VMG) III transport medium is opened over a flame to reduce oxygen. The paper points are placed into the flask (Figs 79 and 80). The flask is sent to an oral microbiology laboratory for anaerobic culture. The total number of subgingival microflora, as well as the percentage of *A actinomycetemcomitans, P intermedius, P gingivalis*, and other black-pigmented *Bacteroides* species, is evaluated. In addition, sensitivity for antibiotics is tested. In this particular pocket, *P gingivalis* represented 85% of the total cultivable subgingival microflora.

Figures 81 and 82 show the periodontal status of the region tested in Figs 77 to 80, during open-flap periodontal surgery that was undertaken to gain access for optimal scaling and root planing.

Figure 83 shows clinical healing 2 years later. Figure 84 shows a radiograph of the alveolar bone before treatment, and Fig 85 shows 2-year postoperative radiograph.

Figs 77 to 80 Slots' paper point technique for obtaining samples for microbial culturing. (Courtesy of G. Heden.)

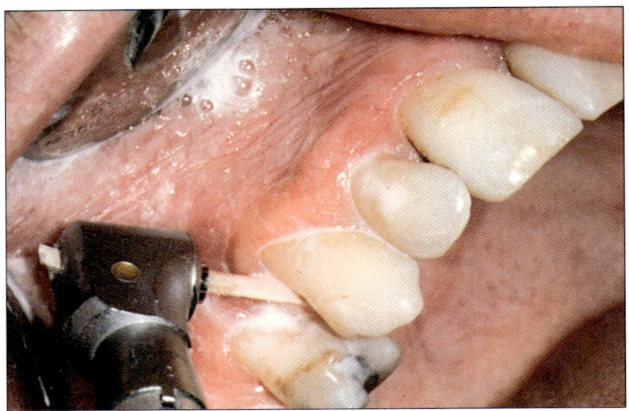

Fig 77 Removal of dental plaque from the gingival sulcus.

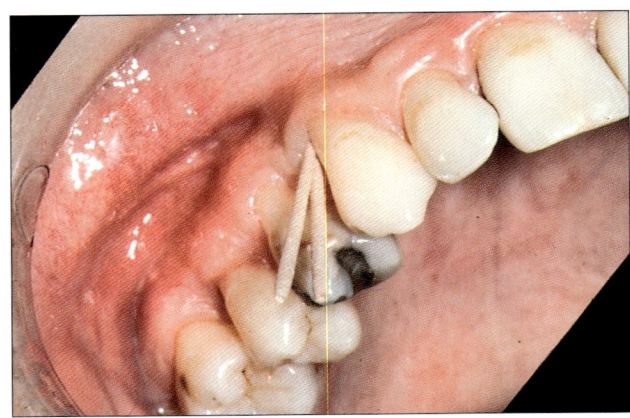

Fig 78 Placement of two sterile paper points to the base of the gingival pocket.

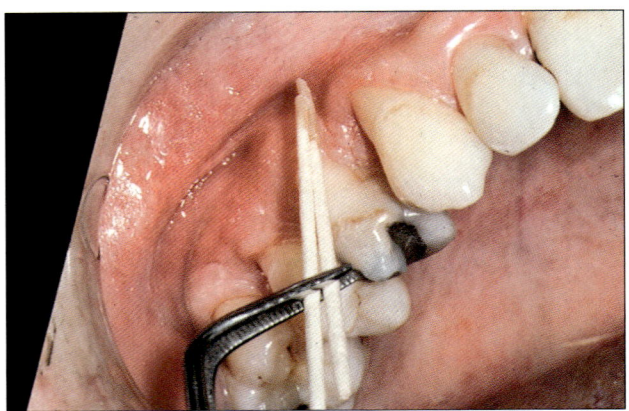

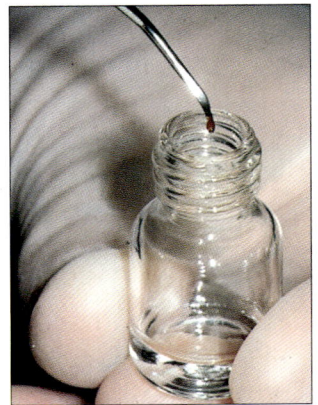

Figs 79 and 80 After they are removed from the gingival pocket, the paper points are placed into a flask containing transport medium.

Although no single microbiologic method can identify all the bacteria in a clinical sample, bacterial culture is capable of detecting the broadest spectrum of periodontal pathogens. However, as mentioned earlier, the range of cultivable microorganisms can be extended through the use of selective media targeted to the specific antibiotic susceptibility and resistance of certain species, as well as through the use of appropriate growth conditions and media nutrients. Culture of subgingival plaque samples on trypticase soy agar containing horse serum, bacitracin, and vancomycin (TSBV) media at 37°C in 5% carbon dioxide, for example, favors the recovery of *A actinomycetemcomitans*. Besides TSBV, a number of selective media have been developed for recovery of periodontal pathogens and oral microorganisms. Overall, when selective media are used, the sensitivity of culture is approximately 10^4 to 10^5 for target species. Although the technique has been refined by the use of the spiral plater (a semiautomated means of distributing dispersed plaque bacteria onto agar media), selective media, improved anaerobic chambers, and better-defined and expedient methods for the identification of cultivable species, such as enzyme

Figs 81 to 85 Periodontal treatment of the patient shown in Figs 77 to 80. (Courtesy of G. Heden.)

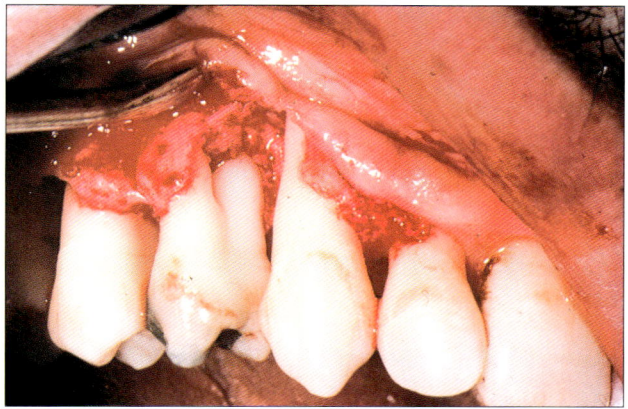 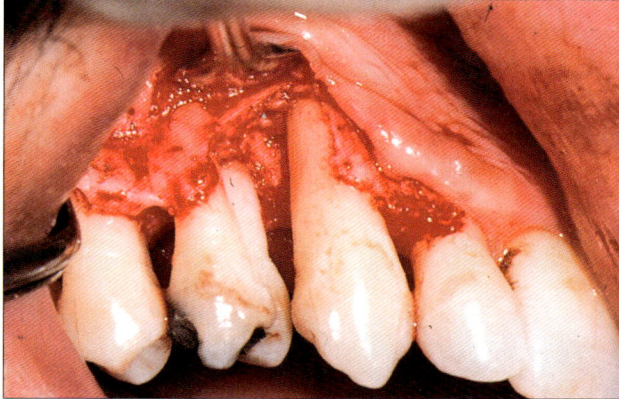

Figs 81 and 82 Periodontal status of the region shown in Figs 77 to 79 during open-flap periodontal surgery, undertaken to gain access for scaling and root planing.

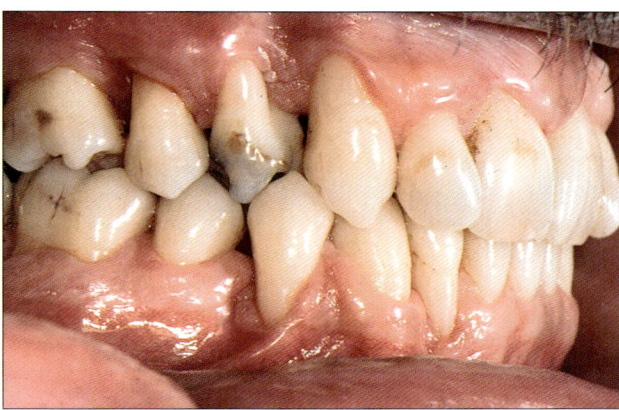

Fig 83 Clinical healing, 2 years after treatment.

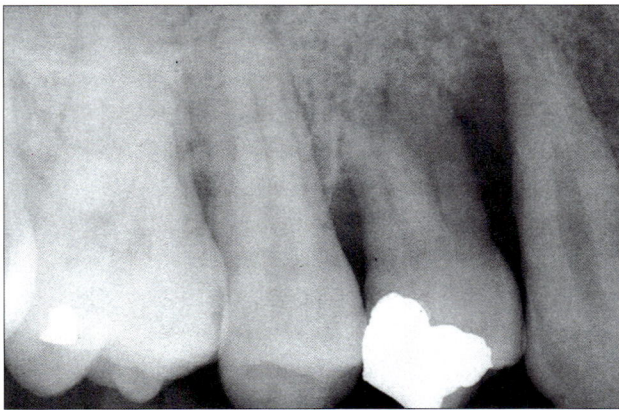 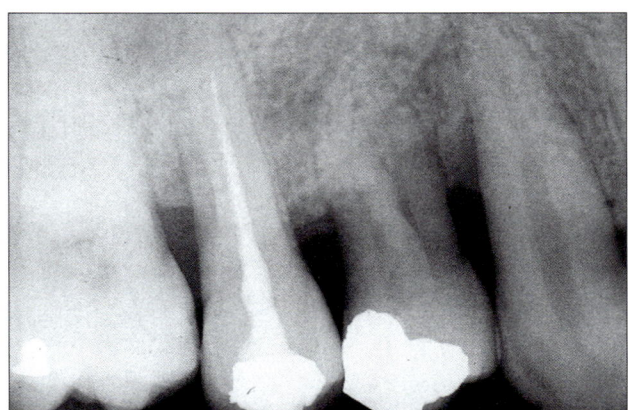

Fig 84 Pretreatment radiograph showing the status of the alveolar bone.

Fig 85 Radiograph taken 2 years postoperatively.

schemes or DNA probes, bacterial culture is still cumbersome, time consuming, and costly.

When used as the gold standard against which other methods are compared and validated, bacterial culture poses several problems. One major problem in comparability is that bacteria in periodontal pockets may be noncultivable: The bacterial cells may already be dead or may be initially viable but unable to survive the accumulated stresses of sampling, sample dispersion, oxygen exposure, and the lack of suitable nutrients in the culture media. Inability to culture bacteria present in the patient's sample can result in a false-negative test.

Nevertheless, not only does bacterial culture permit recovery of the widest range of bacterial species, but it is the method of choice for determining antibiotic susceptibility and resistance—information of great importance in planning treatment of periodontal infections. In the future, techniques in molecular biology, such as the polymerase chain reaction, may facilitate the identification of plasmids and other molecules that serve as the basis for antibiotic resistance, but antimicrobial susceptibility testing by culturing is currently the standard method.

Immunoassays

Immunoassays can exhibit problems with cross-reactivity. In these assays, specificity is usually determined against a large battery of oral and nonoral species, but the reagents may cross-react with a species not included in the battery or with one of the many currently noncultivable bacteria that inhabit periodontal pockets. One advantage of immunofluorescence microscopy in checking for problems of cross-reactivity is the ability to confirm a positive test by a visual examination.

In contrast to bacterial culture, which detects a broad spectrum of bacterial periodontal pathogens, immunoassays are generally targeted toward detecting certain bacterial species or groups of related species. Immunoassays use anti-

bodies—either species-specific polyclonal antisera or a monoclonal antibody—to form antigen-antibody complexes with bacterial antigens and in this way detect the target microorganism.

Immunologic reagents can be used in a variety of test configurations. Immunoassays include immunofluoresence microscopy, membrane immunoassay, and latex agglutination assays. The last two are particularly applicable to clinical practice because they require no instrument and may be completed in the office within 30 minutes. The reagents can also be used to detect pathogenic bacteria in other oral sites, such as in infected root canals, and to spatially localize periodontal pathogens in a bacterial plaque mass to study the distribution of such species in plaque and on root surfaces.

Several other configurations are used for the immunologic detection of periodontal pathogens in clinical samples. One such configuration is the particle concentration fluorescence immunoassay, which uses polystyrene beads as a substrate. The beads are coated with the species-specific antibody and then reacted with a prepared clinical sample. The fluorescent signal and, consequently, the relative number of target bacteria are determined with a fluorimeter. Wolff et al (1991) developed a modification of this method that uses bacterial cells rather than polystrene as the solid phase, together with different monoclonal antibodies, each specific for lipopolysaccharide from different species of periodontal pathogens. The resulting assay exhibits 97% to 100% sensitivity and 57% to 92% specificity, depending on the target species, and has a detection limit of 10^4 target cells in a mixed culture.

Nucleic acid-probe assays

Nucleic acid-probe assays use a piece of DNA or RNA—either a whole genomic probe, a cloned probe, or a synthetic oligonucleotide probe—to hybridize to complementary nucleic acid sequences in the target microorganism. The advantage of these procedures is that the microbial cells in the samples need not be viable. However, the procedures do not allow antibiotic sensitivity testing, and the range of species identified is limited by the number of DNA probes or specific antisera available.

Nucleic acid–based assays include nucleic acid hybridization performed on colony lifts or in dot-blot or slot-blot assays. The probe nucleic acid, usually DNA, is hybridized, under critical temperature and ionic strength conditions, with DNA that has been extracted from plaque bacteria in the patient sample and bound to a suitable substrate, such as a nitrocellulose membrane. Probe DNA, which hybridizes to the bacterial DNA, can be detected by a radiolabel or by a color reaction (Chuba et al, 1988). Paired probe and culture comparisons suggest that DNA probes are often superior to bacterial culture for the detection of periodontal pathogens (Papapanou et al, 1997a; Savitt et al, 1988).

A commercial laboratory in the United States, Omnigene, offers several reference laboratory DNA probe tests for semiquantitative detection of up to six different periodontal pathogens from individual sites or from subgingival plaque samples pooled from several sites (French et al, 1986).

More recently, MicroProbe Corporation has developed an in-office nucleic acid–probe assay for the semiquantitative detection of periodontal pathogens. The bacterial cells in patient plaque samples are lysed by heating in the presence of detergent. The extracted DNA is placed into the first well of a multiwell cassette and then placed into a machine with a programmable robotic arm.

The key to the assay is a small bead on which is bound synthetic oligonucleotides, which are unique in that they hybridize with the species-specific sequences of 16S ribosomal RNA present in multiple copies in the bacterial cell. The presence of multiple copies increases the sensitivity of the assay. A synthetic oligonucleotide probe developed to *B forsythus,* for example, demonstrated 100% sensitivity and 100% specificity compared with bacterial culture for detection of this organism directly from patient subgingival plaque samples (Moncla et al, 1991). In addition,

16S ribosomal RNA contains sequences that are conserved as well as hypervariable regions. Amplification of these hypervariable regions can differentiate individual bacterial strains within the same species.

Synthetic oligonucleotide-coated beads with different specificities, such as for *A actinomycetemcomitans, P gingivalis,* or *P intermedia,* are mounted into a plastic credit card–shaped carrier that, in turn, is attached to the robotic arm. The operator starts the machine and the arm moves the carrier with the beads up and down through a series of solutions in the cassette. This 1-hour process essentially replicates in the office all the steps in nucleic acid hybridization that occur in the laboratory assay. At the completion of the assay, the bead color changes from white to blue if the target sequences are detected, thereby indicating the presence of that bacterium in the patient's sample.

Several DNA probe kits have been developed in recent years. DMD evaluates the quantity of *A actinomycetemcomitans, P gingivalis,* and *P intermedia* separately. Pathotek measures the total combination of these three pathogens in one sample. The test samples have to be sent to a special laboratory (Omni-Gene) for analysis. The results are received after 10 to 12 days.

Recently a rapid, chairside colorimetric DNA probe (Affirm) has been introduced for the analysis of *B forsythus* and *P gingivalis* from plaque samples. Tanner et al (1994) reported that the Affirm DNA probe was comparable to anaerobic culture techniques for identification of *B forsythus* and *P gingivalis.*

"Checkerboard" DNA-DNA hybridization

The "checkerboard" DNA-DNA hybridization technology was developed by Socransky et al (1994) to be used in studies of oral microbiota. The method facilitates rapid processing of large numbers of plaque samples with respect to a multitude of species. Bacterial viability is not essential. It is therefore useful not only in clinical practice but particularly in epidemiologic research. Hence, checkerboard hybridization technology is expected to increasingly replace laborious culture techniques in such studies (Komiya et al, 2000; Papapanou et al, 1997a, 1997b; Ximénez-Fyvie et al, 2000).

In brief, the checkerboard DNA-DNA hybridization technique by Socransky et al (1994), modified by Haffajee et al (1997), is carried out as follows: Baseline subgingival plaque samples are taken using individual sterile Gracey curettes or paper points from the mesiobuccal aspect of each tooth, up to 28 teeth per subject. The samples are placed in separate Eppendorf tubes, the cells are lysed, and denatured DNA is fixed in individual lanes on a nylon membrane using a Minislot (Immunetics, Cambridge, MA). A "Miniblotter 45" apparatus is used to hybridize digoxigenin-labeled whole genomic DNA probes at 90 degrees to the lanes of the plaque sample DNA. Bound probes are detected using phosphatase-conjugated antibody to digoxigenin and chemiluminescence.

Signals are evaluated visually by comparison with the standards at 10^5 and 10^6 for the test species on the same membrane. They are recorded as: 0 = Not detected; 1 = Less than 10^5 cells; 2 = About 10^5 cells; 3 = About 10^5 to 10^6 cells; 4 = About 10^6 cells; 5 = More than 10^6 cells. The sensitivity of this assay was adjusted to permit detection of 10^4 cells of a given species by adjusting the concentration of each DNA probe to provide the same sensitivity of detection for each species. Failure to detect a signal was recorded as 0, although, conceivably, counts in the 1 to 1,000 range could have been present.

Since 1995, the checkerboard technique has been available as a standard oral microbiology test for up to 18 suspected species of periopathogens at the Department of Oral Microbiology, University of Gothenburg. Checkerboard analyses for salivary samples and evaluation of antibiotic sensitivity are also under development.

Case reports

Subgingival microbial sampling is carried out separately from every single site, using sterile paper points. The following three cases illustrate application of such checkerboard techniques in clinical practice before and after treatment of patients who are very susceptible to periodontitis.

Case 1. A 16-year-old girl had aggressive periodontitis localized to two single sites: the mesial aspects of the maxillary and mandibular right first molars. Retrospective bitewing radiographs from the Public Dental Health Service at the age of 14, 15, and 16 years show very rapid, progressive alveolar bone destruction at these sites (Figs 86a to 86c). Probing depth and clinical attachment loss were 9 mm and 6 mm, respectively, at both sites. The patient was otherwise healthy according to her medical history, and no similar pattern of periodontitis was found in her parents or her brother.

According to the initial checkerboard test, these two sites exhibited the highest value for *A actinomycetemcomitans* ever measured in Sweden (Fig 87). After repeated nonaggressive debridement to mechanically remove the subgingival biofilms, tetracycline fibers were applied subgingivally for 10 days. Optimal gingival plaque control was established by self-care, supplemented by PMTC at needs-related intervals and intermittent chlorhexidine mouthrinses.

Five months after the initial examination and treatment, reevaluation showed that the probing depths had decreased from 9 to 5 mm at the maxillary molar and from 9 to 6 mm at the mandibular molar. The examined sites were negative for *A actinomycetemcomitans,* according to both the checkerboard technique (Fig 88) and laboratory culture. The radiographs confirmed new bone formation in the infrabony defects (Fig 89).

Case 2. A 62-year-old female smoker (more than 20 cigarettes per day for more than 40 years, or 40 to 50 pack years) suffered from advanced, untreated periodontitis. Complete-mouth radiographs were taken at the first visit in September

Figs 86a to 86c Sequential bitewing radiographs revealing rapid, progressive destruction of alveolar bone at the mesial surfaces of the maxillary and mandibular right first molars in a teenaged girl. (Courtesy of G. Heden.)

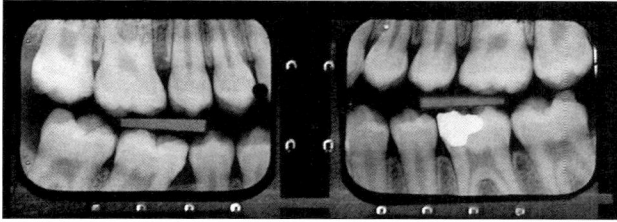

Fig 86a Bone loss at 14 years.

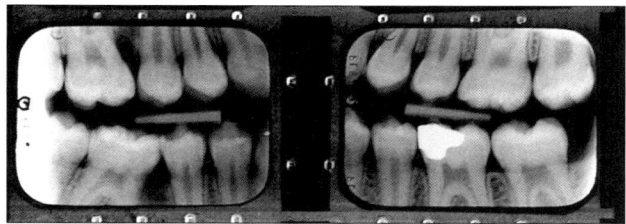

Fig 86b Bone loss at 15 years.

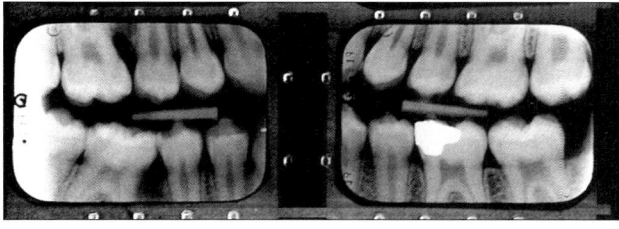

Fig 86c Bone loss at 16 years.

1995 (Fig 90). According to her medical history, she was otherwise healthy.

Anaerobic culture revealed that the 12-mm-deep mesial pocket of the maxillary left canine (tooth 23) contained more than 15 million bacteria (13% *P gingivalis* and 25% *B forsythus*). The 10-mm-deep distolingual pocket of the mandibular right second premolar (tooth 45) contained 3.5 million bacteria (45% *P gingivalis*).

After initial diagnosis, case presentation, education in self-care (including so-called "full-mouth disinfection"), scaling, root planing, debridement, PMTC, extraction of untreatable teeth (both maxillary lateral incisors, both maxillary first premolars, and both mandibular second molars), and hemisection of the maxillary left first molar (furcation involved), regenerative therapy using enamel matrix derivative (Emdogain) was carried out on the mesial surface of tooth 23. During the week before regenerative therapy, a temporary prosthesis was made for the maxilla and the pock-

et on the mesial aspect of tooth 23 was treated twice by debridement and application of metronidazole gel (25%).

Three months later, a permanent maxillary fixed partial denture was constructed, and the patient was enrolled in a needs-related gingival plaque control program. She stopped smoking after treatment. Two and a half years after treatment the probing depth was less than 3 mm, and the site was negative to DNA probe (checkerboard) analyses for *P gingivalis, B forsythus, A actinomycetemcomitans, P intermedia, T denticola*, etc, indicating that the four sites examined were healthy (Fig 91). Figure 92 shows complete-mouth radiographs more than 5 years after the initial therapy. The deep, combined one- and two-wall lesion on the mesial surface of tooth 23 had healed. Figures 93 and 94 show close-ups of tooth 23 before treatment and more than 6 years later, respectively.

PATIENT DATA				DNA SAMPLE -PERIODONTITIS	Lab no
Born, sex	Family name		Given name	Previous lab no in this sampling	
81 12 22 Female				Time for sampling 97 - 08 - 21 kl 11.30	Arr.date 97-08-26
				Reply will be mailed to *(appropriate address)*	

Fill in the formula clearly

Diagnosis - clinical data

Previous treatment		Clinical status	
☐ none	☐ tetracycline	☐ general periodontitis	☐ implants
X depuration	☐ other antibiotics	☐ recurrency	Localized early onset periodontitis (16M and 46M).
☐ surgery	which	☐ treatment control	

	Site 1	Site 2	Site 3	Site 4	Site 5	Site 6
Site	16	46				
Pocket depth	9	9				
P. gingivalis	0	0				
P. intermedia	0	0				
P.nigrescens	0	0				
B. forsythus	0	0				
A.actinomycetemcomitans	5 X	5 X				
F. nucleatum	4	0				
T. denticola	0	0				
P. micros	3	2				
C. rectus	3	2				
E. corrodens	4	4				
S. noxia	0	0				
S. intermedia	3	5				

$5 => 10^6$
$4 = 10^6$
$3 => 10^5$
$2 = 10^5$
$1 = < 10^5$
$0 =$ no reaction

Price: 400 SEK	X The highest value for A.a so far in Sweden.

UNIVERSITY OF GOTHENBURG - DEPT OF ORAL MICROBIOLOGY

Fig 87 Results of the initial checkerboard DNA probe analyses from mesial sites of maxillary (16) and mandibular (46) right first molars.

PATIENT DATA			DNA SAMPLE -PERIODONTITIS		Lab no
Born, sex	Family name	Given name	Previous lab no in this sampling 97 08 21		
81 12 22 Female			Time for sampling 98 - 01 - 27 kl 16.30		Arr.date 98-01-28
			Reply will be mailed to *(appropriate address)*		

Fill in the formula clearly

Diagnosis - clinical data

Previous treatment   **Clinical status**

☐ none   **X** tetracycline   ☐ general periodontitis   ☐ implants

X depuration   ☐ other antibiotics   ☐ recurrency   Localized early onset periodontitis (16M and 46M).

☐ surgery   which ...Acticite-fibre............... **X** treatment control

	Site 1	Site 2	Site 3	Site 4	Site 5	Site 6
Site	16	46				
Pocket depth	5	6				
P. gingivalis	0	2				
P. intermedia	0	4				
P.nigrescens	0	5				
B. forsythus	0	3				
A.actinomycetemcomitans	0	0				
F. nucleatum	0	3				
T. denticola	0	2				
P. micros	0	2				
C. rectus	0	0				
E. corrodens	0	0				
S. noxia	0	0				
S. intermedia	3	4				
$5 => 10^6$ $4 = 10^6$ $3 => 10^5$ $2 = 10^5$ $1 = < 10^5$ $0 = $ no reaction						

Price:

400 SEK

UNIVERSITY OF GOTHENBURG - DEPT OF ORAL MICROBIOLOGY

Fig 88 Results of the 5-month posttreatment checkerboard DNA probe analyses.

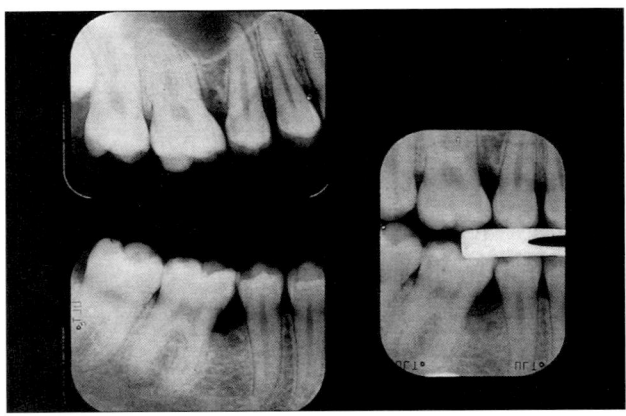

Fig 89 Radiograph taken 5 months after treatment, confirming formation of new bone in the infrabony defects. (Courtesy of G. Heden.)

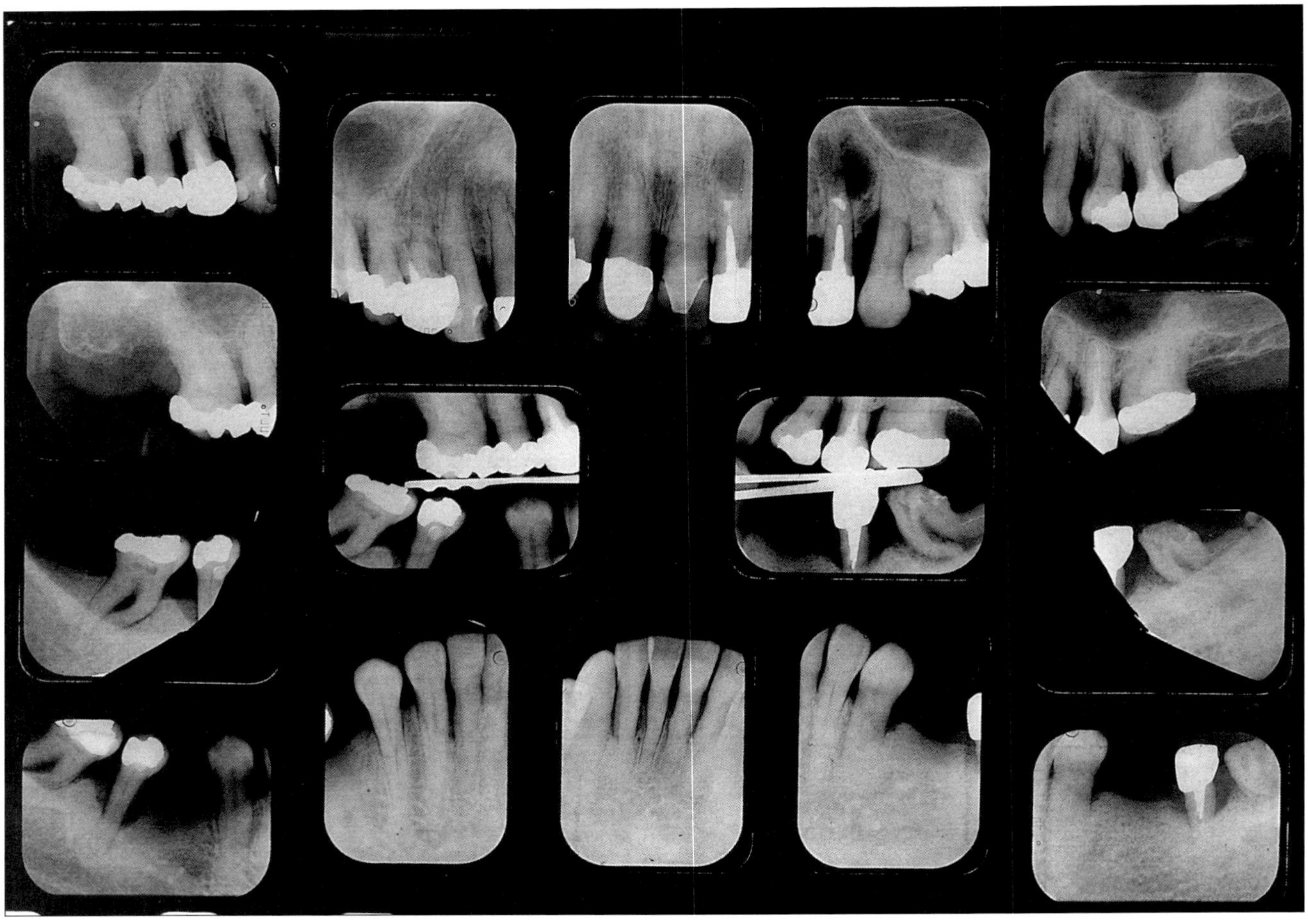

Fig 90 Pretreatment complete-mouth radiographs of a 62-year-old female smoker who suffered from advanced untreated periodontitis. Observe the advanced loss of alveolar bone at the mesial surface of the maxillary left canine (23).

PATIENT DATA

Born, sex	Family name	Given name
33 03 25 Female		

DNA SAMPLE -PERIODONTITIS | Lab no

Previous lab no in this sampling
95 10 31

Time for sampling
98   -   03   -   03   kl 16.30

Arr.date
98-03-04

Reply will be mailed to
(appropriate address)

Fill in the formula clearly

Diagnosis - clinical data

Previous treatment

☐ none

☒ depuration

☒ surgery

☐ tetracycline

☒ other antibiotics

which ..25% Metronidazol-gel
....

Clinical status

☒ general periodontitis

☐ recurrency

☒ treatment control

☐ implants

Localized early onset
periodontitis (16M and 46M).

	Site 1	Site 2	Site 3	Site 4	Site 5	Site 6
Site	23 M	45 M	16 M	13 M		
Pocket depth	3 MM	4 MM	4 MM	3 MM		
P. gingivalis	0	0	0	0		
P. intermedia	0	0	0	0		
P.nigrescens	0	0	0	0		
B. forsythus	0	0	0	0		
A.actinomycetemcomitans	0	0	0	0		
F. nucleatum	0	0	0	0		
T. denticola	0	0	0	0		
P. micros	0	0	0	0		
C. rectus	0	0	0	0		
E. corrodens	0	0	0	0		
S. noxia	0	0	0	0		
S. intermedia	0	1	1	1		
$5 => 10^6$ $4 = 10^6$ $3 => 10^5$ $2 = 10^5$ $1 = < 10^5$ $0 =$ no reaction						

Price:
400 SEK

UNIVERSITY OF GOTHENBURG - DEPT OF ORAL MICROBIOLOGY

Fig 91 Checkerboard DNA probe analyses performed 2.5 years after treatment, revealing that the examined sites are healthy.

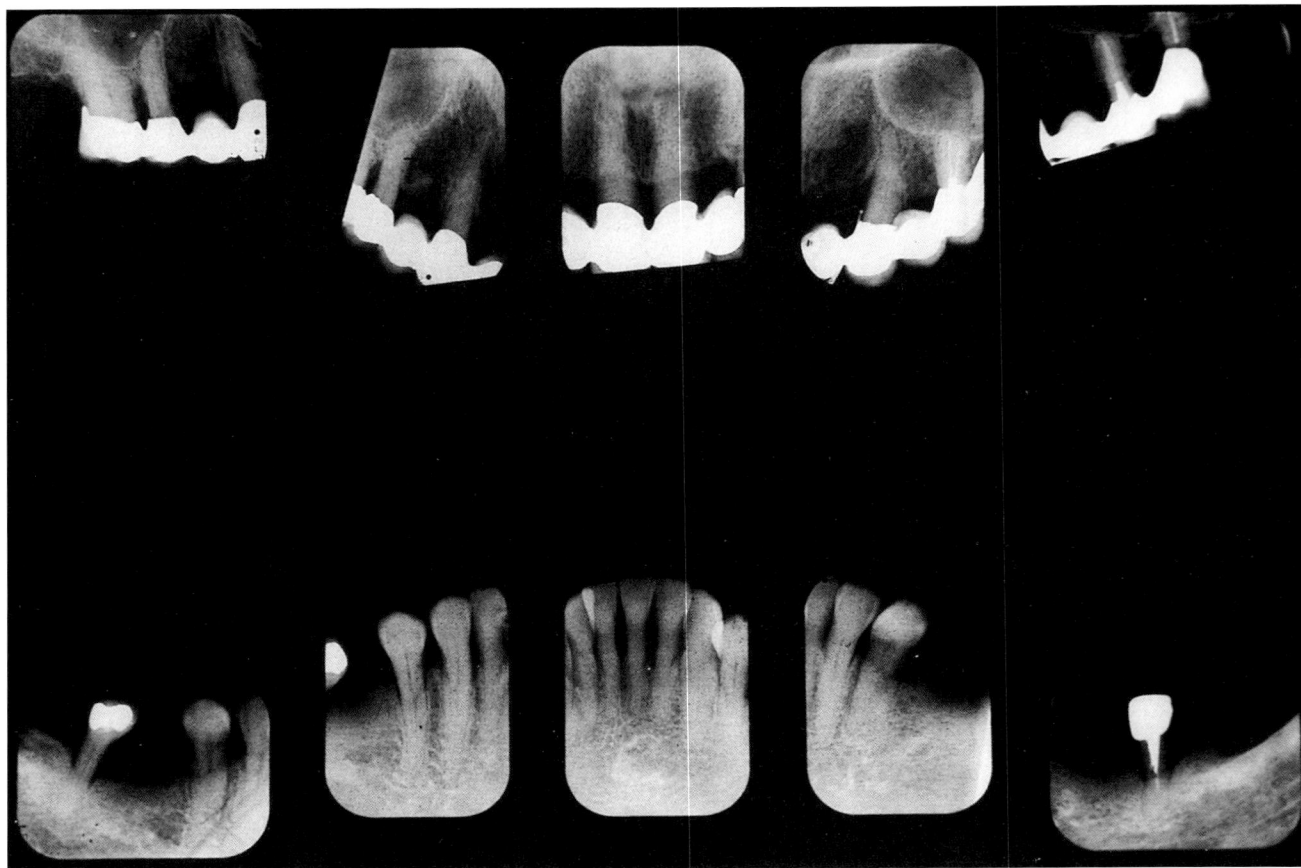

Fig 92 Complete-mouth radiographs 5 years after initial therapy. The patient had stopped smoking after treatment. Notice the succesful arrest of alveolar bone loss.

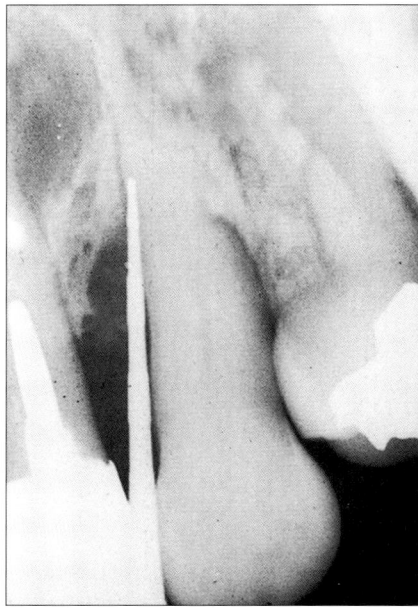

Fig 93 Close-up of tooth 23 with a periodontal probe inserted in the one- and two-wall bone destruction before regenerative therapy.

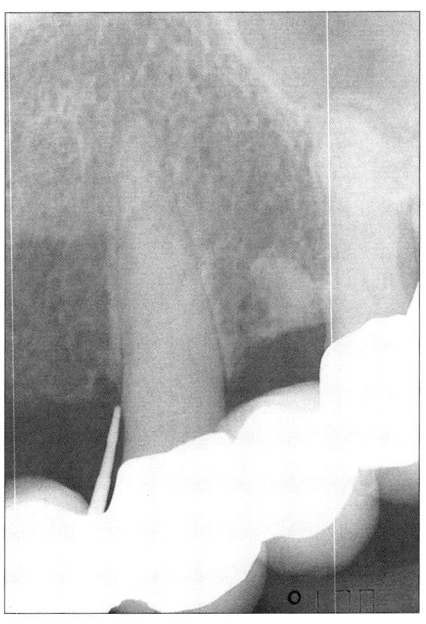

Fig 94 The long-term outcome of regenerative therapy verified with a periodontal probe to the bottom of the shallow pocket (< 3 mm) more than 6 years after treatment.

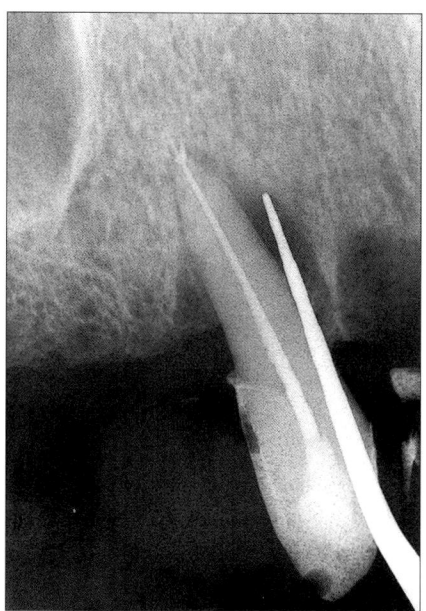

Fig 95 Pretreatment radiograph of the maxillary right canine (September 1997). The inserted periodontal probe illustrates the advanced alveolar bone loss that extends almost to the apex at the mesial and palatal surfaces.

Case 3. A 58-year-old male smoker (more than 20 cigarettes per day, or more than 40 pack years, ie, one pack per day for more than 40 years) had very advanced, untreated periodontitis for his age but was otherwise healthy according to his medical history. Only 20 teeth remained, of which 11 were untreatable and had to be extracted. In the maxilla, only the canines, central incisors, and the left second premolar could be retained; in the mandible, only the two canines and the second premolars could be saved.

After initial diagnosis, history taking, case presentation, education in self-care, scaling, root planing, debridement, and extraction of untreatable teeth, temporary prostheses were constructed. The prognosis for the maxillary right canine was highly questionable, as disclosed on the radiograph, which was taken with a periodontal probe inserted mesiolingually, almost to the apex (Fig 95). The probing depths were 14 mm mesially, 8 mm lingually, 8 mm distally, and 4 mm buccally. Checkerboard DNA probe analyses from the examined sites are shown in Fig 96. Because the canine was the most posterior tooth on the maxillary right side, it was a key tooth for construction

of a fixed prosthesis, and it was therefore decided to make every effort to save this tooth.

After optimal plaque control, including so-called "full-mouth disinfection," and repeated debridement to eliminate all subgingival biofilms, regenerative therapy was carried out. The technique involved flap surgery, debridement, chemical conditioning of the root surface with ethylenediaminetetraacetic acid gel, and the use of an enamel matrix derivative (Emdogain gel). To optimize the healing potential, the patient stopped smoking, and systemic metronidazole plus amoxicillin were administered starting 2 days before therapy (400 mg metronidazole and 375 mg amoxicillin, 3 times per day for 10 days) on the basis of the checkerboard DNA probe analyses (see Fig 96).

Because dramatic healing was achieved after only 5 months, a fixed prosthesis was constructed. Figure 97 shows the checkerboard DNA probe analyses, repeated 6 months after treatment. Figure 98 shows a control radiograph, taken after placement of the prosthesis, in which the periodontal probe indicates the mesial level of attachment 6 months after periodontal treatment, including regenerative therapy. Probing depth

		Site 1	Site 2	Site 3	Site 4	Site 5	Site 6

PATIENT DATA
Born, sex   Family name   Given name

40 11 08 Male

DNA SAMPLE -PERIODONTITIS   Lab no

Previous lab no in this sampling

Time for sampling
97 - 08 - 07 kl 16.30   Arr.date
97-08-08

Reply will be mailed to
(appropriate address)

Fill in the formula clearly

Diagnosis - clinical data

Previous treatment

☐ none   ☐ tetracycline   **Clinical status** ☒ general periodontitis   ☐ implants

☒ depuration   ☐ other antibiotics   ☐ recurrency

                                  Heavy smoker.

☐ surgery   which ....   ☐ treatment control
               ....

	Site 1	Site 2	Site 3	Site 4	Site 5	Site 6
Site	13 M	25 M	43 M	11 M		
Pocket depth	14 MM	6 MM	7 MM	6 MM		
P. gingivalis	5	5	5	5		
P. intermedia	2	2	2	2		
P.nigrescens	2	0	3	3		
B. forsythus	5	5	5	5		
A.actinomycetemcomitans	1	1	1	1		
F. nucleatum	4	0	0	4		
T. denticola	5	5	5	5		
P. micros	3	3	3	3		
C. rectus	1	1	2	1		
E. corrodens	0	0	0	0		
S. noxia	0	0	0	0		
S. intermedia	3	4	4	4		
$5 => 10^6$ $4 = 10^6$ $3 => 10^5$ $2 = 10^5$ $1 = < 10^5$ $0 = $ no reaction						

Price:
400 SEK

UNIVERSITY OF GOTHENBURG - DEPT OF ORAL MICROBIOLOGY

Fig 96 Results of pretreatment checkerboard DNA probe analyses showing the highest scores ($5 = 10^6$) for *P gingivalis* as well as *B forsythus* and *T denticola* in all four examined sites. Lower counts of *A actinomycetemcomitans* also were found in all sites. In particular, *B forsythus* is more frequently found in smokers than nonsmokers.

PATIENT DATA			DNA SAMPLE -PERIODONTITIS	Lab no

PATIENT DATA
Born, sex   Family name   Given name

40 11 08 Male

DNA SAMPLE -PERIODONTITIS   Lab no
Previous lab no in this sampling
97-12-?
Time for sampling
98   -   03   -   12   kl 15.00   Arr.date
98-03-13

Reply will be mailed to
(appropriate address)

Fill in the formula clearly

Diagnosis - clinical data

Previous treatment   **Clinical status**

☐ none   ☐ tetracycline   ☒ general periodontitis   ☐ implants

☒ depuration   ☒ other antibiotics   ☐ recurrency

☒ surgery   which *systemic Metronidazol +*   ☒ treatment control
                       amoxycillin

	Site 1	Site 2	Site 3	Site 4	Site 5	Site 6
Site	13 M	25 M	43 D	11 M		
Pocket depth	2 MM	1 MM	2 MM	2 MM		
P. gingivalis	1	0	1	0		
P. intermedia	2	0	3	0		
P.nigrescens	2	0	3	0		
B. forsythus	1	0	2	1		
A.actinomycetemcomitans	1	0	0	0		
F. nucleatum	2	0	3	0		
T. denticola	0	0	1	0		
P. micros	1	0	2	2		
C. rectus	0	0	1	0		
E. corrodens	1	0	1	0		
S. noxia	0	0	2	0		
S. intermedia	2	1	2	1		

$5 => 10^6$
$4 = 10^6$
$3 => 10^5$
$2 = 10^5$
$1 = < 10^5$
$0 =$ no reaction

Price:
400 SEK

UNIVERSITY OF GOTHENBURG - DEPT OF ORAL MICROBIOLOGY

Fig 97 Results of checkerboard DNA probe analyses 6 months after periodontal therapy, showing very significant reduction of the most important periopathogens, but not complete elimination.

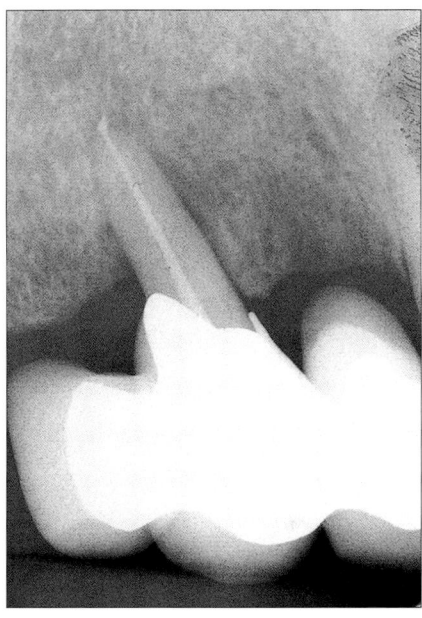

Fig 98 Radiograph taken after placement of a fixed partial denture and 6 months of regenerative therapy. The periodontal probe reveals that almost 100% of the alveolar bone loss at the mesial surface was arrested.

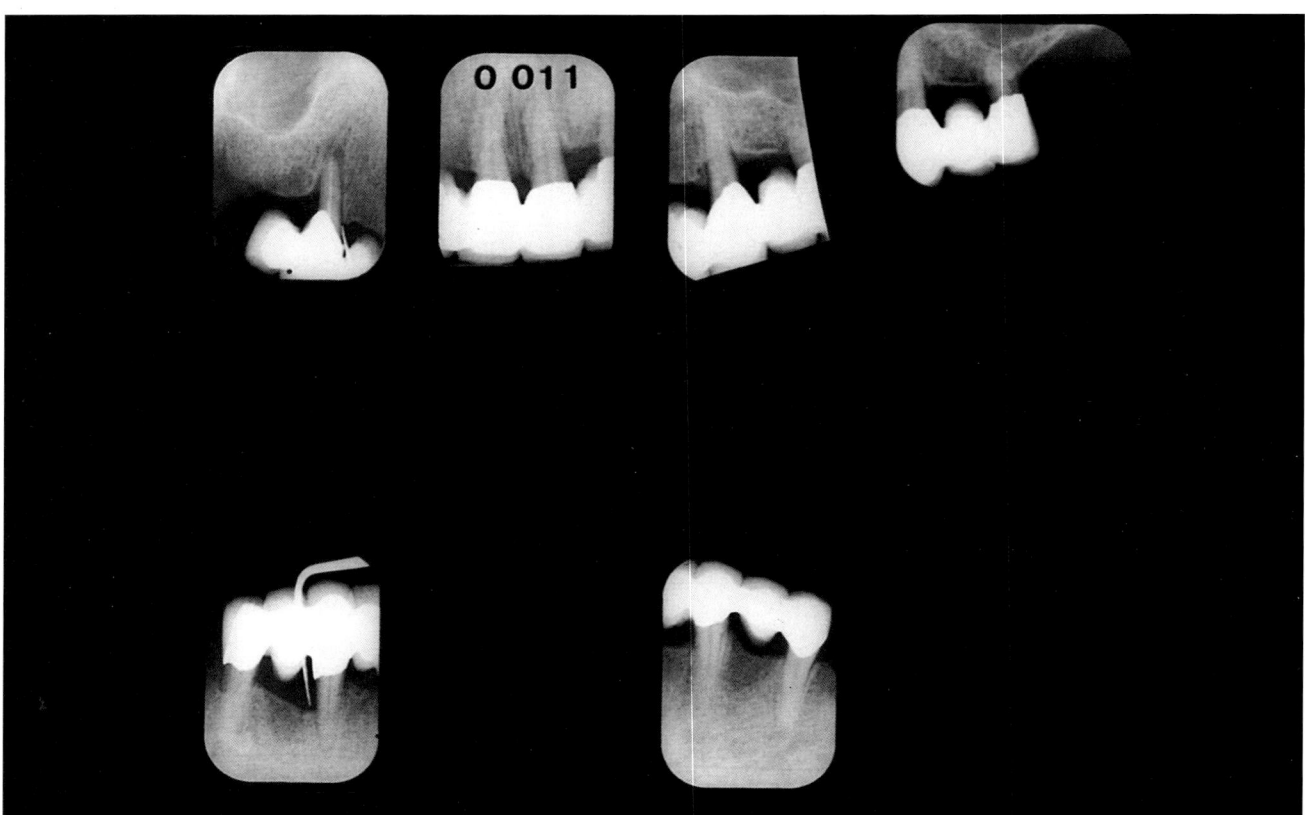

Fig 99 Complete-mouth radiograph more than 3 years after therapy.

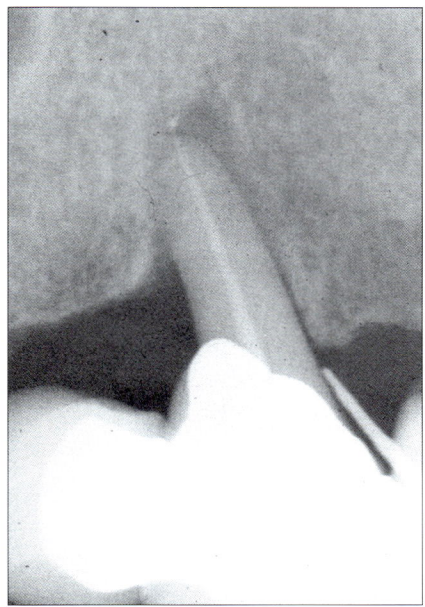

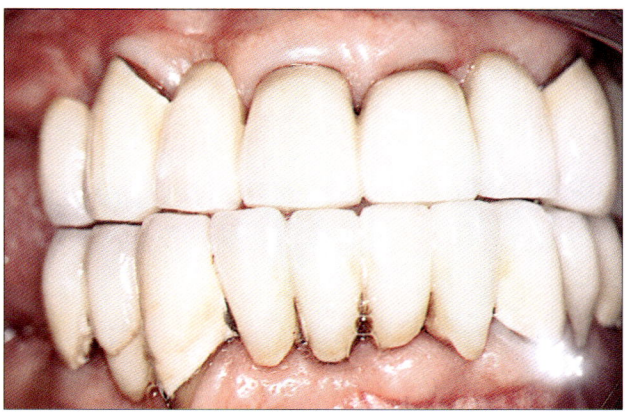

Fig 101 Excellent gingival conditions are still maintained more than 3 years after periodontal therapy, in spite of the initially high counts of periopathogens shown in Fig 96. The maintenance program was based on established excellent self-care habits and need-related intervals of PMTC.

Fig 100 Radiograph with inserted periodontal probe showing that the arrested alveolar bone loss was maintained 4 years after regenerative therapy.

had decreased from 14 to 2 mm. This result was maintained 3 to 4 years later, as shown in the full-mouth radiographs in Fig 99 and close-up in Fig 100. Figure 101 shows the excellent gingival conditions that exist more than 3 years after treatment.

Enzymatic microbial tests

In addition to immunologic and nucleic acid–probe methods for the rapid detection of periodontal pathogens, several enzyme assays are available. In general, these tests do not detect specific bacterial species but indicate the presence of enzymes destructive to periodontal tissue; there enzymes are produced by a group comprising mainly, but not exclusively, periodontal pathogens.

The enzymes used for assay include collagenase, peptidases, trypsinlike enzymes, neutral proteases, and elastase. Collagenase, for example,

is produced by a variety of bacteria as well as host cells. In periodontal applications, bacterial collagenase can be differentiated from host collagenase by gel electrophoresis, but this has limited applicability as a clinical assay. A clinical collagenase assay has been developed in which a patient's sample is incubated with a suitable substrate and the presence of collagen is indicated by a color reaction.

A group of periodontal pathogens, including *B forsythus, P gingivalis,* and *T denticola,* produce this enzyme, as do certain *Capnocytophaga* species that are not usually found to be periodontopathic. The enzyme is detected by degradation of a synthetic substrate, benzoly-DL-arginine-2-naphthylamide (BANA), in a colorimetric assay; a blue-black color on the reagent card indicates a positive test. This assay shows 55% to 73% agreement with paired enzyme-linked immunosorbent assay for *P gingivalis* and *T denticola,* and 51% to 70% agreement with clinical parameters: bleeding on probing, probing depth, and clinical assessment.

Advantages and limitations of current methods for detection of periodontal pathogens

Comparing cultures and other types of microbiologic assays is like comparing apples and oranges. Culture assays measure bacterial cells, or colony-forming units, whereas immunoassays and nucleic acid probes measure antigens and nucleic acid sequences, respectively. Loesche et al (1992) examined the issue of comparability of different microbiologic assays by testing 204 plaque samples for four species of periodontal pathogens by culture, immunoassay, DNA probe assay, and the BANA test. Least accurate was bacterial culture, which had accuracy values of 61% to 79%. The DNA probes were the most accurate assay, exhibiting accuracy values of 88% to 96%.

In a recent study, Papapanou et al (1997b) reported reasonable agreement between checkerboard DNA-DNA hybridization and culture techniques for analysis of the composition of the subgingival microflora in 70 subjects. Although the checkerboard method revealed significantly higher bacterial counts for the majority of species, the culture technique offered the advantage of detecting unexpected species.

The benefits and limitations of different oral microbiology methods are summarized in Table 6. Zambon and Haraszthy (1995) also compared current methods for detection of periodontal pathogens (Tables 7 and 8).

Although assays for bacteria in dental plaque samples measure the presence and number of target organisms directly, there is a major shortcoming: These methods can detect target species only when present in the patient sample. Because there may be more than 100 different subgingival sample sites in the fully dentate mouth, it is difficult to obtain a representative sample. The absence of a target pathogen from the mesiobuccal surface of one particular tooth does not mean that the pathogen is not present at the distobuccal surface of the same tooth or at other surfaces of other teeth in the same mouth.

To overcome the problem of obtaining representative samples, several studies have examined methods that will determine with reasonable confidence that a patient is not infected with a cer-

Table 6 Advantages and limitations of different oral microbiology methods*

Method	Specificity[†]	Sensitivity[†]	Cost	Time
Selective culture	++	+++	US $20–$30	10–12 d
Nonselective culture	+++	++	US $20–$30	10–12 d
Microscopy	+	++	?	Immediate
Immunofluorescence	++	++	?	Immediate
DNA probe	++	+++	US $30–$50	
DMD				10–12 d
Pathotek				10–12 d
Affirm				Immediate
Immunoenzymatic assay (ELISA)				
Evalusite	++	++	US $25–$35	Immediate
Enzymatic (Perioscan)	++	++	?	Immediate

*Modified from Dahlén (1994).
[†]Scale, + to +++, with + = lowest specificity/sensitivity and +++ = highest specificity/sensitivity.

Table 7 Comparison of current methods for the detection of periodontal pathogens*

Test	Advantages	Disadvantages
Phase-contrast and darkfield microscopy	Detects bacterial shape, size, and motility Detects bacteria associated with health and disease Detects microbial shifts	Cannot distinguish individual bacterial species
Bacterial culture	Gold standard Detects broadest spectrum of bacteria in a sample Determines antibiotic sensitivity and resistance	Expensive Time-consuming Reference laboratory test Cannot detect noncultivable bacteria
Immunoassays and nucleic acid probe assays	Targeted to specific microorganisms Rapid Relatively inexpensive Office or reference laboratory test	Possible cross-reactivity Cannot determine antibiotic resistance or sensitivity May require expensive instrumentation
Polymerase chain reaction	Targeted to specific microorganisms Rapid The most sensitive assay	Requires expensive instrumentation Reference laboratory test
Enzyme assays	Targeted Rapid Inexpensive	Detect bacterial groups rather than individual species

*From Zambon and Harazthy (1995). Reprinted with permission.

Table 8 Methods for the identification of bacterial pathogens in periodontal infections*

Method	Limit of detection	Detection of nonviable species	Time
Bacterial culture		No	1–3 wk
Nonselective	10^4–10^5		
Selective	10^3		
Immunologic methods	10^4	Yes	Minutes to hours
Particle concentration fluorescence immunoassay	10^3		
DNA probe	10^2	Yes	1–48 h
Enzyme assay			
BANA	10^4	No	15 min
Polymerase chain reaction	10	Yes	2–4 h

*From Zambon and Harazthy (1995). Reprinted with permission.

tain periodontal pathogen. The findings suggest that different species of periodontal pathogens necessitate different sampling schemes. To determine at 95% confidence that a subject is not infected with *A actinomycetemcomitans*, 25 or more subgingival samples must be negative. For *P gingivalis* and *B forsythus* six or more random sites or three or more sites with clinical probing depths greater than 5 mm must be negative. For *P intermedia* four or more sites with clinical probing depths greater than 5 mm must be negative. These values are based on prevalence rates of 11% for *A actinomycetemcomitans*, 44% for *P gingivalis*, 48% for *B forsythus*, and 54% for *P intermedia* in adult populations. The prevalence of these pathogens and the number of necessary samples in other patient populations, such as those with refractory periodontitis or adults with aggressive periodontitis, have not been determined.

Indications for testing for periodontal pathogens

There is general agreement that microbiologic tests for periodontal pathogens are not indicated in all patients, but certain indications have been proposed: patients with aggressive periodontitis; patients with refractory disease; patients about to undergo extensive prosthetic, implant or regenerative therapy; and patients with cardiovascular disease.

Aggressive periodontitis

Patients with aggressive periodontitis should always be regarded as high-risk patients. Microbial analyses of the subgingival microflora both before treatment and for evaluation of the effect of treatment are therefore indicated.

Refractory periodontitis

As defined by the American Academy of Periodontology, patients with refractory periodontitis are those who, despite appropriate therapy, continue to experience loss of connective tissue attachment and alveolar bone. Determining the composition of the subgingival biofilm and, more importantly, the antibiotics that would be useful in treating the periodontal infection is crucial to the successful management of these patients. Because these patients may have had previous empirical antibiotic therapy, resulting in antimicrobial resistance and the emergence of novel periodontal pathogens such as enteric species or yeasts, bacterial culture and antibiotic sensitivity tests are the assays of choice.

Screening prior to extensive prosthetic or implant therapy

The cost involved in microbiologic tests for periodontal pathogens probably limits their application to conditions for which the test results are particularly useful. Microbiologic tests have been proposed for treatment planning of new patients, selecting an appropriate recall interval, and monitoring periodontal therapy, but such routine use for those with chronic periodontitis, although valuable, may have less economic impact than would limiting these assays to patients who are about to undergo complex rehabilitation: extensive restorative dentistry or implant dentistry.

By including examination of the subgingival microflora in treatment planning, it is possible to limit the risk of adverse sequelae of infection by periodontal pathogens and to enhance a favorable clinical outcome (Dahlén et al, 1996; Mombelli et al, 2000; Nieminen et al, 1996). This increased risk has been demonstrated in several studies. In a prospective study by Machtei et al (1997), it was shown that the odds ratio for further attachment loss in sites infected by *B forsythus* and *P gingivalis* were 7.5 and 6.0, respectively. These species are also important in failing dental implants

(Leonhardt et al, 1992, 1999; Rosenberg et al, 1991). Microbiologic testing should therefore be used in patients prior to extensive restorative and implant therapy and during supportive periodontal therapy.

Regenerative therapy

It is important for the outcome of regenerative therapy that the site be as free of infection as possible. Analysis of the subgingival microflora may be indicated. In particular, microbiologic monitoring may enhance the success of so-called guided tissue regeneration. These procedures result in the adherence of numerous, predominantly gram-negative bacteria to the expanded polytetrafluoroethylene membranes, including many species of periodontal pathogens. The presence in the healing site of at least two of these species, *A actinomycetemcomitans* and *P gingivalis*, seems to inhibit successful repair or regeneration (Demolon et al, 1993; Nowzari and Slots, 1994; Ricci et al, 1996; Wang et al, 1994). Therefore, microbiologic testing prior to and during healing of guided tissue regeneration, combined with appropriate antimicrobial treatment, should enhance clinical success.

Cardiovascular diseases, diabetes mellitus, and other risk factors

Recent longitudinal studies have shown the odds ratio for onset of heart infarct and stroke to be 2.5 to 3.0 times higher for patients with several deep, infected pockets than for patients with good periodontal health. The odds ratio associated with periodontal disease was a little higher than that associated with smoking (Beck et al, 1996).

In addition, it was shown that the need for insulin in diabetic patients can be reduced significantly by successful treatment of infected periodontal pockets (Grossi et al, 1997). Microbial evaluation of treatment outcome may therefore be indicated in patients with diabetes, cardiovascular diseases, and other risks.

CONCLUSIONS

Both gingivitis and periodontitis are caused by microorganisms; ie, both are infectious diseases. The microorganisms colonize the gingival region of the tooth surfaces, supragingivally as well as subgingivally, forming dentogingival plaque, a so-called biofilm. In diseased pockets the microorganisms also extend subgingivally, without attaching to the tooth surfaces, and may invade the periodontal tissues.

Role of the oral environment

The oral cavity has more than 400 species of resident bacteria, but only a few have the ability to colonize a newly cleaned tooth surface. The density of bacteria is about 1,000 times higher in plaque than it is in saliva. About 1 mm³ of plaque may contain more than 200 million bacteria. The oral cavity offers several specific environments (habitats) with different ecosystems, and each habitat has a microflora of specific composition; ie, there is considerable variation in the composition of the microflora, not only between supragingival and subgingival sites but also among different tooth surfaces.

Formation of plaque biofilms

Supragingivally, the tooth surfaces are covered by the so-called pellicle (2 to 10 μm thick), comprised mainly of glucoproteins from the saliva. During the first few hours after mechanical cleaning, bacteria that resist (physiologic) detachment from the pellicle-covered tooth surfaces start to proliferate and form small colonies of morphologically identical organisms. These pioneer colonizers are mainly streptococci (*S sanguis*) and *Actinomyces* species. After 24 to 48 hours, continuous plaque has formed along the gingival margin. The thickness increases dramatically from day 2 to days 3 and 4.

Undisturbed plaque accumulation reaches its maximum after 1 week, at so-called stagnant areas of the tooth crown (gingivally and interdentally).

Meanwhile, the assortment of bacteria in the plaque biofilm increases: There is gradual transition from the "harmless normal microflora," dominated by gram-positive, facultatively anaerobic streptococci and some rods (*Actinomyces*), to gram-negative anaerobic rods. Nonattaching spirochetes may be present in the gingival sulcus.

Experimentally, it has been shown that within 2 to 3 weeks this mixed, nonspecific plaque biofilm will result in clinically visible gingivitis. Because of the swollen gingival margin, the gingival sulcus will deepen, creating an environment that favors the growth of anaerobic, gram-negative rods. If, however, the plaque is removed at least every second day, no gingivitis will develop. Similarly, established gingivitis will heal within 7 to 10 days, if the gingival plaque is removed regularly at least every second day.

Undisturbed gram-negative anaerobic microflora in the gingival crevice will eventually result in loss of periodontal support, directly or indirectly, in individuals susceptible to periodontitis, exposing the root surfaces to the growth of a subgingival biofilm. In addition, nonattaching motile bacteria such as spirochetes will grow in the most apical portion of the periodontal pocket. Some of the subgingival microflora may also invade the periodontal soft tissues.

Amount of plaque

At clinical examination, measurement of the volume and location of plaque discloses only where the patient has cleaned inadequately, despite extra effort on the day of the dental appointment. It does not reveal the age of the plaque, the rate of accumulation, or the patient's habitual standard of oral hygiene. It is therefore important to understand the difference between plaque indices, which are static, and the plaque reaccumulation rate, which is dynamic.

Rate of plaque formation

The plaque formation rate varies considerably among individuals as well as among individual tooth surfaces. An understanding of plaque formation rates and patterns is therefore an essential foundation for successful strategies for both primary and secondary prevention of periodontal diseases. These facts were the rationale underlying the development of the Plaque Formation Rate Index (PFRI), which is based on 24 hours of free (de novo) plaque reaccumulation after PMTC. The PFRI should be used as a guideline for establishment of needs-related plaque control habits. Very rapid plaque formers should clean more frequently than slow plaque formers, and cleaning procedures should start with and concentrate on the tooth surfaces where plaque reaccumulates most rapidly (the linguoproximal surfaces of the mandibular posterior teeth and the buccoproximal surfaces of the maxillary posterior teeth).

The plaque formation rate can be reduced by eliminating or reducing gingivitis and gingival exudate; the roughness, wettability, and surface energy of tooth surfaces and restorative materials; the total number of oral microflora; and the intake of sugar, and by increasing salivary flow by chewing (for example, with fluoridated chewing gum).

Nonspecific plaque hypothesis

Three different theories on the etiology of periodontal diseases have been proposed: the nonspecific plaque hypothesis, the ecological plaque hypothesis and the specific plaque hypothesis. The nonspecific plaque hypothesis contends that many of the microorganisms from the heterogenous mixture in plaque biofilms could play a role in the development of gingivitis as well as periodontitis and that these diseases are the result of the overall interaction of the microflora of the plaque biofilms and the host. This hypothesis explains why, in longitudinal human studies, frequent removal and disruption of plaque by self-care, supplemented with needs-related PMTC and subgingival debridement, has been so successful for prevention and control of both gingivitis and periodontitis.

Ecological plaque hypothesis

The ecological plaque hypothesis proposes that a change in a key environmental factor (or factors) will trigger a shift in the balance of the resident microflora and this might predispose a site to disease. The occurrence of potentially pathogenic species as minor members of the resident plaque microflora would be consistent with this proposal. In health, these organisms would be only weakly competitive and might also be suppressed by intermicrobial antagonism, so that they would constitute only a small, clinically unimportant percentage of the plaque microflora. Microbial specificity in disease would be attributed to the fact that only certain species are competitive under the new (changed) environmental conditions.

It is a basic tenet of microbial ecology that a major change to an ecosystem produces a corresponding disturbance in the stability of the resident microbial community. With respect to the etiology of periodontal diseases, this may be exemplified by the following sequences: Undisturbed gingival plaque gradually results in gingivitis, ie, increased edema of the gingival margin (pseudopocket formation) and gingival crevicular fluid secretion. The improved nutritional conditions and lowered redox potential in the gingival sulcus favor subgingival growth of the gram-negative anaerobic microorganisms, among them the most important periopathogens. The ecological plaque hypothesis would therefore explain why surgical elimination of pockets is a successful method for treatment of periodontal diseases, provided that excellent gingival plaque control is established in the postoperative maintenance program.

Specific plaque hypothesis

The specific plaque hypothesis proposes that, of the diverse collection of microorganisms that constitute the resident plaque microflora, only a very limited number are actively involved in disease. This hypothesis, however, fails to explain satisfactorily those occasions when disease is diagnosed in the apparent absence of putative pathogens or when pathogens are present at sites with no evidence of disease. At the 1996 American Academy of Periodontology Workshop, there was consensus that particularly *P gingivalis, A actinomycetemcomitans,* and *B forsythus,* as well as *P intermedia* and *T denticola,* should be considered as true periopathogens, strongly correlated to the etiology of periodontal diseases (American Academy of Periodontology, 1996c). Both *P gingivalis* and *A actinomycetemcomitans* are regarded as exogenic, transmissible periopathogens, and *B forsythus, P intermedia,* and *T denticola* are considered to be opportunistic bacteria.

Several studies have shown a relationship between *A actinomycetemcomitans* and aggressive periodontitis. A recent prospective study (Machtei et al, 1997) showed that periodontal pockets containing *B forsythus* exhibited seven times higher risk for further loss of periodontal attachment than did *B forsythus*–negative sites. It has also been shown that *A actinomycetemcomitans* and *P gingivalis* in particular may invade the periodontal soft tissues, which may partly explain why diseased periodontal pockets sometimes fail to heal when treated by nonsurgical subgingival debridement alone but may respond to mechanical removal of the subgingival biofilm in combination with administration of antibiotics.

Analysis of clinical and laboratory data indicates that the etiology of periodontal diseases is not satisfactorily explained by any of these hypotheses alone but rather by a combination of all three.

Microbial tests

Several methods and techniques are available for detection of subgingival microflora associated with the etiology of the periodontal diseases. For several decades, direct microscopy, particularly darkfield and phase-contrast microscopy, has been used for morphologic studies of the composition of the subgingival microflora, and the motility of the bacteria. High proportions of long rods and motile bacteria, particularly spirochetes, are associated with diseased pockets. The microflora of healthy sites tend to be dominated by cocci and short rods.

For the past few decades, anaerobic culture has been regarded as the gold standard for evaluation of the subgingival periopathogenic microflora. The advantages are that unexpected species may be detected and antibiotic sensitivity or resistance can be evaluated. The main disadvantages are that not all the subgingival microflora are cultivable, and, in order to be cultured, the sampled bacterial species must be viable.

Immunoassay techniques use antibodies—either species-specific polyclonal antisera or monoclonal antibodies—to form antigen-antibody complexes with bacterial antigens and thus detect the target microorganism. Immunoassays include immunofluorescent microscopy, membrane immunoassay, and latex agglutination assays. The last two are particularly applicable to clinical practice, because no instrumentation is required and they may be completed in the office within 30 minutes. However, compared to anaerobic culture, the number of detectable species is very limited.

The most recent and promising techniques for detection of periopathogens are the nucleic acid–probe assays, which use a piece of DNA or RNA—either a whole genomic probe, a cloned probe, or synthetic oligonucleotide probe—to hybridize to complementary nucleic acid sequences in the target microorganisms.

The advantage of these techniques is that the microbial cells in the samples need not be viable. However, to date, the techniques do not allow antibiotic sensitivity testing and the range of species identified is limited by the number of DNA probes currently available. With the new so-called checkerboard DNA-DNA hybridization technology, up to 40 different species in up to 28 teeth per subject have been evaluated. Chairside DNA probe tests are now available.

In addition to immunologic and nucleic acid probe methods for the rapid detection of periodontal pathogens, several enzyme assays are available. In general, they do not detect specific bacterial species but instead indicate the presence of enzymes that destroy periodontal tissue. These enzymes are produced by a group of mainly, but not exclusively, periodontal pathogens.

From a cost-effectiveness aspect, there is general agreement that microbiologic tests for periodontal pathogens are not indicated for all patients but only for those in certain categories: patients exhibiting aggressive or refractory periodontitis, patients about to undergo extensive prosthetic, implant, or regenerative therapy, and patients susceptible to cardiovascular diseases. (For reviews on plaque formation and microflora related to the etiology of periodontal diseases see Axelsson, 1994; Darveau et al, 1997; Haffajee and Socransky, 1994; Lang et al, 1997; Listgarten, 1994; Mombelli, 1996, 1998; Moore and Moore, 1994; Slots, 1999; Socransky and Haffajee, 1997; Tonetti, 1994; Wolff et al, 1994; Zambon and Haraszthy, 1995; Zambon, 1996.)

CHAPTER 2

EXTERNAL MODIFYING FACTORS INVOLVED IN PERIODONTAL DISEASES

It is apparent that destructive periodontal disease is the result of a complex interaction between the subgingival microflora and nonbacterial factors, specifically host and environmental factors. A model for progressive periodontitis based on bacterial, environmental, and host markers is illustrated in Fig 102.

Microorganisms, however, are a prominent feature: Without bacteria, there would be no infection and thus no disease. Bacteria—alone, in a compromised host, or combined with environmental factors that increase the host's susceptibility to bacterial infection—increase the risk for progressive periodontitis.

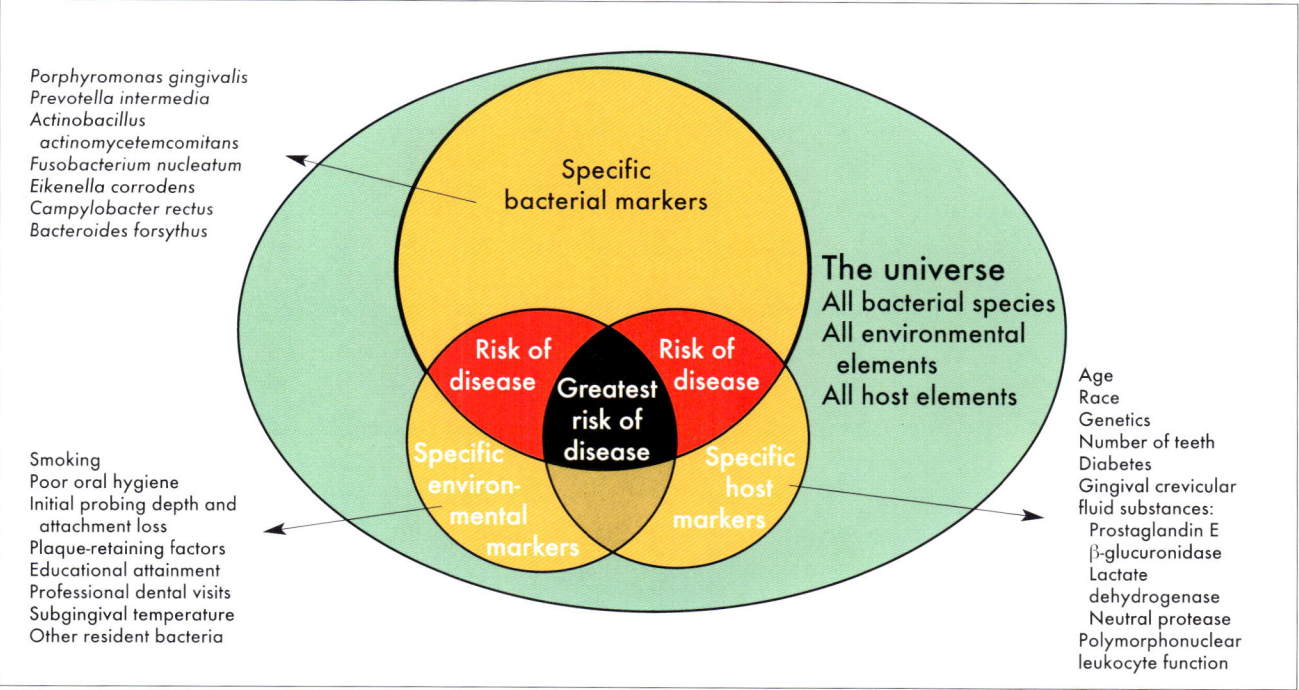

Fig 102 Model for progressive periodontitis based on bacterial, environmental, and host markers. (Modified from Wolff et al, 1994. Reprinted with permission.)

Further investigation is required to evaluate the application of bacterial tests (see chapter 1), combined with environmental and host-based markers, to predict the progression of destructive periodontitis. Progressive periodontitis should be regarded not as a disease for which all individuals harboring a particular bacteria are at equal risk, but primarily as a bacterial infection, causing disease to a limited segment of the population in whom the normal balance between the microorganisms and host is disturbed by an environmental and/or host factor. This will be discussed further in chapter 5, which covers the pathogenesis of periodontal diseases.

DEFINITION OF TERMS

Besides etiologic, preventive, and control factors, many other factors may modify the prevalence, onset, and progression of periodontal diseases. These modifiers may be divided into external (environmental) and internal (endogenous) factors. This chapter will discuss external modifying factors. Internal modifying factors will be presented in chapter 3.

Risk indicators (RIs) are factors that, in cross-sectional studies, have proved to be significantly associated with increased prevalence of a specific disease. Factors that in well-controlled prospective studies have proved to significantly increase the risk for onset and/or progression of a specific disease are termed *risk factors* (RFs) and *prognostic risk factors* (PRFs), respectively.

The RFs and PRFs are often expressed as the *odds ratio* (OR) for onset or progression of a specific disease. On the other hand, *risk markers* (RMs) or *risk predictors* (RPs) are terms used to describe evidence of existing periodontal disease (diseased deep pockets and active lesions), lost periodontal support, and loss of teeth due to periodontal diseases.

Examples of external modifying RIs, RFs, and PRFs for periodontal diseases are smoking, use of smokeless tobacco, irregular dental care, low socioeconomic level, infectious and other acquired diseases, side effects of medication, and poor dietary habits. Smoking and irregular dental care habits are the most important and common factors. Numerous cross-sectional studies have shown that smoking is a very powerful external modifying RI for periodontal diseases. In a multifactorial analytical study, smoking was ranked first (after age) as a risk indicator for periodontal attachment loss (Grossi et al, 1994). After allowing for the greater number of missing teeth in smokers, Axelsson et al (1998) estimated that, among 65-year-old subjects, smokers had lost about 50% more periodontal attachment than had nonsmokers (for review, see Bergström and Preber, 1994).

A recent prospective study showed the risk for further progression of periodontal disease to be about five times higher in smokers than in nonsmokers (Machtei et al, 1997). Compared to nonsmokers, smokers experience significantly impaired outcomes of periodontal therapy, including regenerative therapy (Ah et al, 1994; Tonetti et al, 1995). In other words, smoking is an extremely powerful external modifying risk factor and prognostic risk factor for onset and progression of periodontal disease.

In another recent study, multivariate analyses disclosed that, along with age and the number of teeth, the most consistent markers of periodontal disease experience are educational level and current smoking status (Locker and Leake, 1993b).

In a randomized sample of more than 600 subjects aged 50 to 55 years, those with irregular dental attendance habits had lost almost 50% more periodontal attachment than had regular dental attenders (Axelsson and Paulander, 1994). Other cross-sectional studies have also shown that poorly educated adults (35, 50, 65, and 75 year olds) have more periodontal attachment loss than do subjects with higher education (Axelsson et al, unpublished data, 1990; Paulander et al, 2002). Some infectious and acquired diseases, especially serious diseases, such as ulcerative colitis, Crohn disease, acquired immunodeficiency syndrome

Fig 103 The mean number of remaining teeth in 50- to 55-year-old individuals related to living area, gender, dental care habits (regular care in Public Dental Health Service [PDHS] or in a private practice or no regular dental care), educational level, smoking habits, and tobacco snuffing habits. (From Axelsson and Paulander, 1994. Reprinted with permission.)

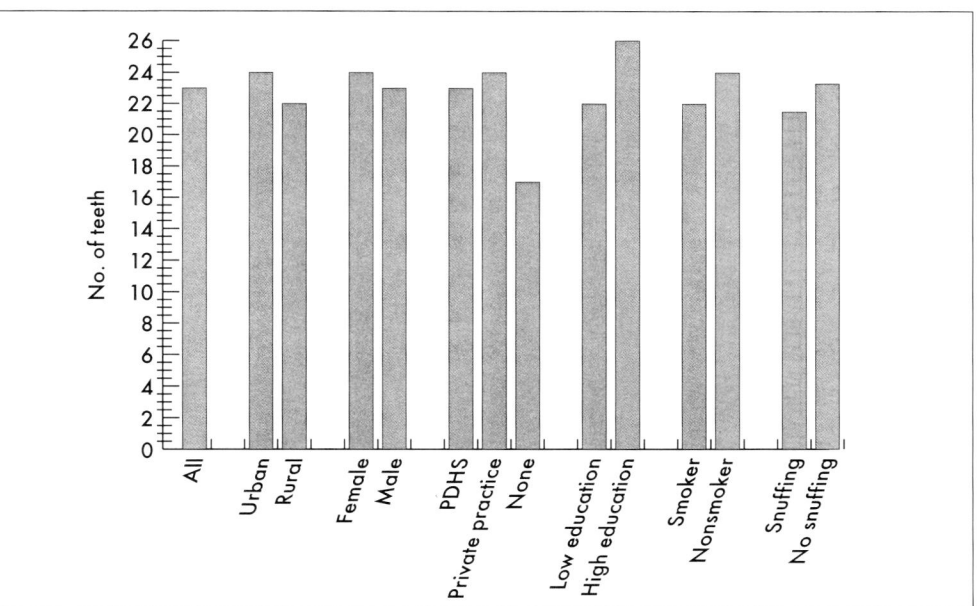

(AIDS), and leukemia, are also high risk factors and prognostic risk factors for periodontal diseases.

Thus, in cross-sectional and longitudinal or prospective studies, several external (exogenous or environmental) risk indicators, risk factors, prognostic risk factors, and background characteristics (so-called determinants: gender, race, living area, etc) have been shown to increase the risk for periodontal disease:

- Use of tobacco products (particularly cigarette smoking)
- Low socioeconomic status (particularly low educational level)
- Poor compliance (particularly poor oral hygiene) and irregular dental care
- Acquired systemic and infectious diseases (particularly infection with the human immunodeficiency virus [HIV])

Figure 103 shows that adults living in urban areas had, on average, 24.0 remaining teeth, while those in rural areas had only 22.0. Third molars were excluded. Women had 1.5 more remaining teeth than did men. Patients receiving regular dental care in private practice or the Public Dental Health Service (PDHS) had 23.8 and 22.5 remaining teeth, respectively; those receiving care sporadically had only 17.0 remaining teeth. People with higher education had 4.0 more teeth than did those with low education. Nonsmokers had 2.0 teeth more than did smokers, and nonsnuffers had, on average, 1.5 more remaining teeth than did snuffers.

Figure 104 shows the mean probing loss of attachment on the mesial surfaces (attachment loss on the mesial surfaces is caused by bacteria, while most buccal attachment loss is a side effect of toothbrushing). The periodontal status of two extreme subsets of subjects was compared: poorly educated, smoking, rural men with irregular dental care habits, and well-educated, nonsmoking, urban women with regular dental care habits. The loss of teeth and periodontal attachment in the men was significantly greater than could be attributed to differences in the composition of the subgingival microflora of the two subsets (Axelsson and Paulander, 1994).

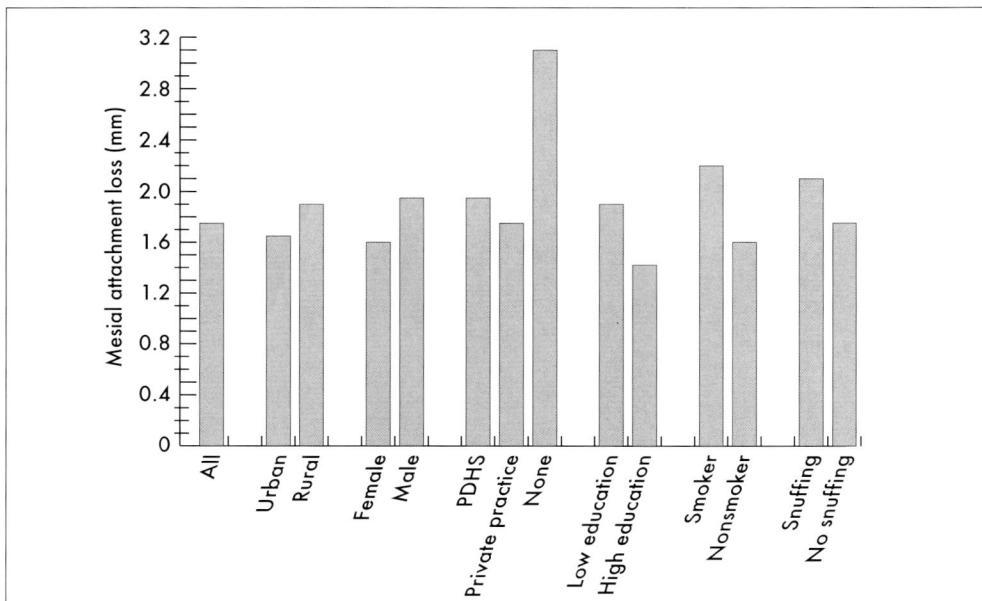

Fig 104 The mean periodontal attachment loss mesially in 50- to 55-year-old individuals related to living area, gender, dental care habits (regular care in Public Dental Health Service [PDHS] or in a private practice or no regular dental care), educational level, smoking habits, and tobacco snuffing habits. (From Axelsson and Paulander, 1994. Reprinted with permission.

ROLE OF TOBACCO PRODUCTS

Tobacco smoking is probably the most widespread (environmental) risk factor for general health. Classic examples of diseases for which tobacco smoking is considered to be a substantial contributing risk factor are lung cancer and cardiovascular disease (US Department of Health and Human Services, 1982). The impact of tobacco on the health status of a population is enormous. In Europe as a whole, tobacco causes almost 400,000 deaths annually from cancer alone; when cardiopulmonary diseases are added, tobacco is responsible for a total of 1 million European deaths annually. The same holds true for the United States. Approximately 20% of all deaths in developed countries are attributable to tobacco (Peto et al, 1992).

Unfortunately, in the developing countries, representing about 70% of the world's population, smoking continues to increase, particularly as an effect of aggressive advertising targeting children and young adults. In industrialized countries, the prevalence of smokers continues to increase among young women, while a significant decrease has been achieved among males (particularly in the United States and northern Europe). On the other hand, the use of smokeless tobacco (snuff) has increased among young males in northern Europe. Tobacco smoking has long been associated with chronic disease, and unquestionably chronic periodontal diseases should now be included among the diseases for which tobacco is a risk.

In populations with relatively high standards of oral hygiene, tobacco use, particularly smoking, is by far the most powerful environmental risk indicator and risk factor for periodontal disease and today is more important than frequent sugar consumption as a risk factor for caries.

Evidence from cross-sectional studies

Data from numerous cross-sectional studies indicate that tobacco use, particularly smoking, is a powerful external (environmental) risk indicator for tooth loss and periodontal diseases. As early as 1947, Pindborg, in a study of 3,600 soldiers, found a significantly higher prevalence of acute necrotizing ulcerative gingivitis (ANUG) and calculus in smokers than in nonsmokers. Herulf (1950) and Schei et al (1959) also presented data supporting a positive correlation between alveolar bone loss and smoking. In the Herulf study (1950), more alveolar bone loss was observed around the anterior than the posterior teeth, indicating a local effect of smoking. The study by Schei et al (1959) was corrected for age and standard of oral hygiene, and the authors concluded that tobacco smoking might exert an effect per se on the periodontal bone and therefore be a complicating factor in the etiology of periodontal disease. This bold and visionary statement was largely ignored for more than 20 years, when the question was readdressed, with similar results (Bergström and Floderus-Myrhed, 1983; Bolin et al, 1986b; Ismail et al, 1983; Solomon et al, 1968). Moreover, recent studies of dentally aware subjects with a high standard of oral hygiene have confirmed an association between tobacco smoking and radiographic bone loss, after the effects of dental plaque and other confounding factors are controlled (Bergström and Eliasson, 1987; Bergström et al, 1991). Ismail et al (1983) found that smoking is a major risk indicator for periodontal disease when they corrected for confounding factors such as age, oral hygiene, sex, and socioeconomic status.

Horning et al (1992) studied a population of 1,783 subjects, ranging in age from 13 to 84 years. Eighty-five percent were males and 39% were current smokers. The odds ratio between smoking and moderate to advanced disease was 1.9 ($P <$ .001). Similarly, after Locker and Leake (1993b) controlled for age and educational level, they observed an odds ratio of 2.9 between smoking and attachment loss in a group of 624 adults older than 50 years (mean age of 62.3 years), 55.4% of whom were female and 95.5% of whom were white. A study by Österberg and Mellström (1986) also confirmed a correlation between the number of lost teeth and total exposure to smoking: The 70-year-old male smokers were missing seven more teeth than were age-matched nonsmokers. Even among a selected group of young adults (20 to 35 year olds) Lindén and Mullally (1994) found that smokers had lost 2.2 ($P < .05$) more teeth than had nonsmokers.

In the aforementioned cross-sectional study of a total of 1,426 subjects, Grossi et al (1994) evaluated different risk indicators for attachment loss. After age, smoking was the most significant risk indicator, followed by diabetes mellitus and the presence of *Porphyromonas gingivalis* and *Bacteroides forsythus*. Smoking had a relative risk ranging from 2 for light smokers to almost 5 for heavy smokers. These associations remained valid after the researchers adjusted for gender, socioeconomic status, educational level, and oral hygiene status, expressed in terms of supragingival plaque accumulation and subgingival calculus. Figure 105 shows the level of probing attachment loss related to a composite value of the number of packs of cigarettes smoked per day, multiplied by the number of years of smoking, ie, the number of "pack years." In a sample of 889 individuals aged 21 to 76 years with mild to advanced periodontitis, Martinez-Canut et al (1995) related the severity of periodontal disease and periodontal destruction to tobacco consumption and age. For subjects of the same age, daily smoking of one cigarette, up to 10 cigarettes, and up to 20 cigarettes increased periodontal attachment loss by 0.5%, 5.0%, and 10.0%, respectively, while each year of life increased periodontal attachment loss by 0.7%. Consumption of 10 cigarettes or more per day seemed to be an important predictor for increased risk of attachment loss.

An analytic epidemiologic study compared tooth loss, probing attachment loss, and Community Periodontal Index of Treatment Needs (CPITN) (see chapter 6) in adult smokers and nonsmokers (Axelsson et al, unpublished data, 1990; Axelsson et al, 1998). The subjects were randomly selected 35, 50, 65, and 75 year olds from the whole county of Varmland, Sweden (n =1,086). Probing attachment loss and the CPITN were measured at all mesial, buccal, distal, and lingual sites (n = almost 100,000). The subjects were stratified into nonsmokers, smokers, and former smokers and nonsnuffers and snuffers.

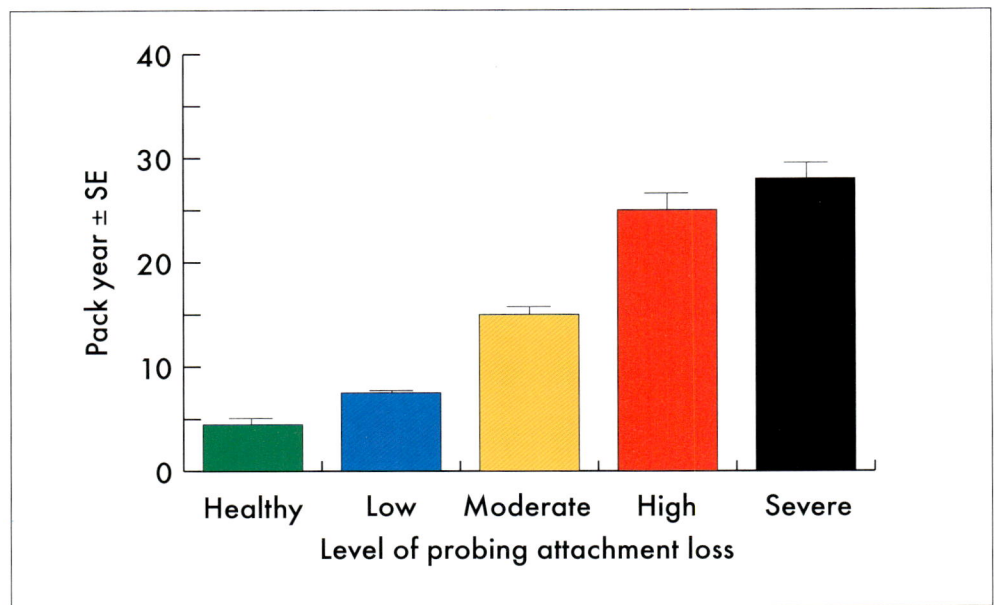

Fig 105 Probing attachment loss in relation to a composite value of the number of packs of cigarettes smoked per day, multiplied by the number of years of smoking (pack years, ie, 20 cigarettes per day for 1 year = 1 pack year). (Modified from Grossi et al, 1994. Reprinted with permission.)

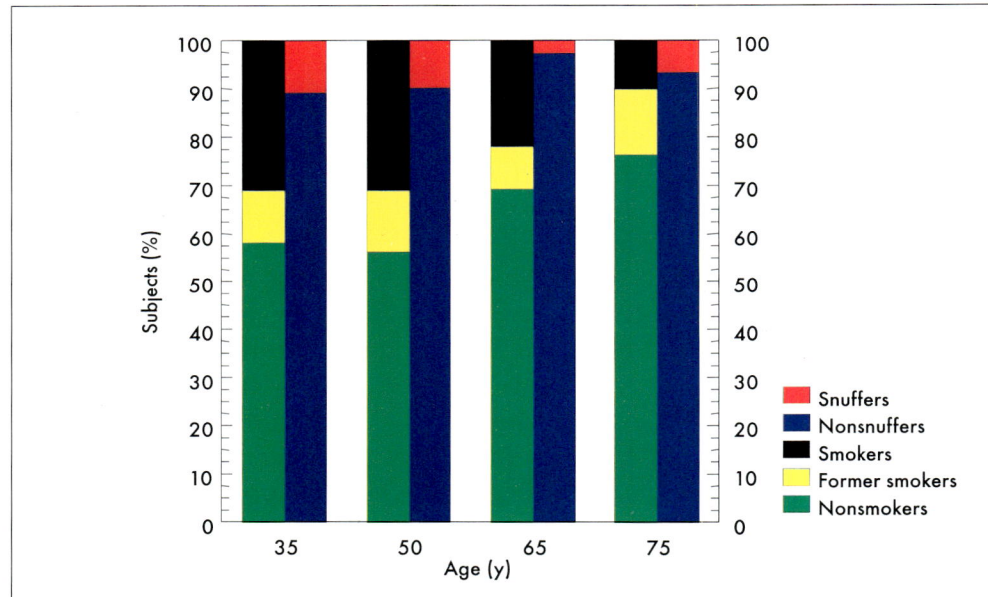

Fig 106 Tobacco habits in 35, 50, 65, and 75 year olds. (From Axelsson et al, 1998. Reprinted with permission.)

The percentages of smokers, former smokers, and snuffers were 30%, 11%, and 11%, respectively, in 35 year olds; 30%, 13%, and 9% in 50 year olds; 21%, 9%, and 3% in 65 year olds; and 6%, 9%, and 4% in 75 year olds (Fig 106). The mean numbers of teeth (third molars excluded) in 35-, 50-, 65-, and 75-year-old smokers versus nonsmokers were 26.0 versus 26.6, 21.8 versus 23.2, 14.2 versus 17.7 and 9.2 versus 15.0 respectively (Fig 107).

Most of the missing teeth were molars and maxillary premolars.

The mean probing attachment losses in smokers versus nonsmokers were 1.1 versus 0.8 mm (P = .001), 2.3 versus 1.5 mm (P = .001), 3.0 versus 2.2 mm (P = .001) and 3.9 versus 2.7 mm (P = .001) in 35, 50, 65, and 75 year olds, respectively (Fig 108). Among poorly educated 50-year-old women, nonsmokers had 50% less probing at-

Fig 107 Mean number of teeth in smokers and nonsmokers. (From Axelsson et al, 1998. Reprinted with permission.)

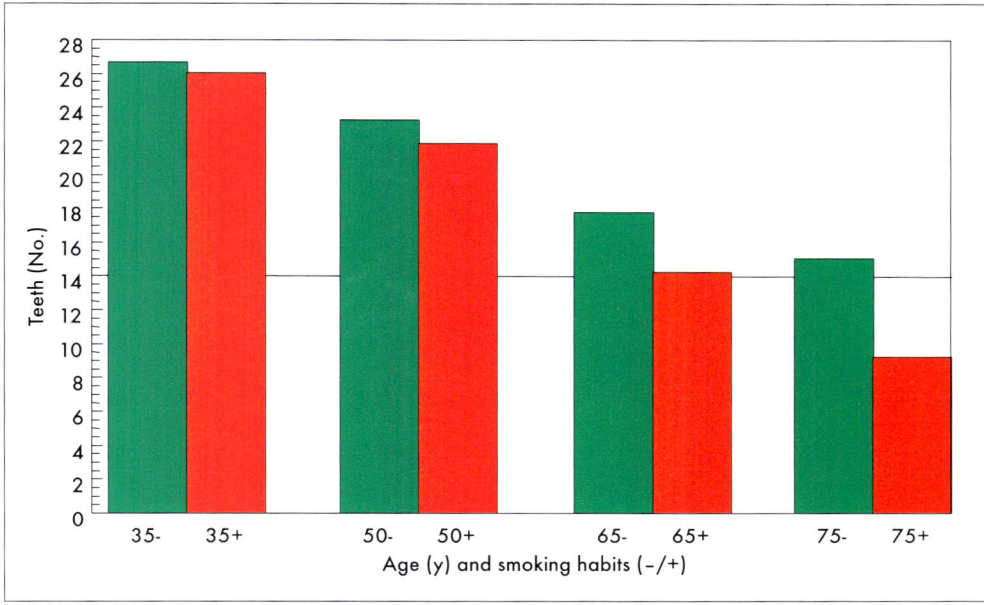

Fig 108 Mean periodontal attachment loss in smokers and nonsmokers. (From Axelsson et al, 1998. Reprinted with permission.)

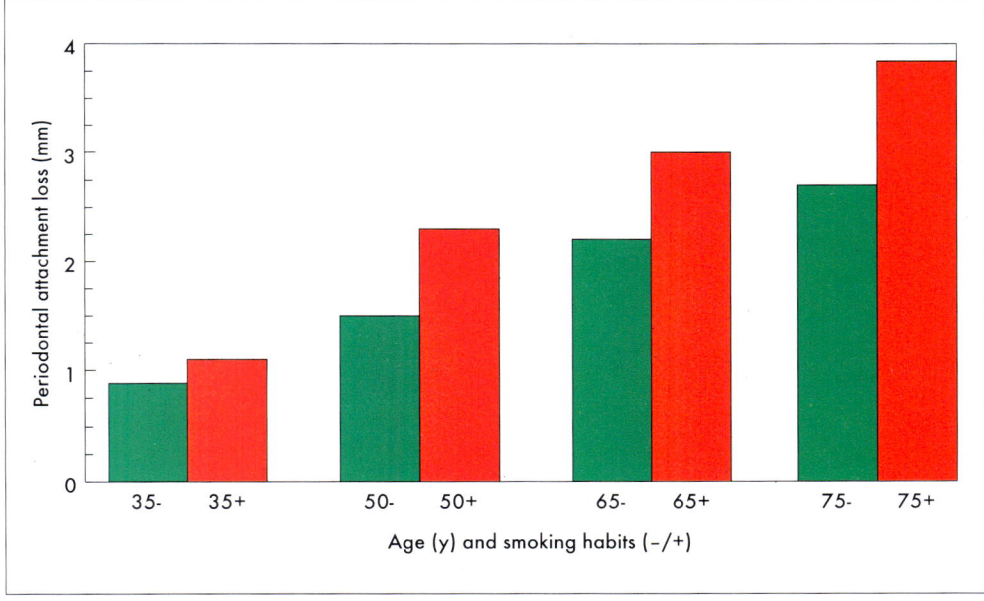

tachment loss than did smokers. The pattern of attachment loss in smokers and nonsmokers on mesial and lingual surfaces is presented in Figs 109 and 110.

The frequency distribution of CPITN scores in smokers and nonsmokers is presented in Fig 111. The patterns of CPITN scores and missing sites on mesial surfaces in 65-year-old smokers and nonsmokers are shown in Figs 112a and

112b, respectively. The highest percentages of CPITN score 4 and missing sites were found on maxillary mesial sites in smokers. On the other hand, smokers had a lower percentage of CPITN score 1 (gingival bleeding on probing) than did nonsmokers. It was also notable that, in this randomized, large-scale analytic epidemiologic study, no differences were disclosed in the oral hygiene, dietary habits, or dental attendance

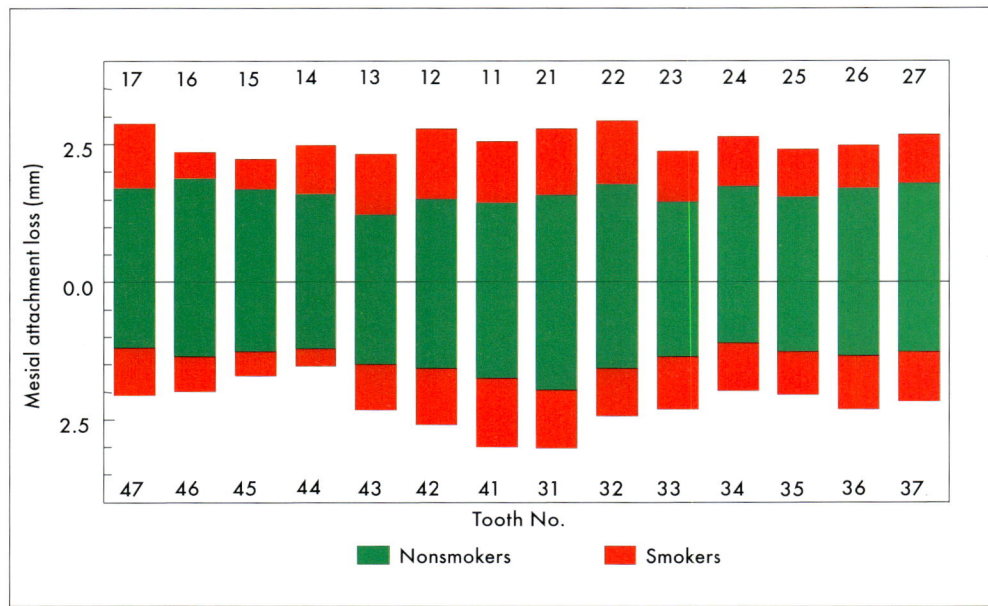

Fig 109 Pattern of mean mesial attachment loss in 50-year-old smokers and nonsmokers. (From Axelsson et al, 1998. Reprinted with permission.)

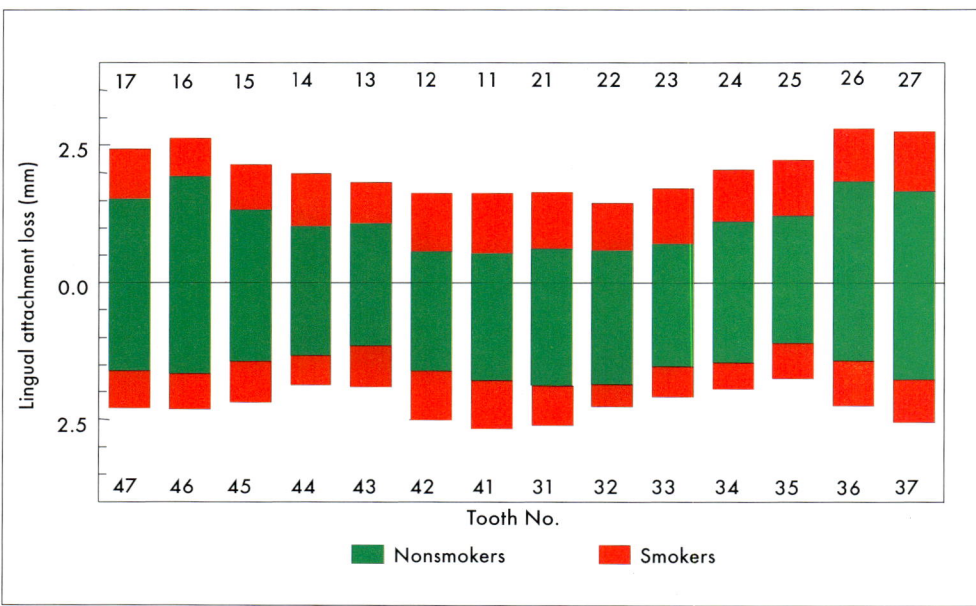

Fig 110 Pattern of mean lingual attachment loss in 50-year-old smokers and nonsmokers. (From Axelsson et al, 1998. Reprinted with permission.)

habits of smokers and nonsmokers. Thus, this study showed that smoking is an extremely powerful environmental (external) risk indicator for loss of teeth, loss of periodontal probing attachment, and periodontal treatment needs, correlated with the total, cumulative exposure to smoking (Axelsson et al, unpublished data, 1990; Axelsson et al, 1998).

In a study of age-matched smokers and nonsmokers, Mullally and Lindén (1996) found that smokers had more than twice as many molars with furcation involvement as nonsmokers (39% and 16%, respectively). Recently, Kerdvongbundit and Wikesjö (2000) also found that long-term cigarette smoking significantly worsens periodontal health, including degree and prevalence of furca-

Fig 111 CPITN scores in smokers and nonsmokers. (From Axelsson et al, 1998. Reprinted with permission.)

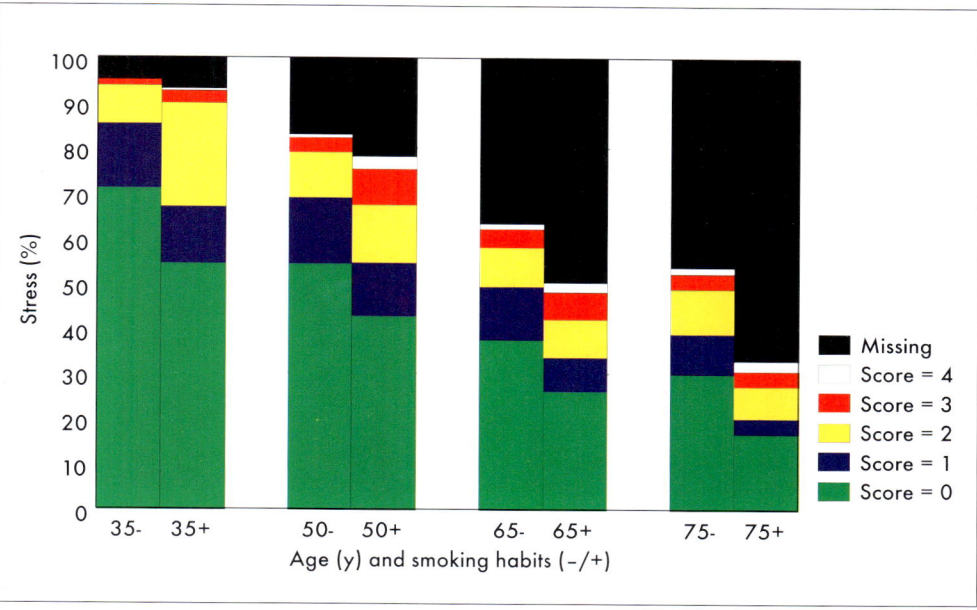

tion involvement in molar teeth. It has also been shown that the severity of attachment loss is directly related to serum cotinine levels (Gonzalez et al, 1996). As discussed earlier, when alveolar bone loss is used as the outcome measure, smoking is still strongly associated with periodontitis (Schei et al, 1959). Wouters et al (1993) showed that individuals who smoked more than 5 g of tobacco per day had significantly more loss of alveolar bone than nonsmokers and former smokers, as well as individuals who smoked only 1 to 5 g of tobacco per day.

Bergström et al (1991) investigated smoking habits and alveolar bone loss in 210 young Swedish dental hygienists with excellent oral hygiene. The mean alveolar bone loss in smokers (1.71 mm) was significantly greater than that in those who had never smoked (1.45 mm) ($P < .01$). Alveolar bone loss was 2.06 mm in those who smoked more than 10 cigarettes a day and 1.60 mm in those who smoked fewer than 10 a day ($P < .05$).

In a further analysis of the study by Grossi et al (1994) described earlier, bone loss ranged from 0.4 to 8.8 mm. The odds ratio for association of smoking with alveolar bone loss was 1.48 for very

light smokers and increased to 7.28 for heavy smokers (Gonzales et al, 1996; Grossi et al, 1995). The odds ratios for the association of smoking with attachment loss ranged from 2.05 to 4.75. In the cross-sectional study on a randomized sample of almost six hundred 50 to 55 year olds discussed earlier (Axelsson and Paulander, 1994), the odds ratios for association of smoking with attachment loss was as high as 10.9.

Using pocketing as a measure of periodontal destruction, several researchers have demonstrated an association between tobacco smoking and disease (Bergström and Eliasson, 1987; Feldman et al, 1983; Haber and Kent, 1992; Preber and Bergström, 1986). In a case-control study based on a large patient sample, Preber and Bergström (1986a) calculated a relative risk (odds ratio) of 2.1 to 2.4 for smokers. This was further substantiated in a subsequent study (Bergström, 1989), which also showed that the relative risk increased with increasing severity of disease. For severe disease, ie, the most severe 25% of cases, the odds ratio was 6.4.

Haber et al (1993a) conducted a study of subjects ranging in age from 19 to 40 years. A diagnosis of periodontitis was made on the basis of

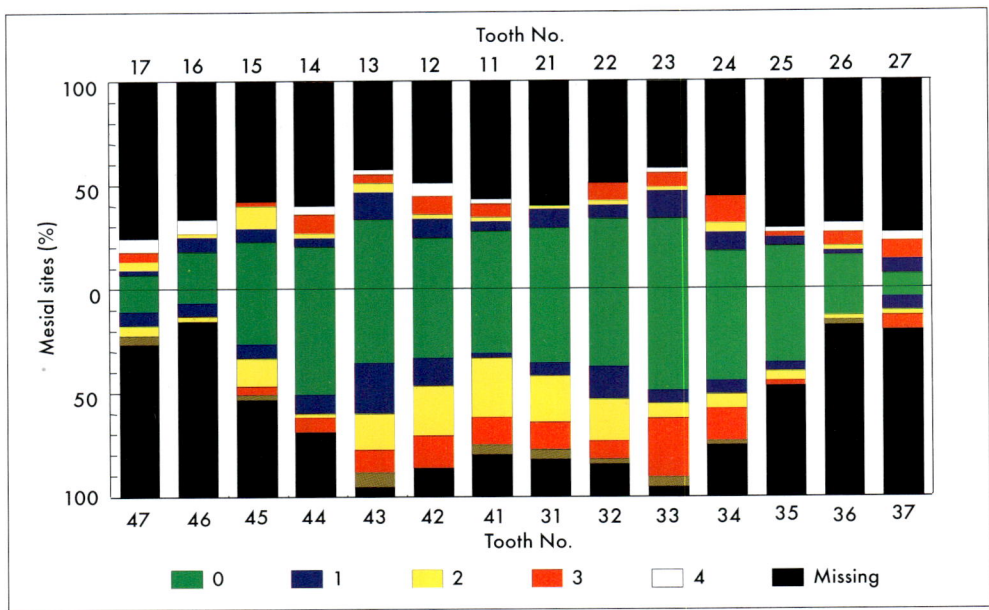

Fig 112a CPITN scores at mesial sites in 65-year-old smokers. (From Axelsson et al, 1998. Reprinted with permission.)

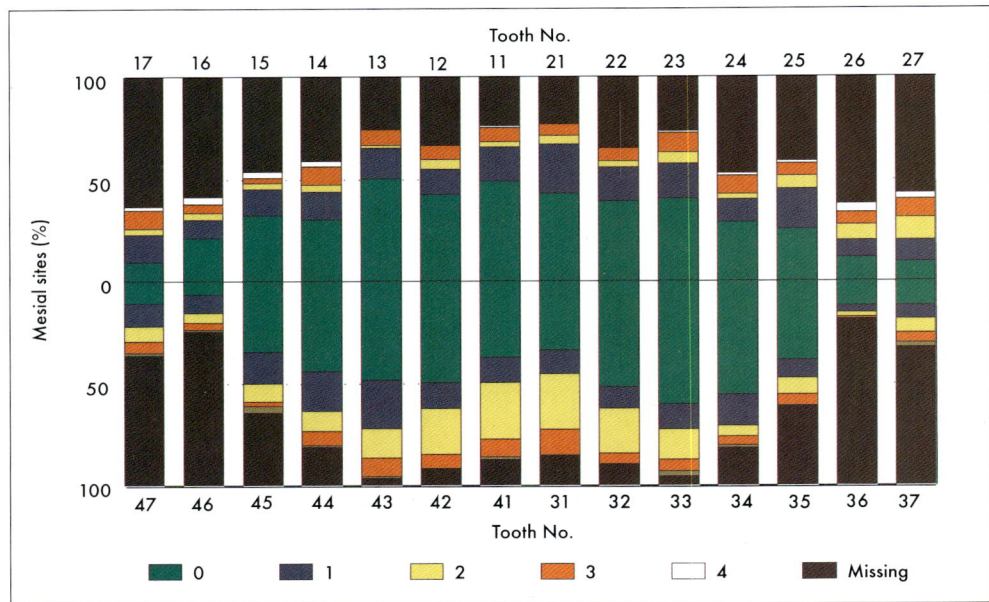

Fig 112b CPITN scores at mesial sites in 65-year-old nonsmokers. (From Axelsson et al, 1998. Reprinted with permission.)

one or more sites with probing depth of 5 mm or more and attachment loss of 2 mm or more. The prevalence ($P < .005$) and severity ($P < .001$) of periodontitis were significantly higher in current smokers than they were in those who had never smoked ($P < .005$). There was also a significant and positive association between the prevalence of periodontitis and heavy smoking. The authors suggested that as much as 51% of the periodontitis observed in the 19- to 30-year-old group, and 32% in the 31- to 40-year-old group was associated with smoking.

Recently, Mullally et al (1999) showed that in subjects with aggressive periodontitis, smokers had significantly more maxillary bone loss than did nonsmokers. In addition, much higher proportions of patients with generalized aggressive periodontitis (GAP) currently smoked (70%), compared with 44% of patients with localized aggressive periodontitis (LAP).

Schenkein et al (1995) studied patients who were 35 years or older who had a history of generalized aggressive periodontitis and who were now experiencing rapidly progressive aggressive periodontitis; smokers had more affected teeth and more attachment loss than did nonsmokers.

In a randomized sample of 547 Swedish subjects aged 20 to 70 years, Norderyd and Hugoson (1998) showed that the odds ratio for severe periodontitis was 11.84 among moderate to heavy smokers, while light smoking (1 to 9 cigarettes per day) was not significantly associated with severe periodontitis.

A study by Stoltenberg et al (1993) showed that after matching for age, sex, plaque, and calculus, the odds of having a mean posterior proximal probing depth greater than 3.5 mm were 5.3 times greater for smokers than for nonsmokers. The prevalence of *P gingivalis, Actinobacillus actinomycetemcomitans, Prevotella intermedia, Eikenella corrodens,* or *Fusobacterium nucleatum* was similar for smokers and nonsmokers. *A actinomycetemcomitans, P intermedia, E corrodens,* and smoking were each associated with increased mean posterior proximal probing depth. However, cigarette smoking was a stronger risk indicator for the presence of a mean probing depth of 3.5 mm than were any of these five common periopathogens.

In another study of patients with so-called refractory periodontitis, it was observed that 90% were regular smokers, compared with the average regional prevalence of smoking of only 21% (MacFarlane et al, 1992). These results are noteworthy, because the patients with refractory disease were well maintained and had a high standard of oral hygiene.

In a recent cross-sectional study, Gunsolly et al (1998) also showed that, compared to nonsmokers, smokers with minimal approximal periodontal destruction had more attachment loss and recession on buccal and lingual surfaces. This was particularly pronounced on the buccal surfaces of the maxillary posterior teeth and the mandibular incisors.

In another recent cross-sectional study, Albandar et al (2000) found that cigar and pipe smoking may have adverse effects on periodontal health and tooth loss that are similar to those associated with cigarette smoking.

Finally, data from the Third US National Health and Nutrition Examination Survey, which studied a randomized sample of individuals aged 18 years and older (n = 12,329), show that the odds of periodontitis (7 or more sites with 4 mm or more attachment loss) for those who smoked 9 or more cigarettes per day or 31 or more cigarettes per day were 2.8 and 5.9 respectively. Among former smokers, the odds ratios declined. It was calculated that 42% of periodontitis cases in the US population were attributable to current cigarette smoking and 11% to former smoking. Among current smokers, 75% of the periodontitis cases were attributable to smoking (Tomar and Asma, 2000). Table 9 presents a review of cross-sectional oral epidemiologic studies related to smoking habits. The association between smokeless tobacco (snuff) and periodontal disease has been addressed in only a few studies (Robertson et al, 1992). The results suggest that smokeless tobacco is associated with an increased risk of gingival recession in areas exposed to the tobacco quid but not with periodontal pocketing or severe forms of periodontal disease. It should be noted, however, that the studies to date are restricted to examination of young people with relatively short-term use of the drug. Further studies are necessary, particularly prospective investigations, on the relationship between long-term use of smokeless tobacco and destructive forms of periodontal disease.

Such a 10-year longitudinal study, in a randomized sample of subjects aged 50 years at baseline, has just been completed and the results are under analysis (Axelsson et al, 2000). The cross-sectional part of the study discussed earlier, in almost 600 subjects aged 50 to 55 years, revealed that, compared with nonsnuffers, snuffers (10%)

Table 9 Review of cross-sectional epidemiologic studies related to smoking habits*

Study	n	Age(y)	Material SEL	Material RAN	Material AG	Material MT	Periodontal AB	Periodontal VAL
Herulf (1951)	535	19–25	X		Int		S	
Massler and Ludwick (1952)	2,577	17–21	X		Int			
Arno et al (1958)	1,246	25–55	X		Int			
Arno et al (1959)	728	21–45	X		Int		S	
Herulf (1968)	700	20–85	X		Int		S	
Bergström et al (1983)	328	39–78	X		Int	S	S	
Feldman et al (1983)	862	?	X		All		S	
Preber and Bergström (1986a)	369	18–70	X		Int			
Österberg and Mellström (1986)	1,377	70		X	Ind	S		
Bergström and Eliasson (1987)	235	21–60	X		Int		S	
Beck et al (1990)	690	65+		X	Int			S
Hansen et al (1990)	144	35		X	Ind			
Goultschin et al (1990)	344	20–70	X		Int			
Bergström et al (1991)	210	24–60	X		All		S	
Horning et al (1992)	1,783	13–84	X		All			
Preber et al (1992)	145	32–74	X		All			
Stoltenberg et al (1993)	189	28–73	X		All			
Haber et al (1993a)	227	19–40	X		Int			
Wouters et al (1993)	723	20–80+		X	Int			S
Lindén and Mullally (1994)	82	20–33	X		All	S		S
Grossi et al (1994)	1,426	25–74	X		All		S	S
Axelsson and Paulander (1994)	572	50–55		X	Ind	S		S
Martinez-Canut et al (1995)	889	21–76	X		All			S
Wiktorsson (1995)	236	44–56	X		All	NS		
Sakki et al (1995)	527	55		X	Ind			
Söder et al (1995)	144	31–40	X		All	S	S	
Mullally and Lindén (1996)	100	35+	X		All	NS		
Axelsson et al (1998)	1,093	35, 50, 65, 75		X	Ind	S		S
Norderyd and Hugoson (1998)	547	20–70		X	Int		S	
Mullally et al (1999)	71	< 35	X		All		S	
Kerdvongbundit and Wikesjö (2000)	120	20+	X		All	S		S
Tomar and Asma (2000)	72,329	18+		X	All			S

*Modified from Axelsson et al (1998). Reprinted with permission.
SEL = Study on selected material; RAN = Study on randomized material; AG = Age group (statistics performed on Int = Age interval; Ind = Indicator age groups; All = All ages simultaneously); MT = Number of missing teeth; AB = Alveolar bone; VAL = Vertical attachment level; HAL = Horizontal attachment level; CPITN = Community Periodontal Index of Treatment Needs; GI = Gingival Index; PD = Probing depth; CAR = Dental caries; PI = Plaque Index; PP = Periopathogens; CP = Caries pathogens; SSR = Stimulated salivary secretion rate; DC = Dental care habits; OH = Oral hygiene habits; DH = Dietary habits; OTH = Other important features; NS = No significant difference; S = Significant difference, nonsmokers being healthier; –S = Reversed significant difference.

disease		Variables								Lifestyle		
HAL	CPITN	GI	PD	CAR	PI	PP	CP	SSR	DC	OH	DH	OTH
		NS										
		S										
		S										-S
		-S			NS							
		NS	NS		-S							
		-S	NS		NS							
					NS							
			NS									
	S											
			S									
						NS						
		NS	S			NS						
			S									
		S	S			NS				NS		
	S											
			S									
				S			S	S				
			S						S	S	S	
		NS	S							NS		
S										NS		
S	S	NS	S	S	NS			NS	NS	NS	NS	NS
S			S									
			S									

had lost on average 1.5 more teeth and about 20% more periodontal attachment ($P < .01$) on the mesial surfaces (see Figs 103 and 104). This indicates that use of smokeless tobacco is also a risk indicator for tooth loss and loss of periodontal support (Axelsson and Paulander, 1994).

Evidence from longitudinal studies

Tooth loss and periodontal attachment loss

A study by Holm (1994) was undertaken to determine whether or not smoking is also a risk factor for tooth loss. A total of 273 individuals were followed for 10 years, during which 93 subjects lost a total of 260 teeth. Individuals younger than 50 years who smoked more than 15 cigarettes per day and men who smoked more than 15 cigarettes per day were found to have the highest relative risk of losing teeth (4.55 and 3.18, respectively) compared with nonsmokers. In the age group younger than 50 years, the proportional attributable risk was also highest (78%) for those smoking more than 15 cigarettes per day. Together with age, the strongest predictor of tooth loss was a combination of high plaque score and smoking. The findings of this study suggest that smokers, especially those younger than 50 years, are a high-risk group for tooth loss. In this age group, 30% of the smokers lost teeth, compared with 3% of the nonsmokers.

Locker et al (1996), in a 3-year longitudinal study, also showed that smokers (over 50 years old) lost 0.8 teeth per individual, while nonsmokers lost 0.4 teeth.

A longitudinal study in US Veterans Administration hospitals in the United States assessed the relationship between periodontal disease and smoking over a 6-year period (Palmer, 1988). The number of teeth lost was higher for cigarette smokers than it was for nonsmokers. Loss of alveolar bone was greater in smokers than it was in nonsmokers, and smokers had more calculus.

There was little evidence of a relationship between gingival inflammation and smoking. In this otherwise valuable study, however, there was very little statistical analysis of the interaction of these variables, which may have confounded the results.

Bolin et al (1993) examined, over a 10-year period, an unselected sample of 349 individuals, each of whom had at least 20 teeth remaining. Age; sex; social class; dental habits; smoking habits; frequency of dental treatment; number of lost teeth; number of carious, missing, or restored teeth; dentures; partial dentures; plaque; calculus; oral hygiene; and interproximal alveolar bone were measured. Stepwise multiple regression analysis showed that, among the factors measured, only two, the initial periodontal index and smoking, predicted alveolar bone loss over the 10-year period. Smokers lost 6% of their alveolar bone and nonsmokers lost 3.9%. Bone loss in subjects who had quit smoking during the 10-year period was 4.4%.

Krall et al (1997) evaluated the rates of tooth loss and smoking status in two populations of systematically healthy men and women in Boston. Among the men, rates of tooth loss and edentulism in relation to cessation of smoking were also evaluated. The subjects were drawn from a group of 584 women (aged 40 to 70 years) and a separate population of 1,231 male veterans (aged 21 to 75 years). In cross-sectional baseline analyses, current cigarette smokers of either sex were missing significantly more teeth than were those who had never smoked or former smokers. Intermediate values were found in former smokers and pipe or cigar smokers. Current male smokers had more teeth with calculus, but the differences in plaque, tooth mobility, probing depth greater than 2 mm, restored and carious teeth, and bleeding on probing in relation to smoking history were not significant.

Prospective observations of 248 women (mean follow-up = 6 ± 2 years) and 977 men (mean follow-up = 18 ± 7 years) revealed that, compared with nonsmokers, men and women who continued to smoke cigarettes had 2.4-fold and 3.5-fold greater risk for tooth loss, respectively. The rates of tooth loss decreased significantly in men who stopped smoking cigarettes but remained higher than rates in nonsmokers (Krall et al, 1997).

In a 3-year prospective study, Beck et al (1995) showed that, among older adults, smokers are significantly more susceptible to loss of periodontal attachment than are nonsmokers. In a recent prospective longitudinal study, Machtei et al (1997) evaluated a large battery of clinical, microbiologic, and immunologic indicators, to try to determine whether the presence at baseline of one or a combination of these variables would correlate positively with increased attachment and/or bone loss (true prognostic risk factors). Following initial screening, 79 patients with established periodontitis were monitored for 1 year. Whole-mouth clinical measurements, plaque, gingival, and calculus indices, and probing depth and attachment level measurements were repeated every 3 months. Changes in crestal bone height were determined by using an image enhancement technique on complete-mouth radiographs taken at baseline and 12 months. Subgingival plaque samples were taken at baseline and every 3 months. Immunofluorescence assays were performed for a battery of target microorganisms. Blood samples were drawn at each visit for quantitative analysis of serum cotinine level.

The overall mean attachment loss and bone loss were almost identical. Mean probing depth showed minimal change over the study period, suggesting that most, if not all, the attachment loss was accompanied by gingival recession. Smokers exhibited greater attachment loss and radiographic bone loss than did nonsmokers. Likewise, the cotinine level showed direct correlation with outcomes of progressive periodontal breakdown. Past severity of periodontal involvement, reflected in the patient's baseline probing depth, attachment loss, and crestal bone height, correlated well with longitudinal changes in the periodontium: The correlation was stronger for crestal bone loss as the outcome variable and somewhat weaker for change in attachment loss. *B forsythus, P intermedia,* and *P gingivalis* were a frequent finding in these patients. Th of these microorganisms at baseline ... ated with further disease progression. Smokers were at five times greater risk for further attachment loss than were nonsmokers. However, subjects harboring *B forsythus* at baseline were at seven times greater risk for increased probing depth (Machtei et al, 1997). When clinical trials are designed or epidemiologic data are evaluated, it is most important to balance for these prognostic risk factors. Treatment strategies should attempt to eliminate or modify these factors.

In a recent 10-year longitudinal study, Bergström et al (2000) showed that 16 out of every 101 smokers exhibited an increase in diseased sites and a decrease in alveolar bone height when compared with nonsmokers and former smokers. In another study, Norderyd et al (1999) reexamined a random sample of adults (n = 361) after 15 to 17 years and found that only 9% of the group that exhibited no alveolar bone loss smoked, while 38% of the group with severe periodontal bone loss (more than 4 mm of bone loss at 6 or more sites) were smokers.

In a comprehensive 10-year longitundinal analytic epidemiologic study, Axelsson et al (2000) evaluated several possible risk factors for tooth loss, periodontitis, and other conditions in a randomized sample of Swedish adults aged 50 to 60 years (n = 426). During the 10-year period, the mean number of lost teeth was 1.2 in smokers (n = 62) and 0.5 in nonsmokers (P = .018). According to Fig 113, there was a significantly higer mean number of mesial sites with more than 2, 3, and 4 mm probing attachment loss in smokers than in nonsmokers per subject per 10 years.

The temporal relationship between cigarette smoking and periodontal disease also has been studied, and the results show that active smoking is associated with a greater increase in probing depth and attachment loss during a 10-year follow-up (Chen et al, 2001).

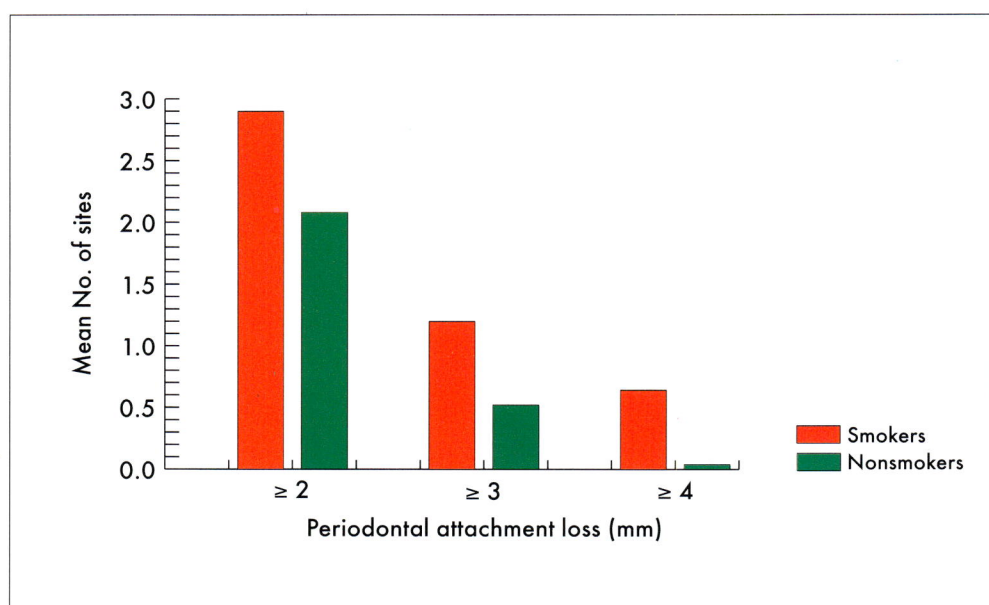

Fig 113 Mean number of mesial sites per individual per 10 years with ≥ 2 mm, ≥ 3 mm, and ≥ 4 mm periodontal attachment loss in smokers compared to nonsmokers (From Axelsson et al, 2000. Reprinted with permission.)

Impaired periodontal healing

Recent longitudinal studies have also shown that smoking significantly impairs the outcome of periodontal treatment. Early short-term studies (12 months or less) have shown healing (probing depth reduction) in smokers to be impaired compared to that in nonsmokers, after both initial nonsurgical and surgical treatment (Preber and Bergström, 1986c, 1990).

A 7-year study by Kaldahl et al (1996) compared four treatment modalities and 3-month supportive periodontal maintenance on a test group of 72 patients. The average reduction in probing depths was 2 mm for nonsmokers and former smokers, and 1 mm for all smokers. Similar differences were also observed for changes in clinical attachment levels: a gain of 1 mm for nonsmokers and no gain for smokers. In addition, the smokers lost more horizontal attachment (furcation involvement). An important finding was the similarity between nonsmokers and former smokers, indicating an improved healing response after cessation of smoking. This has also been reported in the medical literature. By extrapolation, these results suggest that, the longer the follow-up term, the greater the risk of treatment failure associated with smoking.

Ah et al (1994) evaluated the effect of smoking on response to periodontal therapy in a 6-year longitudinal study of 74 adult subjects with moderate to advanced periodontitis, treated according to a split-mouth design involving nonsurgical and surgical periodontal treatment. Clinical data on probing depth, probing attachment loss, gingival recession, etc, were collected at baseline, after initial treatment, 10 weeks after a maintenance program, and annually thereafter. Immediately following active therapy and during each of the 6 years of maintenance, smokers had significantly less reduction in probing depth (Fig 114) and less gain of probing attachment level (Fig 115) than did nonsmokers.

Preber et al (1995) found no differences between smokers and nonsmokers in reduction of Plaque Index, Gingival Index, and subgingival periopathogens (*A actinomycetemcomitans*, *P gingivalis,* and *P intermedia*) after nonsurgical periodontal treatment. Although probing depth was also reduced in both smokers and nonsmokers, the reduction was significantly smaller in smokers than in nonsmokers.

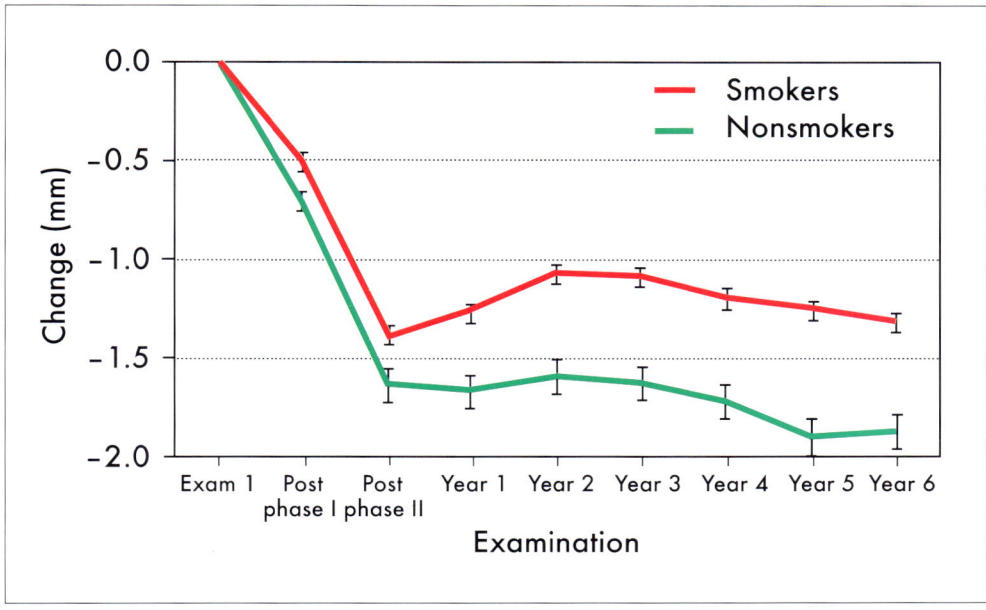

Fig 114 Mean change in probing depth (all modalities and severity categories combined) for smokers and nonsmokers. There was a statistically significant difference between the two groups at every examination after Exam 1 (P < .05). (From Ah et al, 1994. Reprinted with permission.)

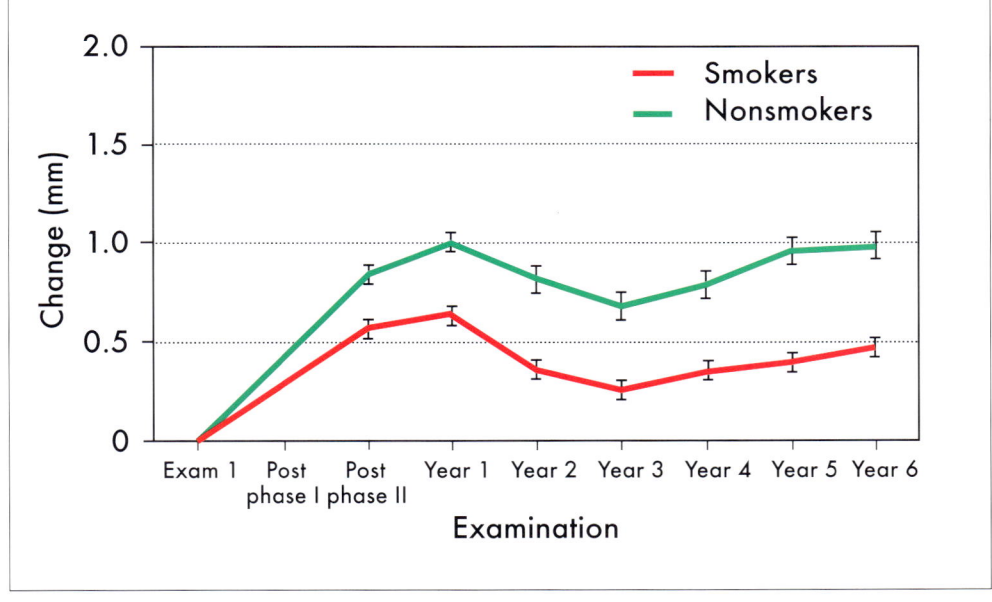

Fig 115 Mean change in probing attachment level (all modalities and severity categories combined) for smokers and nonsmokers. There was a statistically significant difference between the two groups at every examination after Post phase (P < .05). (From Ah et al, 1994. Reprinted with permission.)

Tonetti et al (1995) examined the effect of cigarette smoking on the healing response following guided tissue regeneration procedures in deep infrabony defects. Twenty patients (32 defects) smoked more than 10 cigarettes a day, and 31 patients (39 defects) did not smoke. Clinical measurements were taken at baseline, at membrane removal, and at the 1-year follow-up. The oral hygiene of both groups was good. No significant differences were observed in terms of percentage of tissue gained at membrane removal. At the 1-year follow-up, however, the gain in probing attachment level was significantly smaller in smokers (2.1 ± 1.2 mm) than in nonsmokers (5.2 ± 1.9 mm). A multivariate model, correcting for the oral hygiene level of the patients and the depth of the infrabony component, showed that smoking was in itself a significant factor in determining the clinical outcome. A risk-assessment analysis showed that the risk for poor gain in probing attachment level after guided tissue regeneration was significantly greater in smokers than in nonsmokers. It was concluded that cigarette smoking is associated with a poorer healing response to guided tissue regeneration procedures.

Recently Boström et al (1998) evaluated the 5-year outcome following periodontal surgery in 57 patients who had received regular maintenance care throughout the follow-up period. The study population included 20 smokers, 20 former smokers, and 17 nonsmokers aged 37 to 77 years. The clinical characteristics evaluated were supragingival plaque, gingival bleeding, and probing depth. In the region where surgery was planned, periodontal bone height was evaluated on radiographs. The occurrence of the periopathogens *A actinomycetemcomitans, P gingivalis,* and *P intermedia* and the gingival crevicular fluid levels of tumor necrosis factor-α (TNF-α) were assessed at follow-up.

The Plaque Index was 28.5% at baseline and 32.9% at follow-up, indicating high standards of oral hygiene. The corresponding values for gingival bleeding were 31.7% and 24.9%, respectively, suggesting a low to moderate level of gingival inflammation. In regions treated surgically, mean probing depth decreased significantly from 5.6 to 4.3 mm ($P < .001$) and mean periodontal bone height increased significantly from 62.5% to 67.5% ($P < .001$). In terms of bone height, the outcome was less favorable among smokers than among nonsmokers. There was a predominance of smokers among patients experiencing loss of bone height after 5 years of maintenance. No significant associations were found between treatment outcomes and supragingival plaque levels or subgingival occurrence of periopathogens. The TNF-α levels were significantly elevated in smokers (Boström et al, 1998).

In another recent 5-year longitudinal study, Söder et al (1999) evaluated periodontal treatment comprising initial nonsurgical treatment, systemic administration of metronidazole for 1 week, and scaling and root planing every 6 months for 5 years. The study population consisted of 64 subjects (37 smokers and 27 nonsmokers), mean age 36.3 ± 3.0 years, with severe periodontal disease. After initial scaling and root planing, the subjects were randomly assigned to intervention or placebo groups (400 mg metronidazole each or a placebo administered at 8-hour intervals for l week). The participants underwent an extensive clinical periodontal examination. Gingival crevicular fluid was analyzed for spirochetes and granulocytes. Samples were cultured for *A actinomycetemcomitans, P gingivalis,* and *P intermedia.*

The number of subjects infected with the culture periopathogens and spirochetes decreased during the study. Most patients who harbored spirochetes at the end of the study had had these microorganisms at the beginning of the study. Smokers responded less favorably to periodontal therapy than did nonsmokers. The nonsmokers in the intervention group, who required only nonsurgical therapy, showed statistically significant improvement in the clinical variables after 5 years. At the end of the study, the only subjects with "complete healing," ie, absence of inflamed sites of 5 mm or deeper, were found in the intervention group (Söder et al, 1999).

The data from these longitudinal studies confirm that smoking is an important risk factor and prognostic risk factor for periodontal disease and periodontal treatment efficacy and should be considered a possible contraindication to advanced forms of therapy, such as guided tissue regeneration and implants. Other types of smoking habits, including cigar and pipe smoking, have been shown to have detrimental effects similar to those attributed to cigarette smoking (Albandar et al, 2000; Krall et al, 1999).

Effects of tobacco products on the pathogenesis of periodontal diseases

The strong association betweeen tobacco (particularly cigarette smoking) and the severity of periodontal diseases can be explained by a number of biologic phenomena. Potential molecular and cellular mechanisms in the pathogenesis of smoking-associated periodontal diseases include immunosuppression, exaggerated inflammatory cell responses, and impaired stromal cell functions of oral tissues. There is evidence that tobacco products (especially tobacco smoking) exert both local and systemic effects. More than 6,000 known toxic products from tobacco smoking may together have severe harmful effects on both general health and the periodontal tissues (International Agency for Research on Cancer, 1986).

Local effects

Several findings support the existence of local effects of smoking in the pathogenesis of periodontal diseases. Among these are the patterns of tooth loss, loss of periodontal attachment, recession, and treatment needs (CPITN) in smokers and nonsmokers, discussed earlier (see Figs 109, 110, 112a, and 112b). Other local effects, including plaque retention, nicotine accumulation, and gingival changes, have been identified by numerous studies.

Staining from smoking is both toxic and plaque retentive. In addition, the heat from smoke may have thermal effects. This may explain why smokers have much more attachment loss and recession than do nonsmokers on the lingual surfaces of the maxillary teeth and the mandibular incisors (Axelsson et al, 1998; Haffajee and Socransky, 2001; Kalra et al, 1991; Lannan et al, 1992; Pabst et al, 1995; Selby et al, 1992). Smokers also have significantly more calculus, which is an important factor for retention of plaque (Feldman et al, 1983; Lindén and Mullally, 1994; Pindborg 1947, 1949).

Smokeless tobacco use has long been associated with localized loss of periodontal attachment and oral leukoplakia but not with severe periodontal destruction (Christen, 1970; Christen et al, 1979; Ernster et al, 1990; Johnson and Slach, 2001; Modeer et al, 1980; Robertson et al, 1990). Gingival recession and white lesions of the mucosa are frequent at sites where quids of smokeless tobacco are habitually placed. However, one study that investigated a sample of baseball players in the United States found no greater prevalence of periodontal disease among users of smokeless tobacco than among nonusers (Sinusas et al, 1992).

Nicotine accumulation has been demonstrated on the root surfaces of periodontally diseased teeth (Cuff et al, 1989), and its metabolite, cotinine, has been detected in gingival crevicular fluid and saliva (McGuire et al, 1989). When fibroblasts are exposed to nicotine in vitro, their growth and attachment to root surfaces is impaired (James et al, 1999; Raulin et al, 1988). Fibroblasts have been shown to bind nonspecifically and rapidly internalize nicotine (Hanes et al, 1991). Upon exposure to nicotine, fibroblast cells typically acquire atypical shapes and show the formation of vacuoles; these toxic effects become irreversible at higher concentrations of nicotine. In addition, exposure to nicotine results in decreased protein content and damage to the cell membranes (Alpar et al, 1998). There is also evidence from in vitro studies that nicotine can suppress proliferation of osteoblasts while it stimulates alkaline phosphatase activity (Fang et al, 1991). Together, these effects of nicotine could result in alteration of cellular metabolism, including collagen synthesis, protein secretion, and bone formation, and could have negative implications for periodontal disease susceptibility, wound healing, and the outcome of regenerative therapy (also see Tonetti et al, 1995). These observations may partly explain the role of such products in the progression of periodontitis.

The gingival tissue in smokers tends to be fibrotic and hyperkeratotic with thickened margins; in addition, it manifests minimal erythema and edema compared to that manifested by the gingival tissue of nonsmokers with disease of equal severity and similar plaque volume. Several studies have shown that smokers with periodontal disease have less clinical inflammation and gingival bleeding than do nonsmokers with the disease (Axelsson et al, unpublished data, 1990; Axelsson et al, 1998; Bergström and Floderus-Myrhed, 1983; Bergström, 1990; Feldman et al, 1983; Goultschin et al, 1990; Preber and Bergström, 1985, 1986b). Clinically, this change is of major importance because it may mask serious periodontal disease in smokers.

In a study by Danielsen et al (1990), the rate of plaque accumulation was similar in smokers and nonsmokers, but the increase in gingival vascularity in smokers was only half that in nonsmokers. This may be explained by the fact that nicotine, one of the numerous by-products of tobacco smoke, has a local vasoconstrictive effect, reducing blood flow, edema, and clinical signs of inflammation. There is a similar vasoconstrictive effect not only on peripheral circulation but also on coronary, placental, and gingival blood vessels (Baab and Öberg, 1987).

On the other hand, after an individual has not smoked for several weeks, gingival inflammation becomes more acute, and there is bleeding on brushing. These manifestations may persist for several months. Within about 1 year, the gingival tissue may revert from its thickened, fibrotic appearance to normal anatomy and contour. Recent observations by Hanioka et al (2000) have also shown that smokers exhibit lower function of oxygen sufficiency in healthy gingiva and reduced ability to adapt the function in inflamed gingiva when compared with nonsmokers. This suggests that smokers have functional impairments in the gingival microcirculation.

Dinsdale et al (1997) recently measured periodontal pocket temperature at healthy and diseased sites in smokers and nonsmokers. The mean periodontal pocket temperature was significantly higher in smokers at both healthy and diseased sites.

Smoking also reduces the short-term oxidation-reduction potentials (E_h) in dental plaque: Reduced oxygen levels are associated with a decrease in polymorphonuclear leukocyte (PMNL) mobility and an increase in the proportion of anaerobic bacteria (Palmer, 1988). In untreated deep periodontal sites, cigarette smoking has also been shown to decrease oxygen tension (Loesche et al, 1983; Mettraux et al, 1984), thereby creating a favorable subgingival environment for colonization and growth of gram-negative anaerobic periodontal pathogens.

Zambon et al (1996a) recently examined the association between cigarette smoking and infection with periodontal pathogens to determine whether smokers would be at greater risk for subgingival infection with target periodontal pathogens than nonsmokers. These investigators demonstrated that, in a dose-dependent manner, smokers harbored significantly higher levels of *B forsythus* and were at significantly greater risk of infection with this periodontal pathogen than were nonsmokers.

High PMNL elastase activity in gingival crevicular fluid seems to indicate nonresponders to scaling and root planing (refractory patients). In smokers, increased elastase activity, high levels of prostaglandin E_2 (PGE_2), and high levels of matrix metalloproteinase-8 in gingival crevicular fluid are probably associated with site-specific disease activity and indicate a risk for progression of the periodontal diseases in these sites (Söder, 1998b).

Systemic effects

There are many more known and probably many as yet unknown negative systemic effects of tobacco use, particularly cigarette smoking. However, some important negative effects will be discussed, which together increase susceptibility not only to periodontal diseases but also to many systemic and infectious diseases. Systemic alterations of the host response in cigarette smokers have been evaluated by several investigators.

Smoking exerts effects on both PMNLs and macrophage function (Palmer, 1988). Functional activities of both salivary and tissue PMNLs are reported to be suppressed. The chemotactic as well as the phagocytic functions of the PMNLs are impaired (Eichel and Sharik, 1969; Kenney et al, 1977; Kraal et al, 1977; Lannan et al, 1992; Noble and Penny, 1975). MacFarlane et al (1992) investigated PMNL functions in subjects with refractory periodontitis and periodontally healthy controls; it is notable that 90% of the patients with refractory periodontitis were current smokers. Compared with the controls, the group with refractory periodontitis had significantly impaired PMNL phagocytic capacity, suggesting that, in smokers, PMNL dysfunction may be considered a cofactor in the increased susceptibility to periodontal disease. It also indicates that smoking-mediated PMNL impairment is a characteristic of refractory disease. This was recently confirmed by Söder et al (1998b). Smoking also has major negative effects on the specific immune response. Decreased levels of salivary immunoglobulin A (IgA) and serum immunoglobulin G (IgG) to *P intermedia* and *F nucleatum* have been documented in smokers (Bennet and Read, 1982; Haber, 1994). Furthermore, there are data indicating that T-lymphocyte subset ratios may be altered in cigarette smokers, leading to impaired T-helper cell functions, which would compromise antibody production.

Smoking suppresses production of the IgG2 subclass of immunoglobulin both in patients with periodontitis and in periodontally normal individuals (Haber et al, 1993b; Quinn et al, 1998; Tew et al, 1996). Levels of IgG2 antibody specific for antigens of *A actinomycetemcomitans* are significantly lower in patients with chronic periodontitis and rapidly progressive periodontitis who smoked than in nonsmokers. Because the predominant serum antibody response to antigens of both *A actinomycetemcomitans* and *P gingivalis* is composed of the IgG2 subclass (Ling et al, 1993; Tangada et al, 1997; Whitney et al, 1992), suppression of IgG2 production may be a primary mechanism through which smoking enhances susceptibility to severe periodontitis. However, there is great individual as well as ethnic variation in the capacity to produce IgG2 antibodies in response to carbohydrate antigens, primarily the lipopolysaccharides, from periopathogens.

It has been reported that white young adult smokers have significantly lower levels of serum IgG2 than do their nonsmoking counterparts, while black young adult subjects are generally not affected by smoking. Thus, white adult subjects who smoked, including those with periodontitis, could experience more attachment loss than black adult subjects, and smoking would be associated with lower serum IgG2 levels in white adults, but not in black adults.

This hypothesis was recently tested by Quinn et al (1998). The patient's smoking status was established from serum cotinine levels, determined by radioimmunoassay. Serum IgG subclass levels were determined with radial immunodiffusion. White smokers, both those with and those without chronic periodontitis, had greater mean attachment loss per site than did their nonsmoking counterparts. Furthermore, white smokers with chronic periodontitis and their age-matched controls (white smokers without periodontitis) had substantially less IgG2 in their serum. In marked contrast, no increase in periodontal destruction or significant decrease in serum IgG2 levels in black smokers with chronic periodontitis or their age-matched controls was detected. However, IgG1 and IgG4 levels were reduced in smoking black subjects with chronic periodontitis. IgG3 was the only subclass in adults that was unaffected by smoking. IgG2 can be a good opsonin and may help control periodontitis-associated bacteria in adults. Although a cause-and-effect relationship has not been established, there was a striking association between a smoking-related decrease in serum IgG2 levels and an increase in periodontal destruction in white subjects (Quinn et al, 1998).

High titers of serum IgG2 reactive with *A actinomycetemcomitans* are present in patients with aggressive periodontitis and it appears that antibodies against *A actinomycetemcomitans* may be protective. Smoking is associated with increased disease severity in individuals with GAP, but is not associated with disease severity in patients with LAP. Furthermore, smoking is associated with reduced serum IgG2 levels in black patients with GAP but not in those with LAP, and smoking does not appear to increase the risk for periodontal breakdown in patients with LAP (Tew et al, 1996). Based on this selective effect of smoking, Tangada et al (1997) hypothesized that smoking would be associated with a reduction of specific IgG2 reactive with *A actinomycetemcomitans* in black patients with GAP but not black patients with LAP. In addition, they examined IgG2 responses to carbohydrate antigens from nonperiodontal pathogens, including *Haemophilus influenzae* type b oligosaccharide antigen and the *Streptococcus pneumoniae* antigen, phosphocholine. Smoking status was assessed from serum cotinine levels, and IgG2 specific for *A actinomycetemcomitans, H influenzae* type b, and phosphocholine was assessed. The study revealed that smoking was correlated with a dramatic reduction in serum IgG2 anti–*A actinomycetemcomitans* in smokers with GAP but not in smokers with LAP. In contrast, anti–*H influenzae* type b IgG2 and antiphosphocholine IgG2 were not affected in those with GAP or LAP. In short, these results indicate that smoking is associated with a reduction in serum IgG2 anti–*A actinomycetemcomitans* in black subjects with GAP, but IgG2 reactive with other antigens may not be reduced in smokers with GAP.

Studies by Payne et al (1996) demonstrate that nicotine upregulates monocytic release of PGE_2 and interleukin-1 (IL-1) in response to lipopolysaccharide and may contribute to the increased periodontal tissue destruction observed in smokers. In the presence of vasoconstriction and the hyperkeratotic response to physical heat and chemical stimuli, this could account for the paradoxical clinical presentation of severe pocketing and bone loss without dramatic clinical signs of inflammation. Payne et al (1994) also showed that the combination of smokeless tobacco and lipopolysaccharide in vitro potentiates the release of PGE_2 and IL-1β compared to lipopolysaccharide.

In an in vivo study, Poore et al (1995) examined the effect of smokeless tobacco on gingival inflammation, assessed clinically and biochemically by gingival crevicular fluid levels of PGE_2, IL-1α, and IL-1β. These variables were compared in users of smokeless tobacco and control subjects, matched for plaque and probing depth levels, who did not use tobacco. Both Gingival Index and the concentration of PGE_2 in gingival crevicular fluid were significantly ($P < .05$) greater at smokeless tobacco placement sites than at sites in control subjects. The aforementioned longitudinal study by Söder et al (1998b) revealed that, compared to nonsmokers, smokers had elevated levels of PGE_2, metalloproteinase-8, and PMNL-elastase in the gingival crevicular fluid. Recently Bernzweig et al (1998) presented data indicating that nicotine and smokeless tobacco stimulate peripheral blood mononuclear cells to secrete PGE_2; however, they cannot further activate mononuclear cells extracted from gingiva, possibly because the cells were previously exposed to maximal stimulation in the periodontitis lesion.

Smoking decreases intestinal absorption of calcium and may thereby affect osteoblast function and increase bone loss in otherwise healthy postmenopausal women and in older men (Daniell, 1976; Hollenbach et al, 1993). However, the direct relationship between smoking-related osteoporosis and periodontal disease is unclear. It is estimated that smokers are exposed to two to three times more toxic oxygen free radicals than are nonsmokers (Kalra et al, 1991).

A toxic effect of tobacco on endothelial cells has been reported as evidenced by increased levels of the procoagulant von Willebrand factor (VWF) after exposing epithelial cells to nicotine and by increased levels of VWF in smokers compared to nonsmokers (Blann and McCollum, 1987). Thus, smoking-induced endothelial damage may operate as the initial event in the impaired healing response observed in smokers. Following endothelial compromise, adhesion and migration of competent cells to the healing site may be impaired. Figure 116 summarizes how and where smoking may interact as a modifying risk factor in the pathogenesis of periodontal diseases. In addition, it is well-known that smokers exhibit much higher prevalence of cardiovascular diseases, cancer (particularly lung cancer), allergic diseases,

Fig 116 Schematic illustration of how and where smoking may interact as a modifying risk factor in the pathogenesis of periodontal diseases. PMNLs = Polymorphonuclear leukocytes. (Courtesy of R. Page.)

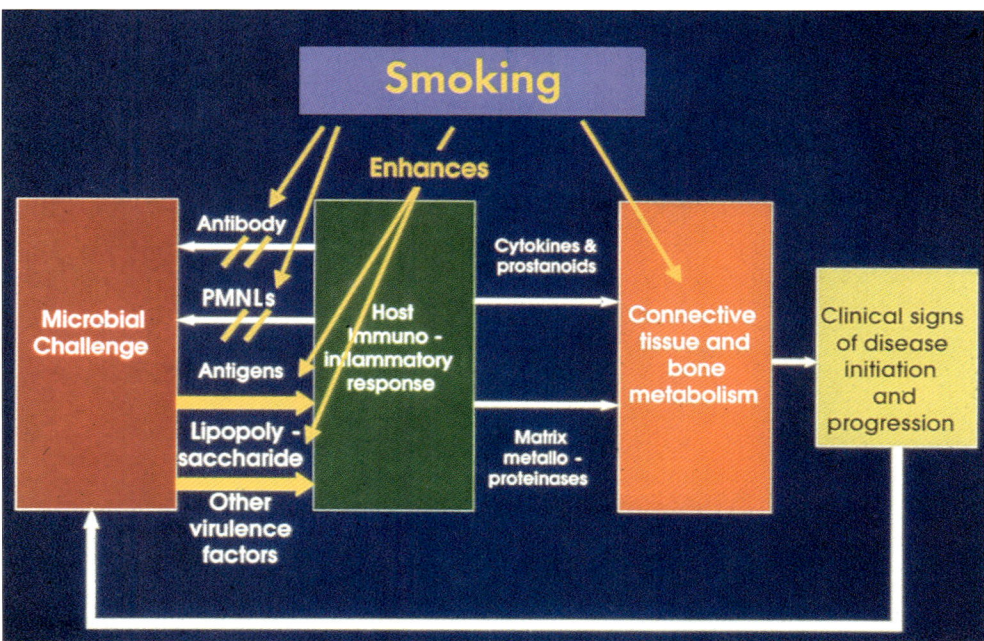

and infectious diseases, which together increase susceptibility to periodontal diseases as well.

In conclusion, the role of tobacco, particularly smoking, as a powerful external (environmental) risk indicator, risk factor, and prognostic risk factor for periodontal disease has been extensively studied in numerous cross-sectional, case-control, longitudinal, and intervention studies. These studies used representative population samples or selective groups long associated with increased use of tobacco. In many of the studies, multivariate analyses showed that smoking was an independent risk factor for periodontal disease, after the analysis controlled for oral hygiene, plaque, calculus, and socioeconomic and demographic factors.

It appears that the risk for periodontitis is considerable if an individual uses tobacco products, with estimated odds ratios of 2.5 to 7.0 or even greater for smokers. A meta-analysis of data from a number of studies examining the effect of smoking on loss of periodontal tissue support (Papapanou, 1996) confirmed smoking as a risk factor for the disease, but with a lower odds ratio (2.8). However, approximately half the periodontitis observed in individuals younger than 33 years is thought to be smoking related, with the odds ratio

for the presence of established periodontitis and smoking being 14.0 or greater (Lindén and Mullally, 1994; Schenkein et al, 1995).

Further support that smoking is a risk factor for periodontal disease is provided by studies in which the frequency of smoking or the consumption of a certain quantity of cigarettes over a period of time has been positively correlated with increasing levels of risk of periodontal disease observed among current smokers (see Fig 105). Disease expression is more severe among current smokers than former smokers, while the risk is lowest in those who have never smoked. In refractory periodontal disease, characterized by low plaque scores and poor healing response to periodontal therapy, smoking may also be an important factor; most individuals with refractory periodontitis are heavy smokers. Smoking delays healing and impairs the quality of repair after periodontal therapy, nonsurgical, surgical, and regenerative therapy. Smoking also increases the risk for progressive periodontal attachment loss and tooth loss in patients with generalized aggressive periodontitis.

Compared to nonsmokers, smokers generally have more severe attachment loss in the anterior

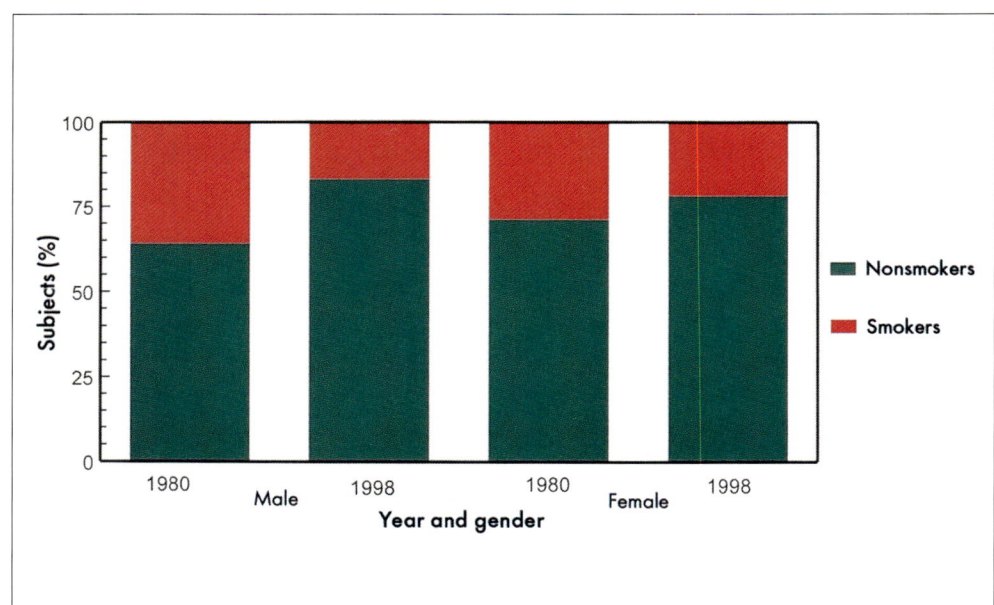

Fig 117a The reduction in the number of smokers among the male and female Swedish population from 1980 to 1998.

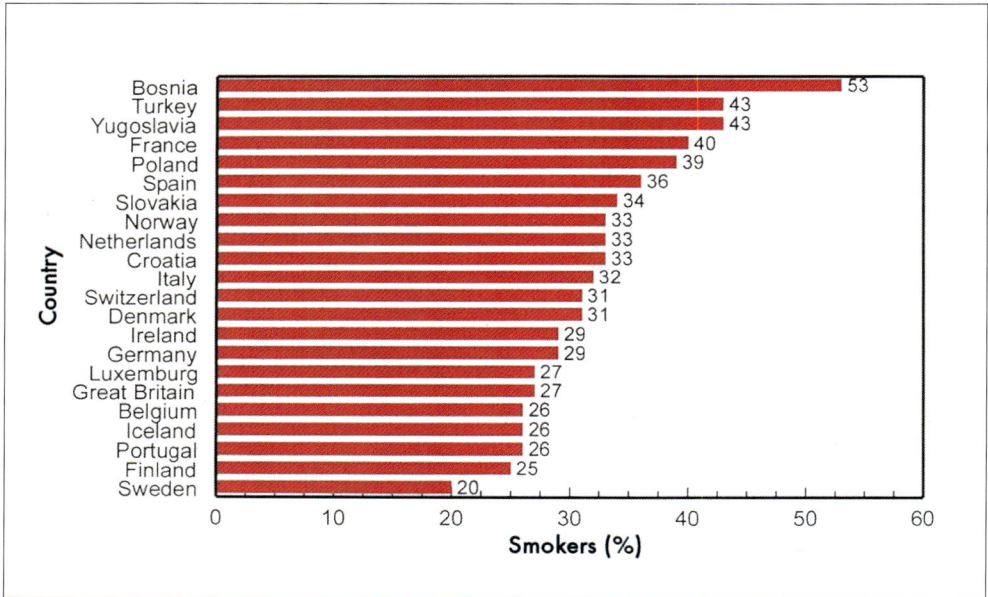

Fig 117b The percentage of smokers in different European countries in 1998.

region, especially the palatal aspects of the maxillary anterior teeth, than around posterior teeth, confirming that smoking also has severe local effects on the pathogenesis of periodontal disease. There are also new data showing that adults who have used smokeless tobacco (snuff) for several years have lost more teeth and periodontal attachment than have nonsnuffers (Axelsson and Paulander, 1994). In the study by Kornman et al

(1997a), smoking and genetic factors (particularly genetic interleukin-1β polymorphism) together identified more than 85% of individuals with enhanced susceptibility to severe periodontitis. Because genetic factors are unchangeable, to reduce the global prevalence and severity of periodontal diseases, it is important that smokers be encouraged to stop smoking and that children and young adults be dissuaded from starting to smoke. Given that nicotine is addictive, and studies have shown that the smoking debut occurs as early as 12 to 14 years of age, preventing children and young adults from starting to smoke would be the most cost-effective measure, from a long-term perspective. Apart from the effect on prevention and control of periodontal diseases, there would be a positive effect on other serious systemic conditions, such as cardiovascular diseases, cancer, allergies, infectious diseases, and prenatally acquired diseases.

However, much remains to be done. The total world consumption of cigarettes continues to increase. In 1997, about 6 billion cigarettes were consumed; this represents approximately 1,000 cigarettes per person per year, including every individual in the world, from newborn babies to 100 year olds. This is not only a health problem but also a serious global pollution problem. According to the World Health Organization's goals, the prevalence of smokers should have been less than 20% of the population by the year 2000. So far only in Sweden do smokers compose less than 20% of the population (19.7% in 1998, 17% males and 22% females) (Fig 117a). Among smokers in Sweden, 23% smoked 15 or more cigarettes per day. The highest percentages of smokers in Europe are found in Bosnia (53%), Turkey (43%), Yugoslavia (43%), France (40%), Poland (39%), and Spain (36%) (Fig 117b). Consumption of cigars, pipe tobacco, and smokeless tobacco is also high (for reviews on the role of tobacco use, particularly cigarette smoking, as a modifying risk factor for periodontal diseases, see Axelsson et al, 1998; Bergström and Preber, 1994; Haber et al, 1993a; Haber, 1994; Page and Beck, 1997; Salvi et al, 1997a; Tonetti, 1998).

ROLE OF LOW SOCIOECONOMIC STATUS

Socioeconomic factors related to high periodontal disease experience are low eduction, low in-

come, and geographic isolation (Fox et al, 1994). The cumulative effect of these factors can clearly be seen in the elderly. Historically, the high-income classes have always been interested in oral hygiene and have been able to afford dental care. Urban residents also have better access to dental care than do those living in rural areas (Fox et al, 1994). In Scandinavia, the welfare policy has managed to level out these differences, at least among those younger than 40 years (Helöe et al, 1988; Hugoson et al, 1986a, 1986b). The percentage of well-educated adults is steadily increasing in every age group, and the difference in net after-tax income between well-educated and poorly educated people is less pronounced. In addition, most adults in Scandinavia today receive regular dental care. Historically, levels of periodontal disease have been related to lower socioeconomic status (SES): Gingivitis and poor oral hygiene are clearly related to lower SES, but the relationship with severe periodontitis in particular is more uncertain. The 1985 to 1986 US national survey (Miller et al, 1987b) found that the prevalence of periodontal attachment loss at all levels of severity was not closely related to household income (Brown and Meskin, 1988). Attachment loss greater than 4 mm and less than 7 mm in at least one site was closely correlated with educational levels. For periodontal attachment loss of greater than 2 mm, the correlation was much weaker because this value was so commonly recorded.

Among other things, SES and gingival health are a function of better oral hygiene among the better educated, and a greater frequency of dental attendance among the more dentally aware and those with dental insurance (who are more likely to be white-collar employees, ie, those with higher education). Although racial and ethnic differences in periodontal status have been demonstrated many times, it is still not clear whether these are true genetic differences or are confounded by SES, a complex and multifaceted variable that can include a variety of cultural factors. Studies comparing populations from developing countries with those from industrialized countries have suggested an association between periodontal disease and nutritional deficiencies in developing countries. However, Ramfjord et al (1968) found that the periodontal condition of young men in India who exhibited clinical symptoms of general malnutrition did not differ from that of well-nourished individuals. A nutritional survey of 700 men in Alaska reported similar findings (Russell et al, 1961). Other studies comparing the periodontal status of individuals in developed and in developing countries of varying levels of socioeconomic status also failed to show a relationship between periodontal disease and nutrition.

Another perspective comes from early studies of periodontal disease in developed countries such as the United States, where it was found that periodontal disease was more severe in individuals of lower socioeconomic status (US Public Health Service 1965, 1979). However, in more recent studies, periodontal status has been adjusted for difference in oral hygiene and smoking habits, and no association between lower socioeconomic status and more severe periodontal disease has been observed (Grossi et al, 1994, 1995).

In all the cross-sectional studies, and in the few longitudinal studies, educational level has proven to be the most important socioeconomic factor related to tooth loss and periodontal diseases.

Evidence from cross-sectional studies

Nikias et al (1977) conducted a cross-sectional study on nearly 1,300 adult members of a prepaid medical group plan in New York City. Oral status indicators were developed, including the number of missing teeth, scores to measure levels of gingival and periodontal disease, Simplified Oral Hygiene Index scores, and ratios of carious teeth. With each of these oral status measures, the interrelationship of economic status, education, and ethnic origin was evaluated. As shown in Table 10, variations in number of missing teeth, oral hygiene levels, and levels of gingival and periodontal diseases were attributed primarily to educational level. Ethnic group differences could be explained in part by differences in economic and educational levels.

A similar epidemiologic survey was carried out by Plasschaert et al (1978) to assess the prevalence

Table 10 Oral conditions by economic status and education*

	Low economic status			Medium economic status			High economic status		
	Grammar school	High school	College	Grammar school	High school	College	Grammar school	High school	College
No. of persons[†]	97	140	31	65	163	94	9[‡]	74	200
Six or more missing teeth (%)	65	61	39	62	50	36	–	54	28
Medium or high gingival and periodontal disease (%)	66	54	48	72	54	39	–	53	37
OHI-S[§] greater than 2.0 (%)	58	46	32	58	33	28	–	51	25
Carious teeth ratio greater than 0% (%)	53	51	71	37	48	43	–	45	38
Ratio of restored teeth less than 100% (%)	68	56	74	48	52	46	–	46	40

*Reprinted from Nikias et al (1977) with permission.
[†]Largest number for each subgroup; actual number is slightly lower for some conditions.
[‡]Number in subgroup too low; percentage not presented.
[§]OHI-S = Simplified Oral Hygiene Index.

and severity of periodontal disease in randomly selected samples of employed populations in the Netherlands. Of the 1,337 persons examined, 19.8% were edentulous. Of the dentate subjects, 61.0% had severe gingivitis in an average of 2.4 segments; 53.0% had 3- to 6-mm pockets, and a further 10.1% had pockets deeper than 6 mm. The prevalence of gingivitis and pocketing increased with increasing age and decreasing levels of education. The average number of teeth missing in 45- to 54-year-old men was 24.2 among the poorly educated and 14.8 among the well educated.

In an interview study among 60-year-old Australians, Slade et al (1993) evaluated the prevalence of edentulism in relation to education level, weekly household income, and prevalence of chronic diseases. The percentage of edentulism was significantly related to educational level but not to the number of chronic diseases.

The New England Elders Dental Study (NEEDS) by Fox et al (1994) is the first to document the periodontal disease status of a probability sample of residents aged 70 to 96 years of an entire US Public Health Service Region. The study disclosed substantially higher estimates of periodontal destruction among older adults than previous national studies would suggest, most likely a consequence of decreasing prevalence of edentulism and increasing numbers of remaining teeth among the elderly.

In the NEEDS study, the degree of periodontal attachment loss (limited = 0 to 3 mm, moderate = 4 to 6 mm, and severe = more than 6 mm) was evaluated in relation to gender, whether one or both arches were dentate, educational status, rural or urban residency, and annual income. The degree of attachment loss was strictly correlated with educational status (Fig 118).

Oliver et al (1991) examined the epidemiologic evidence of periodontitis in relation to socioeconomic variables and dental attendance habits in the employed population (more than 15,000 subjects, 18 to 64 years old) as assessed in the National Institute of Dental Research's *Oral Health of United States Adults 1985-1986 Survey* (Miller et al, 1987a, 1987b). Tables 11 and 12 show

the prevalence of subjects and number of sites with greater than 3-mm attachment loss, greater than 4-mm probing depth, and greater than 3-mm recession in the five different age groups, in relation to years of schooling (Table 11) and annual income (Table 12). It is clear that the prevalence and extent of attachment loss, probing depth, and recession were more closely correlated to different standards of education than to different levels of income. In a second analysis of the same adult survey database, the sample population was divided into deciles according to the prevalence and extent of periodontitis (four sites with greater than 4-mm or two sites with greater than 6-mm probing depths) and evaluated for demographic, socioeconomic, behavioral, and clinical risk factors (Table 13). Among demographic variables, men constituted 88.7% of the most diseased group and 26.1% of the healthiest group. Blacks constituted 10.0% of the sample but 20.7% of the most diseased group and 3.5% of the healthiest group. The strongest difference among socioeconomic variables was education. Those who had not completed high school comprised 43.1% of the most diseased group and only 1.1% of the healthiest group. Income and dental insurance were not significant. The only behavioral variable tested was the most recent dental appointment. In the most diseased group, 37.0% had not been to a dentist in the last 3 years. In the healthiest group, 76.0% had been to the dentist in the last year. Gingival bleeding and subgingival calculus were the clinical explanatory variables tested. The prevalence of gingival bleeding was 10.0% in the healthiest group and 88.4% in the most diseased group. Everyone in the most diseased group had subgingival calculus, but no one in the healthiest group did.

Multivariate analyses provided odds ratios to assess the relative strength of the variables. Subgingival calculus was by far the strongest at 11.1. Advanced age, a lower level of education, and gingival bleeding had odds ratios approaching 2.1. Race, income, insurance, and latest dental appointment were not individually strong predictors. The highest risk profile, a person older than

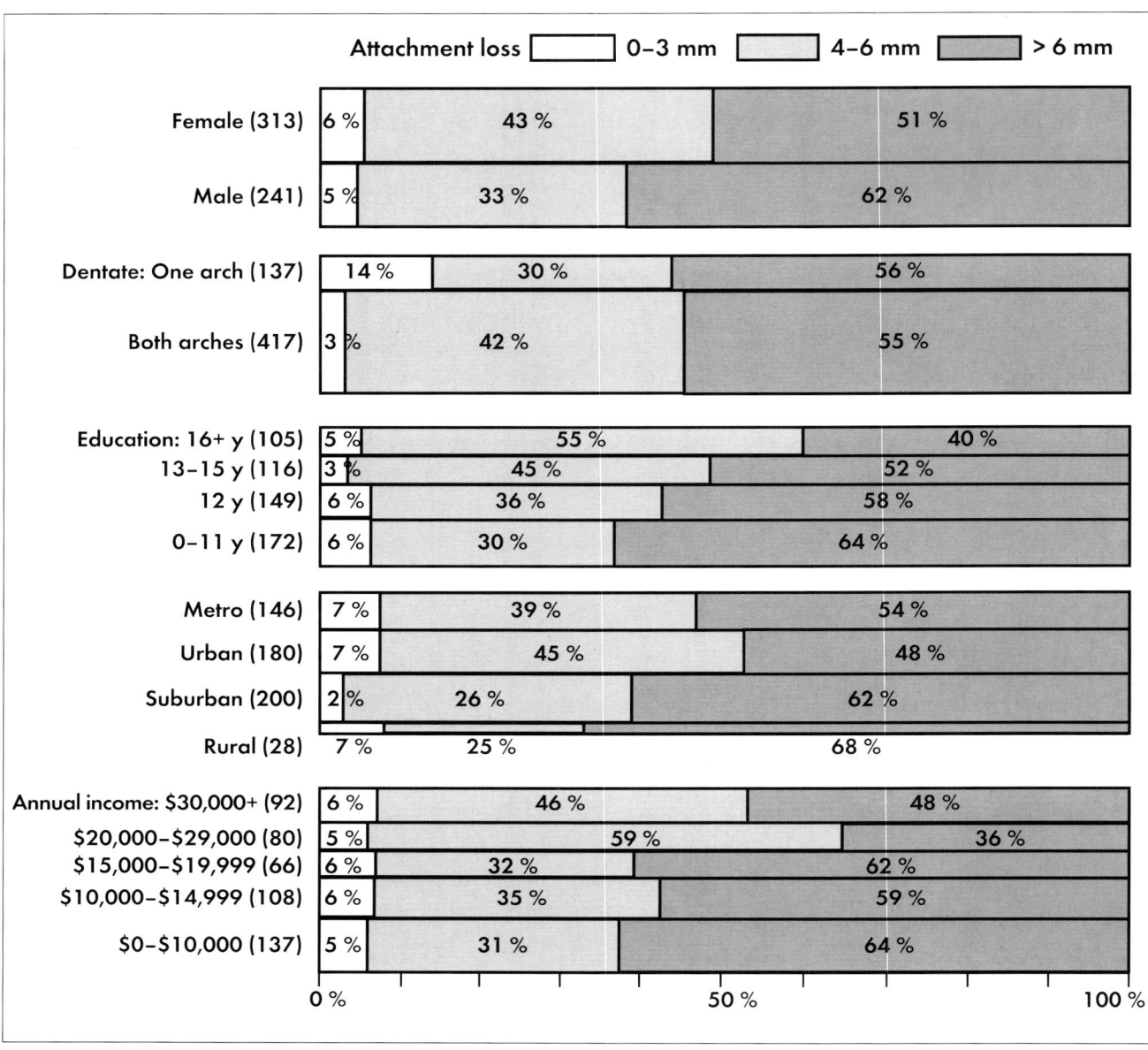

Fig 118 Periodontal attachment loss in relation to gender, remaining dentition, educational level, locale, and annual income. (From Fox et al, 1994. Reprinted with permission.)

34 years with less than 12 years education, subgingival calculus, and gingival bleeding and who had not been to the dentist for more than 3 years, had an odds ratio of 79.1 for the presence of multiple periodontal pockets (Oliver et al, 1998).

In the previously described large-scale analytic epidemiologic study in a randomized sample of 35, 50, 65, and 75 year olds (n = 1,086), representing the whole county of Värmland (Axelsson et al, unpublished data, 1990; Axelsson et al, 1998), the role of educational level on oral health status was also evaluated. Figure 118 shows the percentage of poorly and well-educated subjects in the four age groups, diochotmized into ele-

Table 11 Prevalence and extent of loss of attachment, pockets, and recession, by years of schooling, for employed US adults, 1985*

Age (y)	Schooling (y)	Loss of attachment > 3 mm (%)		Pockets > 4 mm (%)		Recession > 3 mm (%)	
		Subjects	Sites†	Subjects	Sites†	Subjects	Sites†
All	< 12	61	10	26	5	28	5
	12	44	8	15	5	18	5
	> 12	41	7	11	4	15	5
18–24	< 12	27	6	20	3	6	3
	12	16	4	6	3	3	2
	> 12	13	4	3	5	2	3
25–34	< 12	46	8	23	5	10	6
	12	40	7	16	5	10	4
	> 12	31	5	10	4	8	3
35–44	< 12	64	11	33	5	27	4
	12	50	9	22	5	19	5
	> 12	46	7	13	4	15	5
45–54	< 12	76	10	26	4	42	5
	12	68	8	21	4	36	5
	> 12	64	8	16	5	29	5
55–64	< 12	85	10	28	4	54	6
	12	78	11	18	5	53	6
	< 12	75	10	16	4	38	6

*Reprinted from Oliver et al (1991) with permission.
†Half-mouth scores multiplied (× 2) in subjects with one or more sites or pockets. All fractions rounded to nearest whole number.

Table 12 Prevalence and extent of loss attachment pockets, and recession, by income, among employed US adults, 1985*

Age (y)	Income (US$)	Loss of attachment > 3 mm		Pockets > 4 mm		Recession > 3 mm	
		Subjects (%)	Sites (No.)†	Subjects (%)	Sites (No.)†	Subjects (%)	Sites (No.)†
All	< 20,000	41	8	16	5	16	5
	20,000–39,999	44	7	15	5	17	5
	≥ 40,000	43	8	10	4	17	5
18–24	< 20,000	19	4	8	3	4	2
	20,000–39,999	12	4	3	5	2	3
	≥ 40,000	11	5	6	5	1	4
25–34	< 20,000	38	7	13	5	9	4
	20,000–39,999	35	6	13	4	9	4
	≥ 40,000	28	5	8	4	7	3
35–44	< 20,000	57	9	27	5	24	4
	20,000–39,999	48	7	18	5	16	5
	≥ 40,000	43	7	11	4	15	5
45–54	< 20,000	71	9	27	4	38	5
	20,000–39,999	69	9	23	5	34	5
	40,000	62	8	12	4	29	5
55–64	< 20,000	78	10	16	4	42	7
	20,000–39,999	80	10	15	4	47	5
	≥ 40,000	71	11	10	4	42	6

*Reprinted from Oliver et al (1991) with permission.
†Half-mouth scores multiplied (× 2) in those persons with one or more sites or pockets. All fractions rounded to nearest whole number.

Table 13 Demographic, socioeconomic, behavioral, and clinical characteristics of highest and lowest risk deciles*

Variable	Highest risk (%)	Lowest risk (%)
Age: Over 34 years	93.1	17.4
Gender: Male	88.7	26.1
Race: Black	20.7	3.5
Education: < 12 y	43.1	1.1
Income: < US$20,000	33.1	31.7
No insurance	50.7	29.3
≥ 3 y since last dental visit	37.0	5.9
Subgingival calculus	100.0	0.0
Gingival bleeding	88.4	10.0
Probing depth:	20.4	0.4
4 sites > 4 mm or		
2 sites > 6 mm		

*Reprinted from Oliver et al (1998) with permission.

mentary school level (6 to 9 years) and more than elementary school level. In 1988, only 22% of 35 year olds had a low-level education, compared to 72% of the 75 year olds. By extrapolation, in the year 2028, about 80% of the 75 year olds will be well educated. Most adults are already obliged to undergo further training to maintain their increasingly skilled work. There is also growing health awareness as the whole population is increasingly exposed to health information from newspapers, television, and the Internet.

Among the group of 50 year olds (n = 448), there are almost equal numbers of poorly and well-educated subjects. This particular group is larger than the other ages groups because it has been followed longitudinally for 10 years. Hundreds of variables involved in this study are currently under evaluation by multivariate analyses.

Figures 119 and 120 show the 1988 baseline values for the percentage of edentulism (Fig 119) and the mean number of teeth (Fig 120), third molars excluded, among subjects with low education and high education in the four different age groups (Axelsson et al, unpublished data, 1990). Even in 1988, edentulism was clearly rare up to the age of 65 years among the subjects educated beyond elementary school level. Among the den-

tate, the well-educated subjects had significantly more remaining teeth, particularly from the age of 50 years. Although the main reason for missing teeth in the 35 year olds was extraction of premolars during orthodontic treatment, poorly educated subjects had still lost almost one tooth more than had highly educated subjects.

Figure 121 shows the mean loss of probing periodontal attachment on the mesial surfaces in the four age groups. To exclude iatrogenic recession on the buccal surfaces, only the mesial values are presented. With the exception of the 65 year olds, poorly educated subjects had significantly more probing attachment loss than did highly educated subjects. The frequency distribution of sites with CPITN scores 1 to 4 and missing sites in the four age groups is presented in Fig 122. In all age groups, subjects with less education had fewer healthy sites and more missing sites than did those with a high level of education. Particularly among the 35 year olds, poorly educated subjects had more calculus that required removal (CPITN score 2) and diseased 4- to 5-mm pockets (CPITN score 3). The less pronounced differences in existing treatment needs between poorly and highly educated subjects in the other age groups are probably attributable to extraction of the most diseased teeth (particularly molars) in the poorly educated subjects.

In conclusion, this cross-sectional study has shown that low educational level is a powerful risk indicator for tooth loss and periodontal diseases. Multivariate analyses of data from the 10-year longitudinal part of the study will disclose whether low educational level is a true risk factor for tooth loss, periodontal diseases, and dental caries (Axelsson et al, unpublished data, 1990; Axelsson et al, 1998; Paulander et al, 2002).

In the cross-sectional study of a randomized sample of almost 600 individuals aged 50 to 55 years discussed earlier (Axelsson and Paulander, 1994), it was shown that individuals with only elementary-level schooling had lost 7.7 teeth, compared with 3.5 lost teeth ($P < .001$) in individuals with higher educational levels (see Fig 103). Also, individuals with elementary-level schooling ex-

Fig 119 Baseline values for edentulism among subjects with low education (LE) and high education (HE), defined as elementary school (6 to 9 years) and more than elementary school, respectively.

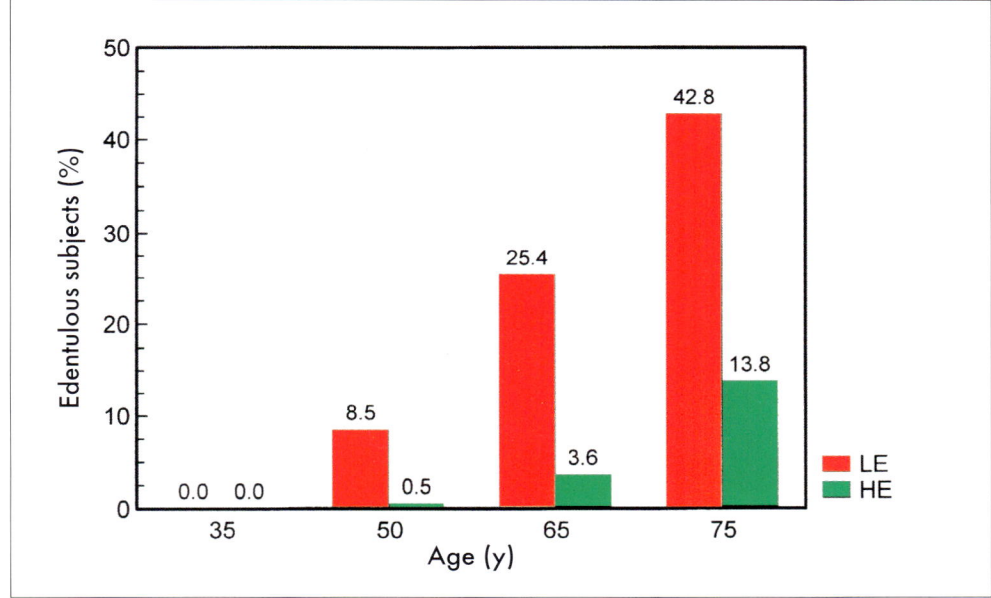

Fig 120 Baseline values for mean numbers of teeth among subjects with low education (LE) and high education (HE), defined as elementary school (6 to 9 years) and more than elementary school, respectively.

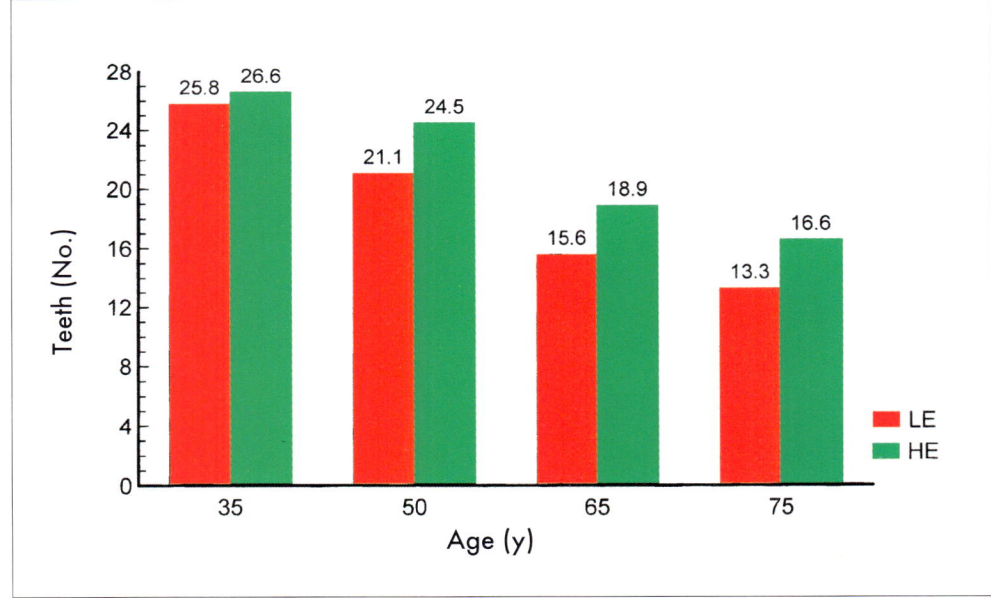

hibited 1.85 mm of periodontal attachment loss on the mesial sites versus 1.4 mm in individuals with higher education levels ($P = .001$) (Fig 104).

In an earlier investigation, Markkanen et al (1985) conducted a large-scale epidemiologic study on a randomized sample of 8,000 subjects representing the Finnish population 30 years and older. Periodontal status was recorded according to the modified Periodontal Treatment Need System (PTNS) in relation to urban or rural region, gender, educational level, and family income.

In age-matched groups, there were limited differences in PTNS between subjects with low and high educational level as well as between those with low and high family income. However, this could be explained by the fact that the percentages of individuals with fewer than four teeth (including edentulous subjects) were 55% among

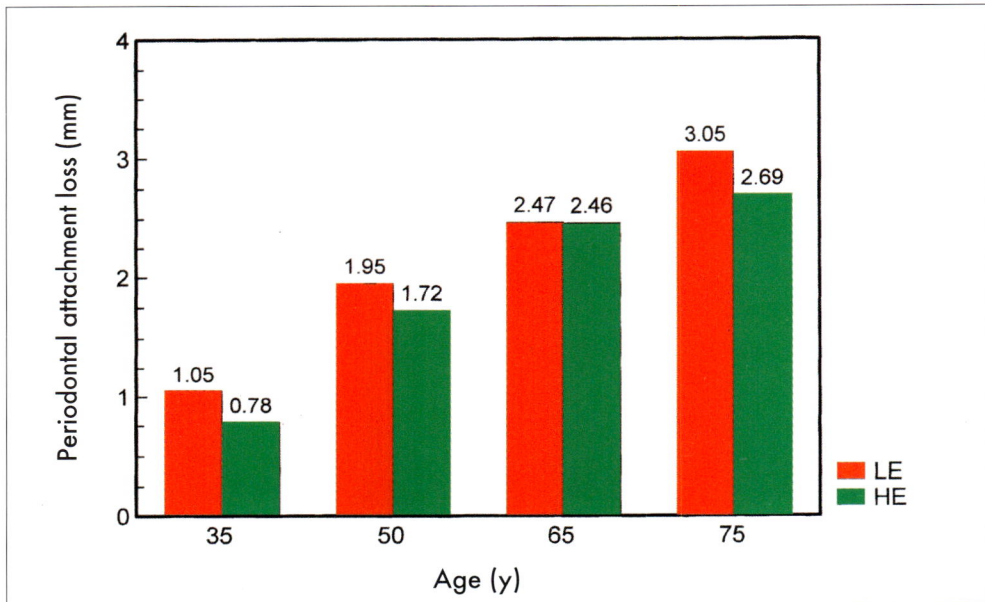

Fig 121 Baseline values for mean periodontal attachment loss at mesial sites among subjects with low education (LE) and high education (HE), defined as elementary school (6 to 9 years) and more than elementary school, respectively.

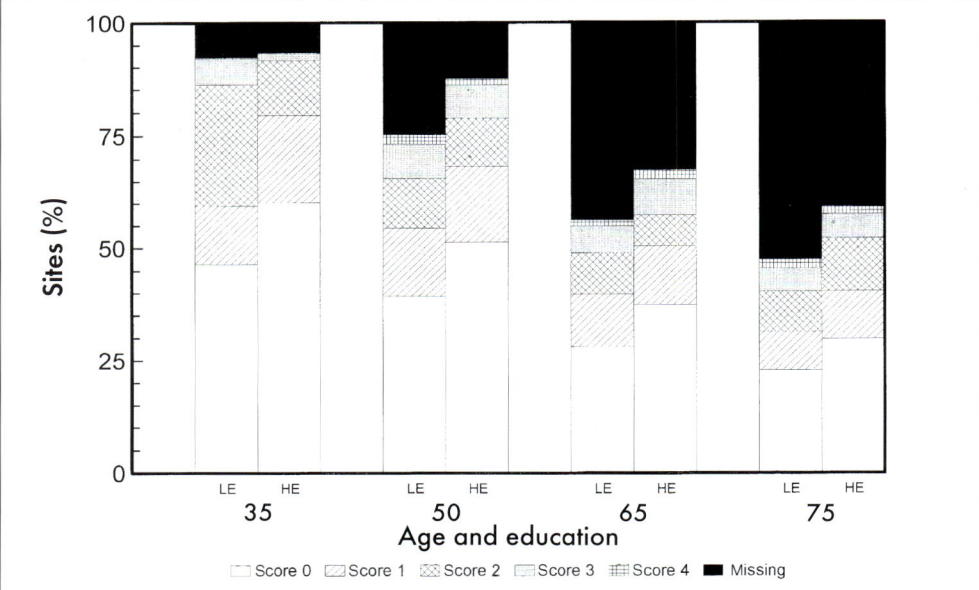

Fig 122 Baseline distribution of CPITN scores among subjects with low education (LE) and high education (HE), defined as elementary school (6 to 9 years) and more than elementary school, respectively.

poorly educated females and only 22% among well-educated females, and 52% and 27%, respectively, among subjects with low and high family incomes.

Evidence from longitudinal studies

As emphasized earlier, most current population-based information about risk factors for periodontitis is derived from cross-sectional studies: They are not risk factors, but risk indicators, which in longitudinal studies may or may not prove to be risk factors. To determine how frequently risk indicators were confirmed as risk predictors or risk factors, Beck et al (1990) compared the cross-sectional findings from the Piedmont (United States) baseline examination with the longitudinal findings from the same study. Table 14 presents risk indicators for serious periodontal disease at baseline and associated odds ratios for blacks, and whether or not the risk indicators appeared as risk factors for attachment loss over 3 years. At baseline, serious periodontal disease was defined as four or more sites with loss of attachment of greater than 5 mm, one or more of which had a probing depth greater than 4 mm. The indicator with the strongest association with serious periodontal disease was an interview item asking whether the subject had experienced bleeding gingiva in the last 2 weeks: The odds of being in the group with serious disease were 3.2 for those who responded affirmatively. However, neither this indicator nor educational level was confirmed in predicting future attachment loss. People who used tobacco had 2.8 times the odds of being in the group with serious periodontal disease, and tobacco use was confirmed as a risk factor with the same odds ratio. The presence of *P gingivalis* was confirmed as a risk factor, as was *P intermedia*. The risk indicator of having had the most recent dental appointment more than 3 years ago was not confirmed as a risk factor and neither were a number of other risk indicators. In this analysis, risk indicators were unlikely to be con-

firmed as risk factors or risk predictors (Beck, 1994b).

To date there are few available data from longitudinal studies on the relationship between periodontal diseases and educational level. In a 10-year longitudinal study based on national data, Eklund and Burt (1994) evaluated risk factors for total tooth loss in the United States. Tables 15 and 16 show the incidence of edentulism related to educational level and family income.

In the previously discussed 10-year longitudinal study of a randomized sample of 50 year olds who were followed from 1988 until 1998, when they were 60 years old (Axelsson et al, 2000), the number of lost teeth (mean = 0.7) and periodontal attachment was very low because more than 95% of the adult population in the county of Värmland, Sweden, receive regular needs-related maintenance care. Figure 123 shows the mean number of lost teeth per individual per 10 years related to smoking habits, Plaque Index, sex, educational level, rural or urban living environment, and regularity of dental care. Because of the aforementioned well-maintained population, only smoking and high Plaque Index were significant risk factors for tooth loss. However, the mean value of lost teeth in individuals with low educational levels was 0.8 compared with 0.6 for those with higher educational levels.

Table 14 Comparison of risk indicators for serious periodontal disease with risk factors for > 3-mm attachment loss over 3 years (bivariate analyses) in blacks*

Baseline individual risk indicator	Odds ratio	Status as risk factor	Odds ratio
Schooling < 8 y	3.1	Not confirmed	
Tobacco use	2.8	Confirmed	2.8
P gingivalis–positive	2.7	Confirmed	2.6
P intermedia–positive	1.9	Confirmed	1.9
Time since last visit to dentist > 3 y	2.7	Not confirmed	
Gingiva bled in last 2 wk	3.2	Not confirmed	
Socioeconomic status below median	1.7	Not confirmed	
Has morning cough	2.2	Not confirmed	
Money meets needs poorly	2.0	Not confirmed	

*Reprinted from Beck (1994b) with permission.

Table 15 Weighted estimates of the 10-year incidence of edentulism, expressed as the percentage of 6,365 US adults, by individual educational level and baseline age, 1971–1975 and 1982–1984*

Age (y)	Educational level		
	< 12 y (n = 2,288)	12 y (n = 2,418)	> 12 y (n = 1,659)
25–34	5.8	3.2	1.0
35–44	14.8	3.6	1.6
45–54	14.7	9.7	3.8
55–64	18.6	9.0	2.0
65–74	16.7	16.1	12.8
All	14.2	6.0	2.5

*Reprinted from Eklund and Burt (1994) with permission.

Table 16 Weighted estimates of the 10-year incidence of edentulism, expressed as the percentage of 6,172 US adults, by baseline family income and age, 1971–1975 and 1982–1984*

Age (y)	Baseline family income			
	< US $5,000 (n = 1,267)	US $5,000–$9,999 (n = 2,093)	US $10,000–$19,999 (n = 2,235)	US $20,000+ (n = 577)
25–34	7.4	2.5	2.6	0.0
35–44	14.7	7.1	4.8	1.1
45–54	19.3	11.5	7.8	1.7
55–64	16.5	14.3	6.5	3.4[†]
65–74	18.4	15.7	12.2	8.2[†]
All	15.1	8.2	5.2	1.7

*Reprinted from Eklund and Burt (1994) with permission.
[†]Coefficients of variation of denominator > 0.15.

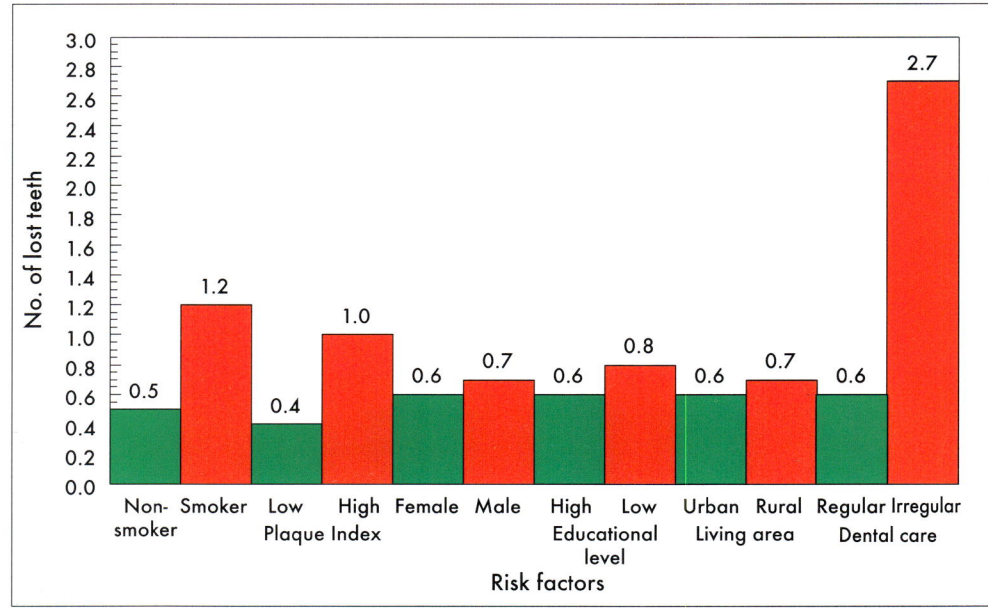

Fig 123 The mean number of lost teeth per individual (50 to 60 years of age) per 10 years related to smoking habits, Plaque Index, sex, educational level, living area, and dental care habits. (From Axelsson et al, 2000. Reprinted with permission.)

ROLE OF LIFESTYLE, COMPLIANCE, AND DENTAL CARE HABITS

Evidence from cross-sectional studies

In a study by Sakki et al (1995), all the 55-year-old citizens of Oulu (a medium-sized Finnish town) were invited to a clinical examination (780 participated). The association of socioeconomic status and lifestyle with periodontal health were analyzed in the 527 dentate subjects. Periodontal pockets deeper than 3 mm were recorded as a percentage of the surfaces at risk. Lifestyle and SES were measured by questions about dietary habits, smoking habits, alcohol consumption, and physical activity.

Lifestyle and SES had an independent association with periodontal health. The less healthy the lifestyle, the greater the periodontal pocketing. Low educational level, low income, and unskilled work (reflecting poor education) were also compared with upper income white-collar work (better education), and men were compared with women (Table 17). In a follow-up of this study it was shown that white-collar workers (well-educated) and women had a healthier lifestyle (oral hygiene and dental attendance habits) than did unskilled workers (poorly educated) and men (Sakki et al, 1998).

Locker and Leake (1993b) examined risk indicators and risk markers for periodontal disease prevalence in 624 adults 50 years and older, living independently in four communities in Ontario, Canada. The data were collected as part of the baseline phase of a longitudinal study of the oral health and treatment needs of this population. Periodontal disease prevalence was assessed in terms of attachment loss, measured at two sites on each remaining tooth. Bivariate and multivariate analyses were used to examine the relationship between a number of sociodemographic, general health, psychosocial, and oral health variables and three indicators of periodontal disease prevalence. These were mean attachment loss, the proportion of examined sites with loss of 2 mm or

Table 17 Distribution of subjects (n = 527) and mean percentage of periodontal pockets > 3 mm in relation to study variables*

Variable	No.	%
Dental health behavior		
Toothbrushing frequency		
Twice a day	311	9.1
Once a day	176	12.4
Rarely	39	26.0
Interval since last dental appointment		
0–2 y	381	9.5
3–4 y	45	14.5
> 4 y	88	17.4
Frequency of dental attendance		
Once or twice a year	277	9.2
Rarely	234	13.8
Never	14	15.0
Lifestyle variables		
Dietary habits: Positive	263	8.2
Moderate	142	12.3
Negative	95	19.1
Alcohol consumption:		
None per 2 wk	258	9.1
1 to 7 times per 2 wk	163	11.3
More than 7 times per 2 wk	105	18.0
Tobacco-smoking habits		
Nonsmoker	282	8.4
Regular, occasional, or former smoker	245	15.3
Physical activity: High	380	10.5
Low	135	14.5
Socioeconomic factors		
Occupational status		
Upper white collar	121	9.4
Lower white collar	187	10.3
Unskilled work	210	14.1
Family income (Fmk)		
> 9,000	242	10.1
6,000–9,000	123	10.4
< 6,000	137	14.9
Vocational education		
University	58	8.9
College	69	10.1
Vocational school	98	13.0
Vocational or other courses	161	12.3
Sex: Male	266	14.5
Female	261	8.7

*Reprinted from Sakki et al (1995) with permission.

Table 18 Associations between periodontal disease indicators and independent variables*

Independent variable		Mean loss (mm) (SD)	Sites with ≥ 2 mm loss (%)	Subjects with severe loss[†] (%)	Odds ratio (95% CI[‡])
Age:	50–64 y	2.8 (1.4)[#]	74[#]	17[#]	3.0[§] (1.6–5.6)
	65–74 y	3.0 (1.3)	79	20	
	≥ 75 y	3.7 (1.6)	87	39	
Education:	High school or less	3.2 (1.4)[#]	79[#]	25[#]	2.2 (1.4–3.5)
	More than high school	2.7 (1.3)	73	13	
Household income:	Can $19,000 or less	3.3 (1.5)[#]	80[¶]	27[‖]	1.8 (1.1–2.9)
	Can $20,000 or more	2.8 (1.4)	74	17	
Residence:	Northern community	3.4 (1.7)[¶]	78	28[‖]	1.8 (1.1–3.0)
	Southern community	2.9 (1.3)	76	18	
Place of birth:	Canada	2.9 (1.4)	76	17[‖]	1.6 (1.0–2.4)
	Elsewhere	3.0 (1.5)	75	25	
Self-rated general health:	Fair/poor	3.3 (1.6)	80[‖]	26	1.5 (0.9–2.5)
	Excellent/good	2.9 (1.4)	76	19	
Limitation in activities of daily living:	Yes	3.2 (1.6)	81[‖]	27[‖]	1.6 (0.9–2.7)
	No	2.9 (1.4)	76	19	
Ever smoked:	Yes	3.2 (1.5)	80[#]	26[#]	2.3 (1.5–3.6)
	No	2.7 (1.3)	72	13	
Current smoker:	Yes	3.7 (1.8)	85[#]	34[#]	2.7 (1.7–4.2)
	No	2.8 (1.2)	75	16	
Flossing frequency:	Less than once per day	3.0 (1.5)[#]	77	22[¶]	2.3 (1.2–4.2)
	Once or more per day	2.6 (1.7)	74	11	
Frequent preventive dental visits:	No	3.4 (1.7)[#]	81[#]	32[#]	2.8 (1.8–4.2)
	Yes	2.7 (1.2)	74	14	
Time since last dental appointment:	> 1 y	3.4 (1.7)[#]	81[¶]	31[#]	2.3 (1.4–3.8)
	< 1 y	2.8 (1.2)	75	16	
Dental attitude scale score:	Median or less	3.1 (1.5)	78	25	1.9 (1.2–2.9)
	More than median	2.7 (1.2)	76	15	
Number of teeth (median = 21):					4.3 (2.7–7.0)
	Median or fewer	3.4 (1.6)[#]	83[#]	31[#]	
	More than median	2.4 (0.9)	70	9	
Carious coronal surfaces:	One or more	3.1 (1.5)[‖]	79[‖]	25[‖]	1.5 (1.0–2.3)
	None	2.8 (1.3)	75	18	
Carious root surfaces:	One or more	3.5 (1.4)[#]	84[#]	33[#]	2.7 (1.8–4.2)
	None	2.7 (1.4)	74	15	

*Reprinted from Locker and Leake (1993b) with permission.

[†]Severe loss defined as mean loss of 3.83 mm or more, representing the upper 20th percentile of the distribution of mean attachment loss.

[‡]CI = Confidence interval.

[§]Odds ratio compares those 75 years and over with those aged 50–64 years.

[‖]$P < .05$; t test and one-way analysis of variance for tests of differences in means; chi-square test for differences in proportions.

[¶]$P < .01$; t test and one-way analysis of variance for tests of differences in means; chi-square test for differences in proportions.

[#]$P < .001$; t test and one-way analysis of variance for tests of differences in means; chi-square test for differences in proportions.

more, and the probability of the subjects' having severe disease, arbitrarily defined as a mean attachment loss in the upper 20th percentile of the distribution.

Mean attachment loss was 2.95 mm, and 76.6% of examined sites had loss of 2 mm or more. In bivariate analyses, the most consistent predictors of periodontal disease prevalence were age, education, income, smoking, dental attendance habits, the number of remaining teeth, the number of carious coronal surfaces, and the number of carious root surfaces (Table 18). In multivariate analyses, age, education, current smoking status, and the number of teeth had the most consistent independent effects (Locker and Leake, 1993b). These data confirm the results of recent US studies indicating that the prevalence of periodontal disease is influenced by social and behavioral factors (Oliver et al, 1998).

In another recent study, Wakai et al (1999) found that poor physical fitness affecting aerobic capacity, foot balance, and reaction was associated with a higher CPITN score. Those associations were independent of other risk indicators such as smoking.

The previously discussed study on a randomized sample of almost 600 adults aged 50 to 55 years in the county of Värmland, Sweden, analyzed the number of remaining teeth and loss of mesial periodontal attachment in relation to urban or rural region, sex, dental attendance habits, educational level, and smoking and snuffing habits (Axelsson and Paulander, 1994). Irregular dental attendance was the most important risk indicator for loss of teeth (see Fig 103) and periodontal attachment (see Fig 104), followed by smoking and a low educational level. Compared to those with regular dental attendance habits, subjects with irregular attendance had lost about six more teeth and almost 50% more periodontal attachment.

The previously discussed study by Oliver et al (1991) on a randomized sample of the employed population in the United States also revealed a considerably better periodontal status in those who had visited a dentist in the past year than in those who visited infrequently. The prevalence and extent of loss of attachment and pockets were higher in those who had not visited a dentist in 3 years or more (Table 19). For example, in subjects older than 35 years, the prevalence of periodontal pockets 4 mm or more in size was 28% in those with irregular dental attendance habits and 16% in those who had seen a dentist in the last year. These cross-sectional studies reveal that irregular dental care is a risk indicator for tooth loss and periodontal diseases.

Evidence from longitudinal studies

Noteworthy in this context is the outcome of a 15-year longitudinal study of adults who visited a dental hygienist at needs-related intervals one to four times per year for education in self-care, professional mechanical toothcleaning, and debridement as indicated (Axelsson et al, 1991). Although the oldest subjects were aged 66 to 85 years at the 15-year reexamination, only 0.2 teeth were lost per individual and the gain in probing attachment was 0.3 mm. During the same period, the adult population in Sweden, receiving traditional regular care, lost an average of 2.0 to 3.0 teeth (Håkansson, 1991).

In the previously discussed 10-year longitudinal study of a randomized sample of 50-year-old individuals who were followed until age 60 (Axelsson et al, 2000), individuals with irregular dental care (< 5%) lost 2.7 teeth, compared with only 0.6 lost teeth per individual in those with regular dental care (see Fig 123).

In the United States, Brown and Garcia (1994) evaluated the relationship between utilization of community dental clinics and the extent and severity of alveolar bone loss in a panel of men followed for more than 6 years. Oral health data were collected by the ongoing Department of Veterans Affairs Dental Longitudinal Study, which began in 1969. The participants were offered regular oral examinations about every 3 years. A variety of oral health conditions were assessed, in-

Table 19 Prevalence and extent of attachment loss, pockets, and recession, in relation to the most recent dental appointment in a sample of employed US adults, 1985*

Age (y)	Time since most recent visit (y)	Loss of attachment > 3 mm		Pockets > 4 mm		Recession > 3 mm	
		Subjects (%)	Sites (No.)	Subjects (%)	Sites (No.)	Subjects (%)	Sites (No.)
All	< 1	43	7	11	4	17	5
	1–2	44	8	16	5	15	5
	> 2	47	9	20	5	8	5
18–24	< 1	13	4	3	4	2	3
	1–2	16	5	7	5	3	2
	> 2	22	4	10	3	5	3
25–34	< 1	30	5	10	4	9	3
	1–2	40	6	14	5	8	3
	> 2	41	7	17	5	11	5
35–44	< 1	47	7	14	4	16	5
	1–2	48	8	18	5	15	4
	> 2	59	10	29	6	22	4
45–54	< 1	64	8	16	4	31	5
	1–2	70	10	25	5	35	5
	> 2	76	10	28	5	39	5
55–64	< 1	75	10	16	4	43	6
	1–2	83	10	25	5	45	6
	> 2	89	12	25	4	60	6

*Reprinted from Oliver et al (1991) with permission.

cluding plaque, calculus, gingival inflammation, probing depth, tooth mobility, clinical attachment level, and alveolar bone loss. Utilization data were extracted from the records of the dental clinics attended by the participants from 1979 through 1988. Neither multivariate modeling nor comparison of high attendance and nonattendance showed that utilization of routine diagnostic and preventive services was predictive of the extent and severity of periodontitis. During the study period of approximately 5 years, the group of subjects not attending routinely for examinations or preventive services received a mean of 1.7 items of dental services of all types. Those attending 1 to 14 times for routine examinations or preventive services received a mean of 19.0 items, mostly services other than diagnosis, prevention, or periodontal therapy. The subjects with high utilization of diagnostic and preventive services received a mean of 35.0 items. Nonutilization of diagnostic and preventive services was associated with minimal utilization of all types of dental services.

Although high utilization of diagnostic and preventive services generated high utilization of restorative and other types of services, it generated very little utilization of periodontal services, and alveolar bone loss in subjects with a high utilization rate was no less than it was in those with low or minimal utilization (Brown and Garcia, 1994). In other words, control of periodontal diseases depends not only on frequency and regularity of dental attendance but also on the quality of diagnosis, prevention, and periodontal treatment provided.

It is disquieting that in the United States, which is acknowledged for its high standards of dentistry, Heins et al (1989) found that partial-mouth probing depths were recorded for only 22% of new patients and 34% of recall patients among

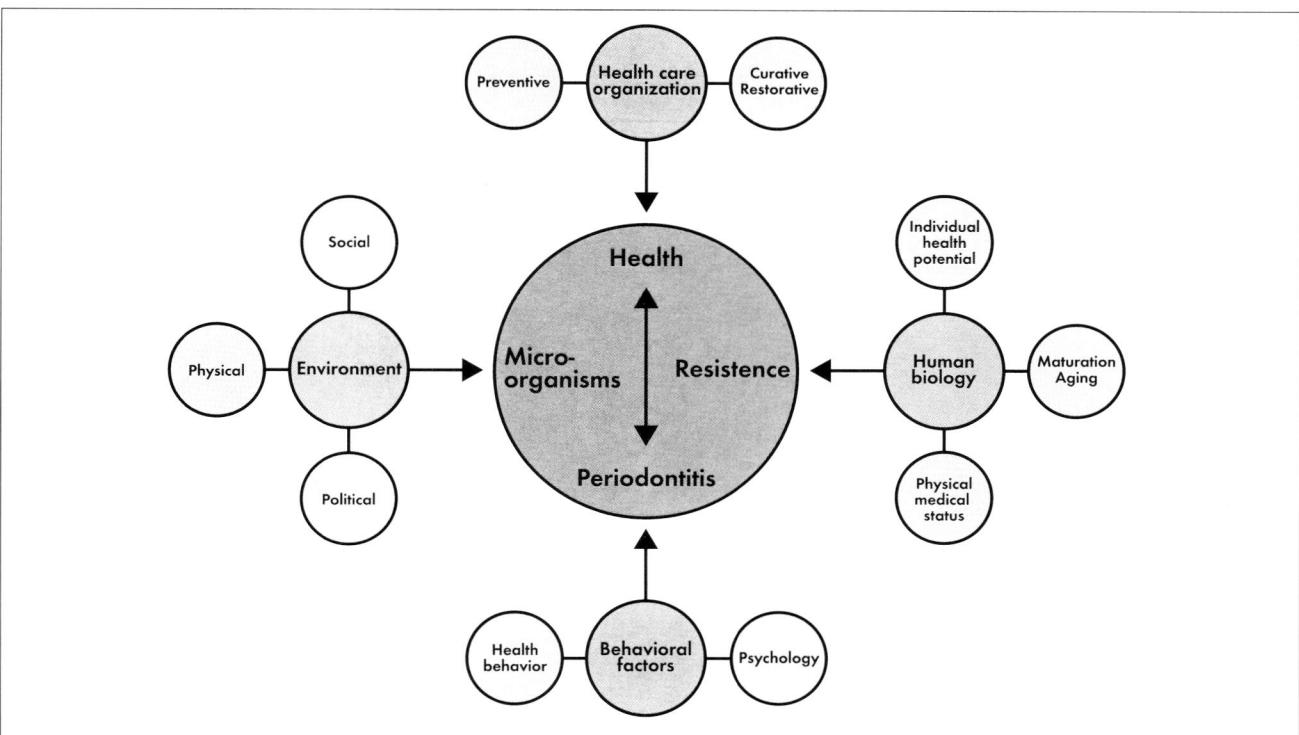

Fig 124 Socioecological model for periodontal diseases, indicating the four main items with subgroups yielding pressure toward changes in the periodontal treatment need over time. (From Hansen et al, 1993. Reprinted with permission.)

general practitioners in Florida. McFall et al (1988) reported the absence of periodontal probing data in patient records from nearly 86% of general practices surveyed in North Carolina. Complete-mouth charting was performed in only a small percentage of general practices in and around Minneapolis and Phoenix. Genco (1992) found that approximately 43% of persons in the Buffalo, New York, area with established periodontitis were untreated and generally unaware that they had periodontal disease, although most had received a dental examination within the previous 3 years. An essential requirement for prevention and management of periodontal disease in the individual patient is the routine recording of the clinical data necessary for accurate diagnosis.

A socioecological model for periodontal diseases, including environmental, behavioral, biologic, and health care variables, has been developed by Hansen et al (1993) (Fig 124). This model

was applied by Hansen et al (1995) in a 15-year longitudinal study for evaluation of possible risk factors for periodontal diseases. Increased periodontal treatment needs were assessed according to the Periodontal Treatment Needs System, in which each quadrant of the mouth is scored according to the most severe condition found. The clinical examination also included registration of oral hygiene status, assessed by the Simplified Oral Hygiene Index. The criteria for the PTNS classification are:

- Score 0—No gingivitis, plaque, calculus, or overhangs (healthy)
- Score A—Gingivitis, but no calculus, and/or overhangs or pockets > 5 mm
- Score B—At least 1 tooth with supragingival or subgingival calculus and/or overhangs, but no pockets > 5 mm
- Score C—At least one pathological pocket > 5 mm

Table 20 Odds ratios for some selected behavioral variables related to an increase in the number of C scores (PTNS) from 1973 to 1988: Results of bivariate analyses*

Group variable	Number	Odds ratio	Confidence interval
Regular physical exercise			
No	42	0.67	0.22-2.00
Yes	39		
Psychological status			
Dissatisfied	9	2.27	0.50-10.00
Satisfied	72		
Smoking			
No	52		
Yes	29	1.52	0.50- 4.55
OHI-S†			
0.00-0.99	25		
1.00-1.99	40	2.44	0.60- 9.94
≥ 2.00	16	1.69	0.33- 8.75
Frequency of toothbrushing			
0-1 times/day	19	0.40	0.08- 1.96
≥ 2 times/day	62		
Interdental cleaning			
No	24	3.06‡	0.99- 9.49
Yes	57		
Alcohol			
No alcohol problems	78		
Alcohol problems	3	2.08	0.18-25.00

*Reprinted from Hansen et al (1995) with permission.
†OHI-S = Simplified Oral Hygiene Index.
‡Significant at 5% level.

Table 21 Odds ratios for some selected environmental variables related to an increase in the number of C scores (PTNS) from 1973 to 1988: Results of bivariate analyses*

Group variable	Number	Odds ratio	Confidence interval
Years of schooling			
< 10 y	26	3.63†	1.17-11.26
≥ 10 y	55		
Economy			
Dissatisfied	7	0.66	0.07-5.89
Satisfied	74		
Social class			
Class 1	11		
Class 2	52	1.61	0.44-5.56
Class 3	18	3.85	0.39-33.30

*Reprinted from Hansen et al (1995) with permission.
†Significant at 5% level.

The subjects comprised a random sample of 35-year-old subjects from Oslo who participated in a survey in 1973 and were reexamined in 1988. The participants attended a structured interview and answered a questionnaire about general health and psychosocial factors. Only small changes in the distribution of subjects in the different PTNS categories were found to have occurred during the 15 years. In 1973, 56.8% were in need of scaling (score B) and 32.1% had one or more deep, inflamed pockets (score C). The corresponding values in 1988 were 54.3% and 30.1%, respectively. A logistic regression model was used to study the associations between risk factors and increased treatment need, as expressed by increase in the number of quadrants with a score of C. A positive association was found for both low educational standard and the absence of interdental cleaning. When the socioecological model for periodontal diseases was used, variables describing the items "behavior" (Table 20) and "environment" (Table 21) were found to be most closely associated with increased need for periodontal treatment.

In another 10-year longitudinal study, Lissau et al (1990) analyzed the epidemiologic relationship between dental health behavior and periodontal disease in young Danes (368 males and 388 females). Indicators of periodontal disease (bleeding and calculus) were measured dichotomously (absence or presence). Periodontal pockets were assessed as normal (0 to 3 mm), shallow (4 to 5 mm), or deep (6 mm or more). Data concerning dental health behavior were recorded for both childhood (1974, at 9 to 10 years of age) and adulthood (1984 to 1985, at 20 to 21 years of age). The information regarding adulthood was obtained through a self-administered questionnaire with items covering regularity of dental attendance, frequency of toothbrushing, and the regular use of interdental cleaning aids. Dental health behavior in childhood (1974) was derived from data on level of plaque, gingivitis, and the number of decayed, missing, or filled surfaces (DMFS).

Determinants of early dental health behavior (plaque and DMFS at age 9 to 10 years) were significant predictors of the pocket index at age 20 to 21 years, and determinants of dental health behavior at age 20 to 21 years (frequency of toothbrushing, use of dental floss, and regularity of dental attendance) were significant predictors of the bleeding index and pocket index. Thus, determinants of dental health behavior both in childhood and in adulthood were significant predictors of periodontal disease in adulthood (Lissau et al, 1990).

Depending on the source of the evidence—cross-sectional, longitudinal, or prospective studies—poor oral hygiene may be considered as a risk indicator, risk factor, and/or risk predictor, respectively. However, the contribution of oral hygiene to overall risk in an individual or a population varies greatly, and may be influenced by:

- Population, social, cultural, medical, dental, and behavioral characteristics
- Oral hygiene practices
- Past and present experience of dental and periodontal diseases
- Methodologic, clinical, and other measurements
- Analytic and statistical strategies

ROLE OF ACQUIRED SYSTEMIC AND INFECTIOUS DISEASES

Role of psychosocial stress

Stress and other personality factors should also be kept in mind. Since the 1940s, numerous efforts have been made to study personality differences and periodontal disease. As early as 1961, Baker et al found patients with various personality problems, hysteria, and hypochondria to be particularly susceptible to periodontal disease. They found a significant correlation between periodontal disease and age, broken home, smoking, marital adjustment, somatization (tendency to develop psychosomatic diseases), and many depressive symptoms. Subjects with high depression scores tended to have higher plaque scores than did nondepressive subjects (Kurer et al, 1995).

According to the 15-year follow-up study by McFall (1982), tooth loss in all age groups receiving maintenance care seemed to follow an irregular cyclic pattern, characterized by periods of sudden periodontal destruction and loss of one or several teeth. In some patients this was associated with changes in systemic health, interruptions in social patterns, and increases in stress.

In a case-control study, Croucher et al (1997) showed that periodontitis was significantly related to the negative impact of life events and the number of negative life events. Literature reviews by both Johnson (1989) and Ballieux (1991) disclosed an association between physical and emotional stress and susceptibility to infections in the oral cavity and upper respiratory tract. The authors also suggested that stressful conditions could influence immune functions, but concluded that more objective markers for stress and periodontal disease were needed to evaluate such a relationship. Moreover, recent data suggest that psychologic stress may contribute to a less favorable response to periodontal therapy (Axtelius et al, 1997, 1998). Genco et al (1999b) estimated a significantly higher risk of having greater clinical attachment loss (OR, 1.7) and alveolar bone loss (OR, 1.68) associated with financial strain in 1,426 subjects after adjusting for age, gender, and cigarette smoking.

The role of psychosocial factors such as physical and mental stress on the extent and severity of inflammatory periodontal diseases has been the subject of a number of recent publications. These studies hypothesized that psychoemotional factors can lead to depression of immune responsiveness to putative periodontal pathogens (da Silva et al, 1995; Freeman and Goss, 1993; Marcenes and Sheiham, 1992; Moss et al, 1996).

Cellular and molecular interactions between the neuroendocrine and immune systems were reviewed by Sternberg et al (1992). Corticos-

teroids are known to exert inhibitory effects on several inflammatory cells, including monocytes and macrophages, PMNLs, eosinophils, and mast cells. According to McGlynn et al (1990), stress-released hormones present in the gingival crevicular fluid may provide a source of nutrients that promote subgingival growth of periodontal pathogens.

Among several possible scenarios, an association between psychosocial factors and endocrine imbalance and lowered host resistance has been used for decades to explain the mechanisms that lead to the clinical picture known as acute necrotizing ulcerative periodontitis. Cogen et al (1983) reported impaired cellular defense mechanisms in stressed patients with acute necrotizing ulcerative periodontitis: Compared with controls, these patients exhibited depressed PMNL chemotaxis and phagocytosis as well as reduced lymphocyte proliferation on stimulation by nonspecific mitogens. Experimental studies in animals also have shown that the recruitment of macrophages stimulated by *P gingivalis* lipopolysaccharide is reduced by stress (Shapira et al, 2000). Exploratory data by Moss et al (1996) indicate that stress, distress, and coping behaviors are associated with increased severity of periodontal tissue destruction. An association between periodontal attachment loss and baseline serum antibody levels to *B forsythus* and smoking status was assessed in individuals with high scores for depression. An important consideration in this context is the fact that psychosocial stress and depression is frequently treated with psychopharmaceutical drugs with side effects such as reduced salivary secretion.

Effect of allergies

Hypersensitivity reactions, or *allergies,* refer to immediate-type inflammatory reactions as a result of allergen-specific binding to the antigen, which usually presents at a cutaneous or respiratory site. Immunoglobulin E–mediated immediate hypersensitivity reactions have not traditionally been associated with periodontal diseases, because bacterial antigens generally stimulate an IgG, IgA, and IgM response and little production of IgE. This is further supported by the relative paucity of mast cells and basophils within the inflamed gingival tissues. However, recent studies have challenged this traditional viewpoint. Grossi et al (1994, 1995) studied a large number of systemic diseases as risk indicators for periodontal disease in a cross-sectional study of residents aged 25 to 75 years in Erie County, New York. Diabetes mellitus was the only systemic disease that was proven to be a risk indicator for periodontal diseases. However, subjects with a history of allergies had less risk of severe attachment and bone loss than did those with allergies. This finding was unexpected, and illustrates how epidemiologic data can generate new hypotheses about fundamental mechanisms of pathogenesis.

The authors suggested that the negative associations between periodontal attachment loss and bone loss are related to the use of antihistamines, which may offer protection against periodontal tissue destruction. Because mast cell concentration is significantly greater in untreated, progressive periodontal lesions than in untreated stable sites, a rise in histamine levels may be expected in sites undergoing periodontal tissue destruction. In subjects suffering from allergies, long-term medication with antihistamines could have an inhibitory function, not only on the release of histamine but also on degranulation of mast cells.

Effect of epilepsy and phenytoin therapy

Epilepsy is a collective term for a class of chronic convulsive disorders characterized by the occurrence of brief episodes (seizures) associated with disturbance or loss of consciousness. These episodes are usually accompanied by characteristic body movements and sometimes by autonomic hyperactivity. Modern antiepileptic drugs prevent about 75% of seizures but do not eliminate the underlying pathologic process causing the cortical cell instability. It is estimated that seizure disorders affect 3% to 6% of the population at large. Epilepsy is therefore the second most prevalent nervous system disorder, after stroke.

Epilepsy may be genetic or the result of trauma, vascular diseases, or the use of some drugs. Approximately 25% to 30% of all institutionalized, mentally retarded persons in industrialized countries suffer from seizure disorders and are therefore prescribed daily, long-term anticonvulsant medication. In most institutions, the medication of choice is phenytoin (Dilantin, Pfizer, New York, NY), and 40% to 60% of patients experience gingival enlargement and overgrowth as a side effect. Anatomically, the contours and pseudopockets associated with the gingival hyperplasia create an environment conducive to accumulation of plaque, formation of calculus, and the subsequent development of caries, gingivitis, and periodontitis. From the standpoints of immunologic changes and plaque accumulation, the significant decrease in levels of salivary IgA reported in patients taking phenytoin may increase the susceptibility of the gingiva to inflammatory stimuli. In addition, other local effects of phenytoin may be expected in patients with poor oral hygiene because constituents of the medicine accumulate in the plaque. Many studies have demonstrated that the severity of phenytoin-induced gingival overgrowth and inflammation varies inversely with oral hygiene standards. If optimal plaque control is maintained, the gingival lesions can be controlled, if not eliminated (Ciancio et al, 1972; Hall, 1969; Navarro and Corell, 1976).

Some people may react more severely than others to phenytoin for genetic reasons. If an individual is genetically susceptible to phenytoin, connective tissue cells (mainly fibroblasts) may be enhanced or inhibited, not only in their protein synthetic activities, but also in their proliferation rates. The latter would lead, with time, to a shift in the fibroblastic subpopulation mixture comprising the connective tissue milieu and, ultimately, to tissue overgrowth.

137

Effect of the human immunodeficiency virus

Impaired immune response will significantly enhance the progression of periodontitis. Therefore it is not surprising that patients with the human immunodeficiency virus (HIV) and those with acquired immunodeficiency syndrome (AIDS) experience a severe, painful, and rapidly progressive form of periodontitis that has been designated *necrotizing ulcerative periodontitis* (Murray, 1994). The occurrence is related to the degree of immunosuppression, as determined by a CD4 lymphocyte count of less than 200 cells/mm^3 (the threshold criterion for diagnosis of AIDS). Recently McKaig et al (2000) showed that in 316 HIV-infected subjects the severity and extent of probing pocket depth, clinical attachment level, and gingival recession vary considerably and are correlated with the degree of immunosuppression, measured by CD4 cell count.

Alterations in the normal cellular immune response may be associated with increased periodontal disease because of modification of normal regulatory mechanisms (Glick et al, 1994; Steidley et al, 1992). Any condition that compromises host defense mechanisms may predispose individuals to severe aggressive periodontitis. Risk factors such as leukemia may also modify the host response in ways similar to those of HIV infection (Glick and Garfunkel, 1992).

In HIV-infected populations, the prevalence of necrotizing ulcerative periodontitis may vary widely, depending on the stage of HIV infection; the duration of seropositivity; the individual's age, level of immunocompetence, lifestyle, and level of care; the use of antiretroviral agents, antifungals, and antibiotics; and other undefined factors.

Early studies on prevalence at the Oral Aids Center at the University of California at San Francisco involved patients seeking dental treatment (Winkler et al, 1986, 1988). Analysis of data derived from these selected populations is likely to overestimate prevalence. Although 100% of the patients seeking treatment at the University of California at San Francisco clinic presented with HIV-associated periodontal manifestations, the original estimate of the prevalence of these lesions during the 1984 to 1988 period was close to 30% (Winkler et al, 1988). Because these early studies represent a period early in the AIDS epidemic, when there was little or no medical intervention, they provide important information about the natural history of periodontal lesions in the HIV-infected population. One medical confounder has been the introduction of antiretroviral therapy. New combinations of medication are continuously being introduced. Combined with early intensified plaque control, these measures will decrease the prevalence of at least the advanced forms of necrotizing ulcerative periodontitis.

As an average based on several studies of HIV-infected individuals in industrialized countries, the actual prevalence of HIV-associated gingivitis is probably between 10% to 15%, and the prevalence of periodontitis may be closer to 5% to 10%. However, the criteria for classification of HIV-associated gingivitis and periodontitis may have varied among different studies. Similar oral manifestations may be found in patients who are HIV negative, for example, in other immunocompromised individuals. It is possible that HIV infection shares pathogenic mechanisms with other systemic diseases or conditions: For differential diagnosis, careful medical history taking and examination are important as a supplement to the detailed oral examination.

The pathogenesis of HIV-associated gingival and periodontal lesions remains unclear. It is well recognized, however, that the development of periodontal disease depends on the interaction between the resident microbiota and the impaired host response. Murray et al (1988) found that HIV-associated periodontitis lesions harbored both typical periodontopathogens and uncommon oral organisms. *Candida albicans* was cultured in a significantly greater percentage of HIV-associated gingivitis and periodontitis sites than it was in control sites (HIV-positive subjects with healthy periodontia).

Zambon et al (1990) reported the presence of subgingival *C albicans* in 62% of subgingival plaque. Because oral candidiasis is a frequent complication of HIV infection, plaque may serve as a reservoir for oral candidal infections. In subjects with HIV-associated gingivitis, treatment with topical antifungal agents results in some resolution of the petechial and red lesions, implicating *C albicans* in the pathogenesis (Murray, 1989). Although no cause-effect relationship has been established between *C albicans* and periodontal lesions, the potential for the involvement of subgingival *C albicans* in HIV-associated periodontitis warrants thorough investigation.

Murray et al (1991) demonstrated the presence of *P gingivalis, P intermedia, F nucleatum,* and *A actinomycetemcomitans* in significantly more HIV-associated periodontitis (80%, 65%, 59%, and 61% of sites, respectively) and gingivitis sites (61%, 70%, 52%, and 52%, respectively) than in HIV-positive healthy and control sites. The microbiota in HIV-associated periodontitis is similar to that of classic periodontitis, but the microbiota in HIV-associated gingivitis differs markedly from that of conventional gingivitis.

The similarity in the prevalence of periopathogens in HIV-associated gingivitis and periodontitis is an unexpected finding and suggests that the HIV-associated gingivitis lesion may be a precursor to the tissue destruction observed in HIV-associated periodontitis. Hence, early detection and treatment of the HIV-associated gingivitis lesion may prevent the rapid and extensive breakdown of periodontal structures associated with HIV-associated periodontitis. Infection with HIV leads to disruption of immune regulation, such as a decrease in the mixed lymphocyte reaction, response to soluble antigens, lymphokine production, specific cytotoxicity, natural killer cell activity, specific immunoglobulin production, and defective chemotaxis of monocytes and PMNLs. Increased polyclonal activation of B cells and hyperresponsive phagocytosis, as well as oxidative bursts and actin polymerization by PMNLs may also occur. The extent of tissue destruction is disproportionate to the relatively low plaque scores of the HIV-infected patients.

It is unclear how the combination of the microbiota and the unregulated responses allow such rapid and extensive tissue destruction. Because the typical chronic phase of inflammation is disrupted by the decrease in number and function of CD4 lymphocytes and macrophages, PMNLs may be forced to play a more active role in the long-term defense of the pocket. The systemic neutropenia common in HIV-positive individuals may be the direct result of increased involvement of PMNLs at localized infected tissue sites, such as the periodontal pocket. The accumulation of hyperresponsive PMNLs at such sites could account for increased host tissue damage. Another possibility in severe HIV infection is an increase in inflammatory mediators such as interleukin-1β at the local site. Pilot studies by Lynch et al (1991) have shown that the amounts of IL-1β in the gingival crevicular fluid were significantly greater at the sites of HIV-associated periodontitis lesions than they were at the sites of HIV-associated gingivitis lesions.

The clinical manifestations of HIV-associated gingivitis and periodontitis are different from those of common gingivitis and periodontitis. The erythema associated with HIV-associated gingivitis is disproportional to the amount of visible supragingival plaque, and the gingivitis fails to resolve completely after plaque removal therapy (Fig 125). As with typical gingivitis, early HIV-associated gingivitis is often a subtle periodontal change and may easily go unnoticed to the untrained eye. Characteristic of HIV-associated gingivitis is an established marginal gingivitis accompanied by petechial or diffuse red lesions of the attached gingiva and oral mucosa. The free gingival margin often presents as a distinct, red line with an increased tendency to bleed. The unique feature is that early HIV-associated gingivitis resists conventional therapy. There is rarely associated pain.

Although many systemic diseases may cause color changes in the oral mucosa, including the gingiva, these changes may be nonspecific and should indicate further diagnostic efforts. The importance of correctly diagnosing HIV-associated

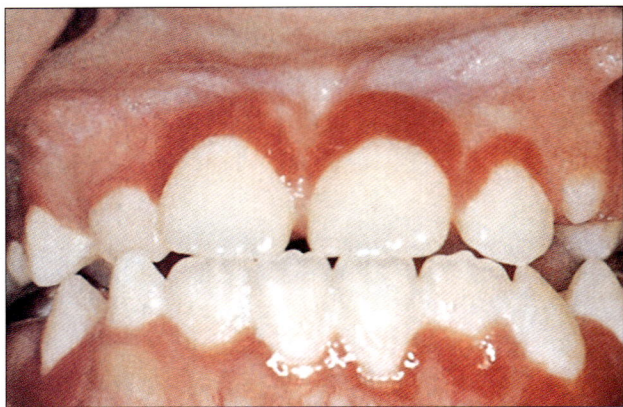

Fig 125 Severe HIV-associated gingivitis in a young boy with AIDS. (From Murray, 1994. Reprinted with permission.)

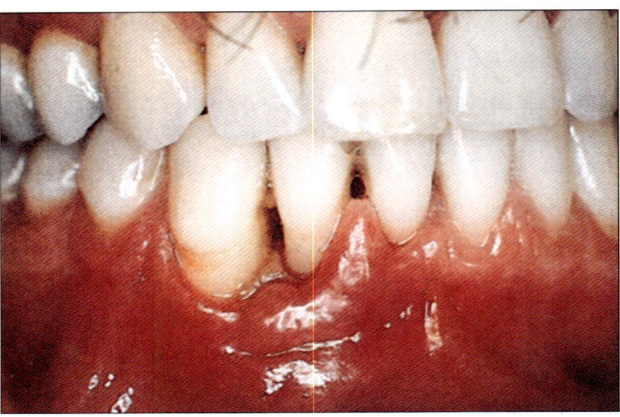

Fig 126 Localized HIV-associated periodontitis with extensive attachment loss and interseptal bone sequestration. (From Murray, 1994. Reprinted with permission.)

gingivitis cannot be underestimated for two reasons. First, this may be the presenting sign of HIV infection and consequently aid in the identification of HIV-positive subjects. Second, HIV-associated gingivitis may be a precursor stage of HIV-associated periodontitis. Consequently, early efforts to arrest HIV-associated gingivitis may prevent progression to necrotizing ulcerative gingivitis and subsequent breakdown of periodontal tissues characteristic of HIV-associated periodontitis.

Because the two conditions have some common clinical features, there is some confusion as to the relationship between acute necrotizing ulcerative gingivitis and HIV-associated periodontitis. Acute necrotizing ulcerative gingivitis has been described in HIV-infected patients, and these individuals generally present classic symptoms of ulceration and necrosis of interproximal gingiva, gingival bleeding, gingival pain, and halitosis (Pindborg and Holmstrupp, 1987).

Periodontitis associated with HIV exhibits the gingival features described for HIV-associated gingivitis and is accompanied by severe pain, gingival bleeding, extensive soft tissue necrosis, severe loss of periodontal attachment, and, in many patients, exposure of bone (Fig 126). A hallmark of HIV-associated periodontitis is rapid and severe attachment loss: More than 90% may be lost

in as little as 3 to 6 months, necessitating extraction of teeth. Soft tissue cratering and interproximal necrosis and ulceration are found in direct relationship to the regions of bone loss. This concomitant loss of soft tissue and bone results in relatively shallow pocket formation.

However, Patton et al (2000) recently presented promising results in 570 HIV-positive patients treated with widespread use of protease inhibitors. Their findings show a reduction in the prevalence of hairy leukoplakin from 25.8% to 11.4% and in acute necrotizing periodontitis from 4.8% to 1.7% as an effect of treatment. In a recent review, Lamster et al (1997) suggest that there is an accelerated rate of chronic periodontitis occurring in HIV-seropositive patients.

The distinguishing feature of patients presenting with HIV-associated periodontitis can be severe pain, localized to the jaws and described as "deep and aching." This pain often precedes the development of the clinically obvious lesion of HIV-associated periodontitis. Most gingival sites with HIV-associated periodontitis bleed on light probing, and 50% of sites show spontaneous bleeding, evidenced by the presence of blood clots at the affected soft-tissue interface (Winkler et al, 1988).

The end result of the rapid bone loss and soft tissue necrosis is severe gingival recession. Although HIV-associated periodontitis occasionally presents as a generalized condition, it is most frequently localized, with areas of severe soft tissue necrosis surrounded by areas of normal tissue (for reviews on HIV-associated gingivitis and periodontitis, see Lamster et al, 1997; Murray, 1994; Salvi et al, 1997a).

- The use of tobacco products (particularly cigarette smoking)
- Low socioeconomic status (particularly low educational level)
- Poor compliance (particularly poor oral hygiene), irregular dental care, and an "unhealthy" lifestyle
- Acquired systemic and infectious diseases

Conclusions

The periodontal diseases are unquestionably infectious. Although bacteria are essential, their presence alone does not result in the development of destructive forms of periodontal diseases. Although undisturbed gingival plaque causes gingivitis in almost 100% of the population, only a minority develop destructive periodontal disease. Apart from the periopathogenic microflora, attachment loss is influenced by external (exogenous, environmental) and internal (endogenous) modifying factors.

Risk indicators are factors that in cross-sectional studies have proved to be significantly associated with increased prevalence of a specific disease. Factors that in well-controlled, prospective studies have proven to significantly increase the risk for onset and/or progression of a specific disease are termed *risk factors* and *prognostic risk factors,* respectively. The risk factors and prognostic risk factors are often expressed as the *odds ratio* for onset or progression of a specific disease. *Risk markers* or *risk predictors* denote evidence of existing or previous periodontal disease (diseased deep pockets and active lesions), lost periodontal support, and loss of teeth due to periodontal diseases.

In cross-sectional or prospective studies, several external RIs, RFs, PRFs, and background characteristics (so-called determinants: gender, race, geographic region, etc) have been shown to increase an individual's risk for periodontal disease:

Tobacco products

Several cross-sectional and some longitudinal studies have shown that, of these external modifying factors, smoking is the most powerful RI, RF, and PRF for periodontal disease. In a recent review, it was estimated that smoking and genetic IL-1 polymorphism together may identify 85% of subjects with enhanced susceptibility to severe periodontitis (Kornman and di Giovine, 1998).

Although periodontitis is initiated by periopathogens, particularly *P gingivalis, B forsythus,* and *A actinomycetemcomitans,* the severity of disease is highly modified by the most powerful RFs and PRFs—particularly genetic IL-1 polymorphism and smoking. Of these two factors, only smoking is modifiable.

In a large-scale, cross-sectional study, smoking was ranked second, after age, as an RI for attachment loss, with a relative risk (odds ratio) ranging from 2, in light smokers, to 5, in heavy smokers. Another large-scale, cross-sectional study, in randomized samples of 35, 50, 65, and 75 year olds, showed that 75-year-old smokers were missing 40% more teeth than were nonsmokers. Among the 65 year olds, after adjustment for the smokers' greater number of missing teeth, loss of periodontal attachment was 50% greater in the smokers than it was in the nonsmokers. A recent prospective study showed that, compared to nonsmokers, smokers were at five times greater risk for further loss of periodontal attachment. In another recent longitudinal study, smokers between the ages of 50 and 60 years lost

2.5 times more teeth and more than 2 times more periodontal support because of periodontitis than did nonsmokers of the same age group. Patients with so-called refractory periodontitis are predominantly smokers (about 90%). The healing response to periodontal treatment, regenerative therapy, and implant therapy is significantly impaired in smokers.

Use of tobacco products (particularly cigarette smoking) has local as well as systemic side effects, which promote the progression of periodontal diseases. (There are about 6,000 known toxic products from cigarette smoking.) The patterns of tooth and periodontal attachment loss in smokers clearly show localized side effects (nicotine staining, thermal effects, several local toxic effects, vasoconstriction, and reduced oxygen levels, which reduce PMNL mobility and increase the proportion of anaerobic bacteria, etc). Smoking affects both PMNL and macrophage functions: The chemotactic and phagocytic functions of the PMNLs are impaired, the specific immune response (salivary IgA and serum IgG2 levels) is reduced, and monocytic release of PGE_2 and IL-1β in response to bacterial lipopolysaccharides is up-regulated.

To reduce the global prevalence and severity of periodontal diseases and other more severe diseases associated with smoking, such as cardiovascular diseases, cancer, and allergies, it is essential that smokers be encouraged to stop smoking and that children and young adults be dissuaded from starting to smoke. On a global scale, this is a daunting task: In 1997, sales of cigarettes were around 6 billion. Because nicotine is highly addictive, preventing children and young adults from starting to smoke would be the most cost-effective measure. As mentioned earlier, only Sweden has met the World Health Organization's goal of reducing the percentage of smokers to less than 20% of the population by the year 2000.

Low socioeconomic status

Of the socioeconomic factors, low educational level has proven to be the most important RI, RF, and PRF. Several cross-sectional studies have shown that poorly educated people are missing significantly more teeth, have significantly greater loss of periodontal support, and have greater periodontal treatment needs, than do those with higher education.

In the US National Study, the increase in incidence of edentulism in 55 to 65 year olds was evaluated over a 10-year period, and was almost 10 times higher in people with fewer than 12 years of education than in those with more than 13 years of education. Other studies have shown that compared to those with a higher standard of education, in poorly educated subjects the odds ratio for further loss of periodontal support ranges from 2 to 3. In another large-scale study, 50 to 55 year olds with only elementary-level schooling had lost 4 more teeth and about 30% more periodontal attachment than had those with higher educational levels.

Lifestyle, compliance, and dental care habits

Although most studies have shown that irregular dental care habits result in an increased risk of lost teeth and periodontal support, regular dental attendance habits do not necessarily guarantee periodontal health. It is also essential that the professional service provided be needs related. Longitudinal studies, based on meticulous plaque control and professional mechanical toothcleaning at needs-related intervals, have shown that, irrespective of the patient's age, tooth loss and loss of periodontal attachment can be prevented.

Because periodontal diseases are infectious, mainly caused by the gingival plaque biofilms, the quality of daily plaque control is of the utmost importance to preventing disease and to maintaining healing after treatment. Poor compliance is therefore a RF and a PRF for periodontal diseases. Several longitudinal studies, using different plaque indices, have shown a strong correlation between oral hygiene status and the outcome of periodontal treatment: Over a period of 10 years, 35-year-old subjects who did not clean interproximally were three times more likely to have extensive periodontal treatment needs than were age-matched subjects who regularly cleaned interproximally.

Acquired systemic and infectious diseases

Some acquired systemic and infectious diseases are also considered to be RIs, RFs, and PRFs for periodontal diseases. Psychosocial stress, administration of phenytoin for epilepsy, HIV infection, and AIDS are the most common. Although it has been hypothesized that psychoemotional stress can lead to depression of immune responsiveness to infectious diseases, and, for example, putative periodontal pathogens, the relationship between stress and periodontal diseases is still unresolved. A side effect of phenytoin administration for epilepsy is gingival enlargement and overgrowth, resulting in the development of pseudopockets. The changed gingival contours create an environment conducive to accumulation of plaque, formation of calculus, and the subsequent development of periodontal disease. A significant decrease in levels of salivary IgA is also reported in patients who are taking phenytoin. Other local effects of phenytoin occur when oral hygiene is poor, because constituents of the medicine accumulate in the plaque. In such patients, excellent gingival plaque control is of particular importance. During the past decade, several studies have shown that patients seropositive to human immunodeficiency virus and those with acquired immunodeficiency syndrome exhibit atypical gingivitis and a severe, painful, and rapidly progressive form of necrotizing ulcerative periodontitis. In HIV-infected populations, the prevalence and the severity of the periodontitis may vary widely, depending on the stage of HIV infection; the patient's duration of seropositivity, lifestyle, oral hygiene standards, and dental care habits; the administration of antiretroviral agents and antibiotics; and other undefined factors. A major goal in management of periodontal conditions in these patients is to prevent progression to the severe, necrotizing ulcerative form of periodontitis. In this context, early diagnosis and optimal mechanical and chemical plaque control by the patient, supported by professional dental care, are very important (for reviews on modifying risk indicators, risk factors, and prognostic risk factors related to periodontal diseases, see American Academy of Periodontology, 1996b; Bakdash, 1994; Beck and Löe, 1993; Beck, 1994a, 1994b, 1995, 1998; Beck et al, 1996, 1998; Bergstrom and Preber, 1994; Brown and Garcia, 1994; Burt, 1996; Curtis, 1991; Ebersole and Holt, 1991; Eklund and Burt, 1994; Genco, 1996; Grossi et al, 1994; Grossi and Genco, 1998; Hart et al, 1994; Johnson, 1991a, 1994; Kinane, 1998a; Kornman and Löe, 1993; Kornman and di Giovine, 1998; Lamster, 1991; Lamster et al, 1994a, 1995b, 1998; Lang, 1991; Locker and Leake, 1993b; Löe, 1994; Machtei et al, 1997; Mandel, 1991; Michalowicz, 1994; Murayama et al, 1994; Murray, 1994; Newman et al, 1994; Offenbacher, 1996; Offenbacher et al, 1991; Oliver and Tervonen, 1994a, 1994b; Oliver et al, 1998; Page and Beck, 1997; Papapanou and Lindhe, 1997; Salvi et al, 1997a; Scannapieco, 1998; Schenkein and van Dyke, 1994; Scully et al, 1991; Tonetti, 1998; Wilton, 1991; Wolff et al, 1994; Yalda et al, 1994).

CHAPTER 3

INTERNAL MODIFYING FACTORS INVOLVED IN
PERIODONTAL DISEASES

The prevalence, onset, and progression of periodontal diseases may be modified by many internal (endogenous) factors. As discussed in chapter 2, *risk indicators* (RIs) are factors that in cross-sectional studies have proved to be significantly associated with increased prevalence of a specific disease. Factors that in well-controlled, prospective studies have proven to increase significantly the risk for onset and/or progression of a specific disease are termed *risk factors* (RFs) and *prognostic risk factors* (PFRs), respectively. The RF and PRF are often expressed as the *odds ratio* (OR) for onset or progression of a specific disease. *Risk markers* (RMs) or *risk predictors* (RPs) are terms used to describe evidence of existing periodontal disease (diseased deep pockets and active lesions), lost periodontal support, and loss of teeth due to periodontal diseases.

Internal RIs, RFs, and PRFs related to periodontal diseases are genetic factors, impaired host factors, chronic diseases, reduced salivary flow and quality, and so on. Most studies of genetic factors have examined the aggressive forms of disease. Family studies suggest that susceptibility to the aggressive forms of disease, particularly in young patients, is influenced, at least in part, by host genotype (Michalowicz, 1993).

In a number of apparently genetically determined syndromes or diseases, there appears to be an associated increased risk for periodontal destruction (Michalowicz, 1994). In most such syndromes or diseases, defects of phagocytic cell function have been described, especially polymorphonuclear leukocytes (PMNLs), but also mononuclear phagocytes.

Recently Kornman et al (1997a) reported a specific genotype of the polymorphic interleukin-1 (IL-1) gene cluster, which in nonsmokers was associated with severity of periodontitis. The presence of the gene cluster was used to differentiate between nonsmokers with severe periodontitis and those with mild periodontitis (odds ratio, 18.9 for persons aged 40 to 60 years). It is estimated that about 30% of most populations exhibit this genotype of IL-1. It was on the basis of these findings that the Periodontal Susceptibility Test (PST) was developed.

Among chronic systemic diseases, type 1 diabetes mellitus is considered to be the most important RI, RF, and PRF for periodontal diseases. It is reported that patients with type 1 diabetes are more susceptible to aggressive localized periodontal destruction, which is initially restricted to first molars and incisors but becomes more widespread and affects other teeth (Novaes et al, 1991; Tervonen et al, 2000). It is generally agreed that the plaque indices in these subjects are similar to those of age-matched nondiabetics, and the severity of any periodontal destruction is unrelated to the amount of gingival plaque. This disease is characterized by a number of defects in host defense systems.

Even in adult studies, a close relationship has been shown between diabetes mellitus and periodontal diseases. This association was valid even after adjustment for age, smoking, socioeconomic factors, plaque, and calculus. Diabetics were twice as likely as nondiabetics to exhibit attachment loss (Grossi et al, 1994).

As mentioned in chapter 2, some infectious and acquired diseases are also high risk factors and prognostic risk factors for periodontal diseases. However, the opposite may also apply: In a recently published 18-year longitudinal study, a direct linear correlation was shown among the number of diseased periodontal pockets, the amount of lost periodontal support, and the risk for development of cardiovascular disease and stroke (Beck et al, 1996). This may be explained in part by the indirect effects of endotoxins (lipopolysaccharides [LPSs]) from the gram-negative, subgingival microflora on the endothelial cells of the blood vessels triggering the release of proinflammatory cytokines. Periodontal disease was a somewhat greater RF for cardiovascular disease and stroke than was smoking, but a slightly lesser RF than were hereditary factors (for review, see Beck et al, 1996).

ROLE OF GENETIC AND HEREDITARY FACTORS

The Global Oral Data Bank (GODB), established by the World Health Organization (WHO), contains a large volume of data based on the Community Periodontal Index of Treatment Needs (CPITN). Globally, the proportion of the population with severe periodontal breakdown is remarkably similar in industrialized and developing societies (Miyazaki et al, 1991b).

In a highly relevant review by Baelum et al (1991), detailed epidemiologic data from several very different ethnic groups were matched with available measurements of periodontal condition in the corresponding subsets of their own detailed records of Kenyan subjects. The mean loss of attachment with age is similar in Kenya, Tanzania, China, Japan, and the United States. On the other hand, highly susceptible populations have been described in the GODB, for example Americans (Wolfe and Carlos, 1987), inhabitants of certain Caribbean islands, Bangladesh, and central Africa, and in a subset of Tamils in Sri Lanka (Löe et al, 1986). However, regardless of nationality, only a minority (10% to 15%) of adults is designated as susceptible to periodontitis and exhibits advanced loss of periodontal support.

In the United States, pronounced epidemiologic differences have been shown among population groups of Caucasian, Negroid, Hispanic, Asian, and Pacific Island origin. In both the United States (Löe and Brown, 1991) and the United Kingdom (Saxby, 1987), ethnic Negroid populations have a 5- to 25-times higher prevalence of aggressive periodontitis. Even in healthy subjects, there are clearly demonstrable racial differences in, for example, the rates of carriage of putative pathogenic bacteria and in polymorph function tests. For details on the epidemiology of periodontal diseases, see chapter 7.

Most studies of genetic risk factors for periodontal disease have concerned the aggressive forms of disease in children on the grounds that, compared to the chronic form found in adults, aggressive disease in young individuals is less likely to result from chronic environmental (bacterial plaque) insults. Furthermore, patients with aggressive forms of the disease probably represent a more homogenous population than do those with chronic periodontitis.

Family studies suggest that susceptibility to the aggressive forms of disease, particularly in young patients, is at least in part influenced by host genotype. Inherited phagocytic cell deficiencies appear to confer risk for aggressive periodontitis in prepubertal children. The prevalence and distribution of aggressive periodontitis in affected families are most consistent with an autosomal-recessive mode of inheritance. Genetic factors also influence the more common chronic periodontitis in adults, but the influence is less pronounced. Although results from family studies suggest that environmental factors appear to be the major determinants of variance in chronic periodontitis, data from twin studies indicate that both genetic and environmental factors influence disease. Furthermore, comparisons between adult monozygotic twins reared together and reared apart indicate that early family environment has no appreciable influence on probing depth and attachment loss in adults.

The Minnesota Twin Periodontal Study (Michalowicz et al, 1991a, 1991b) examined 110 pairs of adult twins, 63 monozygotic and 33 dizygotic (both reared together and reared apart). It was calculated that genetic factors could account for 38% to 82% of the variance in attachment loss, probing depths, and Gingival Index. Updated and additional data from this study show that genetic factors not only contribute to the overall extent of disease, but also may influence the distribution or pattern of disease. To examine the specific influence of genetic factors on disease, the researchers computed the odds of one twin's having disease at a specific site or tooth if the co-twin had disease at the site. Disease sites were defined by probing depths greater than 4 mm and attachment loss greater than 1 mm, or probing depths greater than 5 mm if the cementoenamel junction was immeasurable. For both twin groups (reared together and reared apart), the odds ratios were greater for monozygotic than for dizygotic twins (Michalowicz 1994). The Virginia Twin Study, based on self-reported periodontal disease in an adult population (116 monozygotic and 233 dizygotic pairs of twins out of 4,908 twin pairs; mean age of 34 years) also confirms that the similarities in periodontal disease are significantly greater in monozygotic twins than in dizygotic twins ($P <$ .001) (Corey et al, 1993).

A number of apparently genetically determined syndromes or diseases appear to have an associated increased risk for periodontal destruction. In a few cases, there appears to be a defect that predisposes the periodontal tissues to destruction because of the absence or abnormal regulation of a tissue component necessary for structural integrity, such as the collagen defect of Ehlers-Danlos syndrome and possibly type 1 diabetes. In other syndromes or diseases, defects of phagocytic cell function, especially that of PMNLs, but also that of mononuclear phagocytes, have been described. In diseases such as type 1 diabetes, these phagocytic defects are found in the presence of possible disorders of collagen regulation, such as excess production of collagenase in the gingival tissue. Although there are more data on PMNL dysfunction, it is possible that further studies would also reveal defects of mononuclear phagocytes associated with these syndromes.

When there is only a single metabolic deficiency or the defect is limited to one cell type, such as the PMNL or mononuclear phagocyte, a risk indicator or risk factor is assigned. In other disorders, when the primary defect is either inadequate numbers of PMNLs or defective PMNL function, such as motility or microbial killing, the patient suffers from repeated infections with a variety of bacterial species at a number of sites in the body, including the lungs, skin, gut, and mucous membranes. There are also many case reports of aggressive severe gingivitis and severe periodontal destruction in these patients (Schenkein and Van Dyke, 1994; Suzuki et al, 1984).

Studies showing that stable immune phenotypic characteristics, such as antibody titer, monocyte function, and cytokine production, may result from specific genetic polymorphisms have begun to fuel the search for genes important in susceptibility and resistance to various microbial infections, including periodontitis (for review see Hart and Kornman, 1997).

In humans, studies of inherited variations in the immune system are necessarily complex, and the observed phenotype is usually the result of multiple genetic and environmental influences. This may be especially true for host defenses against gram-negative bacteria and LPSs, in which

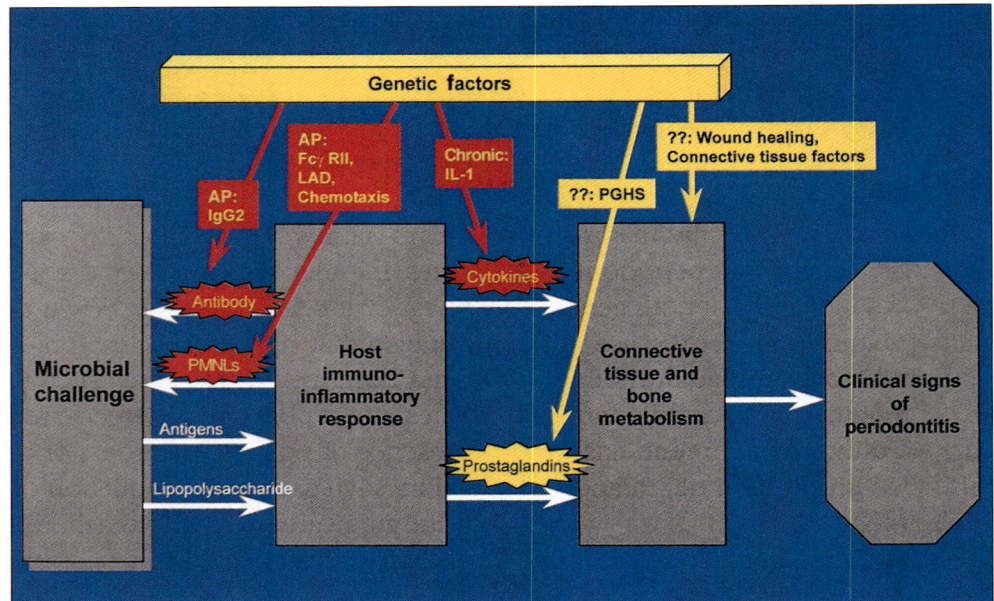

Fig 127 Genetic influences on periodontitis. Shown in red are candidate genetic factors for which there are current data to support a role in periodontitis. Shown in yellow are candidate genetic factors for which there are data to support a role for the biochemical factors in periodontitis but for which there are currently no data associating a specific genetic marker with disease. AP = Aggressive periodontitis; IgG2 = Immunoglobulin G2; IL-1 = Interleukin-1; LAD = Leukocyte adhesion deficiency; PMNLs = Polymorphonuclear lymphocytes; PGHS = Prostaglandin endoperoxide synthase, also referred to as cyclooxygenase. (From Hart and Kornman, 1997. Reprinted with permission.)

Box 5 Genetic traits that may confer enhanced susceptibility to periodontitis*

- Abnormal phagocyte function
- Reduced capacity to produce immunoglobulin G2, chromosome 6
- hFcγRIIa polymorphism
- Tumor necrosis factor-α polymorphism, chromosome 6
- Variable monocyte and macrophage function
- Interleukin-1β polymorphism, chromosome 2q13
- Prostaglandin endoperoxide synthase 1 gene, chromosome 9q32,33

*From Page et al (1997). Reprinted with permission.

---

many cellular and molecular factors are involved. It is likely that genetic polymorphism exists for many of these immunoinflammatory factors. Several immune response traits have been associated with clinical forms of periodontitis, and for some the underlying genetic determinants are known. Although it is unlikely that polymorphism in all of these genetic determinants imparts differential susceptibility to periodontal disease, multiple genes will probably prove to be important in determination of individual susceptibility. The key will be to identify the genetic factors that confer significant clinical risk. In general, a gene may have a potential modifying role in periodontitis if the physiologic processes determined by the gene have been associated with the presence or severity of disease.

Figure 127 illustrates genetic factors in periodontitis and their potential biologic influence. Box 5 lists genetic traits that may confer enhanced susceptibility to periodontal diseases.

Dysfunction of the polymorphonuclear leukocytes

The PMNLs represent a major cellular component of the innate cellular defense system in humans, particularly against bacterial infections. Several genetic defects that affect PMNL function are known to predispose the carrier to microbial infections, and a number of these infections are associated with increased susceptibility to periodontitis.

A defect in PMNL function has been identified and is manifested in approximately 75% of people with localized aggressive periodontitis (Van Dyke and Hoop, 1990). The defect is related to suppressed cellular chemotaxis and possibly to suppressed phagocytosis, although the latter idea remains controversial. In addition, Saunders et al (1995) have demonstrated a defect in intracellular signaling and an abnormality in surface glycoprotein 110. Should these observations prove to be manifestations of a major gene locus, then aggressive periodontitis will be considered to be heterogeneous, because a significant number of patients and families with localized aggressive periodontitis do not manifest PMNL abnormality. Families with generalized aggressive periodontitis in prepubertal children provide the strongest evidence for a genetic role in PMNL function: In a disease known as *leukocyte adherence deficiency (LAD),* there are genetic abnormalities in the transmitting receptors for PMNLs through the vessels, and the PMNLs do not migrate from the vessels. Affected individuals develop severe periodontitis of the primary dentition as soon as the teeth erupt (for details on the role of the PMNLs as the first line of nonspecific defense, see chapter 5).

Reduced immunoglobulin G2 production, chromosome 6

The major serum antibody produced in response to periodontal infection appears to be immunoglobulin G2 (IgG2). The capacity to produce this antibody is genetically determined, and there is marked individual variation. Studies of more than 100 families with aggressive periodontitis have demonstrated a link between disease susceptibility and the human leukocyte antigen region of chromosome 6, which contains the immune response genes (Yang et al, 1996). Segregation analysis of such families has revealed a major locus accounting for approximately 62% of the variance of IgG2 production (Marazita et al, 1994, 1996). Thus, a genetically determined, reduced capacity to produce IgG2 during the course of periodontal infection may in part account for the greater susceptibility to disease.

The bacterial species most strongly related to human periodontitis include *Actinobacillus actinomycetemcomitans, Porphyromonas gingivalis,* and *Bacteroides forsythus* (for details see chapter 1). However, *A actinomycetemcomitans* is particularly associated with the etiology of localized aggressive periodontitis. Patients with periodontitis and periodontally normal subjects vary greatly in their capacity to produce IgG2. Patients with high titers of specific IgG2 antibody and high titers to LPS have significantly less attachment loss than do patients with low titers. Patients with localized aggressive periodontitis have higher titers of specific IgG2 than do those with the generalized form, suggesting that higher titers slow disease progression. These data support the hypothesis that increased serum IgG2 would provide sufficient protection against spread of *A actinomycetemcomitans* to limit the disease to a localized, rather than generalized, form of aggressive periodontitis.

In addition to host factors, environmental factors are capable of modulating IgG2 response. Cigarette smoking is known to reduce serum IgG levels. The effect of smoking on serum immunoglobulin levels is both race specific and serum IgG subclass specific. In a study of African Americans, Quinn et al (1998) reported that levels of IgG2 and IgG4 were reduced in smokers with generalized aggressive periodontitis but were not reduced in smokers with localized aggressive periodontitis or in those without periodontitis. These findings indicate that individual capacity to mount an IgG2 response could be a major indicator of a patient's susceptibility to periodontal disease as well as the eventual severity and progression of disease.

hFcγRIIa polymorphism

The optimal phagocytic efficiency of, for example, localized aggressive periodontitis serum that contains IgG2 antibodies, has been shown to require PMNLs that express Fcγ receptors capable of recognizing this antibody subclass (Bredius et al, 1993). Thus, the effectiveness of antibody in protecting against *A actinomycetemcomitans* appears to be influenced by the serum level of IgG2 and the expression of Fcγ receptors on the PMNL, both of which appear to be genetically determined.

The discovery of polymorphism in the genes for the hFcγRIIA receptor on the phagocytic cells further indicates a possible genetic basis for susceptibility to all forms of periodontitis (Osborne et al, 1994). This polymorphism results in the expression of receptors of high, low, or intermediate affinity. Because the hFcγRIIa receptor is the only one that recognizes bacteria opsonized with IgG2, expression of the low-affinity receptor may be expected to enhance significantly susceptibility to periodontal pathogens and to severe periodontitis, regardless of the capacity of the affected individuals to produce high levels of biologically effective antibody. The genetic polymorphism that defines the FcγRII receptor, therefore, appears to be a promising marker for susceptibility, particularly to localized aggressive periodontitis.

Tumor necrosis factor-α polymorphism, chromosome 6

The proinflammatory cytokines tumor necrosis factor-α (TNF-α) and interleukin-1β (IL-1β), as well as prostaglandins (especially prostaglandin E_2 [PGE_2]), are extremely important in the pathogenesis of periodontitis. The levels of these molecules and of matrix metalloproteinase (MMP) are high at sites of active tissue destruction and low at healthy and successfully treated sites (Söder et al, 1998a). Both IL-1β and TNF-α activate tissue fibroblasts to produce PGE_2 and MMPs. The MMPs are responsible for degradation of the extracellular matrix, and PGE_2, TNF-α, and IL-1β mediate alveolar bone loss in periodontitis. (For details see chapter 5.)

The TNF-α gene has been mapped to chromosome 6: Polymorphism in the gene promoter region results in greatly increased production of TNF-α (Wilson et al, 1995). Individuals expressing this polymorphism manifest greater susceptibility to certain infections. Although this polymorphism is not yet linked directly to susceptibility to periodontitis, there is a strong possibility that such a link exists.

Variable monocyte and macrophage function

Genetic factors may act through the monocyte and macrophage cell types. Macrophage responses are unique for individuals, and variation among individuals is profound and stable over time. For example, low doses of LPSs (12.5 pg/mL) activate production of TNF-α, IL-1β, and PGE_2, and production of these mediators is strongly interrelated. Production of some cytokines may be related to human leukocyte antigen type and to interferon γ regulation. Blood monocytes from subjects designated as susceptible to periodontitis release two to three times more IL-1β and PGE_2 than do those from resistant subjects (see chapter 5).

Fig 128 Cumulative frequency distribution of nonsmokers with 30% or greater mean bone loss (severe) at different ages among genotype-positive and genotype-negative subjects (odds ratio, 18.9; *P* < .001). (From Kornman et al, 1997a. Reprinted with permission.)

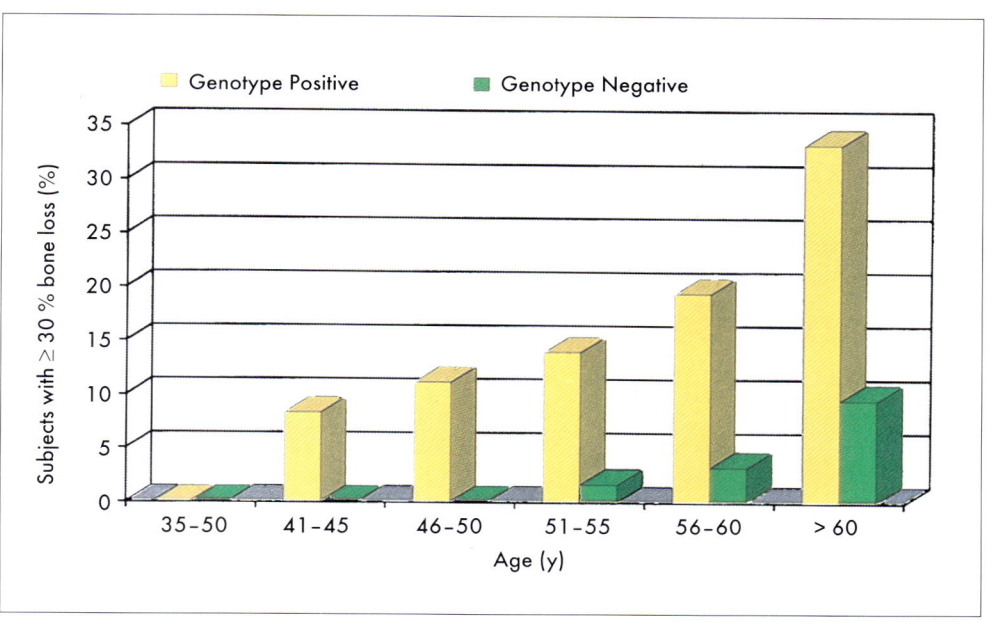

Interleukin-1 polymorphism

Interleukin-1 (IL-1) has the potential to initiate many of the destructive mechanisms involved in periodontitis, including the activation of bone resorption (for review see Tatakis, 1993). Thus it seems reasonable that increased levels of IL-1 in the periodontal tissues could result in a self-destructive, overshooting immunoinflammatory response and a more aggressive destruction of both bone and connective tissue in response to bacterial challenge (for review see Kornman and di Giovine, 1998). For more details on the role of proinflammatory cytokines such as IL-1 in the pathogenesis of periodontal diseases, see chapter 5.

A possible genetic basis for the variation in macrophage response described above was provided by Kornman et al (1997a). They identified from the polymorphic IL-1 gene cluster one genotype that is a major determinant for susceptibility to severe periodontitis. On this basis, a simple test (the PST) has been developed. The test is positive for individuals who are homozygous, and nonsmokers in this group were 18.9 times more likely to develop severe periodontitis by the age of 40 to 60 years than were those with a negative test re-

sult. Figure 128 shows the cumulative frequency distribution of nonsmokers with 30% or greater mean bone loss (severe) at different ages among genotype-positive and genotype-negative subjects. Of those with severe periodontitis, PST-positive subjects and those who smoke constitute 86%. Individuals who are PST positive produce approximately four times more IL-1β than do individuals who are PST negative. Heterozygous individuals produce intermediate amounts of IL-1β.

Recently McGuire and Nunn (1999) evaluated the role of genetic polymorphism of IL-1 and smoking on tooth loss in a selected subgroup of periodontitis patients. This subgroup consisted of 42 patients (1,044 teeth) in maintenance care for 14 years; 16 tested IL-1 genotype positive (IL-1GP). Nine were smokers, and 30 had a history of smoking, with an average of 29.44 pack years.

Both IL-1GP and heavy smoking were significantly related to tooth loss. A positive IL-1 genotype increased the risk of tooth loss by 2.7 times, and heavy smoking increased it by 2.9 times. The combined effect of IL-1GP and heavy smoking increased the risk of tooth loss by 7.7 times (Fig 129). The value of clinical variables traditionally used to assign prognosis was found to be dependent on

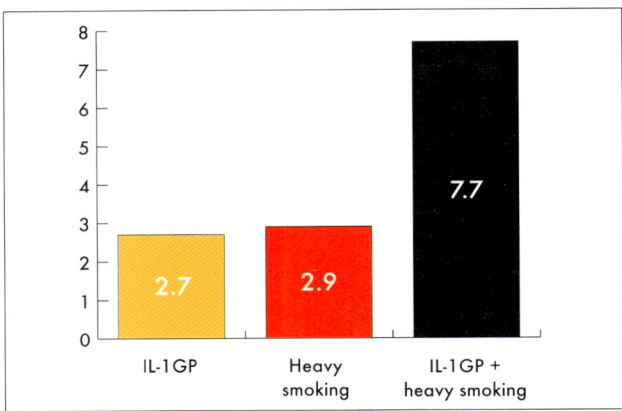

Fig 129 Risk of developing periodontal disease in the presence of various predisposing factors. (Modified from McGuire and Nunn, 1999. Reprinted with permission.)

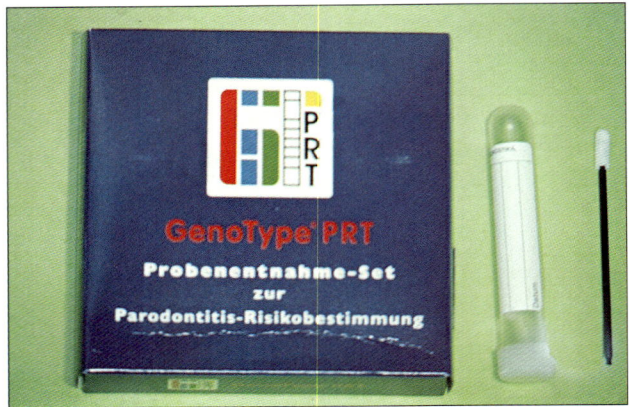

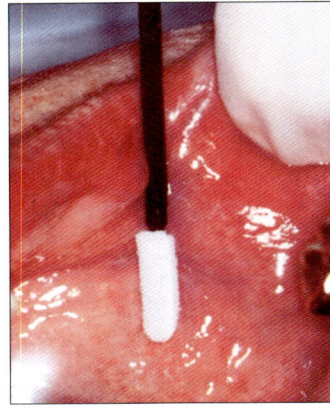

Figs 130 and 131 The PRT test set (Fig 130, *above*) for sampling cell materials for DNA analysis by rotating the soft plastic swab for about 30 to 40 seconds against the oral mucosa on the inside of the buccae (Fig 131, *right*).

IL-1 genotype and smoking status. In the model that included IL-1 genotype and heavy smoking, none of the clinical variables added significantly to the model for tooth loss, while mobility, probing depth, crown-to-root ratio, and percent bone loss added significantly to the model, which included IL-1 genotype in nonsmokers. IL-1GP patients and patients who smoked heavily demonstrated a much worse tooth survival rate when compared to IL-1 genotype–negative patients and nonsmokers, respectively.

In another recent study, Axelsson et al (2001) evaluated the role of genetic IL-1 polymorphism on tooth and alveolar bone loss. A randomized sample of 50 year olds in the county of Värmland, Sweden, were comprehensively examined at baseline for a 10-year longitudinal analytic epidemiologic study. Among the recorded clinical variables were: number of teeth, alveolar bone level, probing attachment level, and periodontal treatment need (CPITN) at surface level. In addition, a detailed questionnaire was filled in regarding oral hygiene, smoking, diet, and other lifestyle habits, as well as other information, such as general diseases, socioeconomic status, and use of medicines. A new periodontal risk test set (PRT) and specific DNA-primer for genetic IL-1 polymorphism was used after the 10-year examination

(Figs 130 and 131). A preview reliability test in 25 subjects showed 100% identical double-test results. A total of 283 subjects were tested for the occurrence of the proinflammatory cytokine IL-1α and IL-1β allele 1 and allele 2 (polymorphic) genes, respectively.

The results showed that 44.5% of the subjects tested positive (PRT+) for genetic polymorphism of IL-1, 32% were heterozygotic PRT+ for IL-1α and IL-1β, and 37% were homozygotic PRT– (Fig 132). More than 95% of the subjects had received regular maintenance care with needs-related intervals during the 10-year period. Therefore, the mean number of lost teeth due to periodontal disease was less than 0.4 per subject per 10 years. During the 10-year period, PRT– nonsmokers, PRT+ nonsmokers, PRT– smokers, and PRT+ smokers lost 0.16, 0.30, 0.43, and 0.95 teeth per subject, respectively (Fig 133a). Figure 133b shows the fre-

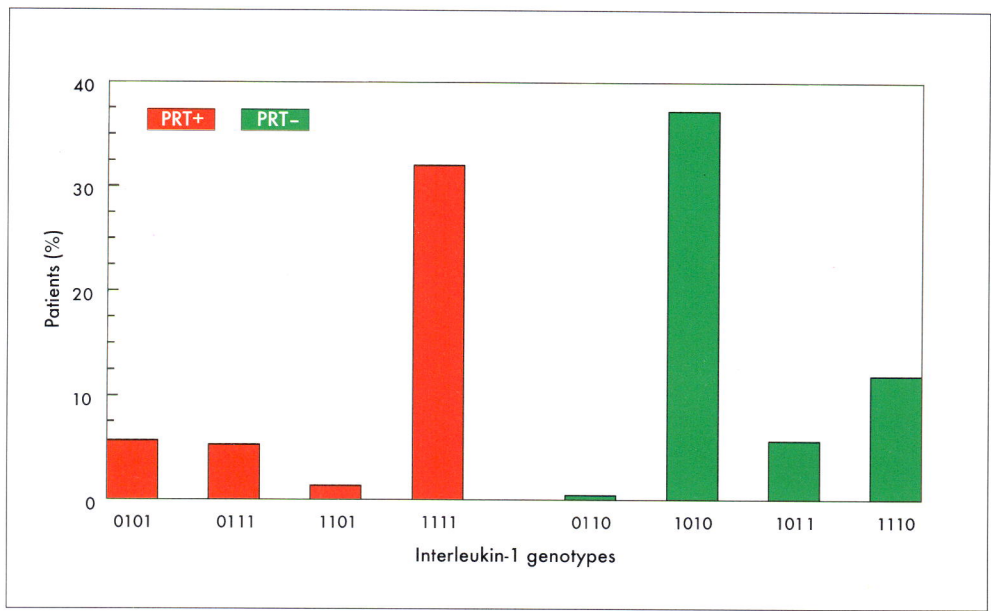

Fig 132 Frequency distribution of Interleukin-1 genotypes. 0101 = Homozygotic polymorphism of IL-1α and IL-1β (allele 2); 0111 = Homozygotic IL-1α (allele 2) und heterozygotic IL-1β (allele 2); 1101 = Heterozygotic IL-1α (allele 2) and homozygotic IL-1β (allele 2); 1111 = Heterozygotic IL-1α and IL-1β (allele 2); 0110 = Homozygotic IL-1α (allele 2) and homozygotic IL-1β (allele 1); 1010 = Homozygotic IL-1α and IL-1β (allele 1); 1011 = Homozygotic IL-1α (allele 1) and heterozygotic IL-1β (allele 1); 1110 = Heterozygotic IL-1α (allele 1) and homozygotic IL-1β (allele 1). (From Axelsson et al, 2001. Reprinted with permission.)

quency distribution of lost teeth in the four subgroups. The mean alveolar bone loss per subject during the same period was 0.26, 0.33, 0.55, and 1.2 mm, respectively, in the four groups (Fig 133c). Figure 133d shows the frequency distribution of different levels of alveolar bone loss in the four subgroups. Among the PRT+ subjects, those with a homozygotic IL-1α polymorphic gene lost more teeth compared with the others (Fig 133e). Thus genetic polymorphism of IL-1 and smoking seem to be synergistic risk factors and prognostic risk factors for not only tooth loss, as was similarly found in the study by McGuire and Nunn (1999), but also for alveolar bone loss. Therefore, PRT+ smokers were regarded as high-risk patients for tooth loss (cut off, > 2 lost teeth) and alveolar bone loss (cut off, > 1.2 mm), while PRT– nonsmokers were selected as non- or low-risk patients for tooth loss (cut off, 0 lost teeth) and alveolar bone loss

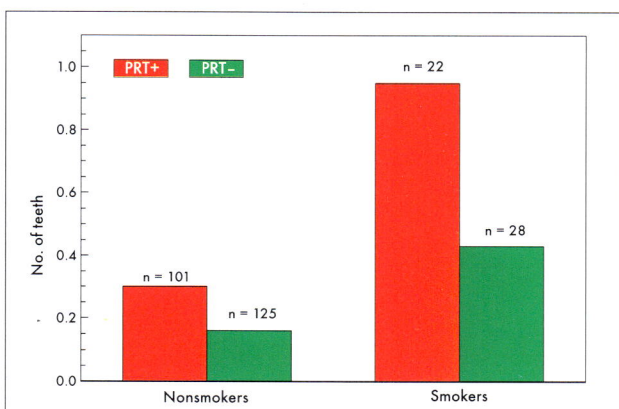

Fig 133a The mean number of lost teeth per subject per 10 years in smokers and nonsmokers testing positive (PRT+) or negative (PRT–) for genetic polymorphism of interleukin-1. (From Axelsson et al, 2001. Reprinted with permission.)

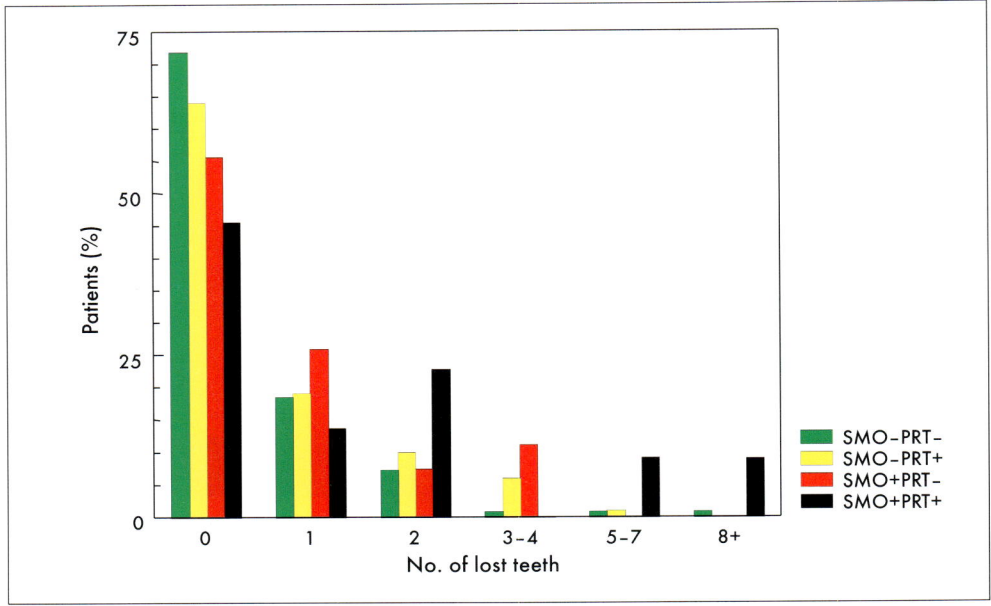

Fig 133b Frequency distribution of lost teeth in nonsmokers testing negative (SMO–PRT–), nonsmokers testing positive (SMO–PRT+), smokers testing negative (SMO+PRT–), and smokers testing positive (SMO+PRT+) for genetic polymorphism of interleukin-1. (From Axelsson et al, 2001. Reprinted with permission.)

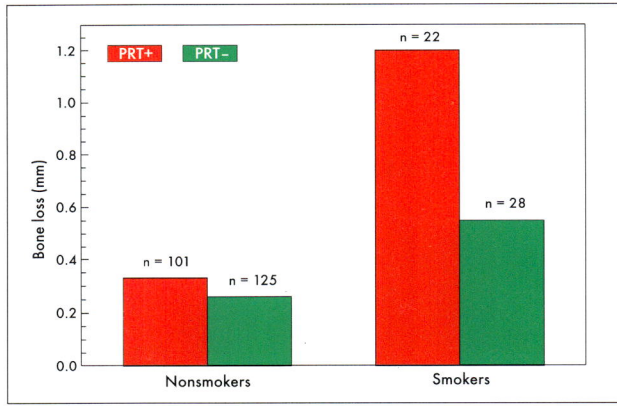

Fig 133c The mean alveolar bone loss per subject per 10 years in smokers and nonsmokers testing positive (PRT+) or negative (PRT–) for genetic polymorphism of interleukin-1. (From Axelsson et al, 2001. Reprinted with permission.)

(cut off, 0.0 to 0.1 mm). Based on these criteria, Figs 134 and 135 show the sensitivity, specificity, and positive and negative predictive values for tooth loss and alveolar bone loss in this random-ized sample of well-maintained subjects. Figures 136 to 140 illustrate tooth loss and alveolar bone loss from 1988 to 1998 in two of the most severe "downhill" smoking subjects who tested positive for polymorphism of IL-1.

Thus, according to Kornman and di Giovine (1998), about 85% of the severe progressive forms of periodontitis may be explained by the above synergistic negative combination of smoking and genetic polymorphism of IL-1, as illustrated in Fig 141. However, out of these two modifying risk factors, only smoking can be successfully prevented. Therefore, even successful regenerative therapy may be possible in heavy smokers with advanced periodontal disease who test positive for poly-morphism of IL-1 if they cease smoking. This is il-lustrated in the two subjects testing positive who previously smoked more than 20 cigarettes per day. After an initial intensive hygiene phase ac-cording to the full-mouth disinfection principles, regenerative therapy with enamel matrix derivate (Emdogain, Biora, Lund, Sweden) was carried out

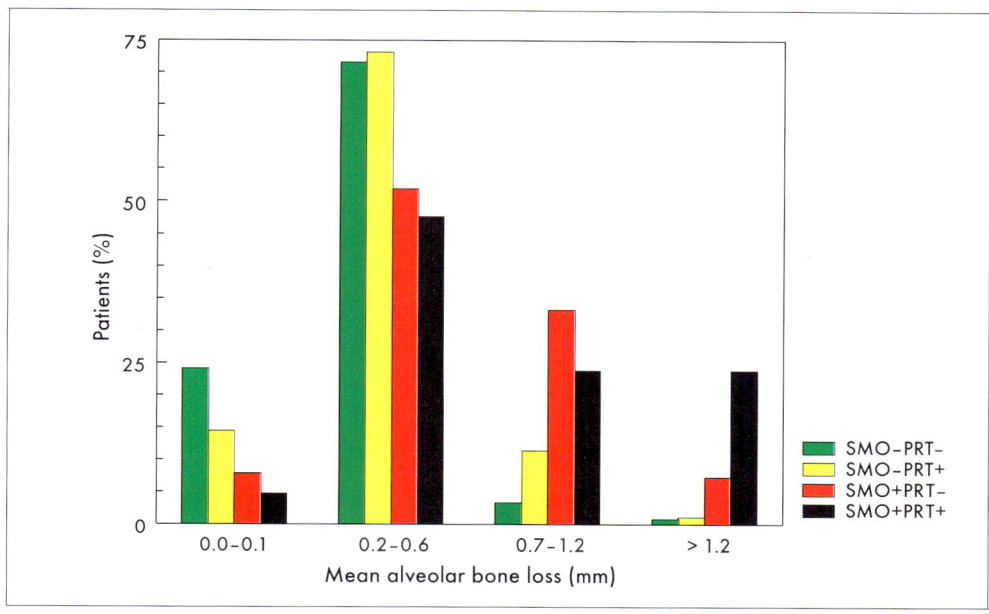

Fig 133d Frequency distribution of mean alveolar bone loss from 1988 to 1998 in non-smokers testing negative (SMO–PRT–), nonsmokers testing positive (SMO–PRT+), smokers testing negative (SMO+PRT–), and smokers testing positive (SMO+PRT+) for genetic polymorphism of interleukin-1. (From Axelsson et al, 2001. Reprinted with permission.)

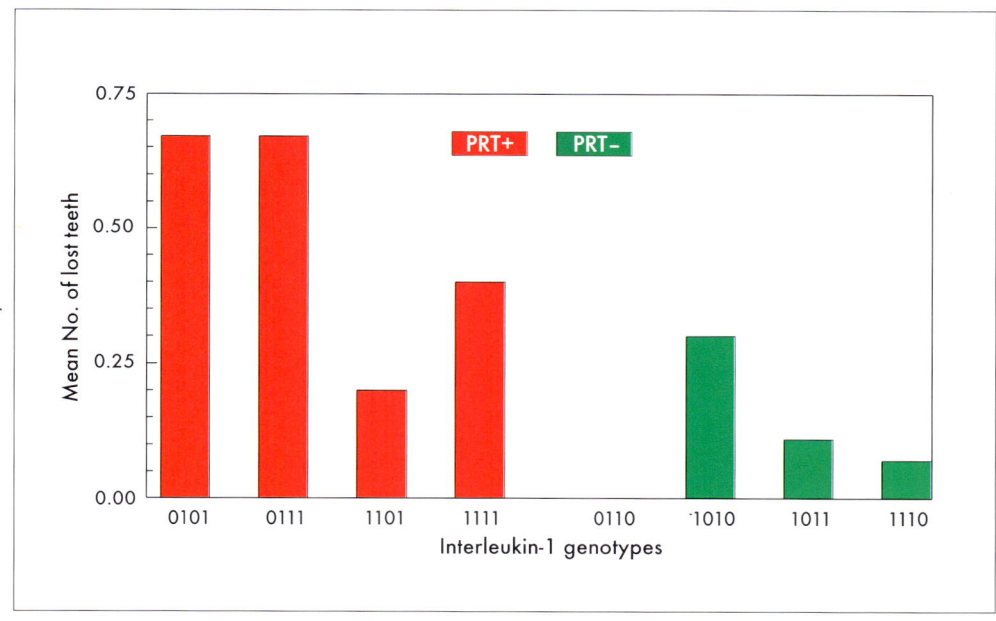

Fig 133e Mean number of lost teeth per 10 years related to different interleukin-1 genotypes (see Fig 132). (From Axelsson et al, 2001. Reprinted with permission.)

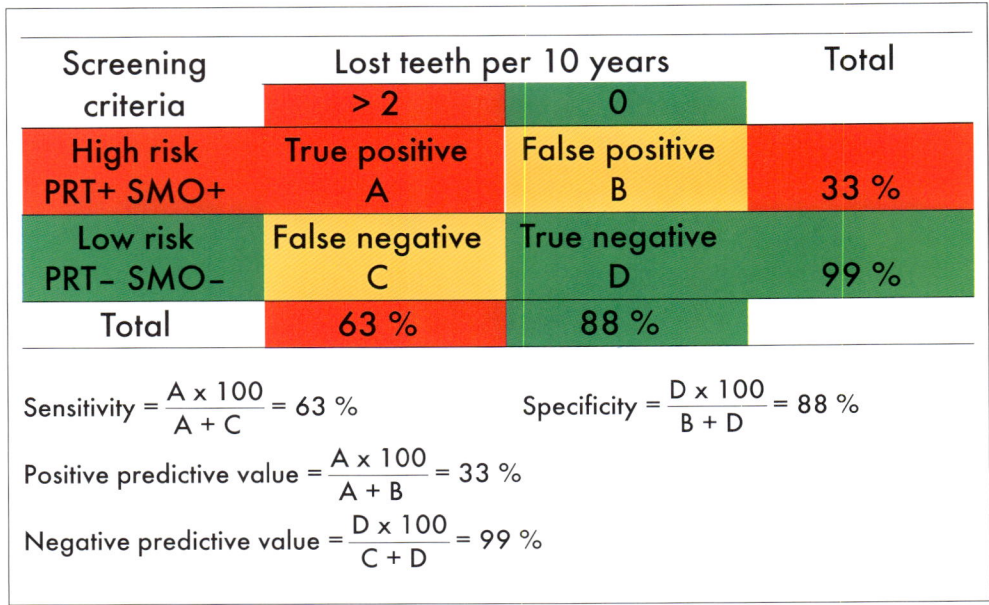

Screening criteria	Lost teeth per 10 years		Total
	> 2	0	
High risk PRT+ SMO+	True positive A	False positive B	33 %
Low risk PRT– SMO–	False negative C	True negative D	99 %
Total	63 %	88 %	

$$\text{Sensitivity} = \frac{A \times 100}{A + C} = 63\% \qquad \text{Specificity} = \frac{D \times 100}{B + D} = 88\%$$

$$\text{Positive predictive value} = \frac{A \times 100}{A + B} = 33\%$$

$$\text{Negative predictive value} = \frac{D \times 100}{C + D} = 99\%$$

Fig 134 Sensitivity, specifity, and positive and negative predictive values for lost teeth due to periodontal disease in smokers testing positive for IL-1 polymorphism (PRT+SMO+) versus nonsmokers testing negative for IL-1 polymorphism (PRT–SMO–). (From Axelsson et al, 2001. Reprinted with permission.)

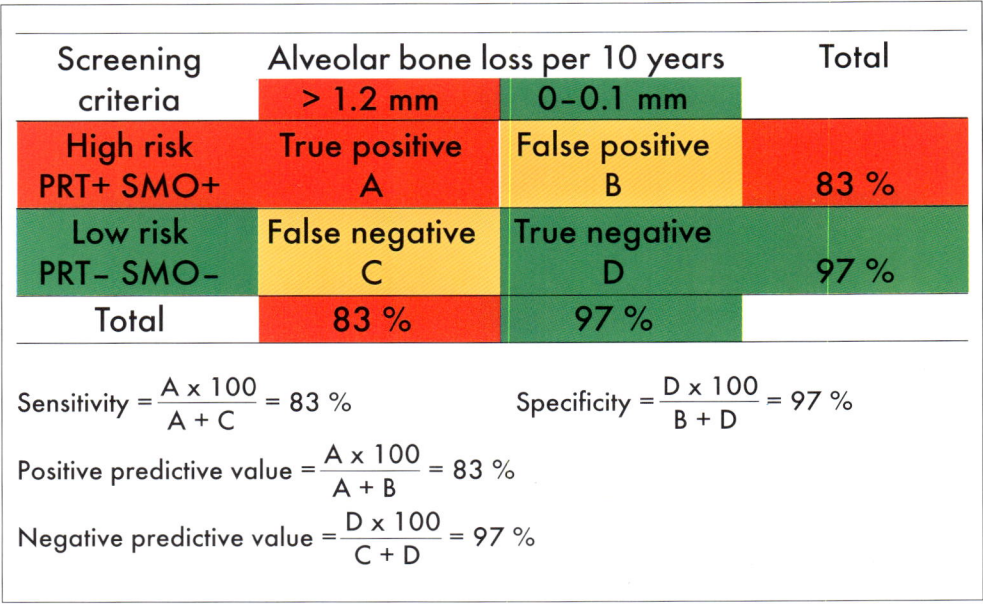

Screening criteria	Alveolar bone loss per 10 years		Total
	> 1.2 mm	0–0.1 mm	
High risk PRT+ SMO+	True positive A	False positive B	83 %
Low risk PRT– SMO–	False negative C	True negative D	97 %
Total	83 %	97 %	

$$\text{Sensitivity} = \frac{A \times 100}{A + C} = 83\% \qquad \text{Specificity} = \frac{D \times 100}{B + D} = 97\%$$

$$\text{Positive predictive value} = \frac{A \times 100}{A + B} = 83\%$$

$$\text{Negative predictive value} = \frac{D \times 100}{C + D} = 97\%$$

Fig 135 Sensitivity, specifity, and positive and negative predictive values for alveolar bone loss in smokers testing positive for IL-1 polymorphism (PRT+SMO+) versus nonsmokers testing negative for IL-1 polymorphism (PRT–SMO–). (From Axelsson et al, 2001. Reprinted with permission.)

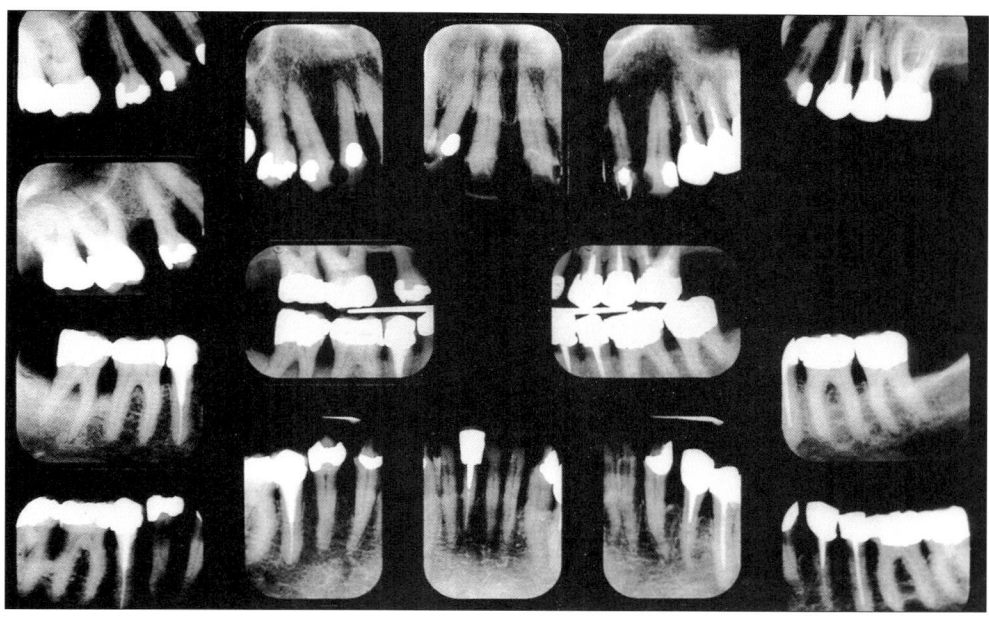

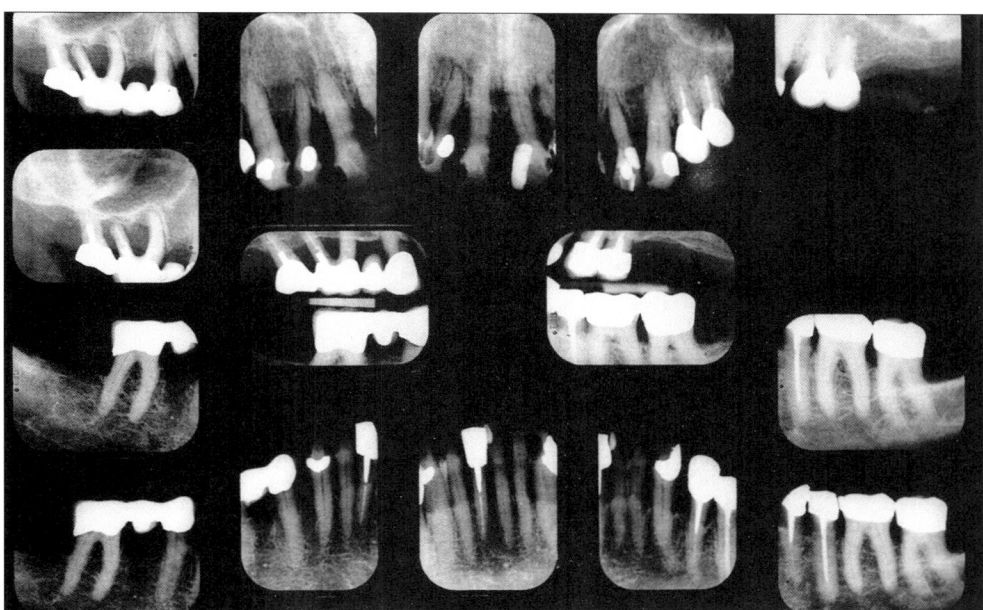

Figs 136 and 137 Full-mouth radiograph of a PRT+ smoker at the age of 50 years (Fig 136, *top*) and 60 years (Fig 137, *bottom*). Observe the severe progression of alveolar bone loss, particularly in the maxillary incisors and the molars on the right side. (From Axelsson et al, 2001. Reprinted with permission.)

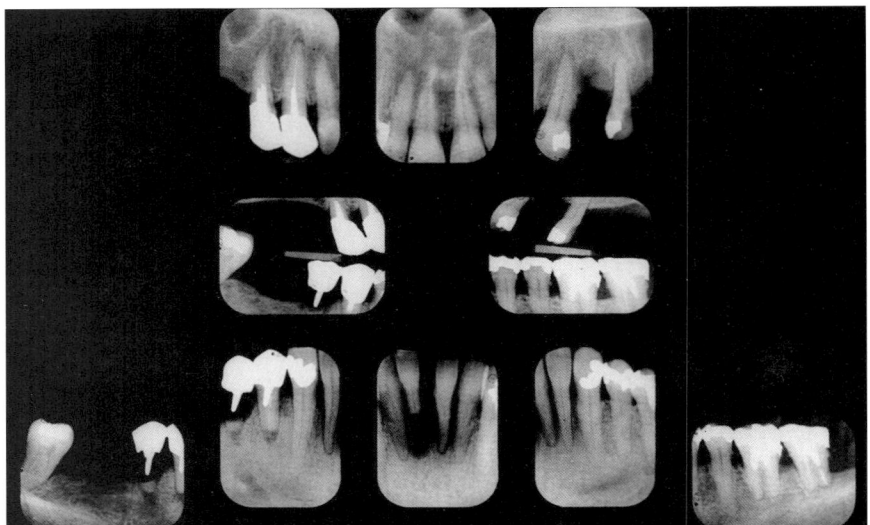

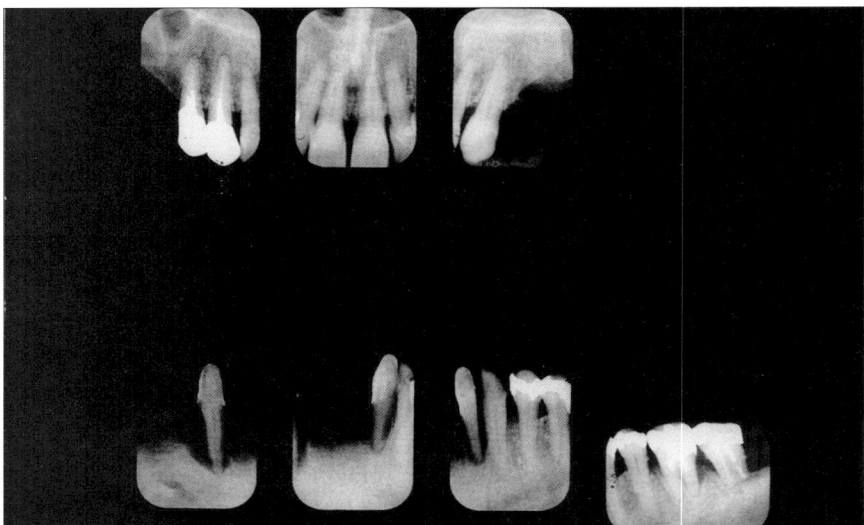

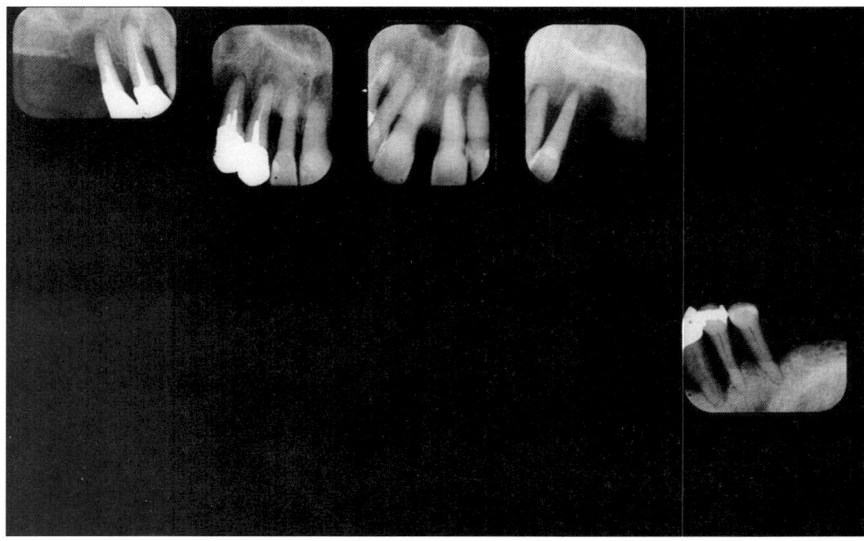

Figs 138 to 140 Full-mouth radiographs of a PRT+ smoker at the age of 50 (Fig 138, *top*), 55 (Fig 139, *middle*), and 60 (Fig 140, *bottom*) years. At the age of 50 years, 12 teeth had been lost and at the age of 60 years, another 11 teeth had been lost, as well as most of the alveolar bone of the few remaining teeth. (From Axelsson et al, 2001. Reprinted with permission.)

Fig 141 Periodontitis as a multifactorial disease. It is estimated that about 85% of severe periodontitis may be explained by the combination of the synergistic negative modifying risk factors smoking and genetic polymorphism of IL-1. (From Kornman and di Giovine, 1998. Reprinted with permission.)

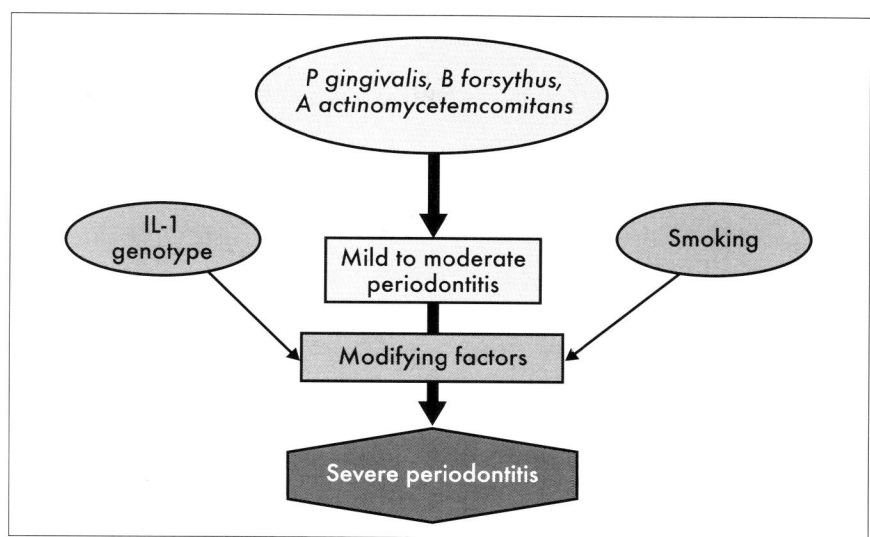

and followed by a comprehensive maintenance care program. As shown in Figs 142 to 149, even advanced periodontitis could be successfully treated within 1 year.

Parkhill et al (2000) also found that smokers testing positive exhibited almost five times higher risk (OR, 4.9) of developing aggressive periodontitis than did smokers testing negative. Recent data also have shown that peri-implantitis and implant failures occur more frequently in smokers testing positive than in smokers testing negative. However, failures occur more frequently in smokers testing negative than in non-smokers testing positive (Gruica et al, 2002). Therefore, smokers should prove cessation of smoking several months before implant therapy is carried out.

Recently Socransky et al (2000) showed that IL-1 genotype positive subjects exhibit significantly higher mean counts of subgingival microbial species related to periodontal disease, such as *B forsythus, Treponema denticola, Fusobacterium nucleatum,* and different *Capnocytophaga* species, than do genotype negative subjects.

Because LPSs from such gram-negative anaerobic periopathogens trigger the release of proinflammatory cytokines such as IL-1, elimination of such microbes from the periodontal pockets is of greatest importance in order to prevent and control periodontal diseases, particularly in patients with genetic polymorphism of IL-1.

Data from more than 12 different countries show that in most populations 30% to 35% test positive for genetic polymorphism. However, only 2% in a Chinese population and about 15% in an African American population tested positive while about 45% of the randomized sample of 60 year olds in the previously discussed Swedish study tested positive (Armitage et al, 2000; Axelsson et al, 2001; Kornman and di Giovine, 1998).

Genetic polymorphic IL-1 tests may be of value for the following patient groups:

- Smokers suffering from periodontitis who want their teeth replaced with implants (contraindication for implants in subjects testing positive who do not cease smoking)
- Patients with severe periodontitis (particularly smokers) who want regenerative therapy (smokers must cease smoking for therapy to succeed)
- Smokers suffering from periodontal disease
- Patients with aggressive periodontitis

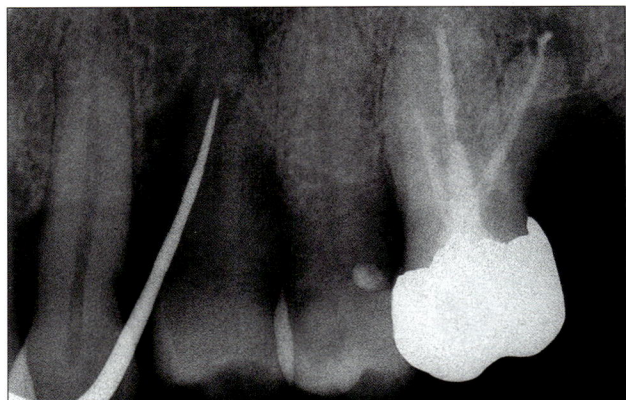

Fig 142 Radiograph with an inserted periodontal probe showing advanced loss of periodontal support along the mesial surface of the maxillary left first premolar in a heavy smoker testing positive for genetic polymorphism of IL-1.

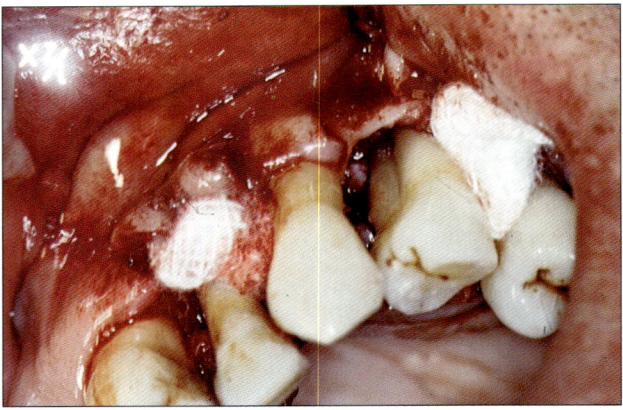

Fig 143 The opened flap shows the deep 2- to 3-wall intrabony pocket along the mesial surface of the maxillary left first premolar after comprehensive but nonaggressive mechanical cleaning and chemical conditioning of the root surfaces with EDTA gel.

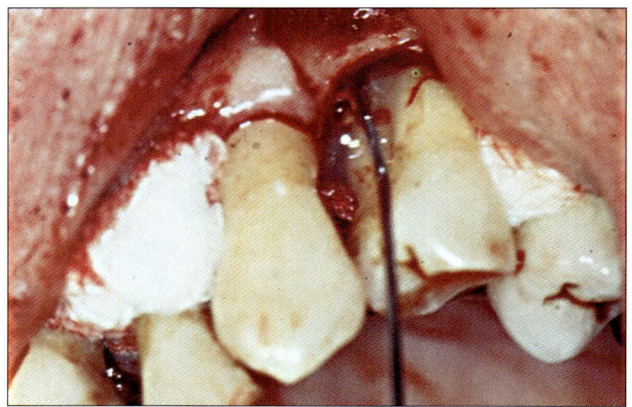

Fig 144 Application of the enamel matrix derivate gel (Emdogain) with a syringe in order to promote regeneration of periodontal support.

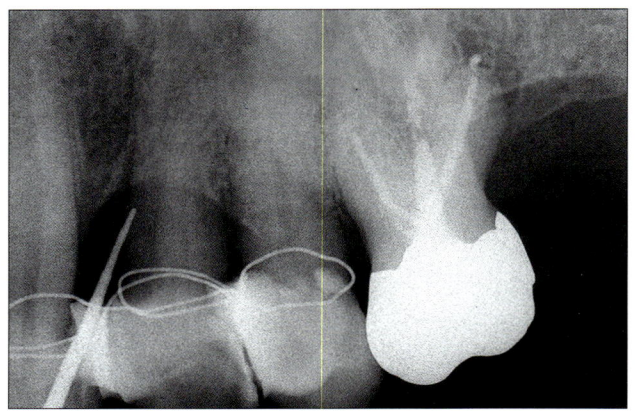

Fig 145 Radiograph with inserted periodontal probe showing considerable new formation of alveolar bone and probing attachment 1 year after the regenerative periodontal therapy.

- Patients with a combination of periodontal diseases and systemic diseases such as cardiovascular disease or diabetes
- Nonsmokers suffering from severe periodontitis

- Children (In the future, screening of children will enable successful primary prevention by prevention of smoking and infection by *A actinomycetemcomitans* and *P gingivalis* in those who test positive.)

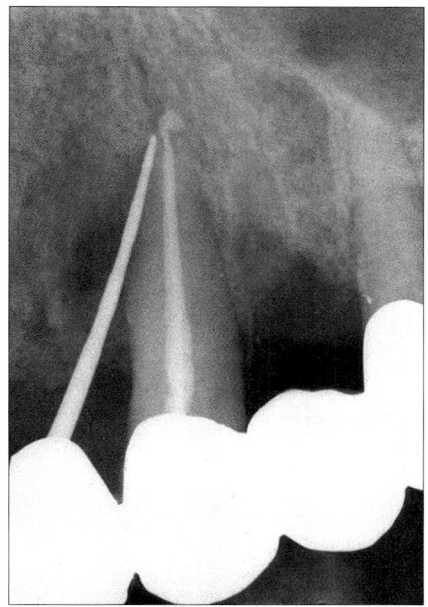 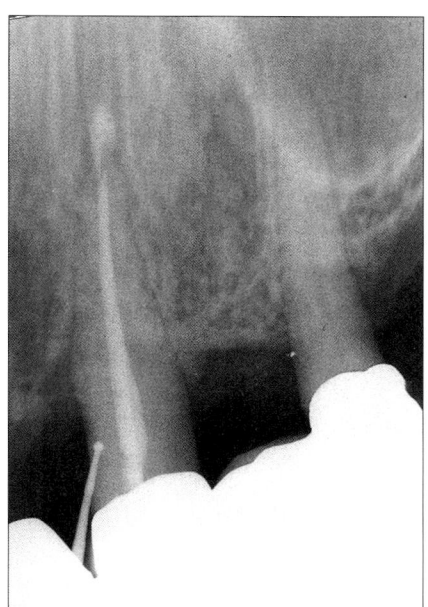

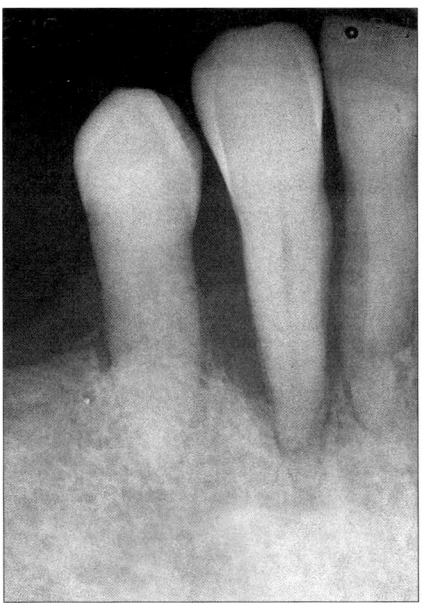 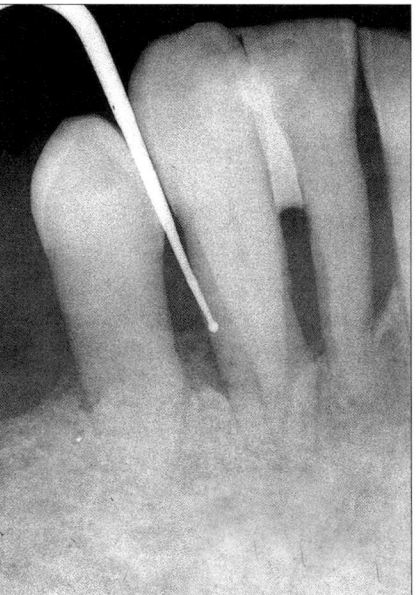

Figs 146 to 149 Radiographs before and 14 months after regenerative therapy of advanced loss of periodontal support on a maxillary left canine (Figs 146, *top left,* and 147, *top right*) and mandibular right canine (Figs 148, *bottom left,* and 149, *bottom right*) in a former heavy smoker testing positive for genetic polymorphism of IL-1.

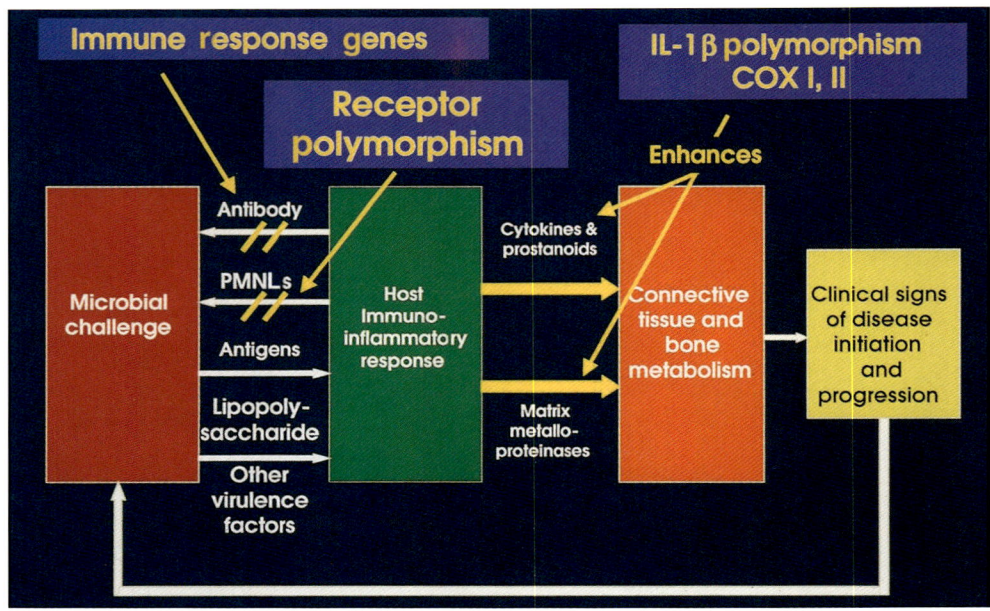

Fig 150 Schematic illustration of how genetic polymorphism of IL-1β and other genetic factors may modify the pathogenesis of periodontal diseases. (Courtesy of R. Page.)

Prostaglandin endoperoxide synthase 1 gene, chromosome 9q32, 33

The observation of the link between susceptibility to aggressive periodontitis and the region on chromosome 9 that encodes for cyclooxygenase l is rudimentary and highlights the importance of PGE_2 in the pathogenesis of periodontitis. This gene encodes for the constitutively produced cyclooxygenase enzyme system responsible for production of PGE_2, the major mediator of alveolar bone destruction in periodontitis. Location and characterization of the gene for cyclooxygenase 2, which is activated by IL-l, particularly in inflammatory diseases such as periodontitis, may have very important implications. Figure 150 illustrates schematically how genetic polymorphism of interleukin-1β and other genetic factors may modify the pathogenesis of periodontal diseases.

These observations on the great importance of genetic factors in the pathogenesis of periodontal diseases point the way to the future, with the development and availability of relatively simple, inexpensive tests of not only the polymorphism in the IL-lβ gene family, but also hFcγRIIa phagocyte receptor affinity, TNF-α, and the capacity to mount an effective IgG2 humoral immune response. It will be possible to test young people and to interpret the results in the context of other potential risk factors, allowing accurate assessment of the risk of periodontitis and differentiating between those who are almost certain to develop periodontitis in later life and those who are not. Susceptible individuals could be monitored, for example, by using DNA probes to detect early colonization by the periodontal pathogens discussed earlier—particularly *A actinomycetemcomitans,* as well as *P gingivalis* and *B forsythus.* When detected, the pathogens could be eliminated easily and inexpensively. In some populations, elimination of periodontitis as a disease of significance may now become a reality.

So far there are no realistic methods to influence genetic susceptibility to periodontal diseases using genetic therapy, but perhaps this will change in the near future as a result of the recent mapping of the human genome. A recent experimental periodontitis study showed that soluble antagonists to IL-1 and TNF-α inhibit loss of attachment (Delima et al, 2001). Thus, "tailor-made" inhibitors of proinflammatory cytokines could be an efficient supplementary method for prevention and control of periodontal diseases in subjects with genetic polymorphism of such cytokines.

Another future method for prevention and control could be the development of efficient vaccines against the most important periopathogens (*P gingivalis*, *A actinomycetemcomitans*, *B forsythus*, *Prevotella intermedia*, and *T denticola*). Thus, the most important etiologic factors are eliminated and the amount of LPSs from these gram-negative microorganisms in the periodontal tissues and the vascular system is inhibited. As a consequence, the release of proinflammatory cytokines (IL-1 and TNF-α) and PGE_2 is reduced, which prevents further periodontal tissue destruction, even in individuals testing positive for genetic polymorphism of such cytokines, and reduces inflammatory reactions in the endothelial cells of the vessels (atherosclerosis). Promising results from vaccination against *P gingivalis* in non-human primates has been presented (Persson et al, 1994). (For reviews on the role of genetics and host factors, see Hart et al, 1994; Hart and Kornman, 1997; Kinane, 2000; Kornman and di Giovine, 1998; and Michalowicz, 1994.

ROLE OF CHRONIC SYSTEMIC DISEASES

Several recent studies have addressed the effect of systemic disorders or diseases on an individual's risk of periodontal disease. As mentioned earlier, Grossi et al (1994, 1995) studied a large number of systemic diseases as risk indicators for periodontal disease in a population of 1,426 subjects, aged 25 to 75 years, in Erie County, New

York. Seventeen conditions were reported frequently enough to allow their assessment as risk indicators for periodontal disease. These included allergy, hives, asthma, hay fever, high blood pressure, arthritis, anemia, cancer, gall bladder disease, mononucleosis, kidney disease, thyroid disease, gout, venereal disease, hepatitis, diabetes, angina, and cataracts. When attachment level was used as the dependent variable, only diabetes mellitus was found to be associated with more severe and destructive periodontal disease.

There is little firm evidence of systemic predisposition to periodontitis, apart from that linked to diabetes mellitus and syndromes associated with PMNL defects (eg, Chédiak-Higashi syndrome, Down syndrome, Papillon-Lefevre syndrome, and the rare condition, Ehlers-Danlos syndrome) (for reviews, see Genco and Löe, 1993; Kinane, 2000; Page and Beck, 1997; Salvi et al, 1997a; Wilton, 1991; Wilton et al, 1988). These reviewers also concluded that type 1 diabetes and acquired immunodeficiency syndrome (AIDS) may exacerbate existing disease. Because the aforementioned syndromes are relatively rare, they were not evaluated in the adult study by Grossi et al (1994, 1995).

Diabetes mellitus

"Diabetes" is a heterogeneous group of metabolic disorders characterized by hyperglycemia (raised blood glucose level) and relative or absolute insulin deficiency. The classification adopted by the WHO Expert Committee on Diabetes Mellitus in 1980 has been generally accepted. A revised version was presented in 1985 (World Health Organization, 1985) (Box 6). There are essential differences among the types of diabetes with respect to prevalence, etiology, pathogenesis, clinical manifestations, and prognosis.

Diabetes mellitus develops from either a deficiency in insulin production or an impaired utilization of insulin. Based on these two conditions, diabetes mellitus can be divided into two main

Box 6 Classification of diabetes mellitus and allied categories of glucose intolerance*

- Type 1 diabetes mellitus
- Type 2 diabetes mellitus
  - Nonobese
  - Obese
- Malnutrition-related diabetes mellitus (MRDM)
- Other types of diabetes associated with certain conditions and syndromes:
  - Pancreatic disease
  - Disease of hormonal etiology
  - Drug-induced or chemical-induced conditions
  - Abnormalities of insulin or its receptors
  - Certain genetic syndromes
  - Miscellaneous
- Impaired glucose tolerance (IGT):
  - Nonobese
  - Obese
  - Associated with certain conditions and syndromes
- Gestational diabetes mellitus (GDM)
- Previous abnormality of glucose tolerance
- Potential abnormality of glucose tolerance

*Modified from World Health Organization (1985). Reprinted with permission.

types: type 1 (formerly insulin-dependent) and type 2 (formerly non–insulin-dependent) (see Box 6). Type 1 diabetes mellitus is caused by destruction of the insulin-producing β cells of the pancreas. The pathophysiology may involve an autoimmune or virtually mediated destructive process (Atkinson and Maclaren, 1990; Szopa et al, 1993; Yoon, 1991). In theory, β cells are destroyed when genetically predisposed individuals are subjected to a triggering event, such as viral infection, that induces a destructive autoimmune response. Onset is often abrupt and the condition may be unstable and difficult to control (Rees and Otomo-Corgel, 1992). Type 2 diabetes mellitus results from defects in the insulin molecule or from altered cell receptors for insulin and represents impaired insulin function (insulin resistance)

rather than deficiency. However, insulin production may be diminished later in the disease and insulin supplementation may become necessary. Onset of symptoms is generally gradual and patients are less likely to develop ketoacidosis. Patients with type 2 diabetes mellitus are often obese and their glucose intolerance typically can be improved with control of diet and body weight. Additionally, agents to control glucose levels are often required (Rees, 1994).

Diabetes is a global, increasing public health problem (World Health Organization, 1985); there are approximately 45 million diabetics in Europe and the United States alone. There are marked regional and ethnic variations in prevalence: Eskimos have the lowest prevalence, and the highest in the world, around 35%, is reported for Pima Indians and certain nonwhite inhabitants of the Pacific area. There are also differences within Europe. Sweden has one of the highest prevalences: about 3% to 4% of the population is affected.

For children younger than 15 years, Finland and Sweden have the highest incidences of type 1 diabetes mellitus in the world (29 and 24 children per 100,000, respectively). The risk of developing diabetes is 30 times greater for a Swedish child than for a Japanese child (Blom and Dahlquist, 1985).

In most studies of prevalence, no distinction has been made between type 1 and type 2 diabetes mellitus. Because patients with type 2 diabetes mellitus constitute 85% to 90% of all diabetics, the total figures in such studies essentially reflect the prevalence of type 2 diabetes mellitus.

The prevalence of diabetes increases drastically with age, because of the high prevalence of type 2 diabetes mellitus in old age. Generally, there is a slight female dominance. Some important characteristics and differences between type 1 and type 2 diabetes mellitus are presented in Table 22.

Insulin regenerates glucose metabolism and is essential for transport of glucose through the cell membrane into the cytoplasm. It is the most important anabolic hormone in the body. The

Table 22 Most important differences between type 1 and type 2 diabetes mellitus*

Characteristic	Type 1	Type 2
Age of onset	Usually before the age of 30 y	Usually after the age of 30 y
Seasonal incidence of onset	Mostly in winter months	No seasonal preponderance
Family history of diabetes	Uncommon	Common
Haplotypes	HLA B8, B15, B18, DR3, DR4	No preponderance
Islet cell antibodies	Present at onset	Absent
Phenotype	Thin	Obese
Speed of onset	Rapid	Slow
Symptoms	Severe	Mild or absent
Ketoacidosis	Prone	Resistant
Serum insulin	Low or absent	Raised, depressed, or low
Treatment	Insulin	Diet, sulfonyl urea, sometimes insulin

*From Bloom and Ireland (1980). Reprinted with permission.

energy-sparing effect constitutes an increased glucose uptake, most evident in the muscles, liver, and adipose tissue. In the muscles and liver, glucose is stored as glycogen, which, when necessary, is converted back to glucose, stimulated by hormones such as glucagons, cortisol, and adrenaline. Insulin preserves the depot of triglycerides in adipose tissue. In the muscles, insulin stimulates the uptake of amino acids and increases the synthesis of protein.

Diabetes is diagnosed when the level of fasting blood sugar is 6.7 mmol/L or greater. Usually a combination of a fasting blood glucose test plus a 2-hour test after glucose loading and an oral glucose tolerance test is used. New diagnostic guidelines allow use of a casual (nonfasting) plasma glucose for diagnosis and restrict routine use of the oral glucose tolerance test (American Diabetes Association, 1997). The casual plasma glucose test provides a simple screening tool because fasting is not required.

The old, insensitive evaluation of urine glucose levels has been replaced by self-monitoring blood glucose instruments for patient self-assessment. The glucated hemoglobin assay measures the amount of glucose irreversibly bound to the hemoglobin molecule. Glucometers are commonly used by diabetic patients for home monitoring of their blood glucose levels using a single drop of blood from a finger stick. This procedure is of interest to the dental practitioner because it is simple, relatively inexpensive, and sufficiently accurate to serve as an in-office screening device for patients suspected to have diabetes and to monitor blood sugar levels of known diabetic patients during prolonged treatment procedures to discover possible hypoglycemia.

The clinical symptoms reflect the severity of the hyperglycemia. In type 1 diabetes mellitus, the symptoms are usually very obvious, eg, polydipsia, polyuria, considerable weight loss, lassitude, blurred vision, pruritus, paresthesia, muscle cramping, and susceptibility to infection. Gastrointestinal symptoms such as nausea, vomiting, and abdominal pain may gradually appear. Untreated, the condition leads to metabolic ketoacidosis, coma, and death.

Long-term complications

With insulin treatment and a normalized blood glucose level, the diabetic usually lives for many years without any symptoms. However, over time, a number of serious complications arise, threatening the quality of life and survival (Bloom and

Ireland, 1980). The development and progression of these complications are related to the degree and duration of hyperglycemia, with the involvement of almost every tissue in the body (Diabetes Control and Complications Trial Research Group, 1993; Reichard, 1990).

Macroangiopathy (disease of the macrocirculation). Macroangiopathy is caused by an atherosclerotic process similar to that occurring in nondiabetics, but in diabetics macroangiopathy occurs at a younger age, is more extensive, and accelerates more rapidly. It frequently culminates in fatal or disabling complications such as myocardial infarct, stroke, intermittent claudication, or gangrene of the lower extremities.

Microangiopathy (disease of the microcirculation). Microangiopathy affects the arterioles, capillaries, and venules in all vascular areas but particularly those of the retina and glomerulus. Microangiopathy is characterized by a thickening of the basement membranes and a proliferation of endothelial cells. It appears to be specific to diabetes.

Retinopathy. Retinopathy implies a risk of serious visual impairment and blindness. The fundamental elements are venous dilation, microaneurysms, hemorrhage, hard and soft exudates, macular edema, and new vessel formation. Severe fibrous reactions in the vitreous body may cause retinal detachment. After 20 years of type 1 diabetes mellitus, most diabetics have retinopathy of varying severity. Diabetes is the most common cause of blindness before the age of 65 years.

Nephropathy. About 40% to 50% of diabetics have nephropathy with a risk of renal failure and uremia. An early sign of renal involvement is microalbuminuria. A rise in blood pressure follows. Untreated, microalbuminuria may progress to clinical proteinuria and ultimately to renal failure.

Neuropathy. The etiology is not clear, but neuropathy is probably not solely an effect of the an-giopathy; a direct metabolic effect is also considered important. Many are symptoms resulting from general neuropathy. Sensory, motor, and autonomic nerves are all affected.

Impairments associated with periodontal diseases

In addition to the aforementioned systemic and local complications related to the degree and duration of hyperglycemia, diabetics exhibit some other impairments that result in increased susceptibility to infectious diseases such as periodontal diseases.

Impaired host response. Defects in polymorphonuclear leukocyte function have been considered a potential cause of bacterial infection in the diabetic. Several studies have found diminished chemotaxis, adherence, and phagocytosis of peripheral blood leukocytes in diabetic patients (Bagdade et al, 1978; Hill et al, 1974; Kjersem et al, 1988; Leeper et al, 1985; Mowat and Baum, 1971). Molenaar et al (1976) extended PMNL dysfunction studies to include nondiabetic, first-degree relatives of diabetics and found that they also had a decreased chemotactic index. A number of studies indicate that the abnormalities in PMNL functions can be corrected by insulin therapy. The origin of the defects is unclear: Both cellular mechanisms in PMNL cells and noncellular mechanisms stemming from the direct effects of serum factors such as glucose and insulin on PMNLs have been hypothesized. The pathologically thickened basement membranes may also contribute to the impaired migration of leukocytes from blood vessels.

It has been shown that, compared to diabetics with mild periodontitis or nondiabetics with severe or mild periodontitis, diabetics with severe periodontitis exhibit depressed chemotaxis of peripheral blood leukocytes. McMullen et al (1981) found decreased PMNL chemotaxis in patients with a family history of diabetes and severe periodontitis and concluded that there was a genetic origin to the PMNL defect. Bissada et al (1982) reported that diabetic patients with severe periodontitis exhibited less phagocytic activity of peripheral blood PMNLs than did nondiabetic patients with localized periodontitis. The phagocytic activity of PMNLs in the gingival sulcus was less than that of peripheral blood PMNLs, and, irrespective of diabetic state, activity at diseased sites was less than that at healthy sites.

The association among diabetes, abnormal PMNL function, and periodontal disease may be explained by (1) impairment of PMNL function as a result of bacterial infection associated with periodontal disease; or (2) primary impairment of the PMNL response, predisposing these patients to periodontitis. Cutler et al (1991) were the first to report a case of a patient with type 1 diabetes in whom PMNLs showed decreased chemotaxis and phagocytosis of a putative periodontal pathogen, *P gingivalis,* isolated from a site of periodontal destruction. It has also been shown that the chemotactic response is gradually reduced as the duration of diabetes and hyperglycemia increases (Golub et al, 1982).

Although in vitro tests may not disclose PMNL defects in most diabetics, there are several possible explanations for altered PMNL function in vivo in the diabetic with periodontitis. In diabetics, impaired PMNL function may be a consequence of a periodontitis-associated bacterial infection: Local LPS may alter oxidative burst capacity to impair killing. It is also possible that elevated levels of PGE_2 in gingival crevicular fluid, which are associated with diabetes, may lead to depressed production of opsonic antibody in the pocket because PGE_2 is a potent inhibitor of plasma cell antibody production (for details, see chapter 5).

Polymorphonuclear leukocyte function is also influenced by systemic levels of lipids, especially unsaturated fatty acids and triglycerides, which can impair phagocytosis and killing. Insulin has a marked effect on both glucose and lipid metabolism. The metabolic state of diabetes also causes hyperlipidemia and has such dramatic effects on lipid metabolism that some investigators have proposed that diabetes be regarded primarily as a dysfunction of lipid metabolism, with a secondary influence on glucose pathways (Abbate and Brunzell, 1990). Even in the absence of diabetes, hyperlipidemia has been associated with impaired PMNL function and exaggerated monocyte function.

Thus, although diabetes is a familial trait in which genetically determined components of the host response may enhance susceptibility to periodontitis, there are several plausible mechanisms by which metabolic irregularities may mediate the increased severity of disease expression.

Impaired inflammatory response. Individuals with refractory, aggressive, and diabetes-associated periodontitis are regarded as high-risk patients. It has been suggested that they have an abnormal monocytic phenotype—a monocyte-positive trait—that increases susceptibility to severe forms of periodontal disease (Offenbacher et al, 1993, 1994). Exaggerated monocytic inflammatory responses to LPS (endotoxin) challenge from gram-negative bacteria have been shown in type 1 diabetic patients, evidenced by abnormal secretion of proinflammatory mediators such as IL-1β, PGE_2, and TNF-α. It has been proposed that this increased monocytic secretion in response to LPS challenge is regulated by genes in the human leukocyte antigen (HLA) regions HLA-DR3/4 and HLA-DQ (Reinhardt et al, 1991).

Investigators have also postulated a potential relationship between HLA-associated autoimmune disease such as diabetes mellitus and increased monocytic secretion of TNF-α (Pociot et al, 1993). As discussed earlier in this chapter, genetically distinct interindividual differences have been reported in endotoxin-stimulated human monocytic secretions of inflammatory mediators such as IL-1, TNF-α, and PGE_2.

These findings suggest that in persons with diabetes, a genetically determined monocytic hypersecretory phenotype may be responsible for the exaggerated inflammatory response to a gram-negative bacterial challenge. On the other hand, monocytic upregulation that results in en-

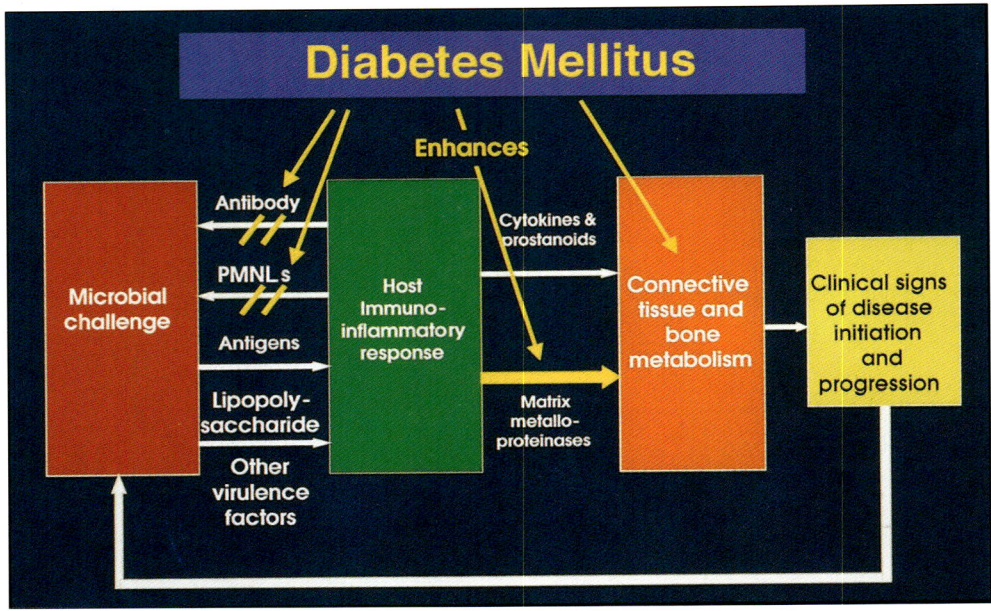

Fig 151 Schematic illustration of how diabetes mellitus may modify the pathogenesis of periodontal diseases. (Courtesy of R. Page.)

hanced secretion of inflammatory mediators can be induced by high lipid levels and by occupancy of monocytic receptors for advanced glycation end products (AGEs). With respect to the risk for periodontitis, it is therefore important that the patient with diabetes not only be metabolically well controlled but also be assessed for genetic risk factors. Promising phase-2 studies are underway for evaluation of a glutamic acid decarboxylase (GAD)–based vaccine against type 1 diabetes mellitus in latent autoimmune diabetes in the adult (LADA) patients.

Impaired collagen metabolism and bone matrix component production. The properties of human collagen change during aging and with the metabolic abnormalities of diabetes mellitus. Collagen is the predominant component of the gingival connective tissue, accounting for approximately 60% of connective tissue volume and 90% of the organic matrix of alveolar bone. Altered collagen metabolism would be expected to contribute to progression of periodontal disease and impaired wound healing in diabetic patients.

A number of studies have reported that cellular proliferation and growth are diminished and that collagen synthesis by skin fibroblasts is reduced under hyperglycemic conditions (Goldstein, 1984; Lien et al, 1984; Seibold et al, 1985; Weringer and Arquilla, 1981). In a series of studies on collagen metabolism in experimentally induced diabetes, Golub and coworkers found that diabetes impaired the production of bone matrix components by osteoblasts, decreased collagen synthesis by gingival and periodontal ligament fibroblasts, and increased gingival collagenase activity (Golub et al, 1978; Schneir et al, 1981). Existing data show that periodontal ligament cells from patients with long-standing type 1 diabetes mellitus have a reduced ability to form mineralized tissue and an altered response to growth factors (Hobbs et al, 1999). This suggests a less favorable response to periodontal treatment and maintenance. Figure 151 illustrates schematically how diabetes mellitus may modify the pathogeneses of periodontal diseases in different ways.

The fact that diabetes produces an increase in gingival collagenase under germ-free conditions indicates that the increase is endogenously mediated and can be independent of bacterial factors. Consistent with these findings are the increased collagenolytic activity in crevicular fluid and the decreased synthesis of collagen by gingival fibroblasts in persons with diabetes. Because of the impaired chemotaxis and phagocytozing capacity of the PMNLs in those with diabetes, connective tissue is the site of PMNL accumulation and collagenase release. This may explain why diabetes enhances the degradation of newly synthesized, less completely cross-linked collagen, a phenomenon that may contribute to poor wound healing.

Advanced glycation end products. In a hyperglycemic environment, numerous proteins, including collagen, undergo a nonenzymatic glycosylation process to form AGEs. The formation of AGEs plays a central role in diabetic complications. AGE formation alters the function of numerous extracellular matrix components. These alterations have an adverse effect on target tissues, especially affecting collagen stability and vascular integrity.

Monocytes, macrophages, and endothelial cells posses high-affinity receptors for AGEs. AGE binding to macrophage and monocyte receptors may induce a hyperresponsive cellular state, resulting in increased secretion of IL-1, insulin-like growth factor, and TNF-α, while endothelial cell binding results in precoagulatory changes leading to focal thrombosis and vasoconstriction (Brownlee, 1994; Esposito et al, 1992; Kirstein et al, 1992; Lalla et al, 2000; Nishimura et al, 1998). Clinically, diabetic subjects with periodontitis have significantly higher gingival crevicular fluid levels of both IL-1β and PGE$_2$ compared with nondiabetic controls matched for periodontal disease severity (Salvi et al, 1997a).

Lalla et al (2000) treated diabetic mice with soluble receptor for advanced glycation end products (sRAGE), which binds ligand and blocks interaction with, and activation of, cell-surface RAGE. Although the mice were infected with the well-known periodontal pathogen *P gingivalis*, the treatment resulted in a decrease in the level of proinflammatory cytokines and matrix metal-

loproteinases in the gingival tissue and a reduction in the alveolar bone loss in a dose-dependent manner. This suggested that the AGEs, which result from hyperglycemia, could contribute to the pathogenesis of periodontal diseases in diabetes (Lalla et al, 1998) and that the blockage of these products could reduce the loss of periodontal tissue.

AGE-mediated events are of primary importance in the pathogeneses of diabetic complications such as retinopathy, nephropathy, and atherosclerosis. They may also be involved in tissue changes within the periodontium. Therefore, diabetic patients with poor glycemic control and elevated AGE production are more susceptible to increased tissue destruction (Salvi et al, 1997b).

AGEs detected in the gingival tissues of diabetic patients have also been shown to increase oxidant stress in these tissues compared with the tissues of nondiabetic subjects (Salvi et al, 1997b). This enhanced oxidant stress may be responsible for the vascular injury common to diabetic complications. Figure 152 illustrates a hypothetical model of inflammatory tissue destruction induced by AGEs in diabetic patients.

Reduced salivary secretion rate. Thorstensson et al (1989) showed that, compared with nondiabetics, both subjects with long-established diabetes and those with recently diagnosed diabetes have lower stimulated salivary secretion rates and greater salivary glucose content.

Altered subgingival microflora? Although in a few earlier studies an association was proposed between diabetes-associated changes in the periodontium and a specific gram-negative microbial flora, recent data have failed to demonstrate that the microflora of diabetics differs significantly from that of nondiabetic patients with periodontitis (Mandell et al, 1992). Mashimo et al (1983) reported high levels of *Capnocytophaga* species in periodontal sites of young individuals with type 1 diabetes mellitus. Sastrowijoto et al (1989) reported that levels of *P intermedia* were significantly greater in diseased sites than in healthy peri-

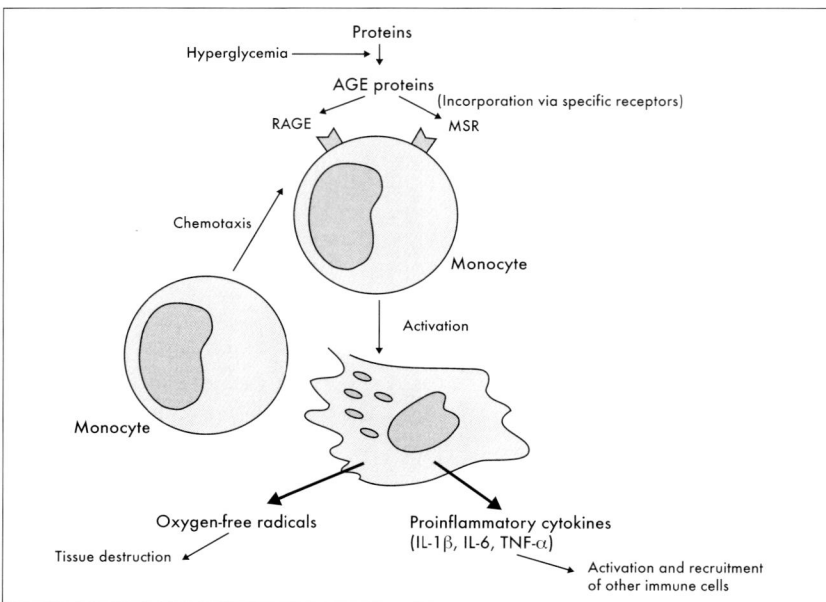

Fig 152 Hypothetical model of inflammatory tissue destruction induced by AGE in diabetic patients. When body proteins are exposed to a high concentration of glucose for a long time in vivo, they are nonenzymatically glycated and structurally modified to become what is termed AGE. Monocytes are chemotactic to AGE and take up this protein via specific receptors termed RAGE or MSR. Monocytes thus activated produce oxygen-free radicals that are destructive to tissues and proinflammatory cytokines, which further exacerbate inflammatory tissue destruction. (From Nishimura et al, 1998. Reprinted with permission.)

odontal sites in subjects with type 1 diabetes mellitus. In this study, *P gingivalis* and *A actinomycetemcomitans* were detected in similar proportions to those found in patients with chronic periodontitis.

However, several subsequent studies have failed to demonstrate that periodontal pathogens in the diabetic flora are unique to diabetic patients. In a group of poorly controlled diabetics, Mandell et al (1992) investigated the microbial composition associated with periodontally diseased sites: The bacterial patterns in the diseased sites of diabetics were similar to those of healthy controls with chronic periodontitis. At these sites, *P gingivalis* and *P intermedia* were detected in proportions similar to those at sites in systemically healthy chronic periodontitis patients. In a group of patients with type 2 diabetes mellitus, Zambon et al (1988) found *P intermedia, Campylobacter rectus,* and *P gingivalis* to be the three predominant periodontal pathogens in the subgingival flora. Thus, it seems that periodontal pathogens in the oral flora of diabetic individuals are not unique and are essentially similar to those found in systemically healthy patients with chronic periodontitis.

However, in a more recent study by Thorstensson et al (1996), the subgingival microflora and serum antibody response were examined in long-term type 1 diabetics and age- and sex-matched nondiabetics. The bacterial species studied *(A actinomycetemcomitans, C rectus, Capnocytophaga* species, *Eikenella corrodens, F nucleatum, P gingivalis,* and *P intermedia)* were recovered in diabetics as well as in nondiabetics. Compared to nondiabetics, significantly more diabetics in both age groups (40 to 49 years and 50 to 59 years) harbored *P gingivalis*. In the diabetics, *P gingivalis* occurred as often at sites with deepened periodontal pockets (> 4 mm) as at sites with shallow pockets (< 4 mm). In the nondiabetics, the presence of *P gingivalis* was associated with deepened periodontal pockets. The serum antibody titers for most antigens showed similar patterns in diabetics and nondiabetics.

Altered medical status in diabetic patients with severe periodontitis

In a recent study by Thorstensson et al (1996), the aim was to define a population of diabetics exhibiting an increased risk of developing severe periodontitis by comparing the medical status of two groups of diabetics, one with little or no periodontal disease and one with severe periodontal disease. The study comprised two parts, a baseline study and a follow-up study. The subjects were 39 selected case-control pairs: adult, long-term type 1 diabetics matched according to sex, age, and duration of diabetes. One subject of each pair (the case) had severe periodontal disease while the other (the control) had gingivitis or only minor alveolar bone loss.

The median age of the case patients was 58 years (range, 36 to 70 years) and that of the control patients was 59 years (range 37 to 69 years). The median duration of disease in cases and controls was 24 and 25 years, respectively. The median follow-up time was 6 years. The following medical variables were registered: weight, insulin dose, systolic and diastolic blood pressure, vibratory threshold, triglycerides, total cholesterol, high-density lipoprotein cholesterol, creatinine glycated hemoglobin (HbA_1), proteinuria, electrocardiogram, retinopathy, stroke, transient ischemic attacks, angina, myocardial infarct, heart failure, hypertension, intermittent claudication, foot ulcer, death, cause of death, and smoking habits.

In the follow-up study, significantly higher prevalences of proteinuria and cardiovascular complications such as stroke, transient ischemic attack, angina, myocardial infarct, and intermittent claudication were found in the case group, suggesting an association among renal disease, cardiovascular complications, and severe periodontitis. These findings are in agreement with those of the longitudinal study by Beck et al (1996), which showed the odds ratio for onset of myocardial infarction and stroke in patients with severe periodontitis to be slightly higher than that for regular, heavy smokers. These studies indicate the need for close cooperation between the diabetic specialist and the dentist in monitoring the diabetic patient.

Effect of periodontal treatment on metabolic control of diabetes

Recently, Grossi et al (1997) assessed the effects of treatment of periodontal disease on the level of metabolic control of diabetes. A total of 113 Native Americans with periodontal disease and type 2 diabetes mellitus were randomized into five treatment groups. Periodontal treatment included ultrasonic scaling and curettage, combined with one of the following antimicrobial regimens:

- Topical application of water and systemic doxycycline, 100 mg, for 2 weeks
- Topical application of 0.12% chlorhexidine and systemic doxycycline, 100 mg, for 2 weeks
- Topical application of povidone-iodine and systemic doxycycline, 100 mg, for 2 weeks
- Topical application of 0.12% chlorhexidine and a placebo
- Topical application of water and a placebo (control group)

The following assessments were made before and 3 and 6 months after treatment: measurement of probing pocket depth and clinical attachment level, detection of *P gingivalis* in subgingival plaque, and determination of serum glucose and glycated hemoglobin (HbA_1).

After treatment, all study groups showed improvement in clinical and microbial variables. Compared to the control group, the groups treated with doxycycline showed the greatest reduction in probing depth and subgingival *P gingivalis*. In addition, at 3 months, all three groups receiving systemic doxycycline showed significant reductions ($P < .04$) in mean glycated HbA, nearly 10% lower than the pretreatment value. The authors concluded that effective treatment of periodontal infection and reduction of periodontal inflammation is associated with a reduction in levels of glycated hemoglobin. Control of periodontal infections should therefore be regarded as an important aspect of overall management of patients with diabetes mellitus.

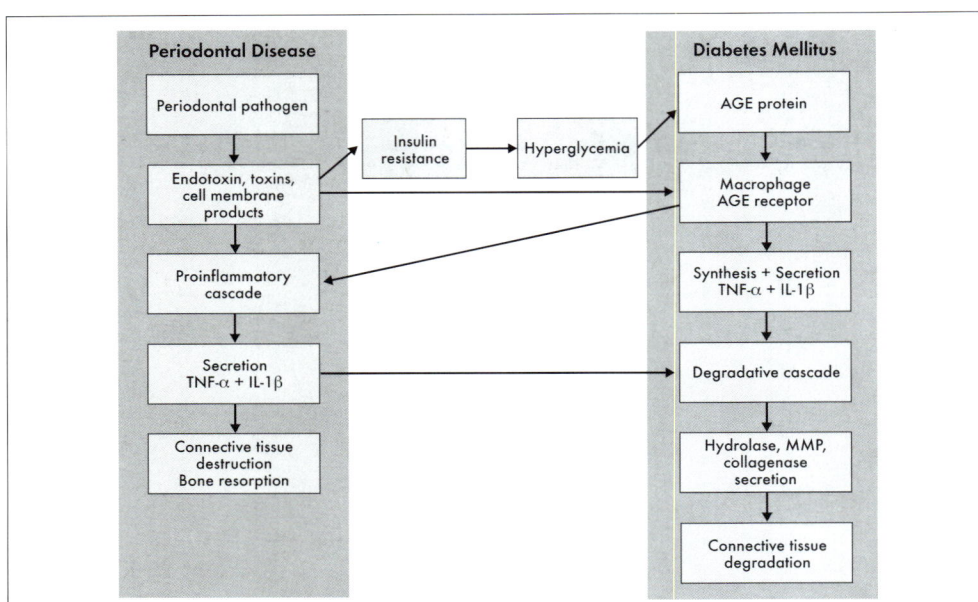

Fig 153 Proposed model for two-way relationship between periodontal disease and diabetes mellitus. (From Grossi and Genco, 1998. Reprinted with permission.)

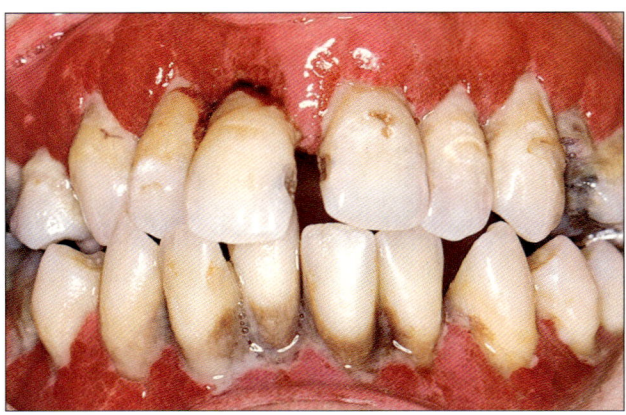

Fig 154 Clinical status, 40 years ago, of a 21-year-old woman with unstable type 1 diabetes, very poor oral hygiene, and an almost complete absence of dental care. Patients with diabetes mellitus usually have impaired host response mechanisms.

In addition, the aforementioned findings show that poorly controlled diabetes mellitus should be regarded as an internal modifying risk indicator, risk factor, and prognostic risk factor not only for vascular diseases but also for infectious diseases, such as periodontal diseases. Thus, diabetes mellitus and periodontal diseases exhibit a two-way relationship. The biologic mecha-

nisms discussed earlier for such a two-way relationship are illustrated in Fig 153.

Figures 154 and 155 show the clinical and radiographic status, 40 years ago, of a 21-year-old woman with unstable type 1 diabetes mellitus, extremely poor oral hygiene habits, and almost total absence of dental care. In spite of the poor quality of the radiographs, it is obvious that few teeth can be saved. This atypical case shows an extreme combination of overwhelming bacterial challenge and internal and external risk factors. However, bacterial challenge alone, even by the most aggressive periopathogens (*A actinomycetemcomitans, P gingivalis,* and *B forsythus*) could not result in such dramatic loss of periodontal support. Individuals with aggressive type 1 diabetes mellitus usually have severely impaired PMNL-cells, a defect in the first line of nonspecific host response, as discussed earlier.

In sharp contrast is the patient shown in Fig 156: An 80-year-old man who, despite massive plaque accumulation and total dental neglect, has no missing teeth, almost no loss of periodontal attachment, and very responsive gingival tissue. The internal (host) factors clearly outweigh the extreme bacterial challenge and other risk factors. It should be emphasized that the conditions of these

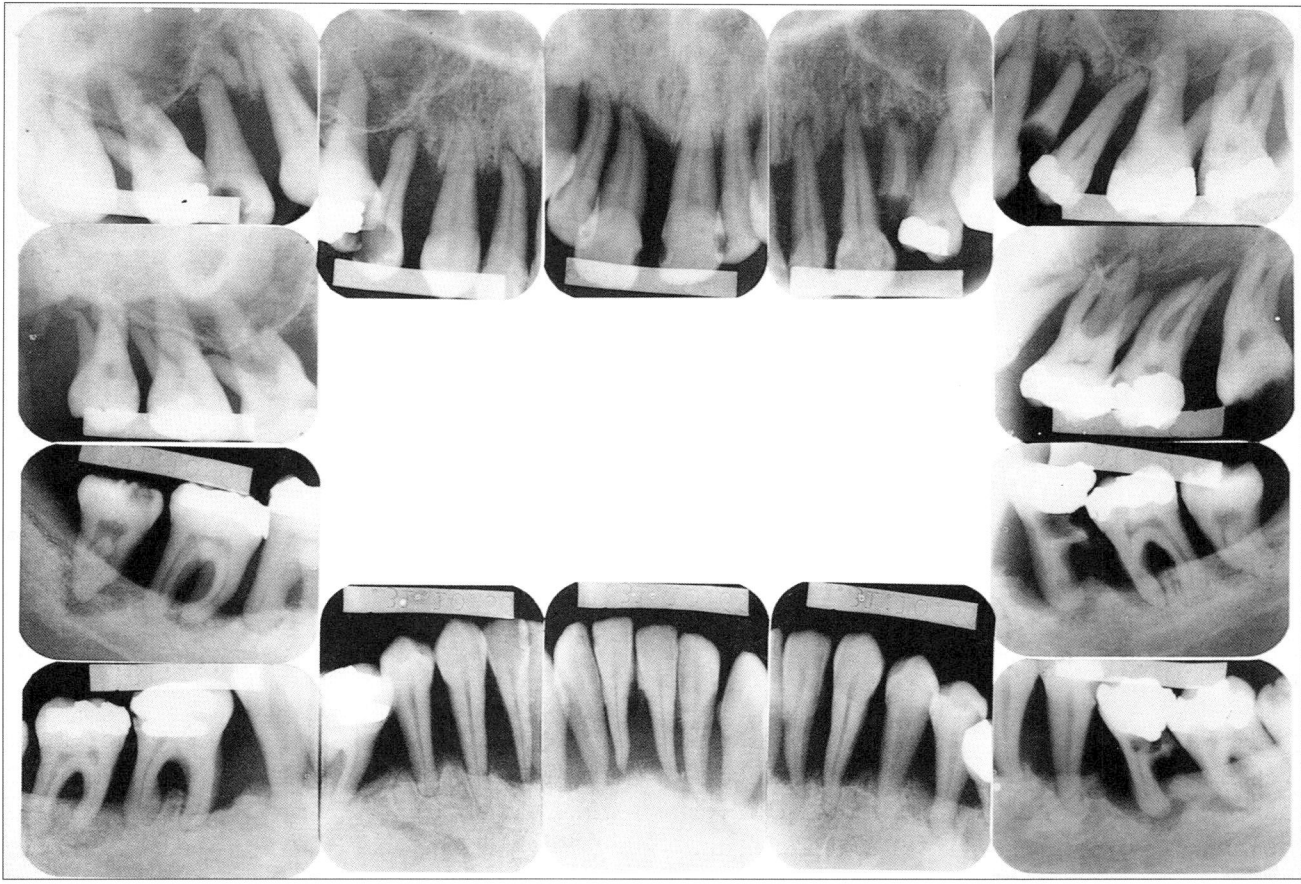

Fig 155 Radiographic status of the woman in Fig 154. Few teeth can be saved.

two patients are extreme, with oral hygiene and dental care standards far below the Swedish norm, even that of 30 years ago.

Figure 157 shows a patient with type 1 diabetes mellitus who, at the age of 40 years, had significantly more periodontal attachment loss than the average for this age group. After successful periodontal treatment and a maintenance program based on high-quality gingival plaque control by self-care and professional mechanical toothcleaning at needs-related intervals no further loss of attachment was recorded; although the internal risk factors persisted, the external causative risk factors had been eliminated.

The short-term response of well-controlled diabetic subjects to nonsurgical periodontal therapy seems to be similar to that of nondiabetic in-

dividuals. Similar improvements in probing depths, attachment levels, and subgingival microbiota have been demonstrated (Christgau et al, 1998; Tervonen et al, 1991). While most diabetic patients may show improvement in clinical variables of periodontal disease immediately after therapy, poorly controlled patients have a more rapid recurrence of deep pockets and a less favorable long-term response (Tervonen and Karjalainen, 1997; Tervonen et al, 2000). Five years after a combination of nonsurgical and surgical periodontal treatment with regular supportive periodontal therapy, diabetic patients had a similar prevalence of sites demonstrating gain, loss, or no change in clinical attachment (Westfelt et al, 1996). Most of the diabetic subjects in this study had moderately or well-controlled glycemia as determined by glycated hemoglobin levels.

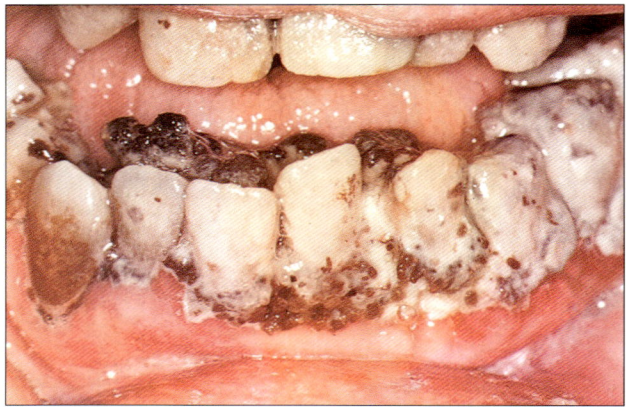

Fig 156 Clinical status of an 80-year-old man with massive plaque accumulation and complete dental neglect. Despite the neglect, he has no missing teeth, almost no loss of periodontal attachment, and very responsive gingival tissue. In this patient, the internal host factors clearly outweigh the bacterial challenge.

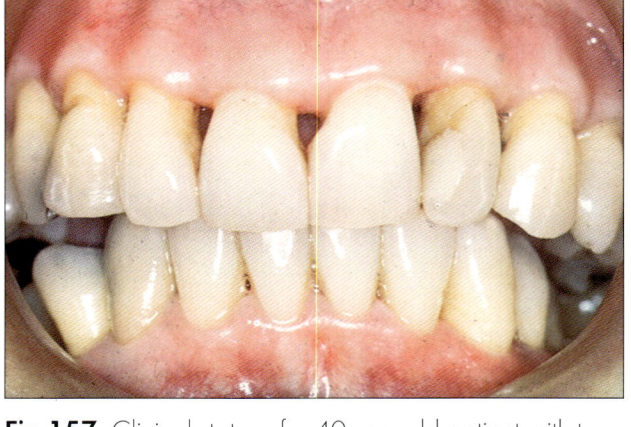

Fig 157 Clinical status of a 40-year-old patient with type 1 diabetes mellitus. This patient has significantly more attachment loss than the average for this age group. After successful periodontal treatment and a rigorous maintenance program, no further loss of attachment has been recorded.

For the most part, treatment of patients with well-controlled diabetes mellitus can be similar to that provided to nondiabetic patients. However, the procedure should be as short, atraumatic, and stress-free as possible. Early morning appointments after a normal breakfast are often preferred because levels of endogenous corticosteroids are generally higher at this time and stressful procedures may be better tolerated. On the day of treatment, patients with type 1 diabetes mellitus may reduce or eliminate the dose of insulin taken prior to the treatment to prevent hypoglycemia during the procedure. The dentist should always know the medication and diet regimen being followed by the patient in advance and should be prepared to handle the complications, such as hypoglycemia or insulin shock, that are most likely to occur. Pretreatment determination of blood glucose levels using the patient's glucometer may aid in prevention of hypoglycemia. Signs of hypoglycemia develop rapidly and treatment should be initiated as early as possible. Early treatment consists of administration of at least 15 g of oral carbohydrates (eg, orange juice).

The combination of mechanical debridement and systemic tetracycline (doxycycline) may pro-

vide a greater positive effect on glycemic control in some patients with diabetes mellitus compared with mechanical debridement alone as discussed earlier (Aldridge et al, 1995; Grossi et al, 1997). For successful management and prevention of extensive periodontal disease in smokers with type 1 diabetes mellitus, cigarette smoking must be discontinued (Moore et al, 1999).

Evidence from cross-sectional and longitudinal studies

Research reporting greater susceptibility to periodontitis in patients with diabetes mellitus extends back more than 60 years (Belting et al, 1964). Whether this is in fact the case has remained controversial until recently. Major obstacles to resolving the issue have included a lack of understanding of the variable and complex nature of both diabetes mellitus and periodontitis, methodological flaws in the studies, small samples, the questionable validity of various indices used to assess periodontal status, and the failure to control covariates, such as the patient's age and the duration of the diabetic state. Nevertheless, today there is evidence that both type 1 and type 2 diabetes mellitus significantly enhance an individual's susceptibility to severe periodontitis. The biologic reasons behind this phenomenon were discussed previously.

During the past decade, both cross-sectional and longitudinal studies have provided evidence confirming the association between diabetes mellitus and periodontitis. In one study, cross-sectional and longitudinal data on the Pima Indians in Arizona, who have the world's highest prevalence of type 2 diabetes but virtually no type 1 diabetes, were compared with data on a group of Danish men, aged 20 to 40 years, with type 1 diabetes (Emrich et al, 1991). In another study, periodontitis in Finnish diabetics was compared to data on similar age groups in the 1985 to 1986 Oral Health of US adults national survey of periodontitis (Oliver and Tervonen, 1993, 1994a, 1994b).

In the large cross-sectional adult study (N = 1,426) by Grossi et al (1994) mentioned earlier, diabetes mellitus was ranked third, after age and smoking, as a risk indicator for severe forms of periodontal disease and was the only systemic disease positively associated with attachment loss. This association remained valid even after adjustments were made for age, smoking, socioeconomic factors, plaque, and calculus. Diabetics were twice as likely as nondiabetics to have advanced attachment loss (odds ratio 2.32). Studies by Glavind et al (1968) and Hugoson et al (1989) have found that periodontitis is more extensive in patients who have had diabetes for many years than it is in diabetics with a shorter history of the disease.

Selwitz et al (1998) assessed periodontal disease outcomes in 9,680 dentate adults aged 30 to 90 years. The study sample comprised individuals who had been previously diagnosed with type 2 diabetes mellitus and individuals who had not been diagnosed with diabetes, all examined in the NHANES III survey in 1988 to 1994 in the US (Albandar et al, 1999). Their findings, adjusted for age, gender, and race/ethnicity, showed that 31% of those with diabetes had ≥ 5 mm periodontal attachment loss; 21% had ≥ 5 mm probing pocket depth; 31.8% had ≥ 3 mm gingival recession; and

13.7% had gingival bleeding, compared with 20%, 8.8%, 22.8%, and 50.4%, respectively, of the individuals without diabetes ($P < .01$). Similarly, those with diabetes had periodontal disease to a significantly higher extent than did those without diabetes. There also is evidence that young people with type 1 diabetes, particularly those with poor glycemic control, have poorer periodontal health than do those without diabetes.

A longitudinal study assessed the risk for alveolar bone loss in a group of Native Americans with poorly controlled type 2 diabetes and in individuals with better controlled diabetes or without diabetes (Taylor et al, 1998). Their results showed that the cumulative odds ratio of showing bone loss over time was 2.2 in the individuals with better controlled diabetes compared with those without diabetes, and 5.3 in the individuals with poorly controlled diabetes compared with those with better controlled diabetes.

These and other studies have shown the following: The prevalence of advanced periodontal disease is substantially higher in individuals with type 1 or type 2 diabetes than it is in nondiabetics. Among the Pima Indian population, there was early onset of bone and attachment loss in those with diabetes, and the rate of progression was almost three times that of nondiabetics. Those with retinopathy were almost five times more likely to have advanced periodontitis than were those without. Edentulousness increased significantly with the duration of the diabetic state and was 15 times more likely in diabetics than it was in nondiabetics.

Patients with uncontrolled or poorly controlled diabetes are at greater risk for periodontitis than are patients with controlled diabetes and those without diabetes. When other variables are controlled, type 1 and type 2 diabetes do not differ with regard to associated risk. Diabetics with a long history of disease are more likely to develop periodontitis than are those with diabetes of shorter duration. Some studies, but not all, have reported greater loss of teeth in diabetics than in nondiabetics. The disclosed association between diabetes and periodontal disease is similar, regardless of whether the presence and severity of the disease are expressed in terms of clinical attachment loss, alveolar bone loss, tooth loss, or probing depth.

Calculus seems to be an important determinant, especially in the Pima Indians: In diabetics, teeth with calculus were much more likely to be severely diseased than were those with little or no calculus. Individuals with poorly controlled diabetes had more calculus than did those with well-controlled disease.

Periodontal therapy improves the periodontal condition and may facilitate metabolic control of the diabetes as previously discussed (American Academy of Periodontology, 1996d; Grossi et al, 1997). A positive observation from most studies is that the risk for severe periodontitis is no greater in patients with well-controlled diabetes than it is in persons without diabetes, especially in the absence of calculus and the presence of excellent dental care and oral hygiene. Patients with well-controlled diabetes generally have on average more teeth than those who have poorly controlled or uncontrolled disease.

Furthermore, as mentioned earlier, the response to periodontal therapy in persons with well-controlled diabetes is as favorable as it is in nondiabetics (Christgau et al, 1998; Grossi et al, 1996; Westfelt et al, 1996). In comparison with such patients, those with severe type 1 diabetes (ie, with poor long-term metabolic control and/or multiple complications) experience more severe and rapid recurrence of periodontal breakdown after periodontal therapy (Tervonen and Karjalainen, 1997). Therefore, to assess the periodontal prognosis and the need for periodontal therapy on an individual basis, the clinician should take into account the diabetic status and the duration of the patient's diabetes (for reviews on the relationship between diabetes and periodontal diseases, see Dennison et al, 1996; Donahue and Wu, 2001; Grossi and Genco, 1998; Grossi, 2001; Iacopino, 2001; Katz et al, 1991; Lamster and Lalla, 2001; Mealy, 2000; Nishimura et al, 1998: Oliver and Tervonen, 1994a, 1994b; Page and Beck, 1997; Salvi et al, 1997a, 1998; Soskolne, 1998; Soskolne and Klinger, 2001; Taylor, 2001; Yalda et al, 1994).

Down syndrome

In children with Down syndrome, the prevalence of periodontal disease is very high, ranging from 50% to 90%. Both the primary and permanent dentitions are affected, and the severity appears to increase with age. Destruction is rapidly progressive and tends to be most severe in the mandibular anterior and maxillary molar teeth, although as the disease progresses other teeth are affected. Compared with other forms of mental retardation, Down syndrome seems to be associated with more severe periodontal disease, suggesting underlying, genetically determined risk factors (for review see Roulard-Bosma and Van Dijk, 1986). This is further supported by observations that, although there are substantial amounts of plaque and calculus, they are not related to the severity of the destruction. Finally, the plaque flora of persons with Down syndrome appears to be similar to that of matched controls, both unaffected people and persons with other forms of mental retardation, indicating that there are probably no virulent bacteria unique to individuals with Down syndrome.

The underlying defects reported in persons with this syndrome include a number of immunologic defects and structural deficiencies of the teeth, which have shorter roots and an excessive rate of gingival collagen synthesis. The reported defects of chemotaxis in PMNLs and mononuclear phagocytes of phagocytosis and microbial killing have not been studied with dental plaque bacteria, but there is no reason to suppose that these deficiencies, demonstrated with organisms such as *Streptococcus pyogenes* and *Candida albicans,* would not also exist for plaque bacteria. Other immunodeficiencies of B lymphocytes are described, including lower levels of IgG and immunoglobulin A in younger subjects and higher levels in older subjects. In the T-lymphocyte lineage, both mitogen- and antigen-induced proliferations are depressed.

It would appear that the multiple deficiencies of the functions of the PMNLs and monocytes may predispose those with Down syndrome to periodontal destruction, but the altered gingival connective tissue may also predispose them to early, rapid destruction. The role of the lymphocyte defects is less clear at present, but the site-specific nature of the lesions would support the concept that phagocytic cell dysfunction is being expressed in the presence of specific bacterial pathogens to cause local destruction.

Papillon-Lefèvre syndrome

Papillon-Lefèvre syndrome is an autosomal-recessive trait that consists of a diffuse palmar-plantar hyperkeratosis and rapidly progressive periodontitis in both the primary and permanent dentitions, leading to loss of the latter in the mid-teens. Some structural abnormalities of the skin and gingival connective tissue, teeth, and periodontal ligament are reported (Nazzarro et al, 1988; Vrahopoulos et al, 1988). Defects of PMNL adherence and chemotaxis have been described (Tinanoff et al, 1986; van Dyke et al, 1984), although microbial killing appeared to be normal.

Mononuclear phagocytosis may be depressed (Preus and Morland, 1987). It is interesting that treatment by a combination of extraction of the affected teeth and tetracycline therapy may reverse the defects of the PMNLs and mononuclear phagocyte. The etiopathogenesis of the periodontal destruction is unknown, but *A actinomycetemcomitans* (Preus, 1989) and *Capnocytophaga* species (Tinanoff et al, 1986) have been incriminated. It is difficult to speculate on the role of the PMNLs in the periodontitis associated with this syndrome, but it would appear that in some cases the peripheral defects of these cells may be induced by bacterial toxins. If there are specific pathogens in the subgingival plaque, such a peripheral defect would be magnified and site-specific destruction would occur. Structural abnormalities, such as thinned cementum, might also place the teeth at particular risk.

Chédiak-Higashi syndrome

This autosomal-recessive syndrome results in abnormal PMNLs, characterized by giant lysosomal granules containing the enzymes that would normally be segregated in the primary and secondary granules. Patients suffer from a variety of pyogenic bacterial infections of the skin, respiratory tract, and mucous membranes, for which the underlying mechanisms are unknown. However, the PMNLs and mononuclear phagocytes have been reported to have deficiencies of chemotaxis, degranulation, and membrane fusion, leading to delayed phagolysosomal fusion and intracellular bactericidal activity, which is probably caused by the reduced content of lysosomal hydrolases in the granules. More recently, a deficiency of the iC3B (MO-1) receptor on the PMNLs has been reported (Cairo et al, 1988).

In patients with this syndrome, severe gingivitis, periodontal disease, and loss of the entire adult dentition at an early age, presumably because of periodontal destruction (Charon et al, 1985), have been reported (Blume and Wolff, 1972; Tempel et al, 1972). The case reports do not contain enough clinical detail about the extent of the periodontal destruction, nor do they make it clear whether all patients with this syndrome are prone to aggressive, severe disease affecting both dentitions. Certainly, a number of patients with the syndrome have excessive periodontal destruction for their age, which will lead to early tooth loss.

Leukocyte adhesion deficiency

This disorder is an inherited autosomal-recessive trait, localized to chromosome 21, and has been described in more than 30 patients (Andersson and Springer, 1987). It consists of two forms, one severe and often leading to death before 1 year of age, and the other in which the patient may survive into adulthood. In the first form, the clinical symptoms are severe; the individual is affected by profound leukocytosis and multiple bacterial infections of many different systems. In the latter form, the infections are intermittent and not all systems are consistently affected. A consistent finding in both forms are destructive periodontitis of the aggressive, generalized prepubertal type, leading to loss of both the primary and permanent dentitions. In contrast to the descriptions of other phagocyte deficiency syndromes, which are often incomplete, the clinical descriptions of the periodontal and gingival conditions in many of these patients are precise (Waldrop et al, 1987).

The periodontal tissues in prepubertal patients with generalized aggressive periodontitis related to adhesion deficiency contain a dense infiltrate of plasma cells and extracellular pooling of antibody. Few lymphocytes are present. Polymorphonuclear leukocytes are seen in large numbers only within the lumen of adjacent blood vessels and are absent from the tissues. In a report of a patient with leukocyte adhesion deficiency (LAD) who was treated by granulocyte transfusion, the histologic picture had changed 12 hours after transfusion, and many neutrophils were observed in the connective tissue and within the pocket epithelial layer (Page et al, 1983).

The molecular basis of the severe syndrome is the complete absence of the three α and β chain complexes—CR3/Mac-1 (CD11b/18), LFA-1 (CD11a/18), and glycoprotein p150,95 (CD11c/18)—on cells of myeloid, monocytic, and lymphoid origin. Because the infections in this syndrome are predominantly bacterial, it is probable that the functions of PMNLs and mononuclear phagocytes are more affected than are the functions of the lymphocytes. It is thus likely that, as risk factors for periodontal destruction, the defects of PMNLs and mononuclear phagocytes also have a greater role than do the defects of the lymphocytes.

The above mentioned glycoprotein complexes are responsible for cellular adherence; their deficiency leads to defective adhesion and leukocytosis because the cells cannot adhere to vascular endothelium and thus cannot enter the tissues. Inflammation is thus severely depressed, and pa-

tients have defects of adherence-related PMNL functions such as aggregation, adherence, spreading, and chemotaxis. Normal PMNLs can upregulate CR3/Mac-1, and p150,95 from secondary and tertiary granule proofs of these molecules, which causes them to become hyperadherent and to aggregate. The absence of this pool in PMNLs of patients with LAD probably accounts for the failure of these cells to marginate in the vessels. Phagocytosis mediated by the CR3/Mac-1 complex is defective, and failure to bind iC3b-coated particles leads to failure of the respiratory burst trigger and possibly defective bactericidal function.

The discovery of this syndrome and the related molecular defects, together with the consistent findings of aggressive, generalized periodontal destruction, highlight the importance of PMNL (and possibly also monocyte) recruitment to the periodontium, where they have a protective role. Because the protective functions of the PMNLs are expressed in the crevice or pocket (Wilton, 1986), the most pronounced and certain failure of this protection must be a failure of the supply of adequate numbers of functional cells. The generalized disease pattern in the periodontium of patients with LAD and the fact that it occurs in all patients distinguishes this type of defect from those in which the expression of the PMNL deficiency is associated with a specific bacterial flora, leading to a site-specific lesion.

Polymorphonuclear leukocyte defects

Studies of host response in periodontal diseases have clearly indicated the polymorphonuclear leukocyte (neutrophil, PMNL) as the key protective cell that, under normal circumstances, limits the pathologic effect of periodontal organisms as the first line of nonspecific defense in the periodontal pocket. The PMNL does not act alone and operates as part of a neutrophil-antibody-complement axis that exerts a protective role against the gram-negative organisms that are important in periodontal diseases. Three lines of evidence support a central role for PMNLs in the host response.

The first line of evidence is derived from clinical studies of naturally occurring disease states involving primary and secondary immunodeficiencies. It has long been recognized that alterations in the number of leukocytes and in the relative proportions of the various white blood cells reflect the body's response to disease. As the predominant phagocyte in blood and inflamed tissues, the PMNL plays a crucial role in the defense process against virulent bacteria. Observations from human and animal disease states demonstrate that defective neutrophil function is associated with the presence of periodontal destruction (Clark et al, 1977; Van Dyke et al, 1983). Periodontal destruction is associated with inherently depressed PMNL function, in conditions such as cyclic neutropenia as well as the chronic systemic diseases discussed earlier: diabetes mellitus, Down syndrome, Papillon-Lefèvre syndrome, Chédiak-Higashi syndrome, and LAD. Neutropenia may also be drug induced. For example, smokers have been shown to have reduced PMNL function (see chapter 2).

Although periodontal destruction has been associated with PMNL dysfunction, individuals suffering from primary lymphocyte disorders, such as hereditary deficiencies in cell-mediated immunity, exhibit no greater severity of periodontitis than do healthy subjects.

The second line of evidence implicating the PMNL as a major protective cell against oral bacterial pathogens is the observation that several periodontopathic bacteria have significant antineutrophil virulence factors. *P gingivalis* and *A actinomycetemcomitans* are leukoaggressive; that is, they produce toxins and other factors that either impair the function of or kill PMNLs.

The third line of evidence for the critical role of PMNLs in periodontal diseases is based on the identification of PMNL dysfunction in several forms of aggressive periodontitis, including localized forms, generalized forms, and forms occurring during prepubescence. A large database and literature support the role of neutrophil ab-normalities in localized aggressive periodontitis (Agarwal et al, 1996; Van Dyke et al, 1982, 1985, 1986, 1988).

These three lines of evidence lead to the conclusions that (*1*) normal PMNL function is an important determinant of host resistance to periodontal destruction and (*2*) impaired PMNL function often results in increased susceptibility to periodontitis (for details on the function of the PMNLs see chapter 5; for reviews on the role of PMNL defects as risk indicators and risk factors, see Dennison and Van Dyke, 1997; Hart et al, 1994; Johnson, 1994; Kornman et al, 1997b; Wilton, 1991).

Ehlers-Danlos syndrome

In this syndrome there is a reduction in or an absence of type III collagen in the skin, parenchymal organs, and blood vessels walls. The collagen defects may arise from a lack of synthesis, decreased rates of synthesis, or abnormal procollagen secretion (Krane, 1983). It may be inherited in an autosomal-dominant or a recessive pattern. Classification is based on the clinical and biochemical features of the disorder: There are 10 variants, types I to X. Type I (gravis) and type IV (ecchymotic) are associated with gingival bleeding, which would presumably be secondary to the vascular and mucosal fragility.

Type VIII, the autosomal-dominant form, results in severe periodontal destruction and a pattern of generalized resorption of the alveolar bone (Stewart et al, 1977). It is not known whether the plaque flora is specific for the condition or whether the plaque levels are disproportionate to the destruction, as reported for patients with type 1 diabetes and Down syndrome. It would appear that, unlike the periodontal effects of the syndromes discussed so far, the periodontal destruction in the type VIII form of Ehlers-Danlos syndrome is related only to the structural and biochemical defects of the connective tissues: No defects of host defense functions have been reported.

Role of Aging

Epidemiologic studies reveal more periodontal disease in older age groups than in younger groups (see chapter 7). Reports of greater plaque development and more severe gingivitis in the elderly than in younger subjects indicate age-related effects. Although the question of why periodontal disease is more severe in the elderly is still open, most studies attribute this to cumulative tissue destruction over a lifetime rather than to an age-related, intrinsic deficiency or abnormality that increases periodontal susceptibility.

There are also significantly more local plaque-retentive factors in the aged dentition (eg, multiple restorations with defects [overhangs], calculus, deep pockets, teeth with furcation involvement, root caries), which may explain the somewhat higher incidence of periodontal disease in the elderly than in younger adults, who have fewer plaque-retentive factors.

However, it is still unclear whether deterioration of host-protective mechanisms, accelerated host-destructive mechanisms, or susceptibility to periodontal infection is altered in the very elderly (those older than 80 years). There may indeed be an increased risk of periodontal disease associated with advanced age, per se. In the elderly, salivary secretion rates (particularly for unstimulated saliva) are reduced, and this may increase the plaque formation rate. Recent studies suggest that, up to the age of 80 years, the rate of periodontal destruction is the same throughout adulthood (Axelsson et al, 1991, 2000).

Therefore, it appears that age, per se, is not an intrinsic risk factor, at least until the age of 70 or 80 years. In a 15-year longitudinal study, the oldest age group (65 to 85 year olds) was as well maintained as the youngest age group (35 to 50 year olds) in a preventive plaque control program by a dental hygienist (Axelsson et al, 1991). The average probing attachment gain per individual per 15 years was 0.3 mm in all age groups.

The association between aging and periodontal status is complicated by the relationship with oral hygiene status. Abdellatif and Burt (1987) evaluated the relative importance of age and oral hygiene status as determinants of periodontitis in an epidemiologic study. They estimated the incidence of disease using age-specific prevalence data gathered from 14,690 dentate Americans, aged 15 to 74 years. The rate of increase in periodontitis with increasing age was much higher, across all age groups, for those with poor oral hygiene. In all age groups, 95% of those with good oral hygiene did not have periodontitis, regardless of age. The odds ratio was 20.52 for the association between oral hygiene status and periodontitis and only 1.24 for the association between increasing age and disease. The researchers concluded that the effect of age on disease progression is negligible when good oral hygiene is maintained.

Interpretation of data that suggest a possible association between aging and periodontal status is further complicated by tooth loss. In most elderly persons, many teeth have been lost, but for unknown reasons, and cannot therefore be considered in assessment of periodontal disease status. In most industrialized countries, the direct or indirect cause of about 70% of tooth loss is dental caries.

Although some published data support the observation that the prevalence and severity of periodontitis increase with increasing age, current evidence from longitudinal studies in which other factors were controlled indicates that the relationship between age and periodontal disease is age associated, rather than a consequence of aging. When higher incidence periodontal disease is found to be related to aging, it appears that the association is caused by other factors. These and other observations have led many authors to question the concept of age as a risk factor whereby the elderly become more susceptible to severe periodontitis than do younger people (Axelsson et al, 1991, 2000).

Periodontitis, especially the aggressive forms that lead to early tooth loss, begins in the young, not in the elderly (Ånerud et al, 1983; Van der Velden, 1991). It is in these individuals, rather than the elderly, that high susceptibility is likely. Notably, bursts of destructive disease activity characteristic of periodontitis have not been reported in the elderly (Page, 1984). Across all ages, there is a close association among good oral hygiene, periodontal health, and tooth retention (Abdellatif and Burt, 1987; Axelsson et al, 1991; Burt, 1994).

ROLE OF LOCAL ORAL CONDITIONS

Plaque-retentive factors

Gingivitis is caused by the gingival plaque (biofilm) and periodontitis is caused by the subgingival periopathogens—particularly in the subgingival biofilm. Frequent removal of gingival plaque by self-care, supplemented with needs-related professional mechanical toothcleaning and removal of the subgingival biofilm by debridement, is therefore essential to the prevention and control of periodontal disease. However, the effect of the different plaque control measures may be seriously impeded by supragingival (Box 7) and subgingival (Box 8) plaque-retentive factors.

Restorations and dental caries

Analytic epidemiologic studies show that, with the exception of the occlusal surfaces of the molars, the highest prevalence of carious and filled surfaces and loss of periodontal attachment occurs on the approximal surfaces of the molars and premolars (Axelsson et al, unpublished data, 1990). In industrialized countries, most approximal surfaces of the molars and premolars in adults 40 years and older are restored (Fig 158).

Early studies in animals (Marcum, 1967; Waerhaug, 1960) and humans (Silness, 1970; Waerhaug, 1975) showed that the most favorable peri-

odontal response is attained when the margins of dental restorations are placed at, or coronal to, the gingival margin. Furthermore, these findings have been corroborated by more recent findings (Kois, 1996).

In the early 1970s, epidemiologic studies in Sweden showed that most approximal restorations of molars and premolars had subgingival defects. In addition, there was a strong correlation between the size of overhangs and loss of adjacent alveolar bone (Björn et al, 1969a, 1970). Sim-

---

Box 7 Conditions that contribute to supragingival plaque retention

- Caries lesions
- Restoration overhangs and defective margins
- Ill-fitting margins of crowns and inlays
- Excess resin cement
- Unpolished restorations
- Resin composite restorations
- Supragingival calculus
- Exposed, unplaned root surfaces

Box 8 Conditions that contribute to subgingival plaque retention

- Rough, unplaned cementum
- Cementum hypoplasia
- Root grooves
- Root resorption
- Calculus
- Iatrogenic effects of subgingival scaling (eg, grooves and exposed dentinal tubules on the root surfaces)
- Restoration overhangs
- Defective and ill-fitting margins of crowns
- Unpolished restorations
- Recurrent caries lesions
- Root caries lesions
- Furcation involvement
- Narrow intrabony defects and deep pockets

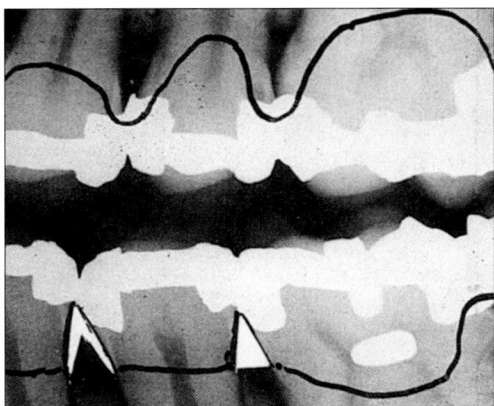

Fig 158 Bitewing radiograph of a 50-year-old Scandinavian. The location of the gingival margin and papillae is marked. Placement of two pointed (wedge-shaped and triangular) toothpicks is illustrated.

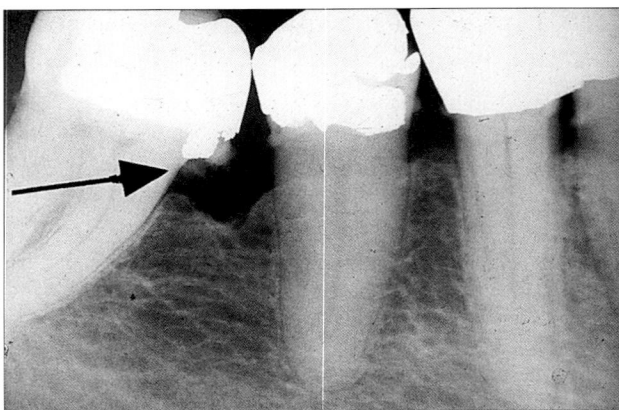

Fig 159 Overhanging restoration (arrow), related to the localized loss of periodontal support.

ilar results have been reported in other studies (Albandar, 1990a; Albandar et al, 1987; Brunsvold and Lane, 1990; Chen et al, 1987; Eid, 1986; Gilmore and Scheiham, 1971; Hakkaranein and Ainamo, 1980; Jeffcoat and Howell, 1980; Keszthelyi and Szabo, 1984; Pack et al, 1990; Rodriguez-Ferrer et al, 1980; Tal et al, 1989).

In particular, subgingival approximal overhangs tend to retain heavy deposits of subgingival plaque and calculus, inaccessible to oral hygiene in a toothbrushing population (Fig 159). In a retrospective study, Jansson et al (1994) evaluated the influence of overhangs on periodontal status and whether any such influence is modified by the patient's oral hygiene level and the degree of radiographic attachment loss. In patients with a mean radiographic attachment loss of less than 5 mm, an overhang was associated with significantly greater loss of attachment. However, in periodontitis-prone patients, a decrease in the influence of marginal overhangs on probing depth and attachment loss was noted as the loss of periodontal attachment increased, ie, as the distance between the overhang and the base of the pocket increased.

Recently, Schätzle et al (2000) showed similar results from a 26-year longitudinal study. Surfaces with subgingival restoration margins showed significantly more periodontal attachment loss than did intact tooth surfaces or supragingivally located restorations (> 1 mm from the gingival margin). However, when the attachment loss resulted in a gradually more coronal location of the former subgingival restoration margins, a "burn-out" effect was observed.

In a study of approximal restorations at a dental school clinic, 62% had marginal overhangs (Pack et al, 1990). Improvement of gingival status usually is attained by correcting the faulty restoration (Rodriguez-Ferrer et al, 1980). However, technically, subgingival approximal overhangs are difficult to remove, and various instruments are available for this purpose. Vale and Caffesse (1979) evaluated the effect of rotary instruments, amalgam knives, and reciprocating triangular diamond points for removing restoration overhangs. Scanning electron micrographs (SEMs) from this study revealed that rotary instruments and amalgam knives resulted in a narrow gap between the tooth surface and the amalgam, caused by fracture of the margin of the restoration (Fig 160). Such a gap will retain bacteria and increase the risk for secondary caries. No fractured margins occurred with the use of the reciprocating

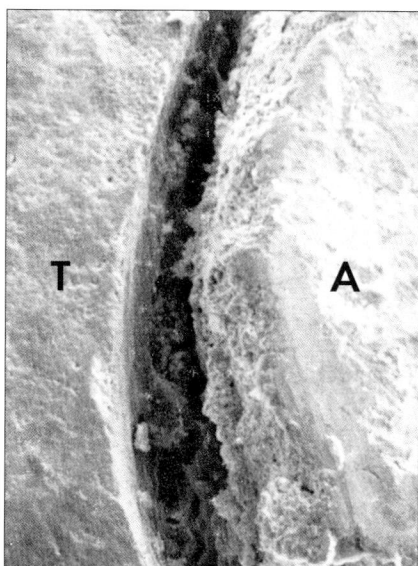

Fig 160 SEM revealing a narrow gap between the tooth surface (T) and the amalgam (A). The gap was caused by fracture of the restoration margin, which arose from the use of rotary instruments and amalgam knives (original magnification ×140). (From Vale and Caffesse, 1979. Reprinted with permission.)

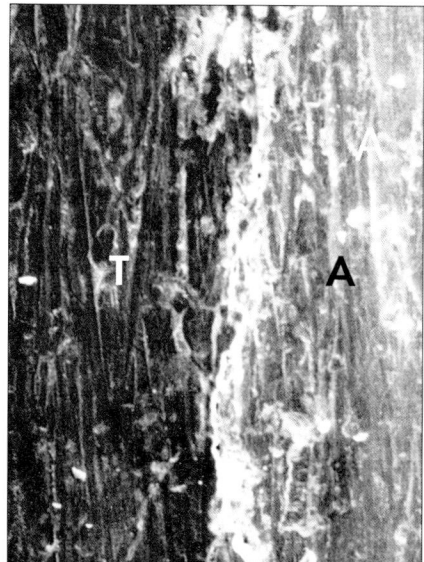

Fig 161 SEM revealing no fracture of the amalgam (A) margin or removal of tooth (T) substance after instrumentation with reciprocating EVA diamonds (original magnification ×140). (From Vale and Caffesse, 1979. Reprinted with permission.)

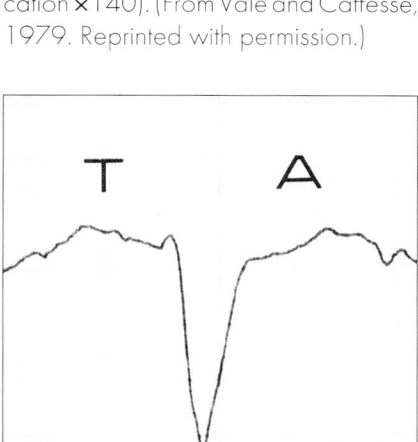

Fig 162 Profilogram after use of rotary instruments. T = Tooth, A = Amalgam. (From Vale and Caffesse, 1979. Reprinted with permission.)

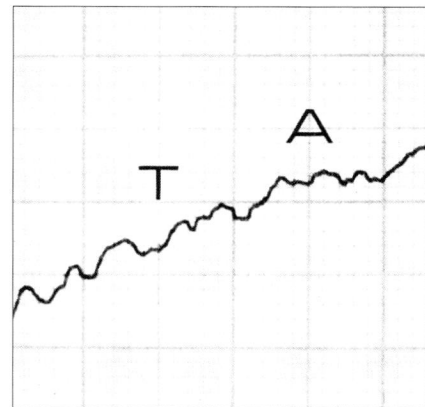

Fig 163 Profilogram after use of EVA reciprocating diamond tips (50 μm). T = Tooth, A = Amalgam. (From Vale and Caffesse, 1979. Reprinted with permission.)

EVA diamonds (Dentatus, Hägersten, Sweden) (Fig 161). The effects were confirmed in profilograms (Figs 162 and 163).

In another study, Spinks et al (1985) showed that removal of overhangs with hand instruments (curettes) or sonic scalers was 2.5 and 5 times

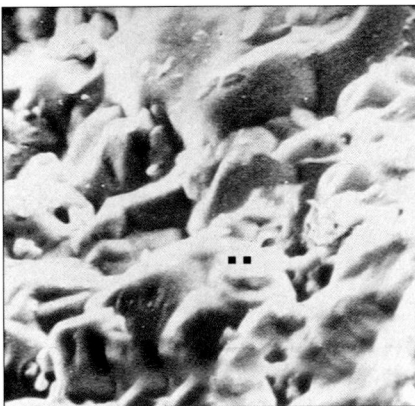

Fig 164 SEM of an unpolished approximal amalgam restoration that has been condensed against a new matrix band. Each black square is equivalent to 50 microbes, which means that each pit on the rough surface can retain hundreds of microbes that are inaccessible to cleaning by toothpicks, dental floss, or dental tape (original magnification ×6,000).

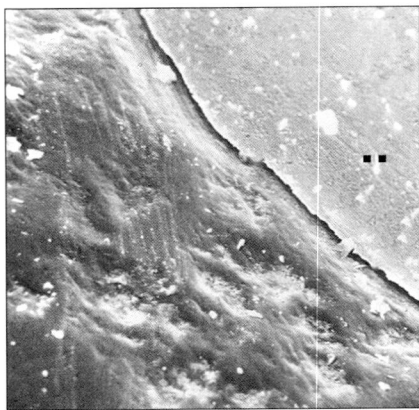

Fig 165 Well-finished and polished approximal amalgam restoration. Each square is equivalent to 50 microbes. The area is now accessible to oral hygiene aids (original magnification ×7,000).

more time consuming, respectively, than the EVA-Profin reciprocating diamond tips (Dentatus). In addition, the sonic scaler resulted in significantly more instances of iatrogenic roughness on the root surfaces apical of the restorations.

A recent 3-year study in Brazilian school children aged 12 to 15 years showed a significant association between the presence of untreated approximal manifest cavitated caries lesions and nondefective and defective approximal amalgam restorations and the progression of alveolar bone loss. There was also a significant correlation between the presence of defective approximal restorations and the incidence of gingival inflammation. An important result of this study was the finding that manifest (cavitated) caries lesions were significantly associated with the development and progression of periodontal disease in adolescents, whereas incipient (noncavitated) caries lesions were not. The other important finding was the effect of the location of the local factor. Albandar et al (1995) employed an analytic model that partitioned the variance according to

the location of the local factor (restoration or caries lesion) at tooth surfaces in adjacent interproximal sites, and showed that local factors on two adjacent teeth will both exert a harmful effect on the periodontal tissue located between these two teeth. Furthermore, the magnitude of the effect on the gingival tissue due to a restoration or caries lesion (cavity) located on the tooth surface closest to the tissue was about twice as much as that of the effect from the local factor located at the adjacent tooth surface. The study indicated that, in adolescents, untreated approximal manifest caries and dental restorations are predisposing factors with a significant negative effect on periodontal health. Young individuals with multiple such sites should be considered at risk of developing destructive periodontal lesions and managed accordingly.

It has been estimated that an unpolished amalgam restoration will retain about 50 times more dental plaque than an optimally finished and polished restoration (Figs 164 and 165). In addition, in vitro studies have shown that optimally finished

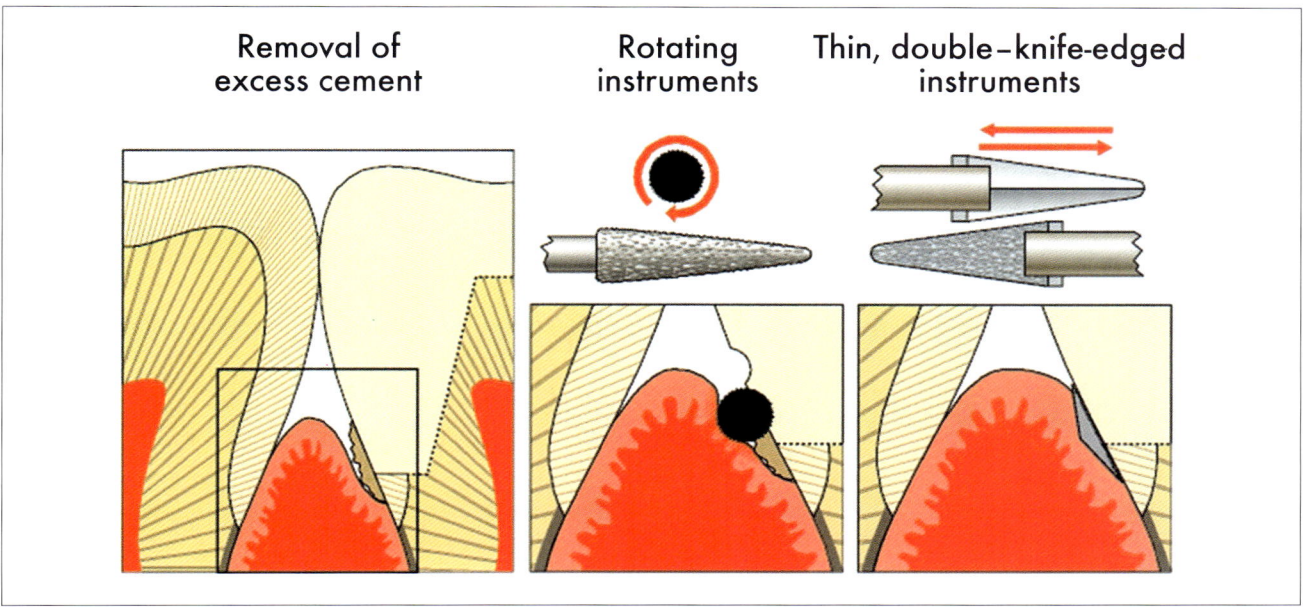

Fig 166 Difference in removal of subgingival excess cement with the use of rotating instruments and thin, double-knife-edged instruments. Observe the risk for horizontal iatrogenic roughness caused by rotating instruments.

amalgam restorations have four times the plaque reaccumulation (wet weight) of intact enamel that has been topically treated with stannous fluoride, because of highly significant differences in surface free energy and wettability (Glantz, 1969). Resin composite materials accumulate much more plaque than does amalgam, porcelain, or gold. The emphasis should therefore be on *prevention instead of extension*. In vivo studies have shown that surface roughness has a greater influence on early plaque formation and plaque composition than does surface free energy (Quirynen et al, 1990).

Early studies by Waerhaug (1960) indicated that the downgrowth of plaque into the subgingival area occurs more quickly on unpolished surfaces of restorations than on enamel or cementum. As mentioned earlier, the margins of almost 100% of approximal restorations on the molars and premolars are located subgingivally (see Fig 158). Traditionally, rotary instruments have been used to finish and polish restorations and remove overhangs. However, in narrow, triangular inter-proximal spaces, the subgingival area is almost inaccessible to rotary instruments. Many subgingival approximal restorations are therefore poorly finished and have persistent overhangs. To prevent and control secondary caries and periodontitis by mechanical gingival plaque control, optimal finishing and repeated polishing are much more important for subgingival approximal restorations than for occlusal, buccal, and lingual restorations.

Reciprocating triangular or V-shaped pointed instruments are more appropriate for narrow triangular interproximal spaces than are rotary instruments. Because of the resilience of the papillae, such reciprocating instruments are effective 2 to 3 mm subgingivally. Profin Lamineer reciprocating, thin, spatulate, or pointed double-knife-edged instruments (Dentatus) are even more useful for finishing, removing overhangs, and recontouring, because they can be used subgingivally between the papilla and the tooth surface (Fig 166). Besides diamond-coated tips in sizes from 15 to 150 μm, tungsten-coated tips are also

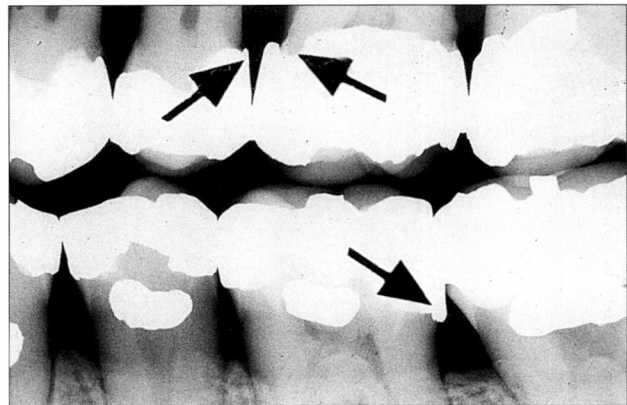

Fig 167 Approximal amalgam overhangs (arrows).

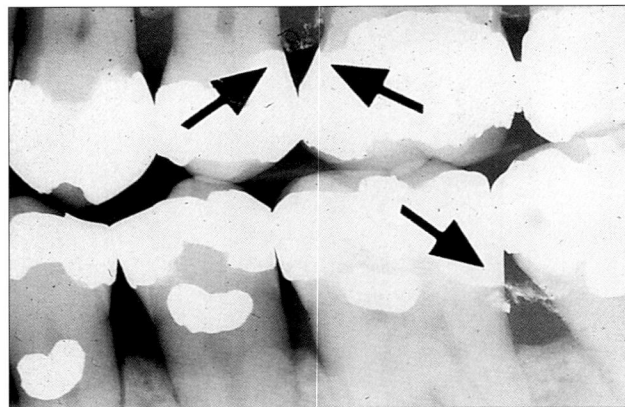

Fig 168 Smoothed margins (arrows), after removal of overhangs with the Profin contra-angle handpiece and a 50-μm diamond-coated reciprocating tip (1.0- to 1.5-mm strokes).

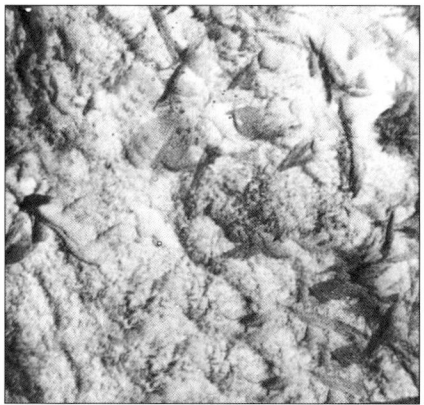

Fig 169 Intact root cementum from an impacted tooth with remnants of collagen fibers (original magnification ×10,000).

available. Tungsten-coated tips do not harm the tooth enamel, root surfaces, porcelain restorations or glass-ceramic restorations and are therefore suitable for final finishing of restorations and removal of excess resin cement.

Figure 167 shows approximal amalgam overhangs that were easily removed with the Profin contra-angle and a 50-μm diamond-coated reciprocating tip (Fig 168). Thereafter the approximal surfaces were finished and polished with less abrasive reciprocating tips, V-shaped pointed plastic tips, and fluoride prophylaxis paste.

Unplaned (intact) root cementum

The root cementum surface is very rough compared to the enamel surface. The cementoenamel junction is another anatomic feature with high plaque-retentive potential (see Fig 30 in chapter 1). The function of the root cementum is to maintain an optimum number of principal collagen fibers, and, in this respect, the rough, large surface is an advantage (Fig 169). However, if the periodontal ligament is destroyed directly and/or indirectly by the gingival microflora, the rough root cementum is a disadvantage, enhancing plaque retention (see Fig 31 in chapter 1). When the gingival plaque extends apically to the cementoenamel junction onto such rough subgingival root cementum, it is very difficult to remove.

Root resorption and hypoplasia

Root cementum resorption and hypoplasia are extraordinary retentive factors for the subgingival

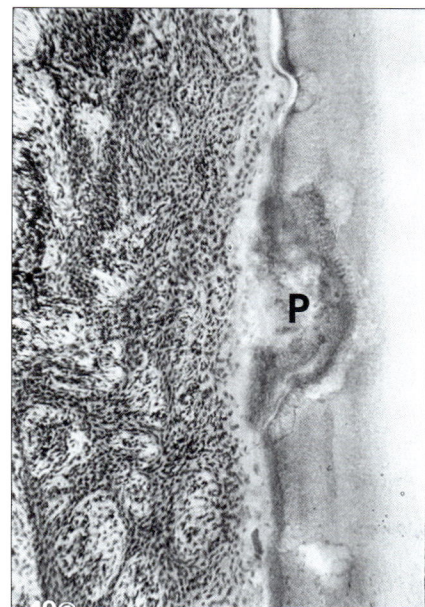

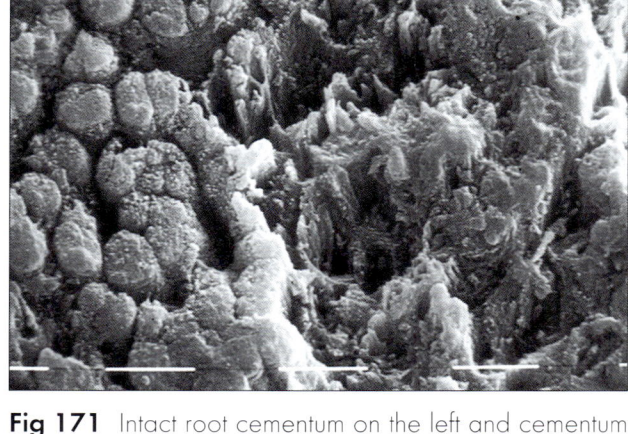

Fig 171 Intact root cementum on the left and cementum hypoplasia on the right (original magnification ×1,500). (From Lindskog and Blomlöf, 1983. Reprinted with permission.)

Fig 170 Subgingival cementum resorption filled with plaque bacteria (P) (original magnification ×100). (From Waerhaug, 1978. Reprinted with permission.)

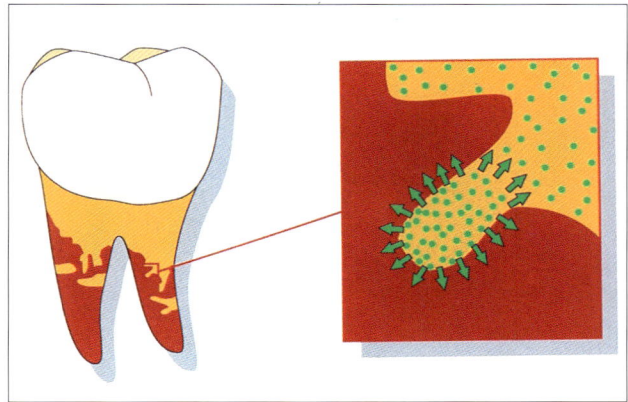

Fig 172 Lateral migration of the biofilm, facilitated by cementum hypoplasia and iatrogenic root grooves from aggressive instrumentation.

microflora (Figure 170). Studies by Lindskog and Blomlöf (1983) have shown that first molars extracted because of advanced, localized aggressive periodontitis exhibit multiple loci of cementum hypoplasia, which may serve as a retentive factor for the subgingival microflora, leading to loss of periodontal support (Fig 171). Adriaens et al (1986, 1988a) proposed that resorption and hypoplasia are important portals of entry for bacteria into root cementum and radicular dentin and demonstrated this in periodontally diseased teeth free of coronal caries.

The root cementum of the first molars and the central and lateral incisors develops at the same time. The predilection of localized aggressive periodontitis for these sites might be caused by cementum hypoplasia, induced for example by overexposure of the cementoblasts to fluoride, in analogy with its effect on ameloblasts in inducing enamel fluorosis.

Ehnevid et al (1995) showed that, in teeth with infected root canals, bacteria and their products could migrate via the dentinal tubules to areas of cementum hypoplasia on the root surface and initiate localized periodontitis. Cementum hypoplasia and iatrogenic root grooves from aggressive instrumentation may also facilitate lateral migration of the subgingival biofilm (Fig 172).

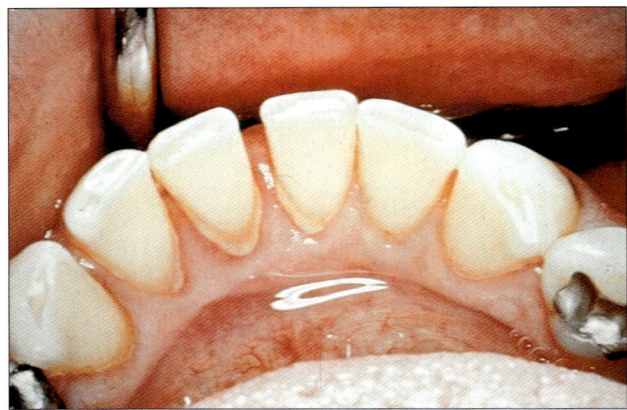

Fig 173a Supragingival calculus on the lingual surfaces of the mandibular incisors. The calculus was formed in the absence of plaque as a result of a high salivary concentration of minerals.

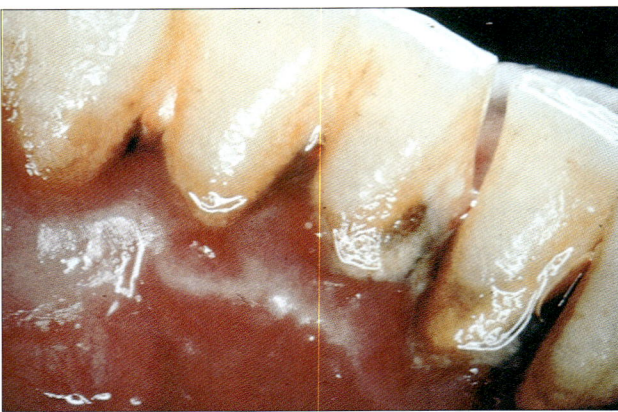

Fig 173b Supragingival and subgingival calculus arising from gingival inflammation at the mandibular incisors. The supragingival calculus and subgingival calculus were formed by minerals derived from saliva and inflammatory exudates, respectively.

Calculus

In individuals with high salivary concentration of minerals, supragingival calculus may form in the absence of dental plaque, especially on the lingual surfaces of the mandibular incisors (Fig 173a). However, if dental plaque results in gingival inflammation, there may be formation of both subgingival and supragingival calculus, by minerals derived from the inflammatory exudates and saliva, respectively (Fig 173b). Localized formation of such plaque-retentive calculus on the linguoapproximal surfaces of the mandibular incisors may explain why attachment loss on these surfaces is greater than the average for the mandibular tooth surfaces (Albandar et al, 1999; Albandar et al, 2002; Axelsson et al, unpublished data, 1990).

The longer the gingival plaque remains in the gingival sulcus, the greater the extent of intracellular and intercellular mineralization at the base of the sulcus, because minerals in the gingival exudates continuously penetrate the plaque (Figs 174 and 175). For optimal gingival plaque control, scaling is therefore a necessary supplement to oral hygiene and professional mechanical toothcleaning.

At the base of diseased pockets there is attached subgingival plaque (biofilms) and nonattaching subgingival microflora (Listgarten, 1976) (see Fig 28 in chapter 1). Subgingival calculus is formed only down to the base of the subgingival plaque biofilm. Calculus is not usually found in the most apical 0.1 to 1.0 mm of the pocket, where most of the motile microflora is located (see Figs 34 and 37 in chapter 1). However, in aggressive forms of periodontitis, subgingival calculus is seldom present. In these advanced and rapid forms of periodontitis, there is normally a very thin, semi-attached layer of subgingival microflora as well as microbes migrating into the connective tissue.

Autopsy studies by Waerhaug (1976) have confirmed the strong relationship between the apical border of subgingival plaque and calculus—the so-called plaque-free zone (0.1 to 1.0 mm wide)—and the coronal border of the periodontal membrane (see Fig 38 in chapter 1). For successful scaling, the instrument must access at least the plaque-free zone, the usual location of the nonattaching microbes.

Subgingival calculus is without question a very important and common plaque-retentive factor in untreated, diseased periodontal pockets. Formed by precipitation of minerals from the gingival exudates, it is much harder and rougher than supragingival calculus, which is formed by minerals from the saliva (Figs 176a and 176b).

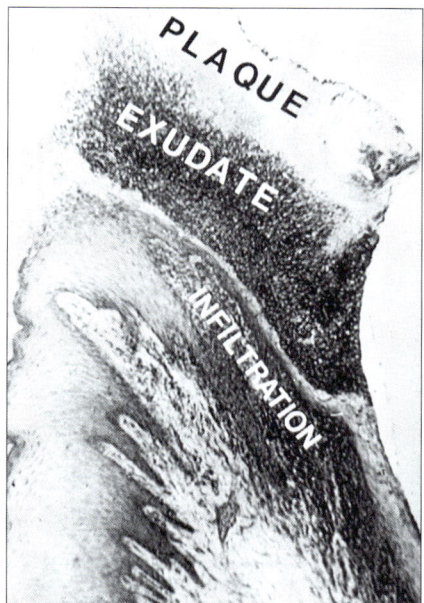

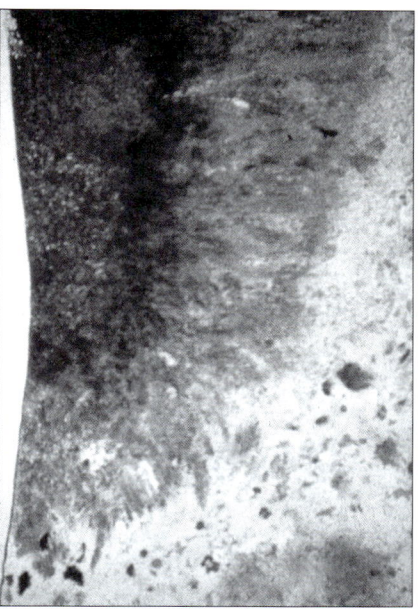

Fig 174 Penetration of the gingival sulcus by gingival exudates (original magnification ×100). (From Waerhaug, 1977. Reprinted with permission.)

Fig 175 The most apical extension of the gingival plaque biofilm is the gingival sulcus. The inner dark part of the plaque is mineralized (original magnification ×400). (From Listgarten, 1976. Reprinted with permission.)

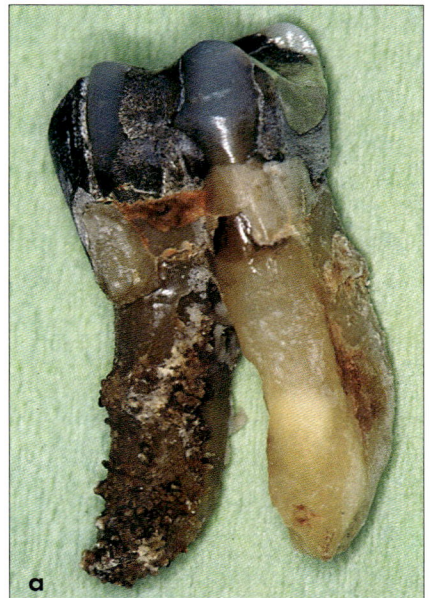

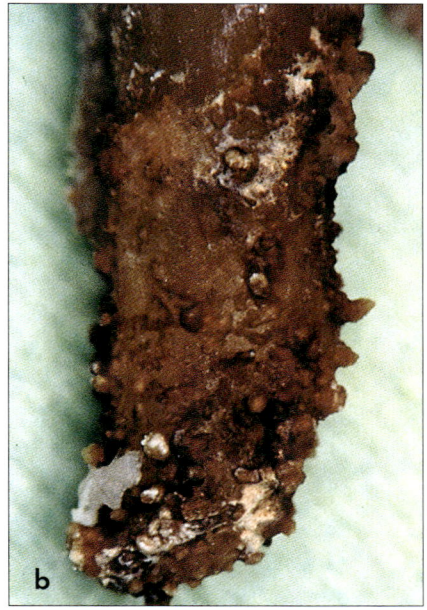

Figs 176a and 176b Excessive, rough calculus formation covering the entire distal root of an extracted, untreatable mandibular first molar.

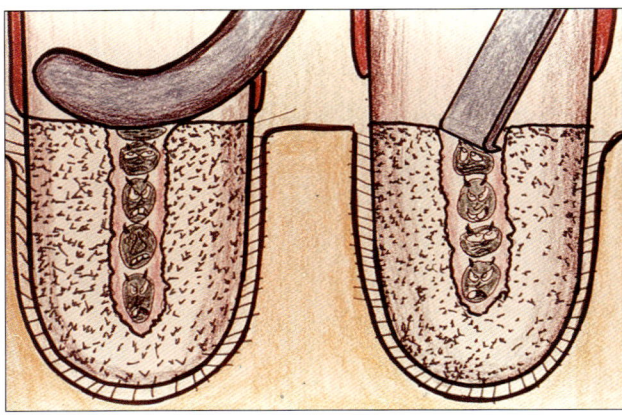

Fig 177 Subgingival microflora migrating apically along root grooves, inaccessible to nonsurgical instrumentation. (Illustrated by J. Waerhaug.)

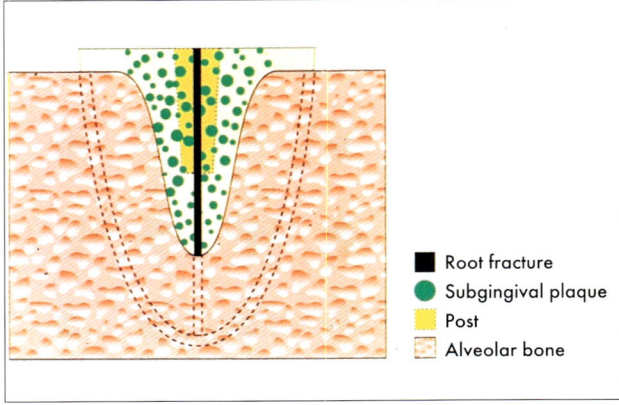

■ Root fracture
● Subgingival plaque
▨ Post
▧ Alveolar bone

Fig 178 Root fracture and resultant alveolar bone loss.

Epidemiologic studies show that populations with high prevalence of gingival inflammation and periodontal destruction also have higher prevalence and extent of dental calculus (Albandar et al, 1996, 1999; Albandar and Kingman, 1999). In addition, longitudinal studies show that dental calculus is associated with a higher rate of periodontal disease progression in adolescents (Albandar et al, 1998), as well as in adults (Albandar, 1990b).

Root grooves and root fractures

Attachment loss is frequently site specific and does not always coincide with the distribution of supragingival plaque. This phenomenon is attributed to a combination of local periopathogenic subgingival microflora and plaque-retentive factors such as root grooves and fractures. Subgingival microflora migrating apically along root grooves is inaccessible to nonsurgical instrumentation (Fig 177).

Nonsurgical periodontal therapy in nonmolar teeth has been reported to be less effective in teeth with root grooves or concavities (Badersten et al, 1987a). Leknes et al (1994) evaluated vertical loss of attachment on grooved and nongrooved approximal surfaces in 103 extracted incisors and premolars. They found, in general, a direct relationship between the location of the groove and the maximum loss of attachment. Attachment loss was statistically significantly greater on grooved surfaces than on nongrooved surfaces.

In a 15-year longitudinal preventive study based on gingival mechanical plaque control in adults, loss of teeth per individual was only 0.2, of which 65% was caused by root fractures in teeth with posts (Axelsson et al, 1991). The root fracture is invaded by microorganisms, resulting in local loss of periodontal support along the fracture (Fig 178).

The deleterious effects of root grooves and fractures are probably plaque related. Grooves and fractures promote plaque growth by providing sheltered areas that are inaccessible to cleaning or to host defense mechanisms. Subsequent bacterial selection and growth may be influenced by anaerobic conditions established within the grooves and fractures (Leknes, 1997).

Iatrogenic effects of subgingival scaling

Successful professional instrumentation of periodontally diseased teeth should completely remove plaque, calculus, and other bacterial components from the tooth surfaces, with little or no

Figs 179 and 180 Results of instrumentation with a rotary diamond tip. The diamond tip removed all the cementum and left deep gouges in the dentin.

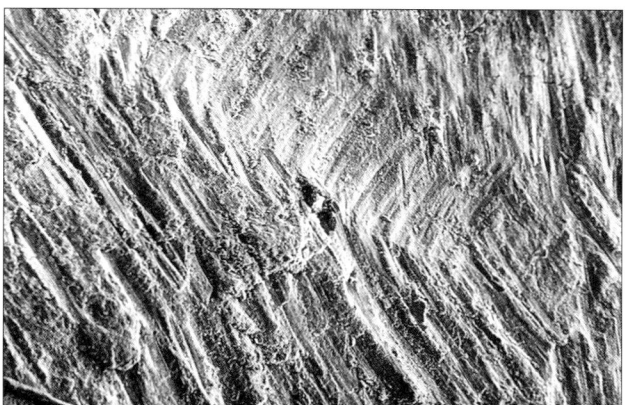

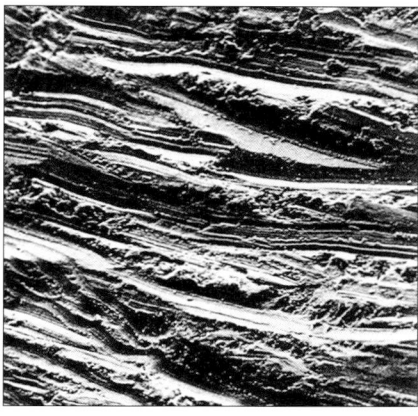

Fig 179 Diamond-treated root surface with typical undulations traversed at right angles by regular instrumental marks (original magnification ×100). (From Meyer and Lie, 1977. Reprinted with permission.)

Fig 180 Typical instrumental marks on the root surface from the diamond particles (original magnification ×200). (From Lie and Meyer, 1977. Reprinted with permission.)

removal of healthy tooth substance and no production of surface roughness. As mentioned earlier, in vivo studies have shown that surface roughness is more important for plaque accumulation and plaque composition than is free surface energy (Quirynen et al, 1990; for review, see Quirynen and Bollen, 1995).

Unfortunately, studies of instruments and methods for scaling, root planing, and debridement have disclosed inadequate cleaning and considerable iatrogenic effects (Jacobson et al, 1994; Jotikastihira et al, 1992; Ladner et al, 1992; Leknes, 1997; Lie and Leknes, 1985; Lie and Meyer, 1977; Meyer and Lie, 1977).

Roughness and loss of tooth substance. The effect of different scaling instruments on calculus removal and side effects such as roughness of the root surfaces and lost tooth substance were evaluated by Meyer and Lie (1977) and Lie and Meyer (1977), using combined SEM and profilograms. In one of these studies a hand curette, Roto-Pro (a specially designed rotary scaling instrument), an ultrasonic scaler (Cavitron, Dentsply, York, PA), and a rotary diamond tip were compared. Calcu-

lus was removed most thoroughly by diamond instrumentation, and the ultrasonic scaler was least efficient. The hand curette, ultrasonic scaler, and Roto-Pro removed about the same amount of tooth substance, whereas the diamond tip removed considerably more.

The diamond tip consistently removed all the cementum and left deep gouges in the dentin (Figs 179 and 180). The use of such aggressive instruments for periodontal scaling is contraindicated. The hand curette resulted in by far the smoothest root surface, while the ultrasonic scaler and the diamond tip caused the greatest roughness, measured with the profilometer. The SEM also showed that the diamond tip resulted in the greatest roughness.

In another study, Lie and Leknes (1985) compared air turbine scalers (Titan-S, Syntex Dental, Audubon, PA; MicroMega Air Scaler, MicroMega, Switzerland; and Calcus, Kollega Konsult, Norway) and an ultrasonic instrument (Cavitron) on medium and maximum power settings. Remaining calculus, roughness, and loss of tooth substance were estimated. The results revealed significant differences with respect to the amount of

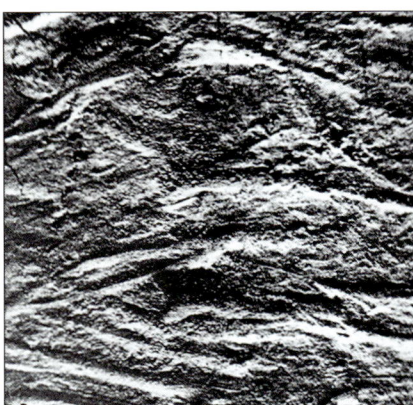

Fig 181 Root surface extensively roughened partially into cementum and partially into dentin by the use of an ultrasonic scaler at maximum power (original magnification ×20). (From Lie and Leknes, 1985. Reprinted with permission.)

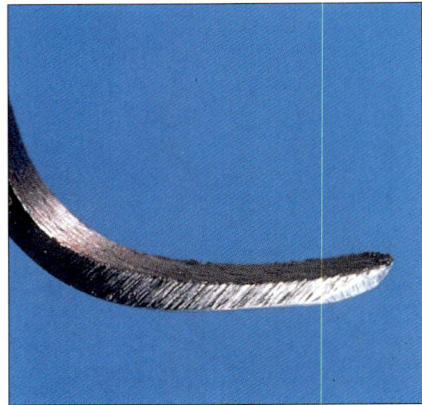

Fig 182 New or resharpened hand curette, exhibiting a rough cutting edge. The roughness of the root surface after scaling and planing is always correlated with the smoothness of the scaling instrument (original magnification ×25). (From Tal et al, 1985. Reprinted with permission.)

remaining calculus: The air turbine scaler, Titan-S, was the most efficient; Cavitron, used on its medium power setting, and Calculus were considerably less efficient than the others. With respect to root surface roughness and loss of tooth substance, Cavitron, on the maximum power setting, proved to be extremely aggressive: Root surfaces cleaned by Cavitron were easily distinguished from all the others. At maximum power setting, the ultrasonic equipment caused considerable roughening of the cementum surface and total removal of cementum in several areas (Fig 181). In vivo, such a rough surface would offer excellent retention for subgingival biofilms and calculus.

The ultrasonic scalers in all of the aforementioned studies generate tip vibration through generation of magnetostrictive power. The latest generation of ultrasonic scaler utilizes the piezoelectric principle of power generation. These different ways of generating tip vibration would be expected to cause differences in clinical performance when the scaler is applied to a root surface, although there are no detailed reports.

Jacobson et al (1994) evaluated different scaling procedures on the untreated root cementum of extracted teeth under standardized conditions. The root surface texture was examined in the SEM after the root was scaled with a new and a resharpened hand curette (McCall 13/14, LM Dental, Finland), an ultrasonic piezoscaler (Amdent 830, Amdent, Sweden), an electromagnetic scaler, and a sonic scaler (Titan-S). The hand curettes were applied to the root surface with a pressure of approximately 500 Pa. Each test surface was exposed to 10 pull strokes. The ultrasonic and sonic scalers were used with 10 back-and-forth strokes (medium power setting) and a pressure not exceeding 50 Pa. Hand and sonic instrumentation produced large grooves and removed cementum, evident at magnification of ×70. Alterations to the root surfaces caused by ultrasonic instrumentation were not detectable at magnifications of less than ×500.

Ritz et al (1991) evaluated the loss of root substance after scaling with various instruments by using a new, precise in vitro method that closely simulated clinical conditions. The instruments tested

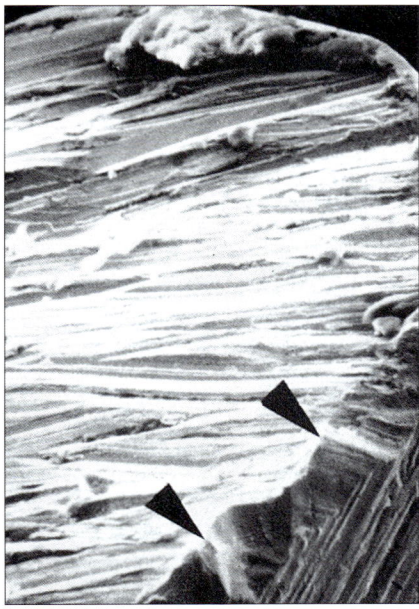

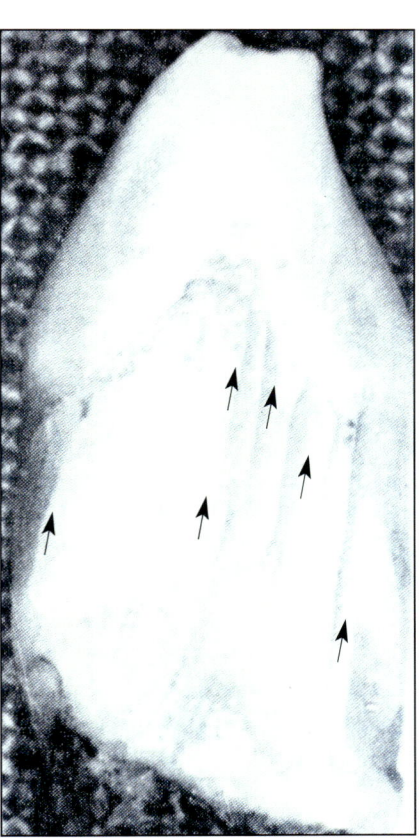

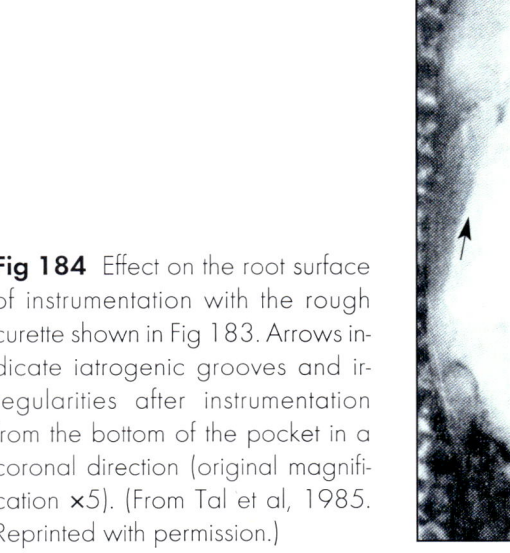

Fig 183 Hand curette with an extremely rough cutting edge. Arrows indicate irregularities near the tip of the instrument (original magnification ×250). (From Tal et al, 1985. Reprinted with permission.)

Fig 184 Effect on the root surface of instrumentation with the rough curette shown in Fig 183. Arrows indicate iatrogenic grooves and irregularities after instrumentation from the bottom of the pocket in a coronal direction (original magnification ×5). (From Tal et al, 1985. Reprinted with permission.)

were an ultrasonic scaler (Cavitron 2002), an air scaler (Titan-S), fine curettes, and diamond burs with a fine grit of 15 μm (Perio-Set No. 415, Intensiv, Switzerland). Each instrument was applied to the root surface for about 15 seconds. The clinical application force was 100 psi for the ultrasonic instrument, air scaler, and diamond burst. The curettes were used with an application force of 500 psi.

The results showed a similar loss of root substance after use of the diamond burs, fine curettes, and air scalers (120, 110, and 95 μm, respectively). With the ultrasonic scaler, the loss was only 12 μm, but it increased to 85 μm if the application force was increased to 400 psi (Ritz et al, 1991). As the average thickness of the root cementum in the coronal third of the root is only 40 to 100 μm, repeated subgingival scaling, also with a hand instrument, will result in complete removal of the root cementum, exposed dentinal tubules, and an hourglass-shaped root. The roughness of such a root surface is correlated with how meticulously the edge of the hand instrument is sharpened (Tal et al, 1985). Figure 182 shows a detail of a hand curette. Although the instrument was new (or resharpened with a fine stone) the cutting edge appears rough. Root surface roughness after scaling and root planing is always correlated with the smoothness of the scaling instrument. Figures 183 and 184 illustrate a hand curette with an extremely rough cutting edge and the corresponding effect on the root surface after instrumentation.

Figure 185 shows a bitewing radiograph from 1980, in a patient who underwent repeated subgingival scaling and root planing during the following 10 years. Note the extensive loss of root substance on the maxillary premolars (Fig 186). In spite of frequently repeated instrumentation, the first molars were extracted because of periodontal disease.

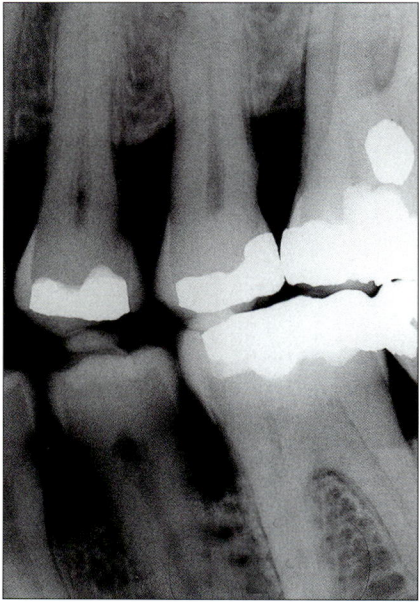

Fig 185 Bitewing radiograph of a patient who underwent repeated subgingival scaling and root planing over a period of 10 years.

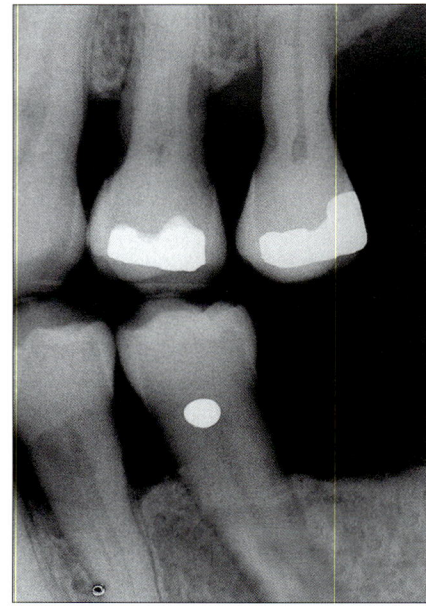

Fig 186 Extensive loss of root surface from the maxillary premolars shown in Fig 185. The first molars had been extracted because of periodontal disease in spite of repeated scaling.

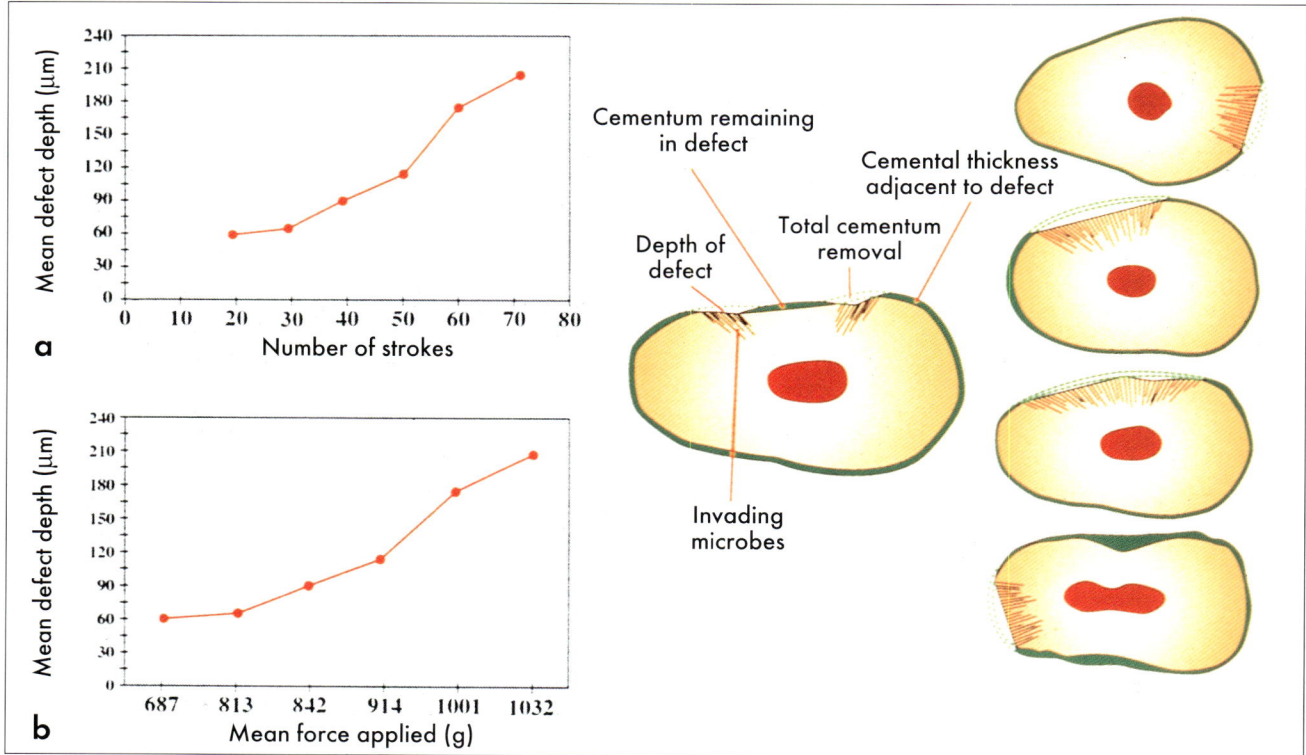

Fig 187 Root surface defect related to the number of curette strokes (a) and force applied to the curette (b). Typical types of root defects formed by the curette during root planing are shown (right). (Modified from Coldiron et al, 1990.)

Using hand curettes on extracted periodontally diseased teeth, Zappa et al (1991) showed that one single stroke at low force (3.0 N) and high force (8.5 N) removed a mean of 6.8 μm and 20.8 μm of the root cementum, respectively.

Coldiron et al (1990) also evaluated the quantitative removal of root cementum by hand curettes. Extracted teeth were used after removal of the periodontal ligament. The results showed that total removal of cementum was generally achieved with a minimum of 20 strokes at exactly the same location on the root surface (Fig 187).

Bacterial recolonization. The consequences of such iatrogenically exposed dentinal tubules were highlighted in studies by Adriaens et al (1986, 1988a, 1988b) that showed that "subgingival microflora may not only invade the subgingivally located dentinal tubules but also the root pulp." The studies investigated the viability and distribution of bacteria within the radicular dentin and pulp of periodontally diseased, caries-free teeth; healthy teeth served as controls. Samples were obtained from the pulpal tissue and from the radicular dentin. Dentinal samples were taken from the interdental surfaces in the subgingival area. Starting from the pulpal side, three to five successive dentinal layers, approximately 1 mm thick, were sampled. The samples were processed and cultured anaerobically.

Bacterial growth was detected in 87% of the periodontally diseased teeth. In 83% of the teeth, bacteria were present in at least one of the dentinal layers. Of the diseased teeth from which pulpal tissue was cultured, 59% contained bacteria in the pulpal samples (see Figs 36a and 36b in chapter 1). The mean bacterial concentrations in the pulpal and dentinal layers ranged from 1,399 to 16,537 colony-forming units per milligram of tissue. These concentrations were 259 to 7,190 times greater than concentrations found in periodontally healthy teeth. It was suggested that the roots of periodontally diseased teeth can act as bacterial reservoirs, not only for recolonization of mechanically treated surfaces, but also for infection of the dental pulp (Adriaens et al, 1986, 1988a,

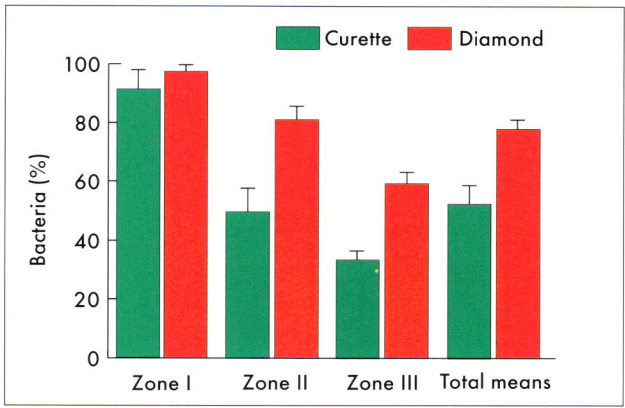

Fig 188 Bacterial recolonization on the cervical (zone I, middle (zone II), and apical (zone III) areas of the root after instrumentation with a hand curette or a rotary diamond point. (From Leknes et al, 1994. Reprinted with permission.)

1988b). These important findings might change current concepts concerning root surface debridement in periodontal therapy from "aggressive" to "nonaggressive" instrumentation.

To evaluate the influence of surface roughness after instrumentation on subgingival microbial colonization, Leknes et al (1994) conducted an experimental animal study. Ten maxillary and ten mandibular subgingival pockets were established in the canine teeth of five beagle dogs. The subgingival root surface areas were debrided by a sharp curette or a flame-shaped, fine-grained, rotary diamond point. The dogs were fed a plaque-inducing diet for 70 days. Specimens from both instrumentation groups were then harvested and prepared for stereomicroscopic and SEM evaluation.

The subgingival root surface areas were divided into three zones: cervical, middle, and apical. The curetted surfaces were smoother and promoted less subgingival colonization than did the diamond-treated surfaces. The difference in bacterial colonization between the two groups was statistically significant in all zones (Fig 188). Bacterial colonization decreased in an apical direction in both instrumentation groups. The study demonstrated that the roughness of the tooth sur-

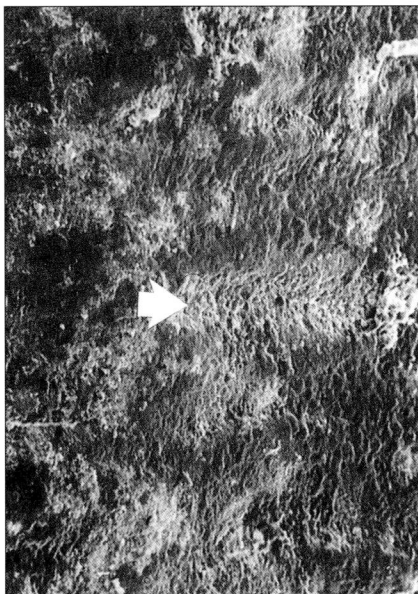

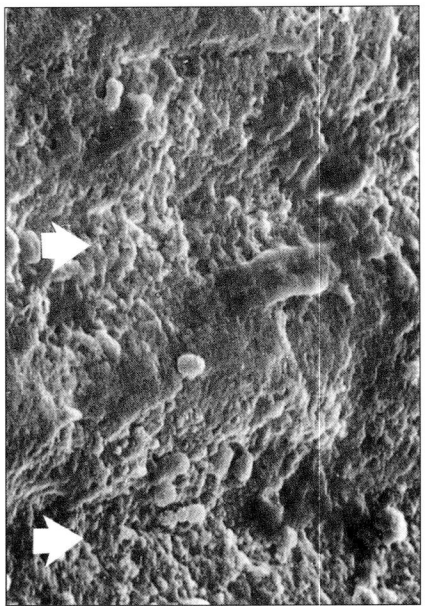

Fig 189 Curetted specimen from zone III. Some isolated cocci are visible *(arrow)*, but considerable parts of the surface are devoid of organisms. Smeared apertures of dentinal tubules are also visible (original magnification ×1,500). (From Leknes et al, 1994. Reprinted with permission.)

Fig 190 Diamond-treated specimen from zone III. Multilayered aggregates of bacteria are located in horizontal instrumentation grooves *(arrows)* (original magnification ×1,500). (From Leknes et al, 1994. Reprinted with permission.)

face after subgingival instrumentation significantly influences subgingival microbial recolonization (Figs 189 and 190).

Studies by Hirsch (1989) also found bacterial penetration of the dentinal tubules of periodontally diseased root surfaces only 10 to 14 days after root planing. There was evidence of chronic pulpitis in 30% of the pulps adjacent to the root-planed area.

In this context, the study by Sbordone et al (1990) on the recolonization of the subgingival microflora after scaling and root planing in patients with periodontitis is notable. After initial clinical and microbiologic examination, each subject underwent a single session of scaling and root planing but received no oral hygiene instruction. Clinical and microbial variables were reassessed after 7, 21, and 60 days. A significant improvement

in probing depth was noted up to 60 days after treatment. The microbial composition of treated sites 7 days after scaling and root planing was similar to that of periodontally healthy sites. At 60 days, none of the variables showed significant deviations from pretreatment levels. The most prevalent anaerobic rods prior to and 60 days after therapy were *F nucleatum*, *P gingivalis*, and *P intermedia*. Similar results were reported by Magnusson et al (1984). The results indicate that, in the absence of excellent gingival plaque control, a single session of scaling and root planing is clearly inadequate for maintenance of a "healthy" gingival microflora.

Aggressive scaling and root planing, with exposure of dentinal tubules, may not only result in invasion of bacteria and their products from the infected periodontal pocket but also have other untoward sequelae. Teeth with infected root canals exhibit more loss of periodontal attachment and alveolar bone than do corresponding vital teeth. Ehnevid et al (1993a) showed that root canal infection can retard periodontal healing. In teeth with periapical lesions, the reduction in probing depth after scaling and root planing was significantly less than for teeth without periapical lesions. It was concluded that the infected root canal serves as a bacterial reservoir for persistent periapical inflammation and marginal inflammation.

The influence of a root canal infection on periodontal status has also been investigated by correlating periapical and radiographic attachment status as well as pocket depth. Teeth with periapical radiolucencies showed less radiographic attachment and deeper pockets than did periapically intact teeth (Jansson et al, 1993). Additional bone loss has also been shown to occur at a higher rate with more advanced radiographic attachment loss (Bolin et al, 1986a; Lavstedt et al, 1986; Papapanou et al, 1989).

In a retrospective study, Ehnevid et al (1993b) showed that, regardless of the extent of radiographic attachment loss, healing after scaling and root planing is significantly impaired over time by the presence of a root canal infection.

In a follow-up experimental study in monkeys, Ehnevid et al (1995) evaluated the extent to which a predefined selection of endodontic pathogens inoculated in the root canal could influence periodontal pathosis and healing in areas of the root covered by or devoid of cementum; root resorption (cementum hypoplasia) was used as a histomorphometric marker. Exposed dentinal surfaces showed significantly larger areas of alveolar bone resorption on infected roots than on noninfected roots; root surfaces covered with intact cementum showed an almost identical distribution of tissue reaction, regardless of the presence or absence of root canal infection. It was concluded that endodontic pathogens and their products are unable to penetrate cementum but can spread via the dentinal tubules to a root surface devoid of cementum (ex-

posed root dentin). This indicates that endodontic pathogens in the root canal can exacerbate marginal infection in areas where the root has been denuded of cementum by aggressive scaling and root planing. The outcome of regenerative therapy may also be impaired.

Experimental studies in both animals and humans have cast doubt on the concept of *diseased root cementum*; ie, the penetration of cementum by bacteria and their endotoxins (Moore et al, 1986; Nakib et al, 1982). Therefore, removal of the cementum is not a prerequisite for successful repair and regeneration of periodontal support, and the resultant exposure of root dentin may allow bacterial invasion of the dentinal tubules (see Figs 36a and 36b in chapter 1).

Nonaggressive subgingival instrumentation. There is a need for a new approach, based on the concept of "nonaggressive" subgingival instrumentation. For rational elimination of subgingival plaque-retentive factors and microflora by scaling, root planing, and debridement, and to minimize iatrogenic defects, a sharp universal curette should be used as a probe for identification of calculus: Whenever located, this calculus should be carefully "lifted away" as a first step. A piezoelectric sonic scaler also could be used for gross scaling, but, for final scaling, root planing, and debridement, the instrument of choice should be as nonaggressive as possible.

Figure 191 illustrates the difference between aggressive and nonaggressive instruments for scaling, root planing, and debridement. Reciprocating PER-IO-TOR instruments (Dentatus), designed with plane load-relieving surfaces between essentially right-angled cutting edges, are examples of nonaggressive instruments: Once the root cementum is planed and thereby clean, no further root cementum will be removed. Different shapes and sizes facilitate access to concave and convex surfaces as well as to furcation areas (Fig 192). The reciprocating instruments are used in the Profin contra-angle handpiece (Axelsson, 1993). Also available are rotary instruments based on the same principle (Fig 193).

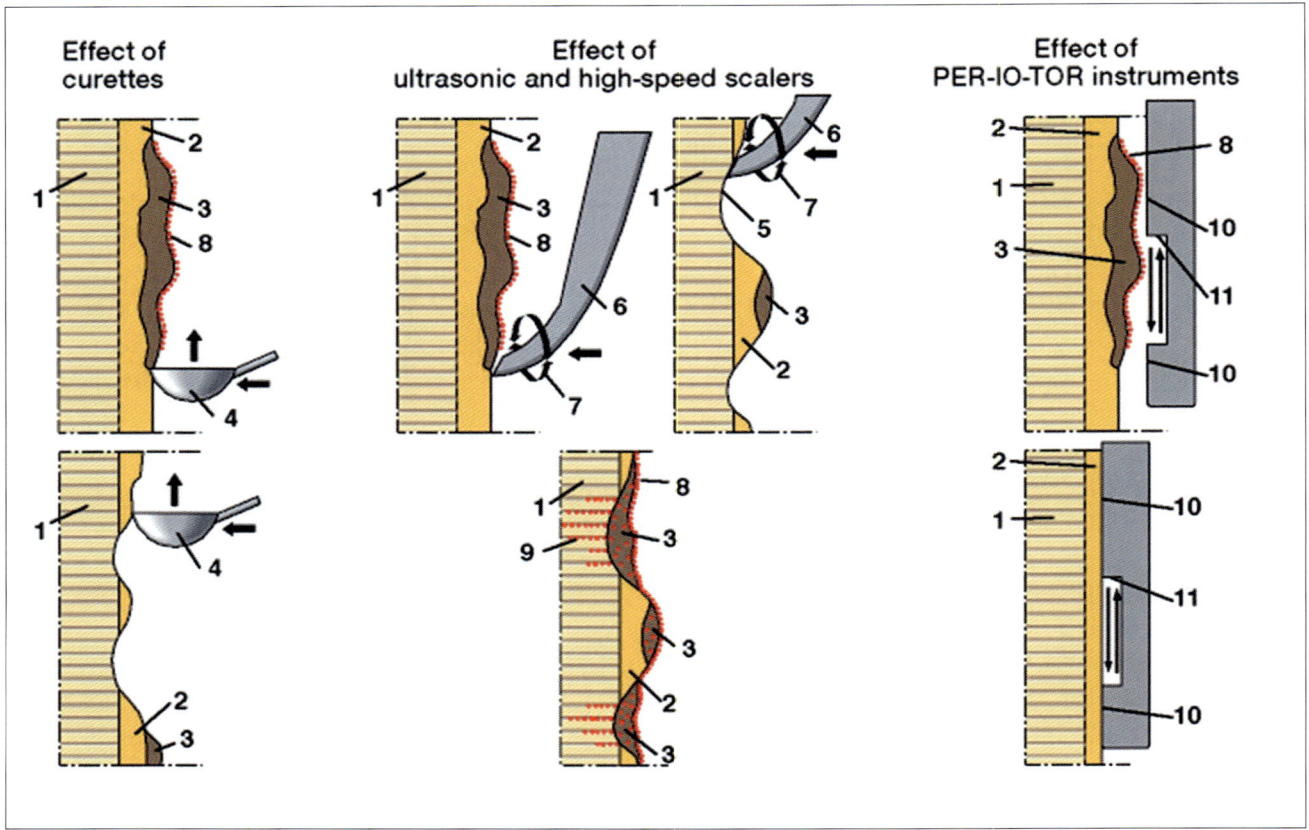

Fig 191 Difference between aggressive and nonaggressive instruments for scaling, root planing, and debridement. I = Root dentin with dentinal tubules; 2 = Root cementum; 3 = Calculus; 4 = Curette hand instrument; 5 = Iatrogenic rough, exposed dentin and dentinal tubules; 6, 7 = Ultrasonic or high-speed scaler; 8 = Subgingival plaque biofilm; 9 = Bacterial invasion of the dentinal tubules; 10, 11 = Principal design of reciprocating PER-IO-TOR instruments.

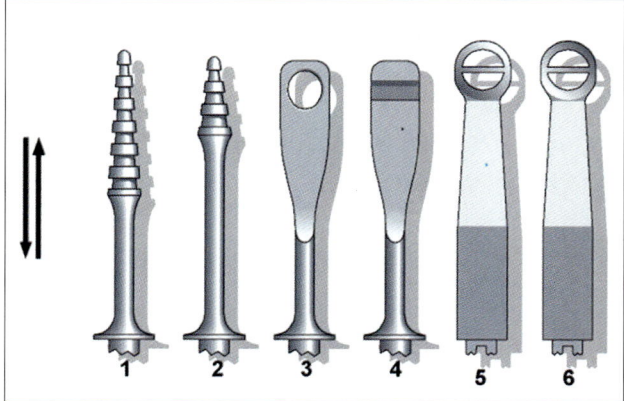

Fig 192 PER-IO-TOR nonaggressive reciprocating instruments. Different shapes and sizes facilitate access on concave and convex surfaces and furcation areas.

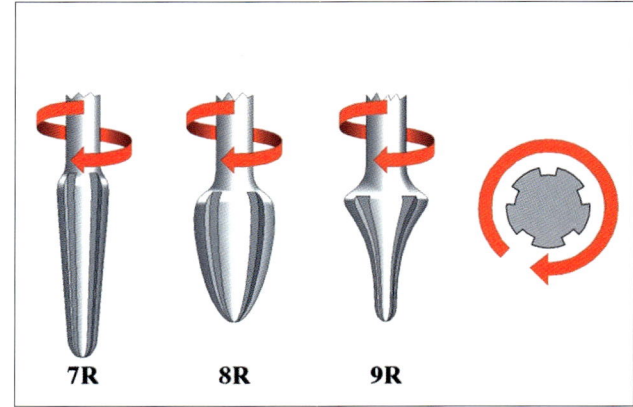

Fig 193 Rotating PER-IO-TOR instruments.

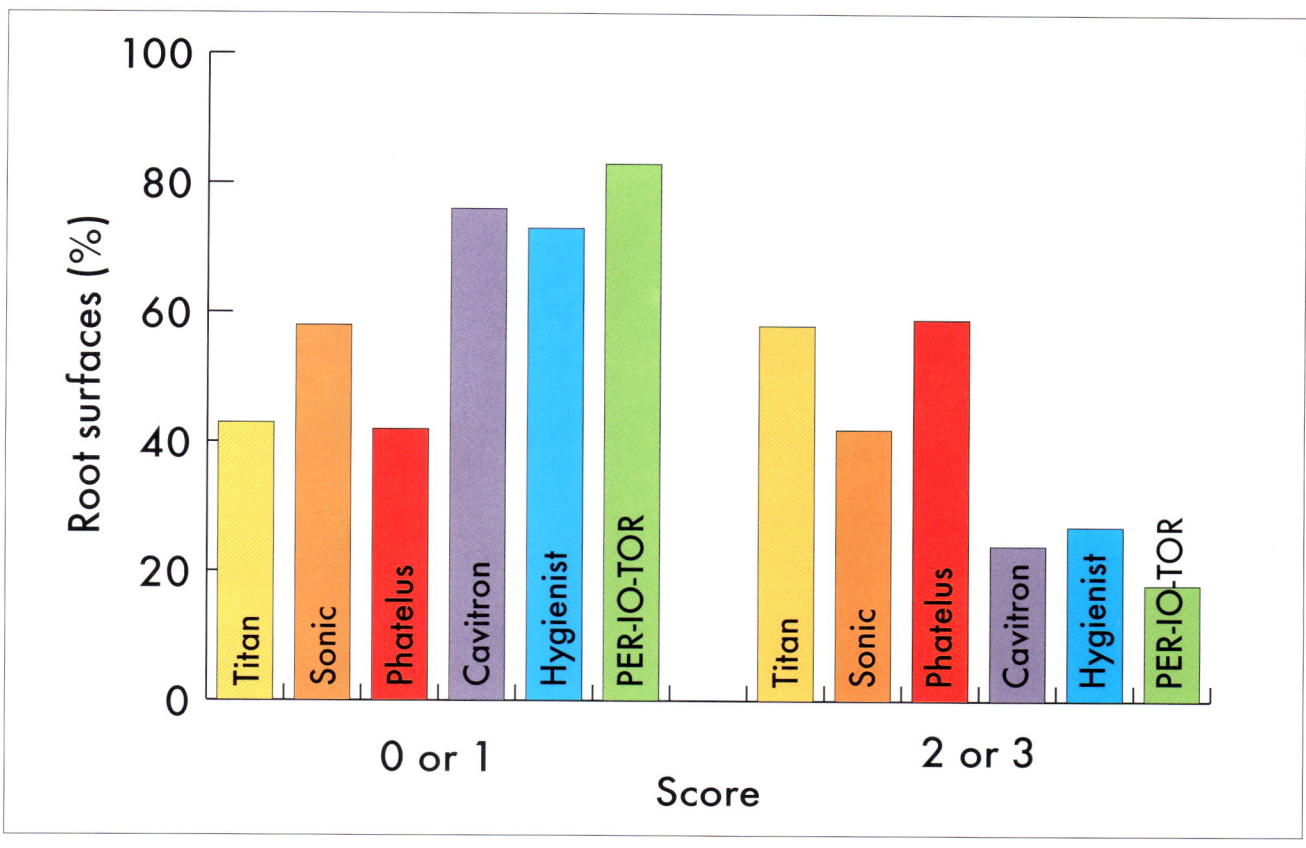

Fig 194 Roughness and loss of tooth substance after instrumentation. 0 or 1 = Smooth or slightly roughened cementum surface; 2 or 3 = Definitely corrugated or completely removed cementum. (From Jotikastihira et al, 1992. Reprinted with permission.)

In an in vitro study, Jotikastihira et al (1992) evaluated root surface roughness and loss of tooth substance after treatment with sonic scalers (Phatelius, Nakanishi Dental, Japan; Sonic Flex, KaVo, Germany; and Titan-S), ultrasonic scalers (Hygienest III, Lysta, Denmark, and Cavitron with TFI-EWPP tip), and a PER-IO-TOR reciprocating instrument (PER-IO-TOR 4, spatula shaped). For evaluation, the Roughness Loss of Tooth Substance Index (RLTSI) (Lie and Leknes, 1985), was applied, according to the following criteria:

0 = There is a smooth and even root surface, without marks from the instrumentation and with no loss of tooth substance.
1 = There are slightly roughened or corrugated local areas confined to the cementum.

2 = There are definitely corrugated local areas where the cementum may be completely removed, although most is still present.
3 = There is considerable loss of tooth substance, with instrumentation marks into the dentin. Large areas of the root are completely denuded of cementum, or there are a considerable number of lesions from instrumentation.

The PER-IO-TOR 4 spatula-shaped instrument, followed by Cavitron with TFI-EWPP probe-shaped tip, resulted in less roughness and loss of tooth substance than did the other instruments used, and were considerably less aggressive than the sonic scalers (Fig 194). In another in vitro study, Mengel et al (1994) evaluated removal of root substance by PER-IO-TOR instruments used

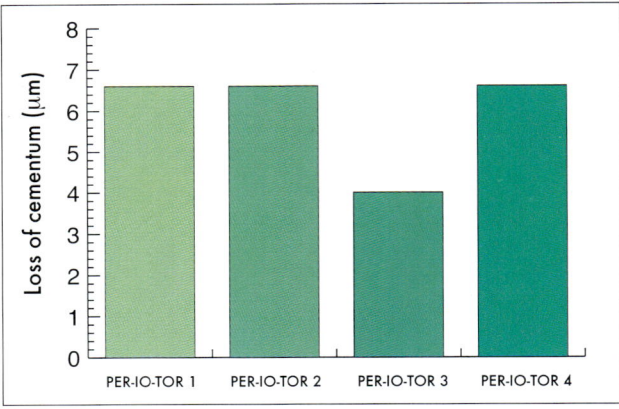

Fig 195 Loss of root cementum after 2 to 3 minutes' scaling and root planing with PER-IO-TOR instruments. (Modified from Mengel et al, 1994. Reprinted with permission.)

Box 9 Goals of subgingival instrumentation

- Attached biofilms and nonattached microflora in the gingival sulcus and the periodontal pockets should be removed.

- Plaque-retentive factors such as calculus, restoration overhangs, and areas of cementum hypoplasia and resorption should be eliminated.

- The root surface should be rendered as smooth as possible: If gingival plaque control should fail, this will allow "nonaggressive" debridement of any reaccumulated subgingival plaque (biofilm).

- To minimize the consequences of subgingival regrowth of microflora, the root cementum should be preserved; removal will expose the dentinal tubules.

- After treatment, it is important to prevent recurrence of infection in the periodontal pocket. Meticulous gingival plaque control and daily oral hygiene should be supplemented, at needs-related intervals, by professional mechanical toothcleaning.

at standardized speeds and application forces. When used nonstop for 2 or 3 minutes, PER-IO-TOR 3 removed on average only 4 µm, and PER-IO-TOR 1, 2, and 4 less than 7 µm of root substance, ie, the approximate amount that has to be removed to plane the rough outer surface of the root cementum (Fig 195). PER-IO-TOR instruments prevent untoward removal of root cementum during root planing and debridement, whereas 10 to 20 strokes with a sharp curette (see Fig 187) or the application of an extra fine, diamond-coated rotary tip for less than 1 second will completely denude the root surface of cementum.

Evidence from the aforementioned studies on the effects of subgingival instrumentation indicate the importance of thorough but careful therapy. Box 9 presents goals of successful instrumentation.

Existing periodontal disease

Evidence of previous periodontal disease, in the form of lost periodontal support—vertical as well as horizontal (furcation involvement)—and deep periodontal pockets, is termed a *risk predictor* and *risk marker,* not a *risk indicator, risk factor,* or *prognostic risk factor.* Markers and predictors of grave risk in teeth with advanced loss of periodontal support (periodontitis complicate) are diseased pockets of 5 mm or more and high gingival crevicular fluid levels of PGE_2 and interleukin-1β. Similarly, sites with grade II furcation involvement and suppuration are markers and indicators of greater risk than are healthy sites with grade I furcation involvement. In other words, local risk markers and risk predictors are not causative factors of periodontal diseases.

Marginal chronic periodontitis does not develop and progress uniformly within the dentition, but it is modified by local anatomic conditions. Local, disease-related modifying factors, such as the presence of vertical destruction, probing depth, and clinical attachment loss, are legacies of previous episodes of destruction of periodontal supporting tissues. The rate of further radiographic attachment loss is significantly higher in sites with vertical destruction than in sites with horizontal destruction (Papapanou and Wennström, 1991). Studies by Bolin et al (1986a), Lavstedt et al (1986), and Papapanou et al (1989) have shown that subjects with radiographically more advanced attachment loss at baseline experience significantly higher rates of further loss than do those with radiographic evidence of mild attachment loss at baseline.

Despite some confusion about the likelihood of disease progression in sites of different probing depths, several recent studies have confirmed the long-standing clinical impression that sites with a previous history of disease are more likely to show future progression than are sites with no history of disease (Albandar, 1990a; Badersten et al, 1990; Grbic and Lamster, 1992; Haffajee et al, 1991a, 1991b, 1991c; Lindhe et al, 1989a, 1989b; Yang et al, 1993). In untreated periodontal pockets, the most obvious influence of preexisting disease on future disease may be the presence of substantial bacterial loads within the pocket. Earlier studies (Loesche et al, 1983, 1985) demonstrated a correlation between probing depth and different bacterial patterns and ecological factors. Although many specific, and as yet undefined, factors may explain this relationship, it does appear that in untreated deeper pockets there is a shift toward a more anaerobic bacterial population. Nevertheless, there is no evidence that such a relationship persists following therapy to eliminate the subgingival plaque: The important issue is whether deeper pockets are more rapidly recolonized after subgingival cleaning.

Provided that a comprehensive maintenance care program is followed, the rate of radiographic attachment loss in marginal periodontitis is reported to be independent of the type of marginal defect (vertical or horizontal) (Pontoriero et al, 1988). However, if only conventional dental care is provided after treatment, the progression rate appears to be significantly higher for sites of vertical destruction than for sites of horizontal destruction (Papapanou and Wennström, 1991). This highlights the importance of an individual periodontal treatment program for the patient susceptible to periodontitis. The objective should be to minimize the influence of marginal plaque in sites at risk: Regardless of the type of defect, the absence of plaque is a prerequisite for periodontal healing (Isidor and Karring, 1986; Nyman et al, 1975; Rosling et al, 1976a, 1976b).

Following periodontal treatment of vertical defects, bone fill and gain of clinical attachment may occur in patients with optimal postoperative oral hygiene (Isidor et al, 1985; Rosling et al, 1976a). If patients are not given an appropriate maintenance care program after treatment, their oral hygiene standards will gradually deteriorate and periodontitis will recur in sites at risk, such as vertical defects (Nyman et al, 1977). However, even very advanced vertical bone destruction can be arrested successfully by regenerative therapy (Emdogain) in the presence of meticulous plaque control before treatment and, most importantly, in the subsequent maintenance program (see Figs 142 to 149; see also Figs 92, 94, 95, 97, 100, and 101 in chapter 1).

The outcome of initial periodontal therapy is also determined by accessibility. For example, in cases of narrow bone pockets and furcation involvement greater than grade I, open flap surgery offers greater accessibility than does nonsurgical treatment.

In a retrospective study, Ehnevid et al (1997) sought a possible relationship between the standard of oral hygiene and reduction in probing depth over time after periodontal treatment of sites with vertical or horizontal destruction. The subjects were a 3-year consecutive referral population of periodontitis-prone patients. Data were collected from complete-mouth radiographs, probing depth registrations, and plaque scores. The analysis was based on a final sample of 3,064 sites in 107 patients. After nonsurgical treatment, sites with vertical destruction had significantly less reduction in probing depth over time than did sites with horizontal destruction. This might be at-

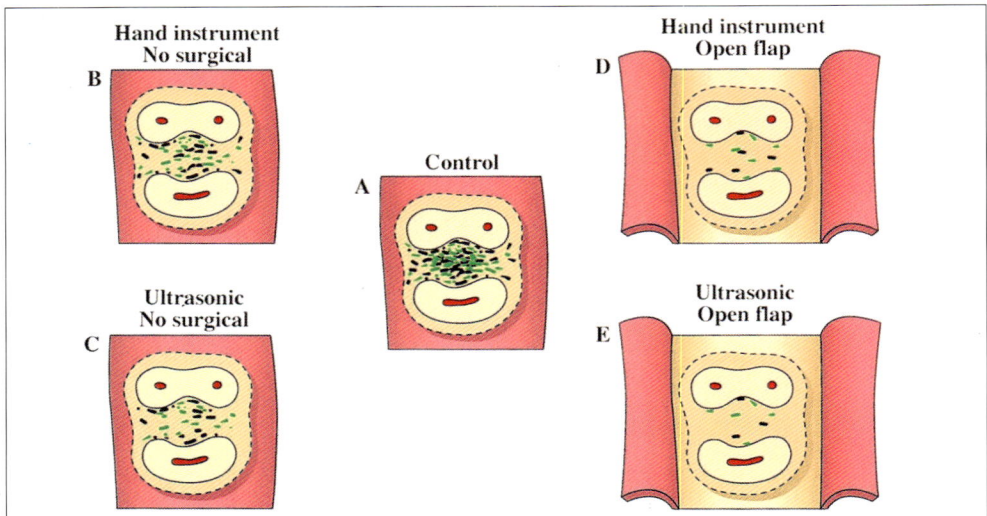

Fig 196 Composite evaluation of the calculus found on the dome surface of all the furcations in each treatment group. (Modified from Matia et al, 1986. Reprinted with permission.)

tributable to the formation of inaccessible lateral pockets (see Fig 172). The importance of maintaining a high standard of oral hygiene was highlighted by the observation of an increase over time in the difference in probing depth reduction between sites with plaque and sites without plaque after nonsurgical treatment of vertical and horizontal defects. In surgically treated teeth, there was no increase over time in the difference in probing depth reduction between vertical and horizontal defects: Osteoplasty and osteotomy limit the surface area available for formation of a long junctional epithelium, which may facilitate recurrence of a periodontal pocket.

Postextraction findings confirm that sites with furcations are less amenable to effective instrumentation, particularly nonsurgical therapy (Caffesse et al, 1986; Saglie et al, 1986a; Stambough et al, 1981; Waerhaug, 1980). This also has been confirmed by microbial monitoring (Loos et al, 1988) and evaluation of postinstrumentation healing responses (Fleisher et al, 1989; Kaldahl et al, 1990; Loos et al, 1989; Nordland et al, 1987). In grade I furcations, instrumentation can successfully eliminate subgingival plaque biofilms and calculus, and recontouring of the tooth crown can eliminate the furcation involvement. However, in grade II and grade III furcations, subgingival mi-

croflora and calculus are almost completely inaccessible to instrumentation.

Matia et al (1986) evaluated the efficacy of scaling molar furcation areas with and without surgical access. Fifty mandibular molars, scheduled for extraction because of severe periodontitis, were selected according to the following criteria:

- Grade II or III furcation involvement
- Probing pocket depth of ≥ 5 mm from the midbuccal and midlingual aspects
- Grade II or III Calculus Index, according to Greene and Vermilion (1960)

Twenty teeth were scaled with curettes; 10 after surgical exposure of the furcation (open scaling) and 10 without surgical exposure (closed scaling). Twenty teeth were scaled with an ultrasonic scaler, 10 after surgical exposure of the furcation and 10 without exposure. The remaining 10 teeth were not instrumented and served as controls.

Immediately after treatment, the teeth were extracted and examined in a stereomicroscope at ×10. Figure 196 presents a composite evaluation of the calculus found on the dome surface of all the furcations of each treatment group. For closed scaling, the mean percentages of calculus were

49.7% (range, 14.5% to 92.9%) in the control group, 37.7% in the curette group, and 34.1% in the ultrasonic group. The lowest values were recorded for open scaling: 2.7% in the curette group and 1.0% in the ultrasonic group.

The results highlight the inadequacy of a closed, nonsurgical approach for calculus removal in grade II and III furcations, regardless of the type of instrument.

Periodontal Disease As a Modifying Factor for Other Diseases or Abnormalities

Relationship between periodontal diseases and both coronary heart disease and stroke

Recent studies have shown that periodontal diseases are risk factors and prognostic risk factors for coronary heart disease (CHD) and stroke (for reviews see Beck et al, 1996, 1998; Kolltveit and Eriksen, 2001; Loesche, 2000; Scannapieco, 1998). The gram-negative microflora and their toxins—particularly LPSs—implicated in the etiology of periodontal diseases also seem to be direct or indirect etiologic factors of CHD and stroke (for reviews see Beck et al, 1996, 1998; Herzberg and Meyer, 1998; Kinane, 1998b; Loesche, 2000; Lowe, 1998).

Much of the published evidence of a causal relationship between periodontal diseases and atherosclerosis is circumstantial and often based on case reports and clinical samples of selected cases referred for medical treatment of diseases associated with atherosclerosis, such as ischemic heart disease, stroke, and myocardial infarction. Without including properly matched controls, an overestimation of a causal association with periodontitis is likely. This is in part due to a relatively high prevalence of periodontal diseases, CHD, and stroke among elderly adults in most countries.

According to Susser (1991), a strict definition of causality implies that the causal factors are directly and actively involved in the disease process. From a more pragmatic point of view, any factor that shows association with the occurrence of a given disease and also demonstrates appropriate sequence and direction may be considered a potential causal factor. Sequence and direction of action have to be estimated empirically or through a longitudinal design.

In epidemiologic research, at least four approaches are valid in the investigation of possible causal relationships: case-control studies, prospective and retrospective cohort studies, and cross-sectional studies with appropriate sample size. In addition, ecological studies may contribute some information. Out of these, case-control studies and prospective cohort (controlled longitudinal) studies have the strongest bearing on causality by studying differences between diseased and nondiseased individuals.

Recently Kolltveit and Eriksen (2001) reviewed the literature published from 1989 through October 2000 in order to evaluate a possible causal association between periodontitis and atherosclerosis. Out of a total of 21 publications retrieved, 14 complied with the following criteria: atherosclerosis or atherosclerosis-related conditions were the outcome variable, the study design was multifactorial, and possible confounders were given proper consideration. In addition, properly selected controls were considered for case-control studies and, for cross-sectional studies, a sufficient sample size was used. Table 23 shows the 14 epidemiologic studies on oral infection (periodontitis) and atherosclerosis that were selected according to the above criteria. Nine studies were prospective longitudinal studies, one was a retrospective longitudinal study, two were case-control studies, and two were cross-sectional studies.

Table 23 Epidemiologic studies selected according to specific criteria for evaluation of possible causal relationship between periodontitis and atherosclerosis*

Author/year of publication	Study design	No. of subjects	Duration (y)	Main conclusions
Syrjänen et al (1989)	Case-control	80		Statistically significant association between bacterial infection (both oral and nonoral) and cerebral infarction
Mattila et al (1989)	Case-control	202		Statistically significant association between oral health and acute myocardial infarction
DeStefano et al (1993)	Prospective	9,760	14	Increased risk (25%) for CHD associated with periodontitis and poor oral hygiene
Paunio et al (1993)	Cross-sectional	1,384		Statistically significant association between missing teeth and CHD
Beck et al (1996)	Prospective	1,147	25	Statistically significant association between periodontitis, CHD, and stroke
Joshipura et al (1996)	Prospective	44,119	6	No association between periodontal disease and CHD, except for subgroup with periodontitis at start
Ridker et al (1997)	Prospective	1,086	14	Plasma biomarker of inflammation shows association with myocardial infarction and stroke
Loesche et al (1998a)	Cross-sectional	320		Statistically significant association between oral health parameters and CHD
Mendez et al (1998)	Prospective	2,073	30	Association between inflammatory conditions and atherosclerosis
Folsom et al (1999)	Prospective	14,700	6–9	Plasma biomarkers of inflammation show association with stroke
Morrison et al (1999)	Retrospective	21,619	21	Statistically significant association between periodontal disease and CHD
Hujoel et al (2000)	Prospective	8,032	10	Slight, but not statistically significant association between periodontitis, gingivitis, and CHD
Wu et al (2000a)	Prospective	9,962	10	Statistically significant association between periodontitis and cardiovascular disease
Wu et al (2000b)	Prospective	10,146	10	Association between plasma levels of cardiovascular risk factors and periodontitis

*Modified from Kolltveit and Eriksen (2001). Reprinted with permission.

Case-control and cross-sectional studies

In a case-control study of patients younger than 40 years with ischemic cerebral infarction, Syrjänen et al (1989) revealed that poor oral health was significantly more likely for men with CHD than it was for controls. Kweider et al (1993) observed significantly higher levels of fibrinogen and leukocytes in 25- to 50-year-old patients with periodontal disease than in age-matched control subjects with healthy periodontal tissues.

In a series of studies, Mattila (1993) and Mattila et al (1993) examined the role of certain infections, among them dental infections, in the pathogenesis of CHD. Adjustments were made for other cardiovascular risk variables. They reported a correlation between the severity of dental infection and the extent of coronary atheromatosis. Individuals with severe dental infection had higher levels of von Willebrand factor antigen, leukocytes, and fibrinogen. Proposed as the underlying mechanism was the effect of bacteria on the cells involved in the pathogenesis of atherosclerosis and arterial thrombosis.

Paunio et al (1993), in a Finnish study of men aged 45 to 64 years, disclosed a relationship between the number of missing teeth and the prevalence of ischemic heart disease, even after controlling for age, hypertension, geographic area, educational level, and smoking. Loesche (1994) also reported an inverse relationship between the number of remaining teeth and a history of CHD and stroke. In older US veterans, those with 15 to 28 teeth and high percentages of teeth with periodontal attachment loss of more than 6 mm were significantly more likely to have a cerebral vascular accident than subjects with fewer teeth and less severe periodontal disease (Loesche et al, 1998a). Based on the above studies, it was proposed that periodontal infections induce low-level bacteremia, elevate white blood cell counts, and expose the host to endotoxins that may affect endothelial integrity, metabolism of plasma lipoproteins, platelet function, and blood coagulation.

Prospective longitudinal studies

The pioneer compelling data were generated by DeStefano et al (1993) at the Centers for Disease Control, from data from the US National Health Studies in adults. The studies were designed to investigate the association between baseline measurements in 1971 to 1974 and subsequent development of specific diseases and conditions. A dental examination was included in the study, which comprised 20,749 subjects aged 25 to 74 years. Because more than 90% of subjects were successfully traced, with a median follow-up of 14 years, this was a prospective study of a national sample of US adults. The main outcome measures

were incidence of mortality or admission to hospital because of coronary heart disease. Adjusted relative risks were estimated, using proportional hazard analysis.

Subjects with periodontitis had a 25% greater risk of coronary heart disease than did those with minimal periodontal disease. After the data were adjusted for age, sex, race, education, poverty index, marital state, systolic blood pressure, total cholesterol level, diabetes, body mass index, physical activity, alcohol consumption, and cigarette smoking, men with periodontitis had a 1.72 relative risk of CHD compared to men without periodontitis. The authors concluded that periodontal disease is associated with an increased risk of CHD, particularly in young men.

In support of these findings is the prospective study of cardiovascular risk by Beck et al (1996). A cohort study was conducted using combined data from the Normative Aging Study and the Dental Longitudinal Study sponsored by the Department of Veterans Affairs, Boston. Mean bone loss scores and worst probing depth scores per tooth were measured in 1,147 men during 1968 to 1971.

Follow-up examination 18 years later disclosed that 207 men had developed CHD, 59 had died from CHD, and 40 had suffered strokes. The odds ratios, adjusted for acknowledged cardiovascular risk factors, were 1.4, 1.6, and 2.1 for bone loss and total CHD, fatal CHD, and stroke, respectively. Levels of bone loss and the percentage of subjects developing total CHD and fatal CHD indicated a biologic gradient between the exposure to periodontal disease and occurrence of CHD. Individuals with a probing depth of more than 3 mm around all teeth were 3.6 times as likely to develop CHD. Those with advanced loss of alveolar bone at baseline had almost twice the incidence of fatal CHD as did those with minimal bone loss.

This study confirmed that periodontal disease is a significant risk factor for coronary heart disease and stroke. In fact, the OR obtained in the logistic model for bone loss scores with total CHD (1.5), is exceeded only by that for cholesterol (1.6). In the model for bone loss with fatal CHD (1.9),

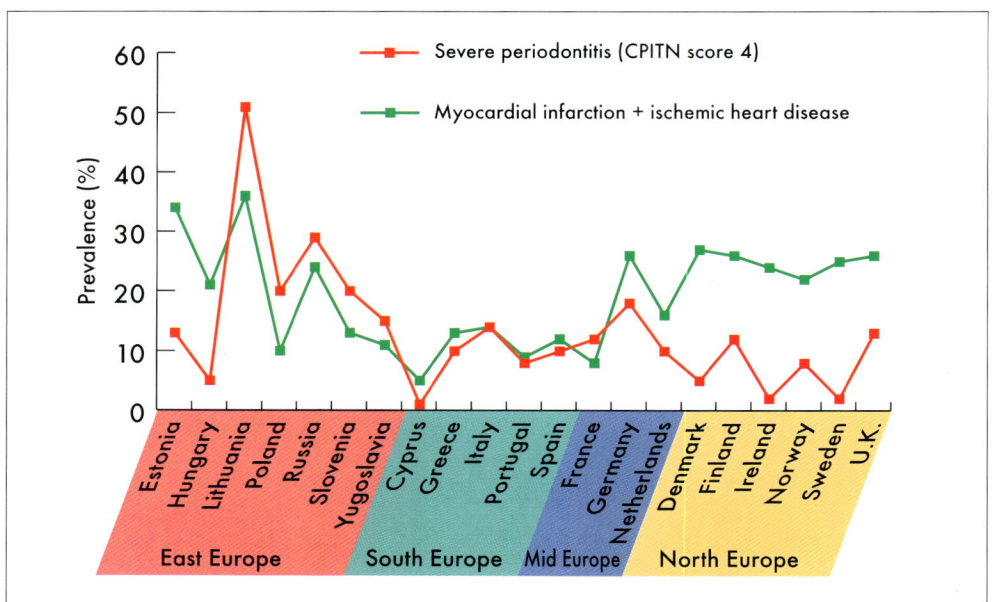

Fig 197 A comparison between prevalence of periodontal disease scored as CPITN score 4 in 35 to 44 year olds and total mortality prevalence from myocardial infarction and ischemic heart disease combined from European countries based on World Health Organization recordings. (From Kolltveit and Eriksen, 2000. Reprinted with permission.)

only smoking approached a similar relationship (1.7). For stroke, the OR for bone loss scores (2.8) was greater than that for smoking (1.6) but substantially less than that for family history of CHD (3.5). Thus, in comparison to more established risk factors, periodontal disease appears to be associated consistently with excess risk for CHD and stroke, at a level warranting further consideration.

In addition to these pioneering prospective longitudinal studies and the other studies reviewed in Table 23, two longitudinal studies have shown that diabetic subjects with periodontal disease are more likely to develop myocardial infarction (odds ratio, 2.7) (Genco et al, 1997) and stroke (Thorstensson et al, 1996) than diabetics without periodontal disease.

Ecological studies

Based on World Health Organization country profiles, prevalence of severe periodontal disease (Ainamo et al, 1982) in 35 to 44 year olds (World Health Organization, 1994) and nonstandardized total mortality rates of myocardial infarction and ischemic heart disease (World Health Organiza-

tion, 1999) were compared in order to study possible associations. With the exception of the northern European countries, including Scandinavia, a conformity of the two distribution curves seems to be present (Fig 197). The low prevalence of periodontal disease in Scandinavia may be explained by a high standard of oral hygiene and well-organized preventive programs while the prevalence of cardiovascular disease may be explained by the relatively high intake of animal fat.

From the extensive prospective studies and the case-control studies reviewed, it may be concluded that a causal association between atherosclerosis-related diseases and prevalence of periodontal diseases is likely. This is supported by the analysis of the ecological data presented in Fig 197. The biologic reasons for an inflammatory origin of atherosclerosis, suggesting microorganisms as the etiologic agent, are discussed below.

Biologic reasons for the relationship

Atherosclerosis has been defined as a progressive disease process that involves the large- to

Fig 198 Hypothetical working model for the biologic basis of the observed association between periodontal disease and atherosclerosis, coronary heart disease, and stroke. (From Beck et al, 1996. Reprinted with permission.)

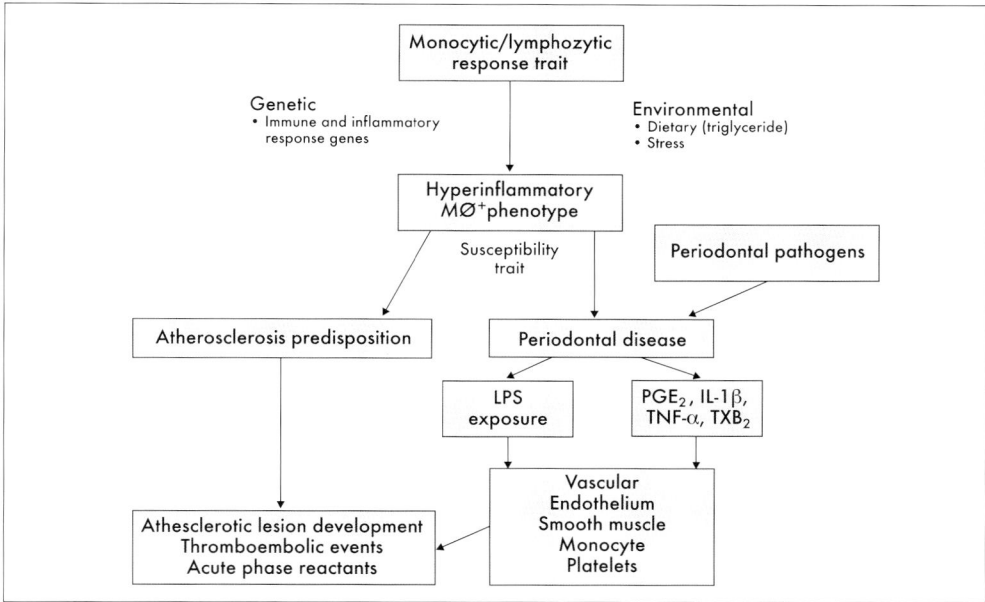

medium-sized arteries. The advanced lesion is the atheroma, which consists of elevated focal plaques on the tunica intima vasorum with a necrotic central core containing lysed cells, cholesterol ester crystals, lipid-laden foam cells, and surface plasma proteins including fibrin and fibrinogen. This central core is associated with a cellular infiltrate with hypertrophic smooth muscle cells, macrophages, and sparse T lymphocytes. The presence of atheroma tends to make the patient thrombosis-prone, because the surface enhances platelet aggregation and thrombus formation. Overall, about 50% of deaths in industrialized countries are attributed to complications from atherosclerosis; coronary thrombosis and myocardial infarction represent about half of these sequelae.

The following RIs, RFs, and PRFs for CHD and stroke have been identified in cross-sectional and longitudinal studies:

- Heredity (positive association)
- Chronic infections (positive association)
- High intake of saturated fatty acids (positive association)
- High body mass index (positive association)
- Physical inactivity (positive association)
- Age (positive association)
- Low educational standard (positive association)
- Gender (higher risk for males)
- Financial status (negative association)
- Tobacco use (positive association)
- Alcohol use (positive association)
- Hypertension (positive association)
- Diabetes (positive association)
- Stress (positive association)
- Social isolation (positive association)

Most of these factors are common to CHD, stroke, and periodontal disease.

Beck et al (1996) have proposed a biologic model to explain the role of periodontal diseases as modifying RIs, RFs, and PRFs for atherogenesis and thromboembolic events (CHD and stroke) (Fig 198).

The model is based on the hypothesis that the presence of a hyperinflammatory monocyte (MØ⁺) phenotype places certain individuals at risk for both atherosclerosis/CHD and periodontitis. Furthermore, it is suggested that certain factors, such as diet, may exacerbate the MØ⁺ phenotype and may thereby contribute to the morbidity of atherosclerosis and periodontal disease status. Periodontal infections may contribute directly to the pathogenesis of atherosclerosis and thromboembolic events by repeated systemic vascular challenges, with bacteremias and bacterial spread of endotoxins, particularly LPSs, antigens such as heat shock proteins (HSPs), and inflammatory cytokines. The principal role of the monocyte response to bacterial challenge as a key regulator of periodontal disease expression is comprehensively discussed in chapter 5.

Biologic effects of bacteremia of periopathogens. Gram-negative anaerobic bacteria, especially black-pigmented species such as *Porphyromonas* and *Bacteroides,* colonize the root surface within the gingival crevice (and periodontal pocket, if present). However, in the depths of infected pockets, the predominant bacteria are nonattaching, anaerobic, motile, gram-negative species. Subgingival bacterial plaque biofilms contain approximately 10^{12} bacteria per gram. In periodontitis, a typical periodontal pocket can harbor about 10^9 bacteria. For details see chapter 1.

The ulcerated pocket epithelium permits direct bacterial contact with both the subjacent connective tissue and the inflammatory cell infiltrate. Periodontal pathogens (particularly *P gingivalis* and *A actinomycetemcomitans*) can invade the periodontal tissues directly, but the loss of epithelial integrity within the periodontal pocket also allows direct bacterial translocation and bacteremia. Recurrent, albeit transient, bacteremias with gram-negative periodontal pathogens are a hallmark of periodontitis. Because bacteremia is induced by scaling and debridement, prophylactic systemic antibiotic coverage is indicated in medically compromised individuals to prevent bacterial endocarditis. However, in the patient with periodontitis, even apparently innocuous procedures, such as toothbrushing and chewing, have been shown to induce a transient bacteremia. The more severe the periodontal inflammatory state, the greater the hematogenous bacterial exposure, in terms of bacterial counts and duration. Thus, periodontitis is a chronic infection that may result in repeated systemic exposure to gram-negative bacteria, LPSs, and other bacterial products.

As mentioned earlier, the absolute majority of the periopathogens are gram negative and anaerobic. These gram-negative anaerobes contain LPSs on their surfaces and, because these organisms may be invasive, they could introduce LPSs directly to the periodontal tissues. If LPSs enter the systemic circulation, it could promote atherosclerosis and thrombosis formation by well-known mechanisms (Libby et al, 1997; Valtonen, 1991). In elderly US veterans it was therefore shown in a logistic regression model that plaques containing *P gingivalis, B forsythus,* and/or *T denticola* (ie, BANA-positive) were statistically associated with a diagnosis of CHD (Loesche et al, 1998a). In a case-control study comparing 97 individuals with myocardial infarction with 233 community controls, increases in *B forsythus* and *P gingivalis* were significantly associated with increased risk for myocardial infarction (Genco et al, 1999a). Odds ratios were 2.99 for *B forsythus* and 2.52 for *P gingivalis* after adjusting for gender, age, pack years of smoking, lifetime alcohol use, and dental plaque scores. These studies show that gram-negative periopathogens can be associated with CHD.

In the past few years, isolates of bacteria from blood have been shown (by either ribotyping, cell wall analyses, or phenotypic profiling) to be identical to strains of the same species isolated from oral sites (Loesche, 1997). A consequence of these transient bacteremias could be plaque bacteria cells depositing on the lining of fatty streaks or atheromas found in the vascular bed. Investigators have found DNA from *Chlamydia pneumoniae* and *Cytomegalovirus* removed at autopsy or during operations for endarterectomies (Blasi et al, 1996; Danesh et al, 1997).

Chapter 1 described how *P gingivalis* and *A actinomycetemcomitans* may invade the pocket epithelium cells and multiply intracellularly, as well as how they may invade the connective tissues (Madianos, 1997; Sandros et al, 1994, 1996).

Recently Progulske-Fox et al (1999) have shown that *P gingivalis* via a specific virulence factor (a hemagglutinin gene [Hag A]) may invade coronary artery endothelial cells and survive intracellularly, which results in an increased degradation of long-lived cellular proteins.

In another recent study, Haraszthy et al (2000) examined 50 human specimens from carotid endarterectomy, finding not only *P gingivalis,* but also other periopathogens. Of the removed atheromas, 30% contained *B forsythus,* 26% contained *P gingivalis,* 12% contained *P intermedia,* 18% contained *A actinomycetemcomitans,* 18% contained *C pneumonia,* and 38% contained *Cytomegalovirus.* In addition, more than 80% of the specimens contained one or more of the above microorganisms. These findings indicate that bacteria from the oral cavity, after gaining access to the bloodstream, can become incorporated into the atheroma and thus may play a role in the development and progression of atherosclerosis leading to coronary vascular disease and other clinical sequelae.

The capture of the dental bacteria in the atheroma could be similar to the mechanism proposed for the involvement of *Streptococcus sanguis* with subacute endocarditis. Among the putative virulence factors of *S sanguis* is a cell-surface protein that can cause platelets to aggregate. Strains positive for this platelet aggregation–associated protein (PAAP) cause extensive vegetative growth on heart valves in animal models, whereas PAAP-negative strains do not (Herzberg et al, 1992). If PAAP-positive strains of *S sanguis* gained access to the bloodstream because of poor oral hygiene, they could cause platelet aggregation and subsequent vascular pathology. Likewise, in periodontal disease, if certain bacteria such as *P gingivalis* and *A actinomycetemcomitans* gained access to the bloodstream, they could cause platelet aggregation. *P gingivalis* also expresses the PAAP cross-reactive antigen (Herzberg et al, 1994), which could be a mechanism for its appearance in the arteromatous plaques (see also Progulske-Fox et al, 1999).

Recently Emingil et al (2000) also showed that there was a significant association between periodontal disease and acute myocardial infarction. Included in the study were 120 patients, 60 with acute myocardial infarction (AMI) and 60 with chronic coronary heart disease (CCHD). Logistic regression analysis showed that the percentage of sites exhibiting bleeding on probing, the number of sites with pocket depths of 4 mm or more, the number of restorations, smoking status, and triglyceride levels were significantly associated with AMI. However, the number of sites with pocket depths of 4 mm or more, the percentage of sites with bleeding on probing, smoking status, total cholesterol, low-density lipoprotein cholesterol, and triglyceride levels were statistically different between AMI and CCHD groups. Therefore, the authors proposed prospective randomized studies in order to determine if periodontal disease is a risk factor in the occurrence of AMI.

Within the periodontium, the monocyte responds to the bacterial LPS (endotoxin) from periopathogens by secreting three key proinflammatory mediators: PGE_2, IL-1β, and TNF-α. These in turn have deleterious effects on the periodontium, eliciting vasodilation and increasing vasopermeability, inflammatory cell recruitment, connective tissue degradation, and bone destruction. The levels of these mediators within the affected periodontium are impressive, and can approach 1 to 3 μmol. For reference, the level of insulin within the pancreas is about 2.2 μmol. Thus, the periodontium may serve as a reservoir of high concentrations of LPS and mediators, with the potential to exert systemic effects.

Accumulating evidence indicates the critical regulatory role of the LPS → MØ → mediator (PGE_2, IL-1β, TNF-α) activation pathway in the pathogenesis of periodontal diseases. With increasing disease severity and during active periods of disease progression, levels of these mediators increase dramatically within the periodontal tissues and gingival crevicular fluid. Compared with those of healthy controls, the peripheral blood monocytes of patients with an MØ$_2$ phenotype secrete 3 to 10 times the amount of PGE_2, IL-1β, and TNF-α in response to LPS in culture.

These same individuals, if infected with *P gingivalis* or another periodontal pathogen, characteristically have extremely high levels of these mediators within the gingival crevicular fluid and severe clinical periodontitis. Anti-inflammatory agents, which block the synthesis or activity of PGE_2 and IL-1β, have been shown to reduce the severity of disease, even in the presence of copious plaque accumulation (Offenbacher et al, 1993). Defining host susceptibility and identifying contributing risk factors for severe forms of periodontal disease may ultimately depend on understanding the genetic and environmental factors that modulate the components of this dominant LPS → MØ → mediator pathway.

There is also increasing evidence of a critical role for the LPS → MØ → mediator pathway in infection-associated atherogenesis and thromboembolism. Intravascular infusion of LPSs upregulates the expression of endothelial adhesion molecules, triggers the release of IL-1β, TNF-α, and thromboxane B_2, initiates platelet aggregation and adhesion, and promotes the formation of lipid-laden foam cells and the deposition of cholesterol within the tunica intima vasorum (Marcus and Hajjar, 1993).

The well-known relationship of elevated levels of cholesterol-binding lipoproteins with CHD also can be related to periodontal disease because LPS would stimulate the production of low- and very low–density lipoproteins, and one of the normal functions of these lipids is to aid in the clearance of LPS from the blood stream (Read et al, 1993). Furthermore, recent studies indicate that elevated triglyceride levels are able to modulate IL-1β production by PMNLs stimulated with *P gingivalis* LPS (Cutler et al, 1999) and inhibit macrophage production of essential polypeptide growth factors, which results in exacerbated tissue destruction and reduced tissue capacity for repair.

Inflammatory cells and mediators (IL-1β, PGE_2, and TNF-α) have a key role in human atherosclerosis and CHD. LPS triggers endothelial expression of IL-1β, favoring coagulation and thrombosis while retarding fibrinolysis (Clinton et al,

1991). Diseased aortas contain large amounts of IL-1β– and TNF-α–secreting monocytes (Pearce et al, 1992). These cytokines have been shown to enhance lipid accumulation within monocytes, especially cholesterol and cholesterol esters. Monocyte cytokines, such as IL-1β, transforming growth factor β, and platelet-derived growth factor, enhance smooth muscle proliferation, presumably leading to thickening of the vessel walls.

Certain periodontal patients, usually those with aggressive forms of periodontitis, have peripheral hyperreactive blood monocytes that secrete 3 to 10 times the normal amounts of PGE_2, IL-1β, and TNF-α when exposed in vitro to LPS (Beck et al, 1996). It is possible that individuals with this hyperactive monocyte phenotype are at risk for both atherosclerosis/CHD and periodontitis. These individuals would overreact to the penetration of gram-negative bacteria from the subgingival biofilms into the periodontium, releasing potentially harmful inflammatory mediators and activated macrophages that might be able to exert an effect on the endothelial lining of large arteries.

Of relevance in this context is the previously discussed study by Kornman et al (1997a), in which about 30% of an adult US population exhibited an IL-1β polymorphism gene. Compared to subjects who were negative for IL-1β polymorphism, they produced roughly four times more IL-β in response to LPS, which resulted in considerably more loss of periodontal attachment. For these subjects, the odds ratio for developing severe periodontitis was 18.9. Recently Kornman et al (1999) proposed a hypothetical model with two different patterns of IL-1 genetic polymorphism, as illustrated in Fig 199.

Systemically, LPS can activate an impressive cascade of inflammatory cytokines, capable of eliciting most of the vascular and coagulation complications associated with atherosclerosis and CHD. It also must be observed that LPS would not need to enter the systemic circulation to have an effect on atherosclerosis. If LPS is retained in the periodontal tissue and degraded, the resulting inflammatory response could provoke the release of cytokines and other inflammatory mediators

Fig 199 Potential models for IL-1 genotype influence on periodontitis and cardiovascular disease (CVD). Model 1 (a): IL-1 genotype pattern 1 directly influences both periodontitis and cardiovascular clinical events. Model 2 (b): IL-1 genotype pattern 2 influences CVDs directly with no influence on periodontitis. (From Kornman et al, 1999. Reprinted with permission.)

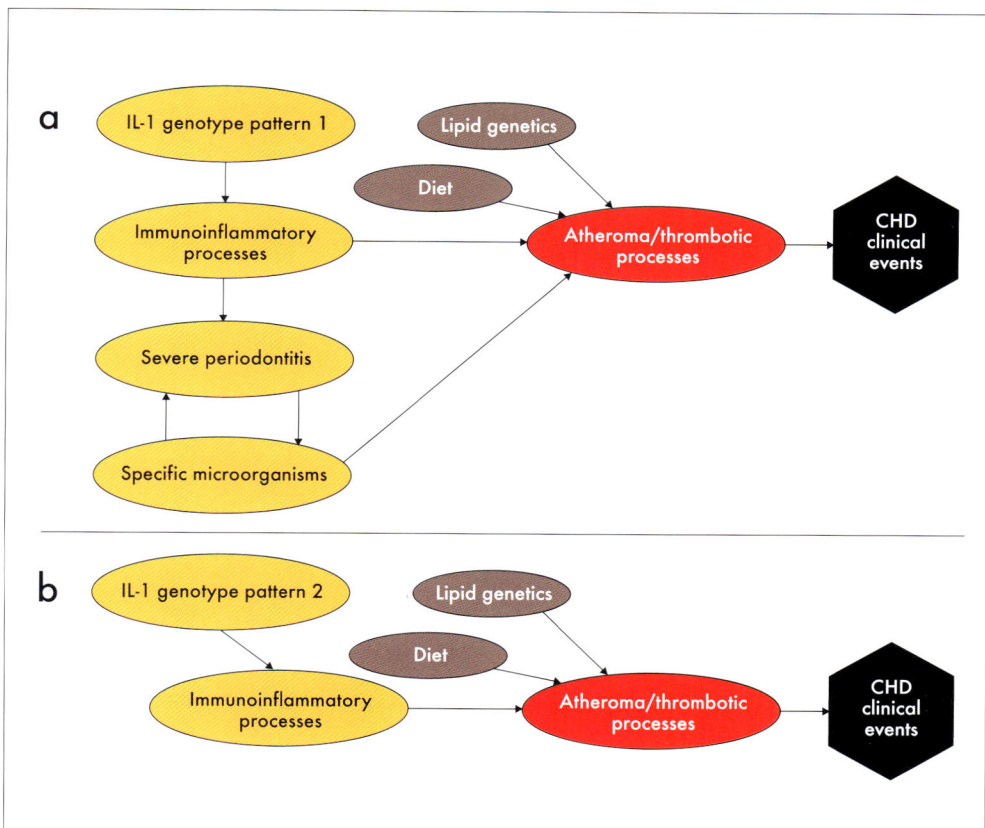

into the systemic circulation. These could have an adverse effect on the lining of the blood vessels or on preexisting atheromas.

Another link between the oral flora, particularly the subgingival periopathogens, and cardiovascular disease may be the presence of HSPs on the bacteria. HSPs are found in all living species and are unique because their amino acid sequences are remarkably conserved (Young and Elliott, 1989). This high degree of homology creates the potential for immunologic cross-reactions between the bacteria and the human host. Many human tissues produce HSPs, including the endothelium lining the vessel wall, which responds to certain stressors like high blood pressure and exposure to LPS by producing HSP 60. Preexisting antibodies against HSPs or HSP-specific T-cells made in response to HSPs on oral bacteria such as *P gingivalis* (Combs et al, 1999) could react with endothelial HSPs and produce

cell damage. HSP-60 expression has been demonstrated in both atherosclerotic lesions and T-cell lymphocytes, which respond to HSP 60 (Xu and Wick, 1996). Elevated serum anti–HSP 65/60 antibodies correlate with a high incidence of both carotid and coronary atherosclerosis (Hoppichler et al, 1996). Saliva contains anti–HSP 65 Ig-A antibodies that can cross-react with human HSP 60 (Schett et al, 1997). These Ig-A antibodies indicate that some members of the oral flora would have HSPs that resemble HSP 60. This autoimmune model involving HSPs could be one link between poor oral hygiene, periodontitis, and cardiovascular disease.

Intervention strategy for prevention and control of cardiovascular diseases

Not until a few years ago was it known that chronic infections, such as periodontal diseases, may be a risk factor and possible causative factor as reviewed in this chapter. Therefore no evidence based on intervention studies is available. However, some trials have been initiated that indicate that antibacterial therapy against chronic infections also could prevent cardiovascular diseases (CVDs).

Two large secondary prevention trials involving azithromycin have been initiated. They are based on findings earlier described that implicate *C pneumoniae* in CVD (Danesh et al, 1997; Saikku et al, 1988) and on a preliminary report that suggests a short course of azithromycin treatment may lower the risk of further cardiovascular events in post–myocardial infarction patients (Gupta et al, 1997). These multicenter studies identify CVD patients and then designate them to a secondary prevention regimen of either placebo or azithromycin for 3 to 12 months. Azithromycin also can have an effect on periodontal anaerobic bacteria (Sefton et al, 1996) so that any positive effects of this preventive approach could reflect a treatment effect on periodontal disease.

This raises the possibility that periodontal disease linked to CVD also should be the focus for prevention and intervention strategies against CVD. Patients with refractory periodontal disease in spite of high standards of self-care and regular nonsurgical maintenance care are likely to be exposing their tissues and blood stream to transient bacteremias, LPSs, HSPs, and inflammatory mediators. In these patients, antimicrobial intervention could be of great value in delaying or preventing the cardiovascular event.

Even without antimicrobial therapy, it has been shown that elderly, dependent-living patients who reported that they saw their dentist/hygienist at least once a year for professional mechanical tooth cleaning and debridement were almost five times less likely to have a stroke than were similarly aged patients who reported that they saw their dentist less frequently (Loesche et al, 1998b).

The previously described evidence that periodontal diseases are risk factors and directly or indirectly etiologic factors for CVD invites well-controlled multicenter studies that will seek to delay or prevent these adverse events by eliminating or controlling periodontal disease.

According to the so-called "full-mouth disinfection" principle (Axelsson et al, 1987; Quirynen et al, 1995), pathogenic microflora should be eliminated from all oral reservoirs. Supragingivally this is performed by the combination of mechanical cleaning of the teeth and dorsum of the tongue, combined with chemical plaque control agents applied by professionals and through self-care. In diseased periodontal pockets, the subgingival microflora should be analyzed (for materials and methods, see chapter 1). Thereafter the subgingival biofilms should be mechanically removed by debridement, supplemented with antimicrobial irrigation (with iodine solution), thereby allowing optimal accessibility for systemic or topical antibiotics to reach remaining subgingival periopathogens. Suitable antibiotics should be selected based on the subgingival microflora analysis. However, in most cases systemic or topical use of doxycycline or systemic use of metronidazole plus amoxicillin should be suitable in selected risk patients.

Unfortunately, periodontal disease is insidious: It is usually painless and has few symptoms, until late in the disease process, when progressive bone loss leads to tooth mobility and migration. Furthermore, diagnosis of the disease requires intraoral radiographs and periodontal probing. These are common diagnostic procedures in dental practice but are rarely applied in medical practice. Thus, physicians, while cognizant of the potential dangers of infection in a patient predisposed to atherosclerosis and infarction, may not identify or detect the presence of periodontal infection, and dentists are not aware that oral infection may contribute to atherogenesis.

Relationship between periodontal diseases and infective endocarditis

Infective endocarditis (IE) is characterized by bacterial infection of damaged heart valves or mural endocardium. Bacteria gain access to the bloodstream and adhere to damaged or otherwise vulnerable endocardial surfaces. Infective endocarditis is commonly, but imprecisely, differentiated into acute or subacute forms, with different clinical manifestations and, frequently, different causative bacteria. Acute bacterial endocarditis (ABE) follows a rapid clinical course (a matter of weeks) and is usually fatal, unless there is intervention in the form of antibiotic therapy. The course of subacute bacterial endocarditis (SBE) is more chronic, and the patient is often unaware of a problem until the onset of a low-grade fever, anemia, and debility. Without treatment, these symptoms may continue for months. Although SBE is preventable in most cases, and is curable in its early stages, it is ultimately fatal in the absence of antimicrobial intervention.

In a comprehensive review of descriptive analytic epidemiologic studies on IE from 1930 to 1996, Drangsholt (1998) found the following:

1. The incidence of IE varies from 0.70 to 6.8 per 100,000 persons per year.
2. The incidence of IE increases 20 times with advancing age.
3. Over 50% of all IE cases are not associated with either an obvious procedural or infectious event within 3 months of symptom development.
4. About 8% of all IE cases are associated with periodontal or dental disease following a dental procedure.

The risk of IE after a dental procedure is probably in the range of 1 per 3,000 to 5,000 procedures. However, it is recognized that dental and other surgical procedures predispose susceptible patients to IE (LaCassin et al, 1995). The most common etiologic agents of SBE are oral streptococci (Bayliss et al, 1983): *S sanguis,* a numerically prominent species of supragingival and subgingival dental plaque, is a prevalent blood isolate from patients suffering from SBE (Kaye, 1994). These bacteria may have an affinity for sterile thrombotic vegetations deposited on cardiac valves. Furthermore, strains of *S sanguis* specifically adhere to and aggregate platelets by a calcium-independent mechanism.

Although most cases of endocarditis are caused by gram-positive species, gram-negative bacteria are also implicated (Geraci and Wilson, 1982). Gram-negative bacteria found in the oral cavity have been isolated from patients with SBE, including a wide variety of putative periodontal pathogens: *Haemophilus aphrophilus, A actinomycetemcomitans, E corrodens, Capnocytophaga* species, and *F nucleatum* (Barco, 1991; Geraci and Wilson, 1982). The underlying mechanisms may be similar to the interactions among *S sanguis, P gingivalis,* and platelets. Thus, individuals with a history of rheumatic fever, atherosclerosis, aortic stenosis, and murmurs, including valve prolapse with regurgitation (ie, those with classic risk factors for SBE), may be at added risk if they also have periodontal disease because of the increased likelihood of bacteremia.

In the aforementioned review of studies on IE (Drangsholt, 1998), it was speculated that dental and oral bacteria, instead of only precipitating bacterial endocarditis, may promote earlier thickening of the heart valves, rendering the heart valve susceptible to later adherence and colonization; a process that is very similar to the previously discussed possible causative relationship between periodontal diseases and CVD. Thus, a new causal model for IE was proposed that includes early bacteremia, which may prime the endothelial surface of the heart valves over a period of many years, and a late bacteremia acting over a period of days or weeks that allows adherence and colonization of the valve, resulting in the characteristic fulminent infection (Fig 200).

The main strategy for prevention of SBE is to limit entry and dissemination of bacteria through the bloodstream. For procedures likely to induce bacteremia, antibiotic prophylaxis is recommended. Thus, most patients with risk factors for

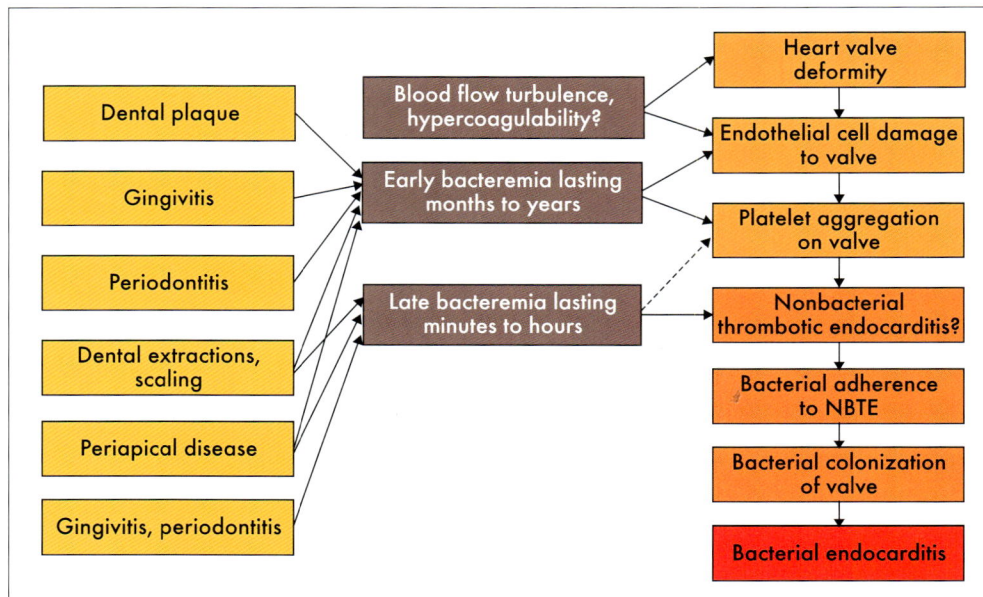

Fig 200 New causal model of endocarditis associated with dental factors. (Modified from Drangsholt, 1998. Reprinted with permission.)

SBE undergoing dental procedures that will induce bleeding should be prescribed antibiotic prophylaxis. However, not all oral bacteria are susceptible to amoxicillin, the current prophylactic antibiotic of choice.

Ultimately, maintenance of periodontal health is desirable to minimize the incidence and degree of bacteremia in IE–susceptible patients. In patients at risk for SBE, it is particularly important to minimize gingival inflammation. This is best accomplished by proper home care, frequent dental recall, and modification of risk factors. Immediately before and during dental procedures (particularly scaling and debridement), irrigation with antimicrobial, bactericidal agents such as povidone-iodine is also recommended to reduce the microbial burden and degree of subsequent bacteremia.

Proper management of such patients, both those at risk and those with cardiovascular disease, requires close collaboration between the attending periodontist and the consulting specialist physician.

Relationship between periodontal diseases and preterm, low–birth weight deliveries

The association between maternal periodontal disease and pregnancy complications is a new, challenging field of research. In the United States, approximately 1 in 10 deliveries results in a preterm, low–birth weight (PLBW) infant (< 2,500 g), usually as a direct consequence of preterm labor or premature rupture of membranes. Preterm low birth weight accounts for more than 60% of infant mortality not associated with congenital anatomic or chromosomal defects.

Risk factors associated with PLBW include high (> 34 years) or low (< 17 years) maternal age, African-American race, low socioeconomic status, inadequate prenatal care, drug abuse, the use of alcohol and tobacco, hypertension, genitourinary tract infections, diabetes, and multiple pregnancies. However, about 25% of PLBW deliveries occur without even a candidate or suspected risk factor.

An association between infection and PLBW delivery has been demonstrated in several studies.

McDonald et al (1991, 1992) showed that vaginal *Bacteroides* colonization was associated with a 60% increased risk of preterm delivery. Inflammation of the extraplacental membrane (chorioamnionitis) has been detected in up to four times as many mothers with preterm deliveries as in those with normal term deliveries (Mueller-Heubach et al, 1990). There is evidence that inflammation in the fetal-placental unit can present without any sign of bacterial infection. These observations support the widely held current opinion that PLBW delivery occurring as a result of infection is indirectly mediated, principally by translocation of bacterial products such as LPSs and by the action of maternally produced inflammatory mediators (Gibbs et al, 1992; Hillier et al, 1988).

Elevated PGE_2 and TNF-α as consistent and reproducible features of PLBW deliveries, even in the absence of any clinical or subclinical genitourinary tract infections, prompted the conclusion by Romero et al (1993) that most cases of PLBW are "probably caused by an infection of unknown origin." Offenbacher et al (1996) hypothesized that periodontal infections, which serve as reservoirs for gram-negative anaerobic organisms, LPS, and inflammatory mediators, including PGE_2 and TNF-α, are a potential threat to the fetal-placental unit. Increased PGE_2 and TNF-α levels as an effect of *P gingivalis* appear to determine the magnitude of the growth retardation response (Collins et al, 1994).

Offenbacher et al (1996) conducted a case-control study of pregnant or postpartum mothers. Cases of PLBW were defined in terms of a mother who gave birth to an infant weighing less than 2,500 g and one or more of the following occurrences: gestational age of less than 37 weeks, preterm labor, or premature rupture of membranes. The controls were all normal-birth weight infants. Assessments included a broad range of known obstetric risk factors, such as tobacco, drug, and alcohol consumption, level of prenatal care, parity, genitourinary infections, and nutrition. Each subject underwent a periodontal examination to determine clinical attachment level.

The results indicated that mothers of PLBW infants and primiparous (firth birth) PLBW infants had significantly more severe periodontal disease than did the mothers of respective normal-birth weight infants. Controlling for other risk factors and covariates disclosed periodontal disease to be a statistically significant risk factor for PLBW, with adjusted ORs of 7.9 for all PLBW deliveries and 7.5 for primiparous PLBW deliveries. The data indicate that periodontal diseases represent a previously unrecognized and clinically significant risk factor for preterm low birth weight in cases of preterm labor or premature rupture of membranes. The odds ratio for periodontal risk (> 7) is more than that for other known obstetric PLBW risk factors, such as smoking (OR of 3 to 5).

Relationship between periodontal diseases and respiratory diseases

The pneumonias are a group of diseases caused by a wide variety of infectious agents, including bacteria, mycoplasma, fungi, parasites, and viruses, resulting in infection of the pulmonary parenchyma. Pneumonia can be life threatening, especially in the elderly and immunocompromised patient. It is a significant cause of morbidity and mortality in patients of all ages. Bacterial pneumonia, a prevalent form of the disease, can arise de novo or as a superinfection of an underlying viral pneumonia and is expected to assume increasing importance because of the continuing emergence of antibiotic-resistant bacteria. Understanding the pathogenesis of and risk factors for bacterial pneumonia is therefore critical to the development of strategies for treatment and prevention of these important and frequently fatal infections.

The pathogenesis of bacterial pneumonia in adults primarily involves aspiration of bacteria that colonize the oropharyngeal region into the lower respiratory tract and the failure of host defense mechanisms to eliminate the contaminating bacteria, which subsequently multiply and cause infection. Thus, the oropharyngeal secretions are directly related to the potential for respiratory infection.

Common respiratory pathogens such as *Streptococcus pneumoniae, S pyogenes, Mycoplasma pneumoniae,* and *Haemophilus influenzae* can colonize the oropharynx and be aspirated into the lower airways. Pneumonia can also be caused by aspiration of oral bacteria, such as *A actinomycetemcomitans* (Yuan et al, 1992, 1994), *Actinomyces israelii* (Morris and Sewell, 1994), *Capnocytophaga* species (Lorenz and Weiss, 1994), *E corrodens* (Joshi et al, 1991), *P intermedia,* and *Streptococcus constellatus.* Studies using careful sampling and strictly anaerobic culture conditions have found that up to 10% of community-acquired pneumonia and 25% of nosocomial pneumonia could be attributed to anaerobic bacteria (Bartlett et al, 1986).

It is also increasingly apparent that potential respiratory pathogens may become established in the oral flora of patients with periodontal disease. Gram-negative bacilli commonly associated with hospital-acquired pneumonia, such as enteric species and *Pseudomonas aeruginosa,* are cultivable from the subgingival flora of periodontally diseased patients (Slots et al, 1988, 1990). The prevalence of staphylococci, Enterobacteriaceae, and yeasts in plaque samples from subjects with periodontitis has been estimated to be as high as 77% (Dahlén and Wikström, 1995); the proportion of these microorganisms in relation to other plaque organisms is usually relatively low (< 1%).

An important observation is that, in periodontal patients, antibiotic therapy is followed by an increase in prevalence of potential respiratory pathogens such as *S aureus,* Enterobacteriaceae, and *Pseudomonas* (Rams et al, 1990). Also of relevance is the study by Scannapieco et al (1992), which found that patients in medical intensive care units, who tend to have poor oral hygiene, often harbor respiratory pathogens in their dental plaque. Following treatment with antibiotics, potential respiratory pathogens adherent to bacteria in the subgingival plaque biofilms of patients with periodontitis may emerge in greater numbers: These bacteria may then be aspirated to cause respiratory disease, especially in patients with compromised defenses.

Subjects at high risk for pneumonia, such as the hospitalized patient, may be more prone to oral colonization by respiratory pathogens following mucosal modification because of prolonged exposure to dental plaque.

This review of new findings about the role of periodontal disease as a modifying risk indicator or risk factor in systemic conditions brings new perspectives to the influence of periodontal heath on the overall health of the individual. Although further research is needed to confirm and expand the aforementioned findings, the data to date imply that periodontal treatment will reduce the risk for these serious systemic conditions. However, recent data on the relationship between periodontal disease and cardiovascular diseases have to be followed up with further studies on lifestyle and genetics (eg, genetic interleukin-1β polymorphism). To a certain extent, diet and other factors may explain the correlation between periodontal diseases and tooth loss, and CVD (Joshipura et al, 1996, 1998). In the near future it should be possible to identify those in whom periodontal therapy might reduce risk and to define appropriate treatment strategies. Such an approach would dramatically merge periodontology into mainstream medicine, with profound implications for the dental profession. In other words, the oral cavity may once again be acknowledged as an integral part of the human body, in health and disease, after being displaced more than a century ago (for reviews on the role of periodontal diseases as a risk factor for other diseases, see Armitage, 2001; Beck et al, 1996, 1998; Beck and Offenbacher, 2001; De Nardin, 2001; Drangsholt, 1998; Garcia et al, 2001; Grossi, 2001; Herzberg, 2001; Iacopino and Cutler, 2000; Jeffcoat et al, 2001; Joshipura et al, 1998; Kinane, 1998b; Kolltveit and Eriksen, 2001; Kornman et al, 1999; Kornman and Duff, 2001; Kuramitsu et al, 2001; Loesche, 2000; Lowe, 2001; Madianos et al, 2001; Offenbacher, 1996; Offenbacher et al, 1998, 1999, 2001; Page, 1998, 2001; Scannapieco and

Mylotte, 1996; Scannapieco, 1998; Scannapieco and Genco, 1999, Scannapieco et al, 2001; Taylor, 2001; Wactawski-Wende, 2001).

Conclusions

The occurrence of attachment loss in an individual is influenced by internal (endogenous, host) modifying factors. Internal modifying RIs, RFs, and PRFs related to periodontal diseases are genetic factors, impaired host factors, chronic systemic diseases, and so on.

Genetic and hereditary factors

Most studies of genetic factors have concerned aggressive periodontal disease—localized and generalized forms found in prepubertal and adolescent children—on the grounds that aggressive disease in young individuals is less likely than the chronic form found in adults to result from chronic environmental (bacterial plaque) insults. Furthermore, patients with aggressive disease probably represent a more homogenous population than do those with chronic periodontitis.

Family studies suggest that susceptibility to the aggressive forms of disease, particularly in prepubertal and adolescent patients, is influenced, at least in part, by host genotype. Inherited phagocytic cell deficiencies appear to confer risk for periodontitis in prepubertal patients. The prevalence and distribution of aggressive periodontitis in affected families are consistent with an autosomal-recessive mode of inheritance. Among genetic traits that may confer enhanced susceptibility to periodontal disease are abnormal function of the phagocytes (particularly the polymorphonuclear cells); reduced capacity to produce IgG_2; interleukin-1, tumor necrosis factor-α, and hFcγIIa polymorphisms; and variable monocyte macrophage function.

Studies have shown that genetic IL-1 polymorphism is an RF for periodontitis. Some recent studies have also shown that genetic IL-1 polymorphism and smoking are synergistic risk factors for periodontal diseases. Most studies show that the prevalence of genetic IL-1 polymorphism is about 30% to 35%. However, the prevalence is very low in China (< 3%) and very high in a Swedish population (45%) (for reviews see Kornman and di Giovine, 1998; Michalowicz, 1994).

Chronic systemic diseases

Of the chronic systemic diseases, both type 1 and type 2 diabetes mellitus seem to be the most important modifying RIs, RFs, and PRFs for periodontal diseases.

Longitudinal studies have shown that diabetes mellitus is an RF and a PRF and that the risk is strongly correlated to the metabolic stability of the diabetes. The chemotactic response of the PMNLs is gradually reduced in relation to the duration of the diabetes and the hyperglycemia. Polymorphonuclear leukocytes accumulate in the connective tissue and their metalloproteinases cause tissue destruction, particularly of collagen.

Other less common, chronic systemic diseases that involve impaired PMNL function, such as Down syndrome, Papillon-Lefèvre syndrome, Chédiak-Higashi syndrome, and LAD, are also strongly associated with advanced progressive periodontal disease, particularly aggressive periodontitis (for reviews see Genco and Löe, 1993; Grossi et al, 1994; Grossi and Genco, 1998; Hart et al, 1994; Mealy, 2000; Michalowicz, 1994; Nishimura et al, 1998; Oliver and Tervonen, 1994b; Salvi et al, 1997a; Soskolne, 1998a; Thorstensson, 1995; Wilton, 1991; Yalda et al, 1994).

Aging

Although aging per se should not be an internal modifying RI, RF, and PRF, all epidemiologic data show that loss of periodontal support is strongly correlated to the age of the population. Rather than an age-related, intrinsic deficiency or abnormality that increases periodontal susceptibility, this is probably an expression of cumulative tissue destruction, including iatrogenic damage, over a lifetime. The elderly also have significantly more local plaque-retentive factors, such as multiple restorations with defects (overhangs, etc), calculus, deep pockets, and furcation involvement; this may explain the somewhat higher incidence than in younger adults, who have fewer plaque-retentive factors. However, longitudinal studies, based on high-quality plaque control, have shown that further loss of periodontal attachment can be prevented in elderly adults just as successfully as it can in younger adults (for review see Abiko et al, 1998).

Local oral conditions

The importance of local RIs, RFs, PRFs, risk markers, and risk predictors should not be underestimated. Several studies have shown that local plaque-retentive factors significantly impede efforts at plaque control, both by the patient and by professionals, resulting in enhancement of localized loss of periodontal attachment and persistence of infectious periodontal inflammation. Local plaque-retentive factors, especially those located subgingivally and along the gingival margin, should be eliminated or minimized at an early stage of treatment.

Well-known plaque-retentive factors are open carious cavities; restoration overhangs; defective restoration margins; unpolished restorations; calculus; rough, unplaned root cementum; cementum hypoplasia; root resorption; root grooves; and iatrogenic effects of aggressive subgingival scaling, such as grooves and exposed dentinal tubules on the root surfaces.

Previous evidence of periodontal diseases, in the form of advanced loss of periodontal support (vertical and horizontal [furcation involvement]) and deep, diseased pockets, is considered a risk predictor and risk marker. Sites with advanced loss of periodontal support and deep, diseased pockets progress much more rapidly than do sites with less pronounced loss and shallow, healthy pockets (for review see Axelsson, 1993, 1994; Ehnevid, 1995; Ehnevid et al, 1995; Jansson, 1995; Kornman and Löe, 1993; Newman et al, 1994).

Periodontal disease as a modifying factor for other diseases or abnormalities

Periodontal diseases also should be regarded as risk indicators, risk factors, and prognostic risk factors for other diseases and abnormalities. Recent longitudinal studies have shown that periodontal diseases are potential RFs and PRFs for coronary heart disease and stroke. In addition, the gram-negative periopathogens and their toxins (particularly LPSs) seem to be direct or indirect etiologic factors of atherosclerosis and subacute bacterial endocarditis.

Periodontal diseases also may adversely affect diabetic metabolic control.

Experimental animal studies and human studies have shown that periodontal diseases may be a risk factor for preterm, low–birth weight infants.

In susceptible individuals, periodontal diseases may also predispose patients to respiratory diseases, particularly pneumonia.

Thus, the objectives of treatment of periodontal disease should not be restricted to the maintenance of healthy periodontal support of the dentition, but also should be seen in a broader perspective: the prevention of untoward effects on systemic health.

CHAPTER 4

PREDICTION OF PERIODONTITIS RISK AND RISK PROFILES

Most children and young adults are periodontally healthy or have gingivitis. Only a small minority of susceptible children and young adults exhibit aggressive periodontitis: In Scandinavia, the prevalence is only about 0.1% to 0.3% of the population. In adults, three groups are discernible in the population: the majority, consisting of periodontally healthy individuals and individuals with gingivitis; a smaller intermediate group with mild to moderate chronic periodontitis (10% to 15%); and a small, high-risk group with advanced, aggressive periodontitis (< 5%).

The proportions may vary significantly in different age groups and populations because the prevalence of gingivitis and mild or moderate chronic forms of periodontitis is strongly correlated with the standard of gingival plaque control and dental care habits. The fact that periodontitis is always preceded by gingivitis and a high prevalence of local plaque-retentive factors explains why the prevalence of mild and moderate chronic periodontitis is higher among elderly adults, even those with low susceptibility, than it is among younger adults.

However, periodontitis is the result of a complex interplay of bacterial challenge, host response, and other modifying factors. Despite extreme variations in oral hygiene standards, the prevalence of aggressive periodontitis in adults is about 5% to 15%, in both industrialized and developing countries.

Thus in populations with very low standards of oral hygiene and dental care, a "whole-population strategy" should be implemented, to reduce periodontal treatment needs in the general population. More cost effective, however, in populations with relatively high or high standards of oral hygiene and well-organized oral health care services, is a "high-risk strategy," ie, targeting risk groups, at-risk and high-risk individuals, and key-risk teeth and surfaces.

DEFINITION OF TERMS

Probability statements

For cost effectiveness, the methods used to select and predict groups and individuals at "true" risk for disease development should be as sensitive as possible. The optimal *sensitivity* for a diagnostic risk test is 100%; ie, of 100 individuals selected as "risk individuals," all are true risk individuals. Similarly, for methods used to select true "nonrisk individuals," *specificity* should be as high as possible; ie, of selected nonrisk individuals, 100% are truly nonrisk.

Usually, the higher sensitivity, the lower the specificity. Thus, the clinician is usually forced to choose a test based on the consequences of making an error. A test method with high sensitivity and low specificity is likely to err in the direction of false positives. For a disease such as periodontitis, the implications are not usually serious when people are incorrectly identified as having active disease: They do not suffer extreme anxiety or undergo radical treatment. They may undergo intensified preventive treatment and incur increased treatment costs.

The consequence of a false-negative result, ie, when a person with disease is incorrectly identified as healthy, is that the disease may progress further before it is diagnosed at a subsequent examination. This may be serious in the case of aggressive disease and of major consequence when there are prolonged intervals between examinations. Thus, for periodontal disease, the consequences of a false-positive diagnosis are less serious than those of a false-negative diagnosis. If a choice is necessary, a highly sensitive test method, with few false-negative diagnoses, is preferable to a highly specific test, which generates few false-positive diagnoses. Alternatively, multiple tests, one highly sensitive and one highly specific, may be combined.

The probability of development of periodontitis, given the result of a test method, is known as the *predictive value*. The positive predictive value is the probability that a patient with a positive test result actually has active periodontitis. Similarly, the negative predictive value is the probability that a patient with a negative test result actually has inactive periodontal disease.

Likelihood ratios can be used to evaluate the performance of a diagnostic test that is dichotomous or has interval properties. In addition, likelihood ratios can be used to calculate the probability of disease after a positive or negative test result.

Sensitivity, specificity, and predictive value are probability statements, representing the propor-

tion of people with disease who have a positive test. Likelihood ratios are based on odds, which is the ratio of two probability values that contain the same information but express it differently. The relationship between the two is expressed in the following formulas:

$$Odds = \frac{Probability\ of\ event}{1 - Probability\ of\ event}$$

$$Probability = \frac{Odds}{1 + Odds}$$

The likelihood ratio for any value of a diagnostic test method is the probability of getting that test result when disease is present, divided by the probability of the result when disease is absent. Thus, likelihood ratios express how many times more or less likely a test result is to be found in diseased test subjects than it is in nondiseased test subjects.

This type of calculation can be done with different values of an interval scale diagnostic test. The resulting distribution of likelihood ratios can then provide the clinician with information on the likelihood of disease for a range of values.

Risk categories

For the clinician, accurate prediction of patients or sites at high risk of developing periodontitis is of fundamental importance. Because of the particular nature of periodontal disease, prediction of disease progression is also important. Diagnostic tests differentiate whether or not a person has a specific disease at the time. *Risk indicators* (RIs) are factors that have proved to be significantly associated with the occurrence of a specific disease, but only in cross-sectional studies. For example, in a cross-sectional study by Grossi et al (1994), smoking was ranked second (odds ratio, 2.0 for light smoker and 4.75 for heavy smoker), after age, as a risk indicator for periodontal disease. Diabetes mellitus was ranked third (odds ratio, 2.3).

Risk factors (RFs), on the other hand, are those that significantly increase the likelihood that people without disease, if exposed to these factors, will succumb to the disease within a specified time interval. Although diagnostic tests and RIs can be evaluated by cross-sectional research designs, longitudinal studies are necessary to confirm RFs.

The term *risk factor* is rather loosely used and can refer to an attribute or exposure associated with increased probability of disease (not necessarily causal); any type of determinant (cause); or a determinant that can be modified. This loose terminology may cause confusion when multivariate aspects of diseases are considered. Use of the term should be restricted as follows: Risk factors are characteristics of the person or environment that, when present, directly result in an increased likelihood that a person will get a disease and, when absent, directly result in a decreased likelihood.

Exposure to a risk factor means that a person has been exposed to or manifested the factor prior to the onset of the disease. There may be continuous exposure, an isolated episode, or multiple exposures over a period of time. Clinicians must recognize that risk factors, like etiologic factors (the periopathogens), are based on the current state of knowledge about a direct relationship: In light of further knowledge, a current risk factor for a specific disease may in the future be excluded. Because periodontal diseases are the result of multiple etiologic factors (different species of periopathogens) and modifying risk factors, removal of a risk factor, such as the cessation of smoking, does not necessarily cure the disease. It should reduce the likelihood of disease development, but, once a person has the disease, removal of the risk factor may or may not result in cure.

Factors that significantly increase the risk of further progression of existing disease are termed *prognostic risk factors* (PRFs). For example, in a prospective study by Machtei et al (1997), smokers were at significantly greater risk than nonsmokers for further attachment loss (odds ratio, 5.4).

Risk markers and *risk predictors* (eg, advanced attachment loss and deep diseased pockets) are usually biologic markers that either indicate disease or disease progression but currently are thought not to be causal or represent historical evidence of the disease, such as the number of missing teeth or past evidence of periodontal disease. If a risk predictor is more strongly associated with the disease than a risk factor, and the risk predictor and risk factor are also associated with each other, then the risk predictor will appear in the multivariate model instead of the risk factor. For example, baseline periodontal status is usually strongly associated with the occurrence of new disease, because it is a measure of past disease and thus is a risk predictor.

Microorganisms are thought to be etiologic risk factors and are also associated with new disease. Microorganisms are also associated with baseline periodontal status because they are partially responsible for this status. Thus, baseline periodontal status may replace microorganisms in the multivariate model. Having a risk predictor in the model results in a prediction model rather than a risk model.

Finally, periodontal diseases have multiple levels of measurement: person, tooth, and site. A person can have disease, although many teeth and even more tooth sites may be disease free. Thus, the same person can have sites with disease onset as well as established sites of disease, exhibiting progression. If the risk factor for disease onset is different than the prognostic factors for disease outcome, established sites should be evaluated under prognosis and not under risk prediction. Currently, however, both types of sites tend to be considered together when risk factors are delineated. In the future it may be useful to consider the two as separate entities.

RISK GROUPS

In addition to etiologic and preventive factors, many other factors may modify the prevalence, onset, and progression of periodontal diseases. Such factors are divided into external (environmental) and internal (endogenous) factors (see chapters 2 and 3).

External modifiers

Examples of external modifying RIs, RFs, and PRFs for periodontal diseases are smoking, use of smokeless tobacco, irregular dental care, low socioeconomic level, infectious and other acquired diseases, side effects of medication, and poor dietary habits. The most important and most common are smoking and irregular dental attendance habits. Numerous cross-sectional studies have shown that smoking is a very powerful external modifying RI for periodontal diseases. In a multifactorial analytic study, smoking was ranked No. 1 (after age) as a risk indicator for periodontal attachment loss (Grossi et al, 1994). Among 65 year olds, it was estimated that smokers had lost about 50% more periodontal attachment than nonsmokers, after adjustment for the greater number of missing teeth in the smokers (Axelsson et al, 1998; for review, see Axelsson et al, 1998; Bergström and Preber, 1994; Tonetti, 1998).

In a recent prospective study, Machtei et al (1997) showed that the risk for further progression of periodontal disease was about five times greater in heavy smokers than in nonsmokers. It has also been shown that the outcome of periodontal therapy, including regenerative therapy, is significantly poorer in smokers than in nonsmokers (Ah et al, 1994; Tonetti et al, 1995). These studies confirm that smoking is not only an extremely powerful external modifying risk factor but also a prognostic risk factor for onset and progression of periodontal disease.

In a study by Locker and Leake (1993b), multivariate analysis disclosed that the most consistent markers for prevalence of periodontal disease were the subject's educational status and current smoking habits, along with age and the number of teeth.

Other cross-sectional studies have also shown that adult subjects (35, 50, 65, and 75 year olds) with low educational level lost more periodontal attachment than did subjects with higher educational level (Axelsson et al, unpublished data, 1990; Paulander et al, 2002). Some infectious and acquired diseases, especially severe diseases such as ulcerative colitis, Crohn disease, acquired immunodeficiency syndrome (AIDS), and leukemia, will also be strong risk and prognostic risk factors for periodontal diseases.

However, the opposite may also apply: In a recently published 18-year longitudinal study, a direct linear correlation was shown among the number of diseased periodontal pockets, the amount of lost periodontal support, and the risk for development of cardiovascular disease and stroke (Beck et al, 1996; for review, see Beck et al, 1998; Kolltveit and Eriksen, 2001; Loesche, 2000; Scannapieco, 1998).

Internal modifiers

Internal RIs, RFs, and PRFs related to periodontal diseases include genetic factors, impaired host factors, chronic diseases, and reduced salivary flow and quality. Most studies of genetic factors in periodontal disease have concerned the aggressive forms of disease. Family studies suggest that susceptibility to the aggressive forms of disease, particularly in prepubertal and adolescent children, is at least in part influenced by host genotype. Inherited phagocytic cell deficiencies appear to confer risk for aggressive periodontitis in prepubertal children. The prevalence and distribution of aggressive periodontitis in affected families are most consistent with an autosomal-recessive mode of inheritance. Comparisons between adult monozygous twins reared together and reared apart indicate that early family environment has no appreciable influence on probing depth and attachment loss in adults. Michalowicz et al (1991a) calculated that 38% to 82% of the variance of attachment loss, probing depths, and gingival index in monozygous and dizygous adult twins may be attributed to genetic factors.

A number of apparently genetically determined syndromes or diseases appear to carry an associated increased risk for periodontal destruction. In a few cases, there appears to be a defect that predisposes the host to destruction of the periodontal tissues because of the absence or abnormal regulation of a tissue component necessary for structural integrity, such as the collagen defect of Ehlers-Danlos syndrome and possibly type 1 diabetes. In other syndromes or diseases, defects of phagocytic cell function have been described, especially polymorphonuclear leukoytes (PMNLs), but also mononuclear phagocytes. In diseases such as type 1 diabetes, these phagocytic defects are found in reduced chemotactic capacity and the presence of possible disorders of collagen regulation, such as excess production of collagenase in the gingival tissues. Although more extensive data are available on PMNL dysfunction, it is possible that further studies will also reveal defects of mononuclear phagocytes to be associated with these syndromes.

Recently Kornman et al (1997a) reported a specific genotype of the polymorphic interleukin-1 (IL-1) gene cluster associated with severe periodontitis in nonsmokers. On the basis of the gene, subjects with severe disease were differentiated from those with mild disease (odds ratio, 18.9 for subjects aged 40 to 60 years). It is estimated that almost 30% of the adult population has this genotype of IL-1. The Periodontal Susceptibility Test was developed on the basis of these findings. Recent longitudinal studies have shown that the combination of smoking and genetic IL-1 polymorphism are synergistic risk factors for periodontal diseases (Axelsson et al, 2001; McGuire and Nunn, 1999). It may be estimated that more than 85% of cases with advanced periodontal disease are disclosed when selection is based on smoking (an external risk factor) and the occurrence of polymorphic IL-1 genes (an internal, genetic risk factor). Screening for subjects potentially susceptible to aggressive periodontitis on the basis of the occurrence of periopathogens *Porphyromonas gingivalis, Bacteroides forsythus,* and *Actinobacillus actinomycetemcomitans* in periodontal pockets will disclose only about 20% of cases.

Of the chronic diseases, type 1 diabetes mellitus is considered to be the most important RI, RF, and PRF for periodontal diseases. Children and young adults with type 1 diabetes are more susceptible to localized aggressive periodontitis, which initially is restricted to first molars and incisors but becomes more widespread, affecting other teeth.

Plaque indices in these subjects are similar to those of age-matched nondiabetics, and the severity of the periodontal destruction, when present, is not related to the amount of gingival plaque. The susceptibility of these diabetic patients to periodontal destruction may be multifactorial and depend on defects of phagocytic cells, such as the PMNLs, and on the vascular and structural defects of the periodontal tissues. There are also reports of changes in the subgingival flora of these patients: Whether this is caused by the diabetic state and might cause the periodontal destruction, or whether it is secondary to the destruction, has not been determined.

Even in adults, a close relationship has been shown between diabetes mellitus and periodontal diseases. In the large cross-sectional study of adults by Grossi et al (1994) discussed earlier, diabetes mellitus was ranked third, after age and smoking, as a risk indicator for severe forms of periodontal disease. It was also the only systemic disease positively associated with attachment loss.

Thus, groups at risk for periodontal diseases constitute primarily smokers and individuals with type 1 or type 2 diabetes, polymorphic IL gene clusters, poor oral hygiene, irregular dental care, and low educational level. For details, see chapters 2 and 3.

Table 24 Criteria for evaluating individual periodontal risk in children, young adults, adults, and the elderly

No periodontal risk (P0; green)

I	Children
I:1	Healthy gingivae
I:2	Excellent oral hygiene habits
I:3	No approximal probing loss of attachment
I:4	No internal or external risk factors or risk indicators

No periodontal risk (P0; green)

II	Young adults
II:1	Healthy gingivae
II:2	Excellent oral hygiene habits
II:3	No approximal probing loss of attachment
II:4	No internal or external risk factors or risk indicators

No periodontal risk (P0; green)

III	Adults
III:1	No diseased periodontal pockets
III:2	Excellent oral hygiene habits
III:3	No approximal probing loss of attachment
III:4	No internal or external risk factors or risk indicators

No periodontal risk (P0; green)

IV	Elderly
IV:1	No diseased periodontal pockets
IV:2	Excellent or good oral hygiene habits
IV:3	Mean approximal probing loss of attachment < 1 mm
IV:4	No internal or external risk factors or risk indicators

Low periodontal risk (P1; blue)

I	Children
I:1	Gingival bleeding index < 10% (CPITN* 1)
I:2	Good oral hygiene habits
I:3	No approximal probing loss of attachment
I:4	No internal or external risk factors

Low periodontal risk (P1; blue)

II	Young adults
II:1	Gingival bleeding index < 10% (CPITN* 1)
II:2	Good oral hygiene habits
II:3	No approximal probing loss of attachment
II:4	No internal or external risk factors

Low periodontal risk (P1; blue)

III	Adults
III:1	Fewer than five diseased approximal pockets > 3 mm (CPITN* 3–4)
III:2	Good oral hygiene habits
III:3	Mean approximal probing loss of attachment < 1 mm
III:4	No internal or external risk factors

Low periodontal risk (P1; blue)

IV	Elderly
IV:1	Chronic periodontitis: fewer than five diseased approximal pockets > 5 mm (CPITN* 4)
IV:2	Good oral hygiene habits
IV:3	Mean approximal probing loss of attachment < 2 mm
IV:4	No tooth loss caused by periodontal disease
IV:5	No internal or external risk factors

Periodontal risk (P2; yellow)

I	Children
I:1	Gingival bleeding index < 20% (CPITN* 1)
I:2	Poor oral hygiene habits
I:3	Internal risk indicators, risk factors, and prognostic risk factors
I:4	External risk indicators, risk factors, and prognostic risk factors (low educational level of the parents, etc)

Periodontal risk (P2; yellow)

II	Young adults
II:1	One to five diseased approximal pockets > 3 mm (CPITN* 3–4)
II:2	Poor oral hygiene habits
II:3	Mean approximal probing loss of attachment < 1 mm
II:4	Internal risk indicators, risk factors, and prognostic risk factors (type 1 diabetes, etc)
II:5	External risk indicators, risk factors, and prognostic risk factors (smoking, low educational level, etc)

Periodontal risk (P2; yellow)

III	Adults
III:1	Chronic periodontitis: more than five diseased approximal pockets > 5 mm (CPITN* 4)
III:2	Poor oral hygiene habits

INDIVIDUAL RISK

The relative risk for developing periodontal disease can be evaluated by combining clinical examination, preventive factors, etiologic factors, the absence or presence of environmental (external) and host-related (internal) risk indicators, risk factors, prognostic risk factors, risk markers, and risk predictors. Periodontal risk increases in accordance with the severity and number of these factors to which the individual is exposed. Criteria for grading individual risk into one of four classes, from no risk to high risk (P0 to P3), have been proposed for children, young adults, adults,

III:3 Mean approximal probing loss of attachment > 2 mm

III:4 Internal risk indicators, risk factors, and prognostic risk factors (type 1 or type 2 diabetes, etc)

III:5 External risk indicators, risk factors, and prognostic risk factors (smoking, low educational level, etc)

Periodontal risk (P2; yellow)

IV Elderly

IV:1 Chronic periodontitis: more than 15 of the approximal sites = CPITN* 4

IV:2 Poor oral hygiene habits

IV:3 Mean approximal probing loss of attachment > 4 mm

IV:4 More than four teeth lost because of periodontal disease

IV:5 Internal risk indicators, risk factors, and prognostic risk factors (type 2 diabetes, etc)

IV:6 External risk indicators, risk factors, and prognostic risk factors (smoking, low educational level, etc)

High periodontal risk (P3; red)

I Children

I:1 Localized or generalized aggressive periodontal diseases (0.1% to 0.3% of the Scandinavian population)

I:2 Very poor oral hygiene

I:3 Most diseased sites infected with bacteria associated with aggressive periodontitis (A actinomycetemcomitans, etc)

I:4 Internal risk indicators, risk factors, and prognostic risk factors, such as genetic IL-1 polymorphism, dysfunction of the PMNL cells, reduced immunoglobulin G2 (IgG2) response, type 1 diabetes, Down syndrome, and leukemia.

I:5 External risk indicators, risk factors, and prognostic risk factors (low educational level of the parents, AIDS, etc)

High periodontal risk (P3; red)

II Young adults

II:1 Localized or generalized aggressive periodontal diseases

II:2 High periodontal incidence (annual probing loss of attachment) and several sites related to aggressive periodontitis

II:3 Very poor oral hygiene

II:4 Most diseased sites infected with bacteria associated with aggressive periodontitis (A actinomycetemcomitans, P gingivalis, etc)

II:5 Internal risk indicators, risk factors, and prognostic risk factors, such as genetic interleukin-1 polymorphism, dysfunction of the PMNL cells, reduced IgG2 response, type 1 diabetes, leukemia, etc

II:6 External risk indicators, risk factors and prognostic risk factors (smoking, low educational level, AIDS, etc).

High periodontal risk (P3; red)

III Adults

III:1 Aggressive periodontitis: high periodontal incidence (annual probing loss of attachment) and several sites with aggressive periodontitis

III:2 More than four teeth lost because of periodontal disease

III:3 Very poor oral hygiene and most diseased sites infected by P gingivalis, B forsythus, and other periopathogens

III:4 Internal risk indicators, risk factors, and prognostic risk factors (type 1 or type 2 diabetes, genetic interleukin-1 polymorphism, etc)

III:5 External risk indicators, risk factors, and prognostic risk factors (smoking, low educational level, AIDS, etc)

High periodontal risk (P3; red)

IV Elderly

IV:1 Aggressive periodontitis (periodontitis gravis and complicata involving most teeth)

IV:2 More than 10 teeth lost because of periodontal disease

IV:3 Very poor oral hygiene; most diseased sites infected by P gingivalis, B forsythus, and other periopathogens

IV:4 Internal risk indicators, risk factors, and prognostic risk factors (type 1 or type 2 diabetes, genetic interleukin-1 polymorphism, etc)

IV:5 External risk indicators, risk factors, and prognostic risk factors (smoking, low educational level, etc)

*CPITN = Community Periodontal Index of Treatment Needs.

and the elderly (Table 24). The colors, from green to red, symbolize escalated risk. The criteria are based on history taking, established clinical diagnostic criteria, and supplementary bacterial sampling and laboratory tests, where indicated.

Recently, all the adult patients (N = >100,000) at the Public Dental Health Service Clinics in the county of Varmland, Sweden, were evaluated according to the four classes of periodontal risk (P0 to P3). Figure 201 shows the frequency distribution of periodontal risk in all the adult patients, 20 to 80 years old. The frequency distributions of no periodontal risk, low periodontal risk, periodontal risk, and high periodontal risk were 61%, 36%,

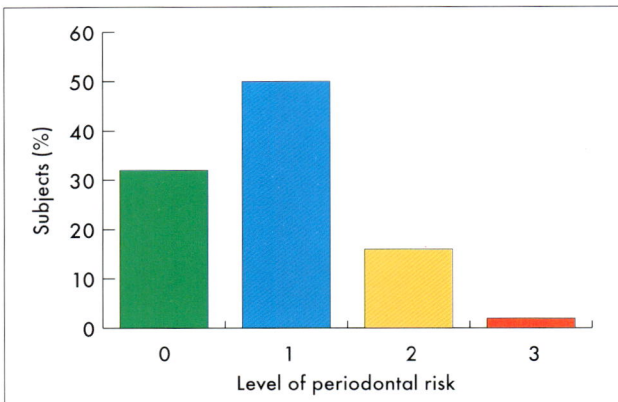

Fig 201 Frequency distribution of periodontal risk in adult patients, aged 20 to 80 years. Results indicated that 32% had no periodontal risk (0); 50% had low periodontal risk (1); 16% had periodontal risk (2); and 2% had very high periodontal risk (3).

2%, and 1%, respectively, in 20 year olds; 24%, 59%, 15%, and, 2%, respectively, in 40 year olds; 11%, 58%, 27%, and 4%, respectively, in 60 year olds; and 12%, 55%, 28%, and 4%, respectively, in 80 year olds.

KEY-RISK TEETH AND SURFACES

An analytic epidemiologic study was conducted in the county of Varmland, Sweden, on randomized samples of more than one thousand 35, 50, 65, and 75 year olds (see chapter 7). The many clinical variables recorded included probing attachment loss (vertical as well as horizontal [furcation involvement]) and the Community Periodontal Index of Treatment Needs (CPITN) at every site (>130,000) (Axelsson et al, unpublished data, 1990; Axelsson, 1998).

In 35 year olds, attachment loss on the distal surfaces of the maxillary first molars was already about twice that of the mesial surfaces, implying greater risk for future furcation involvement on the "inaccessible" distal surfaces. These surfaces should have been targeted for gingival plaque control from early adulthood. Attachment loss on the mandibular central and lateral incisors in 35 year olds may be explained at least partly by local factors, such as plaque retention arising from heavy supragingival calculus formation, abnormal frenum, smoking, crowded and rotated teeth, and iatrogenic side effects from toothbrushing due to very thin alveolar bone.

Treatment of teeth with furcation involvement is much more complicated than is treatment of diseased pockets in single-rooted teeth. Therefore, diagnosis and analytic epidemiology on the pattern of furcation involvement is important. Analysis of the frequency distribution of noninvolved surfaces (score = 0) and furcation-involved surfaces (scores 1 to 3) on the molars and the maxillary first premolars in the 50 year olds revealed that score 2 to 3 was most frequent on the distal surfaces of the maxillary first molars and score 1 was most frequent on the buccal surfaces of the mandibular first molars.

The pattern of disease in the dentition at the surface level is an important basis for planning an efficient preventive strategy, particularly needs-related plaque control measures. The study also evaluated the pattern of CPITN scores 0 to 4 and missing surfaces in the 50 year olds. Scores of 4 were almost negligible. Score 3 was limited mainly to the mesial and distal surfaces of the maxillary molars, ie, the "key-risk" surfaces. The mesial, distal, and lingual surfaces of the mandibular incisors frequently had a score of 2, indicating supragingival calculus to be removed.

This study, in a randomized sample of an adult toothbrushing population, revealed that needs-related plaque control should target the approximal surfaces of the posterior teeth (particularly the maxillary teeth). This should be introduced at the age of 12 to 14 years to prevent the initiation of periodontitis and should also be reinforced in all adults to control periodontitis and limit the treatment need.

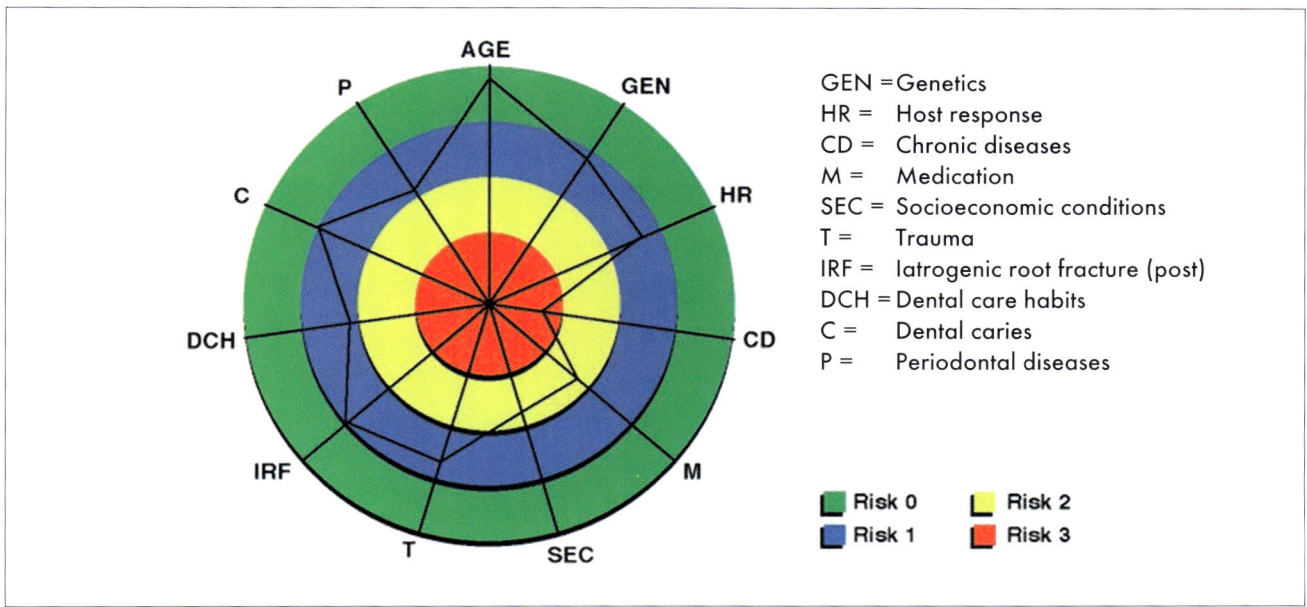

Fig 202 Risk profile for tooth loss.

RISK PROFILES

Risk profiles for tooth loss, dental caries, and periodontal diseases can be presented graphically, by combining symptoms (risk markers) of disease (prevalence, incidence, treatment needs, etc); etiologic factors; external modifying risk indicators, risk factors, and prognostic risk factors (EMRIRF); internal modifying risk indicators, risk factors, and prognostic risk factors (IMRIRF); and preventive factors. This can be done manually or by computer. Degrees of risk, 0, 1, 2, or 3, are displayed in green, blue, yellow, or red, respectively (Figs 202 to 204). The graphs are very useful tools for communication with the patient when discussing the oral health status, etiology, modifying factors, prevention, possibilities, responsibilities, and reevaluations.

Risk profiles for tooth loss

As illustrated in Fig 202, a profile of risk for future tooth loss can be compiled by combining several RIs, RFs, and PRFs. Among these are age, estimated risk for periodontal diseases (P0 to P3), and dental caries (C0 to C3), poor socioeconomic conditions, chronic diseases, iatrogenic root fractures, trauma, genetics and impaired host response, medication, and irregular dental care habits.

In many industrialized countries, elderly people have heavily restored dentitions because of high caries incidence 30 to 50 years previously, when dental treatment comprised "drilling, filling, killing (the pulp), and billing." In such populations, the most frequent reason for tooth loss would be iatrogenic root fractures caused by posts in endodontically treated teeth. On the other hand, in developing countries with very limited oral health care resources, the main reasons for tooth loss would be untreated periodontal diseases and dental caries among elderly people, and untreated dental caries and trauma among young people.

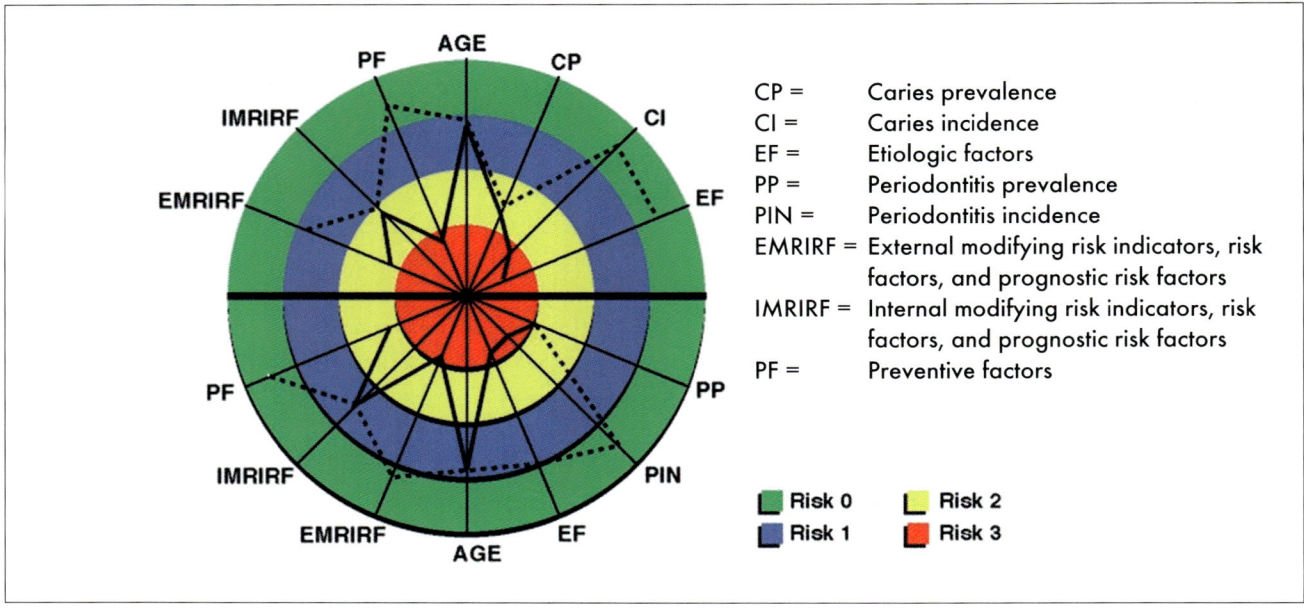

Fig 203 Risk profile for dental caries (*top*) and periodontal diseases (*bottom*). Solid line = C3P3 at baseline; dotted line = C1P1, 2 years later.

Combined risk profiles for dental caries and periodontal diseases

Because some patients may suffer from both dental caries and periodontal diseases, risk profiles can be presented separately or combined. Figure 203 illustrates a combined risk profile from a patient classified, after detailed examination and history taking, as being at high risk for both dental caries and periodontal diseases (C3P3), on the following basis:

- The prevalence of caries and periodontitis were high.
- The incidence of caries and periodontitis had been very high.
- He was exposed to many etiologic factors; both nonspecific (high plaque formation rate and plaque volume) and specific (caries-inducing bacteria and periopathogens such as salivary mutans streptococci, salivary lactobacilli, *A actinomycetemcomitans, P gingivalis, Prevotella intermedia, B forsythus,* and *Treponema denticola*).

- He exhibited many external and internal modifying risk indicators, risk factors, and prognostic risk factors (EMRIRF and IMRIRF) for both dental caries and periodontal diseases. For dental caries the most important EMRIRF were high frequency of intake of sticky, sugar-containing products and medication with salivary depressive side effects. For periodontal diseases, the most important EMRIRF was regular smoking of 10 to 20 cigarettes per day. Of the IMRIRF, the most important for dental caries was reduced stimulated salivary secretion rate (0.6 mL/min) and the most important for periodontal diseases was poorly controlled diabetes mellitus.
- His standard of oral hygiene was very low and his dietary habits were poor. The patient had no preventive dental care habits, and his dental care visits were irregular.

After presentation of the case findings and a session of self-diagnosis, the dentist and patient discussed a treatment strategy based on shared responsibility between the patient and the oral

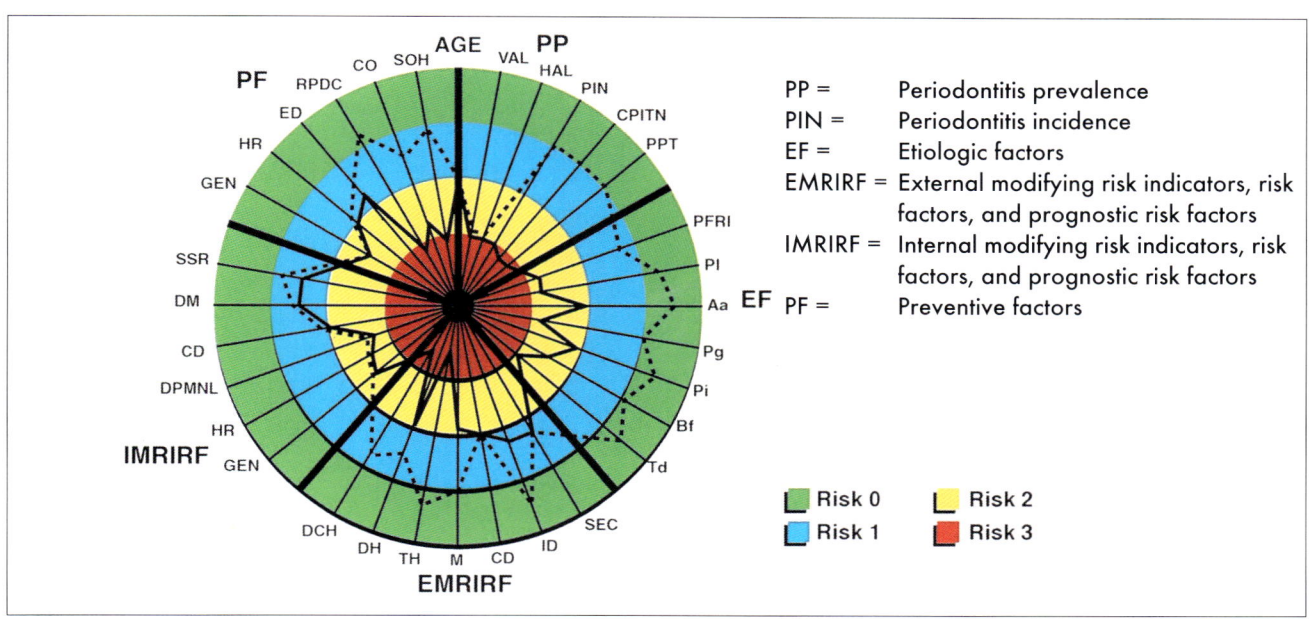

Fig 204 Risk profile for periodontal diseases. Solid line = P3 at baseline; dotted line = P1, 2 years later. See Box 10 for an explanation of abbreviations related to periodontal risk.

health personnel. Two years later, he was classified as a low-risk patient for both dental caries and periodontal diseases (C1P1), on the following basis:

- The etiologic factors had been dramatically reduced (from red to green) by an initial intensive combination of mechanical and chemical plaque control (self-care and professional) and by maintenance of a high standard of plaque control, ie, a dramatic improvement in the most important preventive factors.
- Treatment needs (excavation and restoration of open cavities, scaling, root planing, and debridement of diseased periodontal pockets) and plaque-retentive factors had been eliminated.
- Important EMRIRF had been eliminated. The patient stopped smoking and reduced the estimated daily sugar clearance time by 80%. In addition, there was no further need of medicine with salivary depressive effects. As a consequence of this and regular use of fluoride chewing gum, the salivary secretion rate increased from 0.6 mL/min to 1.0 mL/min.

- His exposure to fluoride had been increased: A new fluoride toothpaste technique was introduced, and fluoride chewing gum was recommended after meals, supplemented by professional application of fluoride varnish.

As a consequence of these preventive measures and the healthier lifestyle, the patient developed no new caries lesions and experienced no further loss of periodontal support (see Fig 203).

Detailed risk profiles for periodontal diseases

A more detailed risk profile is also available for patients at high risk predominantly for periodontal diseases. The risk profile in Fig 204 illustrates graphically how high periodontal risk has been reduced to low risk (from P3 to P1; see Box 10) by improved needs-related plaque control measures, via self-care and supplementary professional

Box 10 Abbreviations related to periodontal risk

Periodontal risk

- P0 = No periodontal risk
- P1 = Low periodontal risk
- P2 = Periodontal risk
- P3 = High periodontal risk

Periodontal diagnosis

- PP = Periodontitis prevalence (experience)
- VAL = Vertical attachment loss
- HAL = Horizontal attachment loss (furcation involvement)
- PIN = Periodontitis incidence (activity)
- PPT = Periodontal pocket temperature

Etiologic factors (EF)

- PFRI = Plaque Formation Rate Index
- PI = Plaque Index (scores and pattern)
- Aa = *Actinobacillus actinomycetemcomitans*
- Pg = *Porphyromonas gingivalis*
- Pi = *Prevotella intermedia*
- Bf = *Bacteroides forsythus*
- Td = *Treponema denticola*

External modifying risk indicators, risk factors, and prognostic risk factors (EMRIRF)

- SEC = Socioeconomic conditions
- ID = Infectious diseases
- CD = Chronic diseases
- M = Medication
- TH = Tobacco habits
- DH = Dietary habits
- DCH = Dental care habits

Internal modifying risk indicators, risk factors, and prognostic risk factors (IMRIRF)

- GEN = Genetic factors
- HR = Host response
- DPMNL = Defective PMNL function
- CD = Chronic diseases
- DM = Diabetes mellitus
- SSR = Stimulated salivary secretion rate

Preventive factors (PF)

- HR = Host response
- ED = Educational level
- RPDC = Regular preventive dental care habits
- CO = Compliance
- SOH = Standard of oral hygiene

treatment. The greater the difference between the solid line and the dotted line, the greater the improvement. The absence of any change suggests that this particular factor cannot be influenced (for example, genetic factors, host response, and some chronic diseases). The patient in question was a 50-year-old man with the following clinical diagnosis and anamnestic data at his initial assessment.

Clinical variables related to periodontal disease

- Eight teeth had been lost because of periodontal disease (four maxillary molars, two maxillary premolars, and two mandibular molars).
- The mean vertical attachment loss (VAL) on the approximal surfaces was 4 mm more than the average for his age group. In addition, several posterior teeth had two- and three-wall infrabony pockets. All of the remaining molars had furcation involvement degree 1 to 2 (horizontal attachment loss [HAL]).
- Retrospective radiographs and diagnoses of vertical attachment loss from the referring dentist showed irregular but advanced loss of periodontal support during the last few years (periodontal incidence [PIN]).
- More than 60% of the approximal sites were diseased, with greater than 5-mm probing depths (CPITN score 4). Purulent exudate was frequent. Analysis of the gingival crevicular fluid (GCF) showed high levels of prostaglandin E_2 (PGE_2), IL-1β, aspartate aminotransferase (AST), and other endogenous metalloproteinases (MMPs), particularly from polymorphonuclear cells (PMNLs), which together indicated active lesions with advanced breakdown of periodontal tissues.
- The periodontal pocket temperature (PPT) was elevated in all pockets deeper than 3 mm, which also indicated active lesions.

Etiologic factors

- He was a very fast plaque former (Plaque Formation Rate Index [PFRI] = 5).
- The standard of oral hygiene was very poor (Plaque Index [PI] = 76%).
- DNA probe analyses from the deepest pockets showed the following values, on a scale of 0 to 5: *A actinomycetemcomitans* (Aa) = score 3 ($>10^5$); *P gingivalis* (Pg) = score 5 ($>10^6$); *P intermedia* (Pi) = score 3 ($>10^5$); *B forsythus* (Bf) = score 4 (10^6); and *T denticola* (Td) = score 5 ($>10^6$).

External modifying risk indicators, risk factors, and prognostic risk factors

- His socioeconomic condition (SEC), including education, was about average.
- He had a history of urinary infection (infectious diseases [ID]).
- He had diagnosed hypertension and had experienced some minor heart infarcts (chronic diseases [CD]).
- He was taking medication (M) for his cardiovascular disease.
- He had smoked more than 20 cigarettes a day since the age of 15 years (more than 35 pack years).
- His dietary habits (DH) were poor, with frequent snacks between meals, sweets, and sweet drinks. His body mass index was high.
- His dental care habits (DCH) were very irregular.

Internal modifying risk indicators, risk factors, and prognostic risk factors (IMRIRFPRF)

- Use of the new Periodontal Susceptibility Test (PST) revealed that he was positive for the polymorphic IL-1 gene clusters; ie, he was genetically impaired. It has been shown that this genetic defect is strongly correlated to increased susceptibility to periodontal diseases.

- His host response (HR) was also reduced because of defect polymorphonuclear leukocyte (PMNL) function, an effect of regular smoking. The importance of aggressive, phagocytozing PMNLs as the first line of nonspecific defense in periodontal pockets should not be underestimated.
- As stated previously, he had a diagnosis of cardiovascular disease, which could be attributable to the presence of several diseased pockets, from which gram-negative microorganisms and their lipopolysaccharides (LPSs) continuously enter the connective tissue and the vascular system. Other contributing factors could be 35 years of smoking, poor dietary habits, hereditary factors, physical inactivity, etc.
- He occasionally experienced symptoms of type 2 diabetes.
- Because of regular medication with saliva-depressive effects, his stimulated salivary secretion rate was low (< 0.7 mL/min).

Preventive factors

- As mentioned, he was genetically impaired.
- Instead of having an effective host response, his first line of defense was impaired because of smoking.
- His educational level was slightly above average.
- He sought preventive dental care (RPDC) only irregularly.
- His compliance (CO) on oral hygiene, smoking, and dietary habits was very poor, resulting in a very low standard of oral hygiene. He used a toothbrush and toothpaste only irregularly (SOH).

During the case presentation, the graphic illustration (see Fig 204) was used as a tool for communication with the patient. Concurrently, the patient was educated in self-diagnosis to confirm the diagnosis of his own oral health status and treatment needs. Thereafter, an agreement was reached by the patient and the oral health personnel with respect to a treatment strategy in which responsibility for the patient's oral health was shared between the patient and the oral health personnel (dentist and dental hygienist) at the clinic. This was followed by an initial intensive preventive period, including education in needs-related plaque control measures, based on self-diagnosis.

The dentist and dental hygienist, working in cooperation, eliminated all supragingival and subgingival plaque-retentive factors. Conservative, nonaggressive methods were used for scaling and root planing to achieve smooth root cementum without exposing dentinal tubules, which would have led to bacterial invasion. The subgingival biofilm and nonattaching microflora were comprehensively removed by nonaggressive debridement and powered irrigation with chemical plaque control agents. During this initial intensive period, the entire oral cavity was treated according to the so-called complete-mouth disinfection strategy: three times in 1 week, the dental hygienist cleaned the tongue and all tooth surfaces (supragingival as well as subgingival) mechanically (professional mechanical toothcleaning [PMTC]) and chemically with chemical plaque control agents (chlorhexidine [CHX]).

Thereafter, the patient practiced needs-related plaque control measures twice a day, based on self-diagnosis and self-evaluation. Plaque disclosure before and after cleaning was performed every day during the first week and weekly thereafter. Needs-related plaque control measures included use of selected mechanical toothcleaning aids and a tongue scraper, as well as a toothpaste that contained triclosan. For the first 4 weeks, the patient also used a CHX mouthrinse twice a day. Because CHX is cationic, the patient was instructed not to use toothpastes containing anions (eg, sodium lauryl sulfate, monofluorophosphate) within an hour before or after CHX rinsing.

The first reevaluation was carried out after 2 months. Thereafter, the patient began a maintenance program tailored to his individual requirements. Maintenance included needs-related intervals of clinical evaluation, PMTC, nonaggressive

debridement of diseased pockets, and control of the oral hygiene standard.

The 1-year recall assessment involved comprehensive clinical examination, digitized computer-aided radiographs, DNA probe analyses, pocket temperature measurement, and gingival crevicular fluid analysis. It was confirmed that only three remaining deep pockets (> 5 mm) exhibited signs of activity: PGE_2, IL-1, and AST levels in gingival crevicular fluid were still high, and pocket temperature was elevated. The levels of *A actinomycetemcomitans, P gingivalis,* and *B forsythus* remained high. Use of millimeter-graded probes in combination with the digitized radiographs disclosed the presence of two-wall infrabony pockets at all three active sites.

At this stage, the patient was highly motivated (prepared to act) and his standard of oral hygiene was excellent. After a "case presentation," including reevaluation of the risk profile, the patient decided to stop smoking if the remaining three active lesions could be healed and arrested by regenerative therapy.

One week before regenerative therapy, any remaining subgingival biofilms were mechanically removed by nonaggressive debridement, followed by comprehensive powered irrigation with iodine solution. Because the sites contained high levels not only of the anaerobes *P gingivalis* and *B forsythus* but also the exogenous pathogen *A actinomycetemcomitans,* a fiber delivering controlled, slow release of tetracycline was inserted into the pockets for 1 week. In addition to the needs-related mechanical plaque control measures and the use of fluoride toothpaste that contained triclosan, the patient began a CHX-rinsing program 1 week before surgery.

Tailor-made miniflap surgery was used both to gain accessibility to the three different periodontal lesions and for regenerative therapy at the one surgical session. After nonaggressive mechanical cleaning of the root surfaces with curettes (used with negative angle) and the PER-IO-TOR reciprocating instruments (Dentatus, Hägersten, Sweden) followed by chemical cleaning and surface conditioning with ethylenediaminetetraacetic acid

(EDTA) gel (PrepGel, Biora, Lund, Sweden), a new matrix-guided regenerative material (Emdogain gel, Biora) was placed on the root surfaces. The miniflaps were resutured.

For the first postoperative month, only chemical plaque control by rinsing twice a day with CHX solution and the use of an extra-soft toothbrush was allowed around the treated sites, to prevent disruption of healing by mechanical trauma, particularly from interdental cleaning aids. After 4 weeks, the patient resumed needs-related plaque control measures and the needs-related maintenance program, based on evaluations, PMTC, and nonaggressive debridement at sites where subgingival biofilms had re-formed, despite the concerted efforts at gingival plaque control by both patient and hygienist.

The second detailed reexamination was carried out after 2 years. At these reexaminations it is most important that the patient be activated in self-evaluation. Digitized radiographs, an intraoral camera, and a lighted mouth mirror are very useful tools for this purpose. The risk profile (see Fig 204) was again used as a tool for communication with the patient, to supplement self-evaluation in the mouth and on radiographs. The dotted line shows how successfully the patient and the dental personnel fulfilled their responsibilities:

- Etiologic factors were dramatically reduced by improved mechanical plaque control and intermittent use of CHX by self-care, supplemented at needs-related intervals by PMTC and debridement.
- The PFRI was reduced from 5 to 2 (indicating that the gingivae had healed, following the establishment of meticulous gingival plaque control).
- The PI was reduced from 76% to 8%.
- The exogenous periopathogens *A actinomycetemcomitans* and *P gingivalis*, as well as the opportunistic periopathogens *B forsythus, P intermedia,* and *T denticola*, were almost totally eliminated.
- The urinary infection and the periodontal pockets healed. The patient stopped smoking and improved his dietary habits. The need for medication for infection as well as for cardiovascular disease was reduced.
- For 2 years, the patient had participated in a needs-related maintenance program, which included regular dental care habits and regular professional preventive care.
- The reduced need for medication for cardiovascular disease eased the saliva-depressive effects of the drugs. Together with changes in dietary habits (increased intake of fiber-rich vegetables, etc), this led to improved salivary function: The stimulated salivary secretion rate increased from < 0.7 to 1.2 mL/min.
- Because the patient stopped smoking, the PMNL function and thereby the host response seemed to improve.
- The patient's educational level, that is, knowledge of dental diseases, self-diagnosis, and self-care, increased considerably over 2 years.
- High motivation, based on self-diagnosis, knowledge, and training resulted in establishment of excellent needs-related plaque control habits and compliance.

The outcome of these efforts and improvement by self-care and needs-related professional preventive treatment was that there was no further loss of periodontal support during the 2-year period. Instead a mean 6-mm gain of vertical attachment was achieved at three sites, as a result of successful regenerative therapy. All periodontal sites were healthy (CPITN = 0), and no increased PPT was observed. Periodontal risk was therefore reassessed: Although the risk lessened, the patient tested positive (PST) for the polymorphic IL-1 gene cluster, and he therefore will continue in a maintenance program, with recall at needs-related intervals. The aim will be to gradually prolong the intervals between recalls.

This example illustrates how useful the risk profile is as a tool for:

- Case presentation and communication with the patient
- Establishment of needs-related self-care habits

- Detailed evaluation of self-care and professional preventive treatment, even in individuals assessed as high risk according to current knowledge

CONCLUSIONS

Risk groups

For cost effectiveness, prevention and control of periodontal diseases should be based strictly on predicted risk. In industrialized countries, with relatively high standards of oral hygiene and well-organized oral health care services, the prevalence of aggressive periodontitis in children and young adults is very low (0.1% to 1%), and aggressive periodontitis affects 5% to 15% of the adult population. A high-risk strategy is appropriate, targeting key-risk groups, individuals, teeth, and surfaces.

In populations with poor oral hygiene standards and limited oral health care resources, most children have gingivitis and most adults have gingivitis and untreated chronic periodontitis. Under these conditions, until the existing treatment needs are met, a whole-population strategy for general oral health promotion should be applied.

The high-risk strategy combines methods with as high a sensitivity as possible (85% to 100%), to select true high-risk groups, individuals, teeth, and surfaces, with methods with a similarly high specificity, to identify true non-risk and low-risk groups, individuals, teeth, and surfaces.

In children and young adults, groups at very high risk for aggressive periodontitis are those with genetic IL-1 polymorphism, type 1 diabetes mellitus, leukemia, human immunodeficiency virus, and syndromes with impaired PMNL functions. The concomitant presence of poor oral hygiene and *A actinomycetemcomitans* increases risk.

In adults, groups at very high risk for more severe forms of periodontal disease are those with genetic IL-1 polymorphism, smokers, and those with unstable type 1 or type 2 diabetes mellitus, impaired PMNL, and AIDS. The combination of poor oral hygiene, irregular dental attendance, and infection with *A actinomycetemcomitans, P gingivalis,* and *B forsythus* increases risk.

Periodontal risk should be evaluated individually as no risk (P0), low risk (P1), risk (P2), or high risk (P3). At "key risk" for periodontal disease are the approximal surfaces of the maxillary posterior teeth.

Risk profiles

Individual risk profiles can be established for tooth loss, dental caries, and periodontal diseases. These are compiled by combining symptoms (risk markers) of disease (prevalence, incidence, and treatment needs), etiologic factors, external and internal risk indicators, risk factors, prognostic factors, and preventive factors. Risk profiles are very useful tools for patient communication, with reference to risk assessment and evaluation of self-care and professional treatment.

Based on risk evaluation and current knowledge, the strategy for needs-related prevention and control of periodontal diseases should be:

- Introduction of regular parental tooth cleaning, from the age of 1 year.
- Establishment of needs-related oral hygiene habits in schoolchildren.
- Development of school-based preventive programs to discourage smoking, from the age of 12 years.
- Early (prepubertal) identification of individuals susceptible to localized and generalized aggressive periodontitis, by regular clinical examination and genetic screening for the polymorphic IL-1 gene family (such a test is now available) and for the capacity to mount an effective immunoglobulin G2 humoral immune response.

Once identified, young high-risk individuals should be examined regularly with DNA probes to identify the exogenous periopathogens *A actinomycetemcomitans* and *P gingivalis* and the opportunistic endogenous periopathogens *B forsythus* and *P intermedia*. Whenever an infection is discovered, it should be eliminated by an initial combination of mechanical cleaning and chemical therapy followed by a needs-related maintenance program.

Young adults and adults may be broadly regarded as two groups: the majority, which includes healthy patients and patients with gingivitis, and a minor group of patients with periodontitis. In the group susceptible to periodontal disease, individual periodontal risk profiles should be evaluated. This involves comprehensive history taking, clinical examination (periodontal attachment loss, treatment needs, PPT, etc), evaluation of the patient's standard of oral hygiene, measurement of the plaque formation rate, DNA probe analyses of the subgingival microflora, evaluation of external modifying risk indicators, risk factors, and prognostic risk factors (particularly smoking habits, infectious diseases, irregular dental care, and low educational level), evaluation of internal modifying risk indicators, risk factors, and prognostic risk factors (particularly polymorphism in the IL-1 gene family and other genetic impairments to immune response), and notation of the presence or absence of type 1 diabetes mellitus and unstable type 2 diabetes mellitus.

Based on the risk profile, the basic strategy should be individualized treatment to eliminate infection by periopathogens and to eliminate or at least reduce modifying risk indicators, risk factors, and prognostic risk factors (particularly smoking) as much as possible. As a consequence, the periodontal tissues will heal.

Initial healing should be maintained by an individualized maintenance program, based on the establishment of meticulous gingival plaque control by self-care, supplemented by needs-related professional mechanical toothcleaning and nonaggressive subgingival debridement. At needs-related intervals, the effect of the maintenance program should be evaluated in terms of probing attachment level measurements, probing depth measurement, radiographs, pocket temperature measurements, gingival crevicular fluid analyses (particularly PGE_2 levels) and DNA microbial probes at susceptible sites. Use of antibiotics (topical or systemic) should be restricted to extremely high-risk patients with aggressive or so-called "refractory" periodontitis and some related systemic diseases, and only after mechanical removal of the subgingival biofilms and identification of pathogens by DNA probe evaluation.

In the near future, it is likely that in selected high-risk periodontitis subjects, specific methods to stimulate cytokines that suppress the immunoinflammatory response (interleukin 10), transforming growth factor-β, and tissue inhibitors of metalloproteinases will be used in combination with optimal reduction of the bacterial challenge. Promising initial results have been confirmed for the use of nonsteroidal anti-inflammatory drugs to retard bone resorption and chemically modified tetracycline (doxycycline) to reduce extracellular destruction. Also promising are the results of a recent 3-year longitudinal study of selected patients with periodontitis who used toothpaste containing triclosan (Rosling et al, 1997a, 1997b). Triclosan has antiplaque as well as anti-inflammatory properties.

Repair and regeneration of periodontal tissues is already a reality. Guided tissue regeneration by use of barriers was introduced in the late 1980s. The most promising method to date is the so-called guided matrix method, which involves the use of enamel matrix derivatives (Emdogain gel). Other combinations of biomaterials are under development (for reviews on risk evaluation for periodontal diseases, see: Axelsson, 1998; Beck, 1994a, 1994b, 1995, 1998; Beck and Löe, 1993; Beck et al, 1996; 1998; Burt, 1996; Genco, 1996; Grossi et al, 1994; Grossi and Genco, 1998; Johnson, 1991a, 1991b; Kornman and di Giovine, 1998; Lamster et al, 1998; Locker and Leake, 1993b; Machtei et al, 1997; Offenbacher, 1996; Oliver et al, 1998; Page and Beck, 1997; Page and Kornman, 1997; Papapanou and Lindhe, 1997; Salvi et al, 1997a; Tonetti, 1998).

CHAPTER 5

CLASSIFICATION AND PATHOGENESIS OF PERIODONTAL DISEASES

CLASSIFICATION OF PERIODONTAL DISEASES

The periodontal diseases range in severity from early inflammation of the gingival margin (Fig 205) to advanced loss of periodontal support (Fig 206) and tooth loss. Traditionally, periodontal diseases have been classified as gingivitis or periodontitis. *Gingivitis* is caused by the oral microflora that colonize the tooth surfaces, forming plaque along the gingival margin. Figure 207 shows the close relationship between the gingival plaque and the inflamed gingival margin. With control of gingival plaque, gingivitis can heal successfully; it is a reversible condition.

In the absence of control of gingival plaque, the inflammation of the gingiva may progress to *periodontitis,* or irreversible loss of periodontal support (destruction of periodontal ligament as well as alveolar bone). Although untreated, infectious, inflamed gingival sites do not always progress to loss of periodontal support, periodontitis is always preceded by gingivitis. Meticulous control of gingival plaque, which maintains gingival health, should therefore also prevent periodontitis. Regeneration of the periodontal lig-

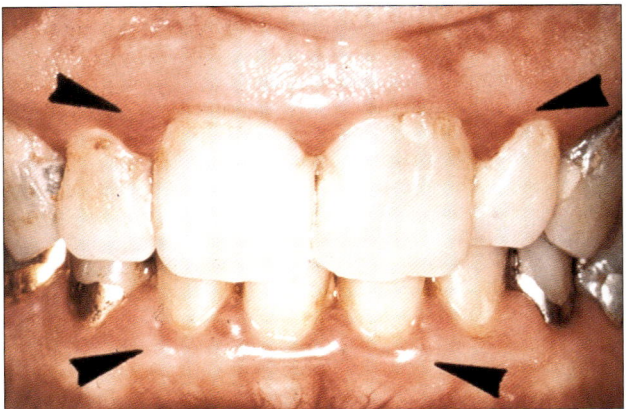

Fig 205 Inflammation of the gingival margin *(arrows)* (gingivitis).

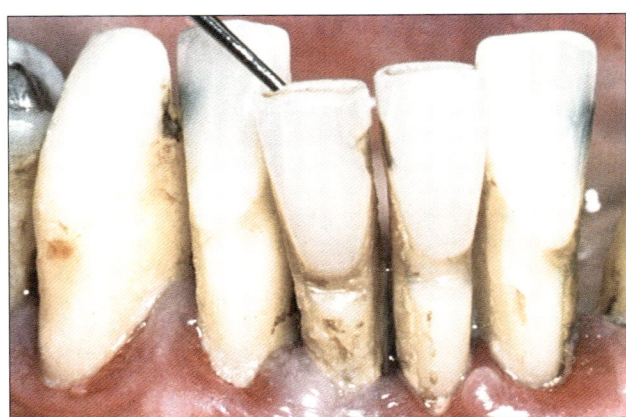

Fig 206 Advanced loss of periodontal support (periodontitis).

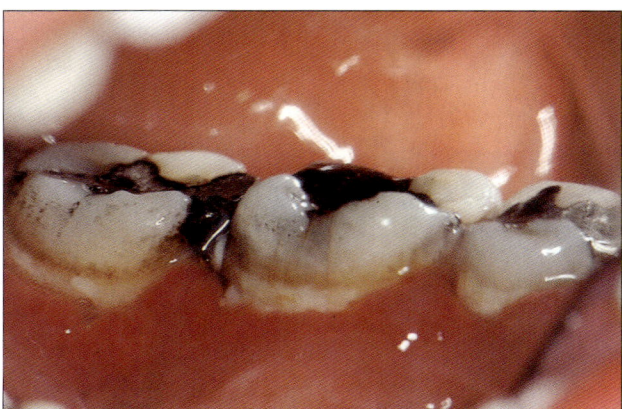

Fig 207 Close relationship between gingival plaque and an inflamed gingival margin.

Box 11 Classification of gingivitis

- Initial gingivitis
- Early gingivitis
- Established or manifest gingivitis
- Acute necrotizing ulcerative gingivitis (ANUG)
- Chronic necrotizing ulcerative gingivitis (CNUG)

Box 12 Classification of marginal periodontitis*

- Localized prepubertal periodontitis (LPP)
- Generalized prepubertal periodontitis (GPP)
- Localized juvenile periodontitis (LJP)
- Generalized juvenile periodontitis (GJP)
- Localized postjuvenile periodontitis (LPJP)
- Generalized postjuvenile periodontitis (GPJP)
- Adult rapidly progressive periodontitis (ARPP)
- Adult (chronic) periodontitis (A[C]P)
- Acute necrotizing (ulcerative) periodontitis (AN[U]P)
- Chronic necrotizing (ulcerative) periodontitis (CN[U]P)
- Adult refractory periodontitis (ARP)

*American Academy of Periodontology, 1989.

---

ament and the alveolar bone can now be achieved by so-called regenerative therapy and excellent gingival plaque control, indicating that plaque-associated periodontitis and other kinds of periodontal attachment loss are not always irreversible.

Gingivitis and periodontitis may manifest clinically in various forms, which serve as the basis for classification. Based on histologic and clinical criteria, gingivitis is classified into several forms (Box 11).

For marginal periodontitis, a classification that takes into account the age of the patient, the pattern of periodontal attachment loss, and the rate of disease progression was used at the individual level during the past decade (Box 12).

Another classification, described by Ranney (1991, 1993) is presented in Box 13. This system includes not only forms of gingivitis and periodontitis other than those caused by gingival plaque (biofilms) but also modifying factors, for example, systemic aggravating factors, general disease states, viral infections, and so on (see chapters 2 and 3).

Recent retrospective studies have shown that most patients diagnosed with localized juvenile periodontitis (LJP) had experienced early loss of periodontal support in the primary dentition (Sjödin et al, 1989, 1993). Based on the data from the 1986 to 1987 survey of US schoolchildren (mean age of 16 years), Albandar et al, (1997) concluded that those that were diagnosed with localized and generalized early-onset periodontitis (EOP) are heterogenous groups comprising rapidly and slowly progressing forms of periodontitis within each classification. In addition, localized forms of periodontitis may become more generalized in young adults. Other studies in adults have shown that the same individual may experience periods of what was termed rapidly progressive periodontitis (RPP) followed by more quiescent or "burned out" phases, at the individual level as well as at the site level (Goodson et al, 1982; Lindhe et al, 1983).

The differential diagnosis of so-called refractory (treatment-resistant) periodontitis and re-

---

Box 13 Classification of periodontal diseases*

Gingivitis	Early-onset periodontitis:
• Gingivitis, plaque bacterial:	Localized early-onset periodontitis:
Nonaggravated	Neutrophil abnormality
Systemically aggravated:	Generalized early-onset periodontitis:
Related to sex hormones	Neutrophil abnormality
Related to drugs	Immunodeficiency
Related to systemic disease	Early-onset periodontitis related to systemic disease:
• Necrotizing ulcerative gingivitis:	Leukocyte adhesion deficiency
Systemic determinants unknown	Hypophosphatasia
Related to human immunodeficiency virus (HIV)	Papillon-Lefèvre syndrome
• Gingivitis, nonplaque:	Neutropenias
Associated with skin disease	Leukemias
Allergic	Chédiak-Higashi syndrome
Infectious	AIDS
Periodontitis	Diabetes mellitus type 1
• Adult periodontitis:	Trisomy 21
Nonaggravated	Histocytosis X
Systemically aggravated:	Ehlers-Danlos syndrome (type VIII)
Neutropenias	Early-onset periodontitis, systemic determinants unknown
Leukemias	• Necrotizing ulcerative periodontitis:
Lazy leukocyte syndrome	Systemic determinants unknown
Acquired immunodeficiency syndrome (AIDS)	Related to HIV
Diabetes mellitus	Related to nutrition
Crohn disease	Periodontal abscess
Addison disease	*Ranney (1991, 1993).

current periodontitis in adults is also often uncertain. Therefore, the first European Workshop on Periodontology (Attström and van der Velden, 1994) recommended the following classification of periodontal diseases:

• Early-onset periodontitis
• Necrotizing periodontitis
• Adult periodontitis

New classification system of periodontal diseases and conditions

The need for a revised classification system for periodontal diseases was emphasized during the 1996 World Workshop in periodontics (Armitage, 1996). As a consequence, the American Academy of Periodontology organized an international workshop in 1999 in order to develop a new classification system. State-of-the-science reviews for each of the outlined classification terms were discussed. The new classification that was agreed upon is shown in Box 14. This most recent classification system was used in the writing of this volume.

Box 14 Classification of Periodontal Diseases and Conditions*

I. Gingival Diseases

A. Dental plaque–induced gingival diseases[†]

1. Gingivitis associated with dental plaque only
   a. without other local contributing factors
   b. with local contributing factors
2. Gingival diseases modified by systemic factors
   a. associated with the endocrine system
      1) puberty-associated gingivitis
      2) menstrual cycle–associated gingivitis
      3) pregnancy-associated
         a) gingivitis
         b) pyogenic granuloma
      4) diabetes melitus–associated gingivitis
   b. associated with blood dyscrasias
      1) leukemia-associated gingivitis
      2) other
3. Gingival diseases modified by medications
   a. drug-influenced gingival diseases
      1) drug-influenced gingival enlargements
      2) drug-influenced gingivitis
         a) oral contraceptive–associated gingivitis
         b) other
4. Gingival diseases modified by malnutrition
   a. ascorbic acid–deficiency gingivitis
   b. other

B. Non–plaque-induced gingival lesions

1. Gingival diseases of specific bacterial origin
   a. *Neisseria gonorrhea*–associated lesions
   b. *Treponema pallidum*–associated lesions
   c. streptococcal species–associated lesions
   d. other
2. Gingival diseases of viral origin
   a. herpesvirus infections
      1) primary herpetic gingivostomatitis
      2) recurrent oral herpes
      3) varicella-zoster infections
   b. other
3. Gingival diseases of fungal origin
   a. *Candida* species infections
      1) generalized gingival candidosis
   b. linear gingival erythema
   c. histoplasmosis
   d. other
4. Gingival lesions of genetic origin
   a. hereditary gingival fibromatosis
   b. other
5. Gingival manifestations of systemic conditions
   a. mucocutaneous disorders
      1) lichen planus
      2) pemphigoid
      3) pemphigus vulgaris
      4) erythema multiforme
      5) lupus erythematosus
      6) drug-induced
      7) other
   b. allergic reactions
      1) dental restorative materials
         a) mercury
         b) nickel
         c) acrylic
         d) other
      2) reactions attributable to
         a) toothpastes/dentifrices
         b) mouthrinses/mouthwashes
         c) chewing gum additives
         d) foods and additives
      3) other
6. Traumatic lesions (factitious, iatrogenic, accidental)
   a. chemical injury
   b. physical injury
   c. thermal injury
7. Foreign body reactions
8. Not otherwise specified (NOS)

II. Chronic Periodontitis[‡]
   A. Localized
   B. Generalized

III. Aggressive Periodontitis[‡]
   A. Localized
   B. Generalized

IV. Periodontiis As a Manifestation of Systemic Diseases
   A. Associated with hematologic disorders
      1. Acquired neutropenia
      2. Leukemias
      3. Other
   B. Associated with genetic disorders
      1. Familial and cyclic neutropenia
      2. Down syndrome
      3. Leukocyte adhesion deficiency syndromes
      4. Papillon-Lefèvre syndrome
      5. Chediak-Higashi syndrome
      6. Histiocytosis syndromes
      7. Glycogen storage disease
      8. Infantile genetic agranuloctosis
      9. Cohen syndrome
      10. Ehlers-Danlos syndrome (Types IV and VIII)
      11. Hypophosphatasia
      12. Other
   C. Not otherwise specified (NOS)

V. Necrotizing Periodontal Diseases
   A. Necrotizing ulcerative gingivitis (NUG)
   B. Necrotizing ulcerative periodontitis (NUP)

VI. Abscesses of the Periodontium
   A. Gingival abscess
   B. Periodontal abscess
   C. Pericoronal abscess

VII. Periodontitis Associated with Endodontic Lesions
   A. Combined periodontal-endodontic lesions

VIII. Developmental or Acquired Deformities and Conditions
   A. Localized tooth-related factors that modify or predispose to plaque-induced gingival diseases/periodontitis
      1. Tooth anatomic factors
      2. Dental restorations/appliances
      3. Root fractures
      4. Cervical root resorption and cemental tears
   B. Mucogingival deformities and conditions around teeth
      1. Gingival/soft tissue recession
         a. facial or lingual surfaces
         b. interproximal (papillary)
      2. Lack of keratinized gingiva
      3. Decreased vestibular depth
      4. Aberrant frenum/muscle position
      5. Gingival excess
         a. pseudopocket
         b. inconsistent gingival margin
         c. excessive gingival display
         d. gingival enlargement
      6. Abnormal color
   C. Mucogingival deformities and conditions on edentulous ridges
      1. Vertical and/or horizontal ridge deficiency
      2. Lack of gingiva/keratinized tissue
      3. Gingival/soft tissue enlargement
      4. Aberrant frenum/muscle position
      5. Decreased vestibular depth
      6. Abnormal color
   D. Occlusal trauma
      1. Primary occlusal trauma
      2. Secondary occlusal trauma

*From Armitage (1999). Reprinted with permission.
[†]Can occur on a periodontium with no attachment loss or on a periodontium with attachment loss that is not progressing.
[‡]Can be further classified on the basis of extent and severity. As a general guide, extent can be characterized as: localized = $\leq$ 30% of sites involved; generalized = > 30% of sites involved. Severity can be characterized on the basis of the amount of clinical attachment loss (CAL) as follows: slight = 1 or 2 mm CAL; moderate = 3 or 4 mm CAL; severe = $\geq$ 5 mm CAL.

Gingival diseases

Most of the earlier classifications of periodontal diseases did not include gingival diseases. In this new detailed classification, two groups of gingival diseases and lesions are described: those that are plaque-induced and those that are not primarily associated with dental plaque.

Dental plaque–induced gingival diseases. Four main types of plaque-associated gingival diseases have been classified. The most common form is gingivitis or inflammation of the gingiva resulting only from gingival plaque. The other three types of plaque-associated gingival diseases are those modified by: *(1)* systemic factors, *(2)* medication, or *(3)* malnutrition. For details on classification of plaque-induced gingival diseases, see Box 14 and Mariotti (1999).

Non–plaque-induced gingival lesions. The classification of non–plaque-induced gingival lesions is presented in Box 14. The definitions of these subcategories are:

1. Gingival diseases of specific bacterial origin: Conditions induced by exogenous bacterial infection other than common components of dental plaque.
2. Gingival diseases of viral origin: Acute manifestations of viral infections of the oral mucosa characterized by redness and multiple vesicles that easily rupture to form painful ulcers affecting the gingiva. These infections may be accompanied by fever, malaise, and regional lymphadenopathy.
3. Gingival diseases of fungal origin: These gingival manifestations of fungal infections are characterized by white, red, or ulcerative lesions associated with several predisposing conditions.
4. Linear gingival erythema: A distinct linear erythematous band limited to the free gingiva mainly as an effect of immunosuppression. The lesion does not predictably respond to plaque removal.

5. Hereditary gingival fibromatosis: A genetically derived fibrotic gingival enlargement.
6. Gingival manifestations of mucocutaneous disorders: Erosions, vesicles, bullae, ulcers, and desquamative lesions of the skin and oral mucous membranes. The lesions may look erythematous, white, or streaked.
7. Gingival manifestations of allergic reactions: Gingival manifestations of immediate or delayed hypersensitivity response.
8. Traumatic lesions: Self-initiated, accidental, or iatrogenic injuries. These may occur as localized gingival recessions, abrasions, ulcerations, and burns. The lesions may be edematous, erythematous, or white in appearance. Combinations of these clinical textures may also occur.
9. Traumatic lesions induced by chemicals: Such lesions can be caused by local application of certain chemicals such as aspirin, cocaine, pyrophosphates, detergents, smokeless tobacco, betel nut, and bleaching agents.
10. Traumatic lesions caused by physical injury: Accidental lesions or the result of inappropriate oral hygiene procedures, inadequate dental restorations, etc.
11. Foreign body reactions: These lesions may occur as acute or chronic inflammation associated with foreign bodies. The lesions can exhibit suppuration and may be red or red/white in appearance. Tattoos may also occur.

For details on classification of non–plaque-induced gingival lesions see Holmstrup (1999).

Chronic periodontitis

Epidemiologic data and clinical experience suggest that the form of periodontitis commonly found in adults can also be seen in adolescents (Papapanou, 1996). Thus the term "adult periodontitis" seems to be inaccurate in spite of the fact that periodontitis is more prevalent in adults and elderly than in adolescents and young adults.

Chronic periodontitis is initiated and sustained by gingival plaque biofilms at any age, but internal (genetics) and external (eg, smoking) modifying factors play an integral role in its pathogenesis.

Chronic periodonitits can be further characterized by extent and severity. Extent refers to the number of sites involved and can be described as localized or generalized. Extent can be classified as localized if 30% or fewer of the sites are affected and generalized if more than 30% of the sites are affected. Severity refers to the mean amount of clinical attachment loss (CAL) for the entire dentition or for individual teeth and sites (slight = 1 to 2 mm CAL, moderate = 3 to 4 mm CAL, and severe = 5 mm or more CAL).

So-called recurrent periodontitis represents a return of periodontitis and is not a separate disease entity. For a variety of identifiable and non-identifiable reasons, not all cases of periodontitis have a successful treatment outcome. Such cases can be referred to as refractory periodontitis, but do not necessarily constitute a separate disease entity. For details on classification of chronic diseases see Fleming (1999).

Aggressive periodontitis (formerly early-onset periodontitis)

The term "early-onset periodontitis" (EOP) was used both in the 1989 classification by the American Academy of Periodontology (see Box 12) and at the First European Workshop of Periodontology in 1993 as a collective designation for a group of dissimilar destructive periodontal diseases that affected young patients (ie, prepubertal, juvenile, and rapidly progressive periodontitis in postjuveniles).

Early-onset periodontitis was classified as either localized (LEOP) or generalized (GEOP). The following criteria were proposed by Tonetti and Mombelli (1997):

- Aggressive localized early-onset periodontitis (Figs 208a to 208c)
  —Attachment loss of 4 mm or more in at least two permanent first molars and incisors (at least one first molar must be affected)

  —Distribution: Attachment loss of 4 mm or more in not more than two teeth other than first molars or incisors
  —Age of onset: between puberty and 25 to 30 years of age
  —Familial tendency
- Generalized aggressive periodontitis (Figs 209 and 210)
  —Attachment loss of 4 mm or more affecting at least eight teeth
  —Distribution: Teeth other than molars and incisors also affected
  —Age of onset: before 35 years
- Aggressive periodontitis associated with systemic diseases (Figs 211a and 211b)
  —Advanced attachment loss, frequently leading to premature tooth exfoliation in children, adolescents, and young adults
  —Age of onset: variable and dependent on nature of systemic condition
  —Distribution: most of the dentition (both primary and permanent)
  —Severe inflammation of both marginal and attached gingiva
  —Association with severe systemic conditions, frequently with a genetic basis, leading to impaired host defense against bacterial infections

However, from data taken from a 1986–1987 survey of US schoolchildren, Albandar et al (1997) concluded that schoolchildren (mean age of 16 years) diagnosed with localized as well as generalized early-onset periodontitis are heterogenous groups, comprising aggressive rapidly and slowly progressing forms of periodontitis within each classification. In addition, localized forms of aggressive periodontitis may become more generalized in young adults (see Figs 208a to 208c and 210).

Several studies have shown that *Actinobacillus actinomycetemcomitans* is the key microorganism in the etiology of what was known as LEOP. *A actinomycetemcomitans* (particularly serotype b) is regarded as an exogenous, transmissible periopathogen and is found in more than 90% of patients diagnosed with LEOP but in few healthy individuals. *A actinomycetemcomitans* is respon-

243

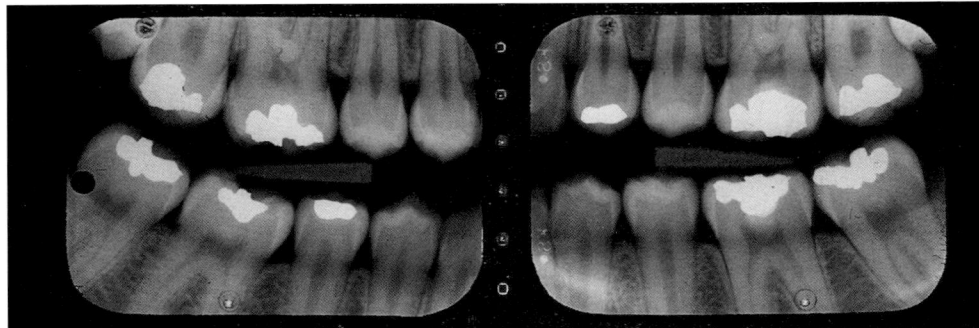

Fig 208a Sixteen-year-old girl with radiographic signs of alveolar bone loss on the mesial and distal aspects of the maxillary right first molar.

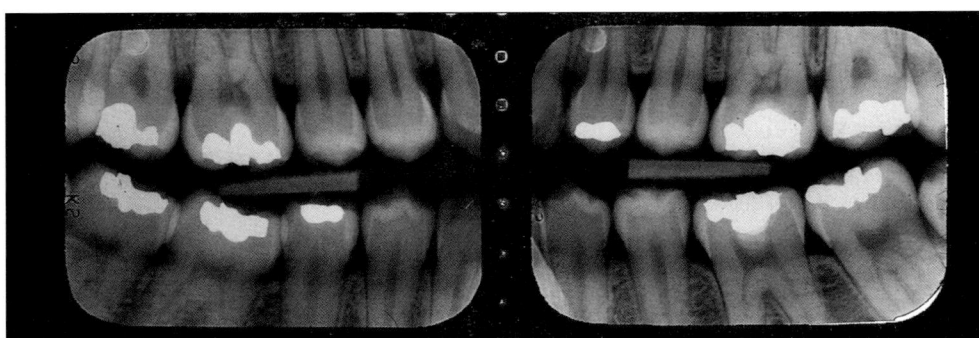

Fig 208b Same patient, aged 18 years, exhibiting a further 2-mm loss of alveolar bone at the same sites.

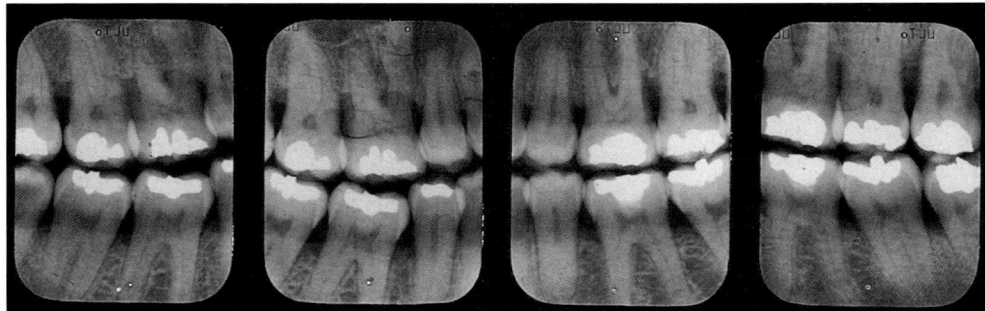

Fig 208c Same patient, aged 22 years, exhibiting advanced loss of periodontal support around all molars and second premolars and furcation involvement of the maxillary first and second molars.

sible for several pathogenic substances, including leukotoxin, which can kill the polymorphonuclear leukocytes (PMNLs), thereby eliminating the first line of defense in the periodontal pocket and allowing *A actinomycetemcomitans* to invade the pocket epithelium as well as the connective tissue. Therefore, a combination of mechanical removal of the subgingival biofilms and systemic use of antibiotics is more efficient than mechanical instrumentation alone. The treament outcome is strongly correlated to how efficiently *A actino-*

mycetemcomitans has been eliminated from the infected sites. Like all other gram-negative bacteria, *A actinomycetemcomitans* releases lipopolysaccharides (LPSs) from the cell walls when it regenerates or dies (for details see chapter 1).

Both systemically, and locally at infected and diseased sites, patients diagnosed with LEOP exhibit very high titers of immunoglobulin G2 (IgG2) with high attachment strength (avidity) against *A actinomycetemcomitans*. This strong IgG2 response could explain why, after an attack

Fig 209 Advanced loss of periodontal support in a patient diagnosed with aggressive generalized early-onset periodontitis. (Courtesy of K. Rateitschak.)

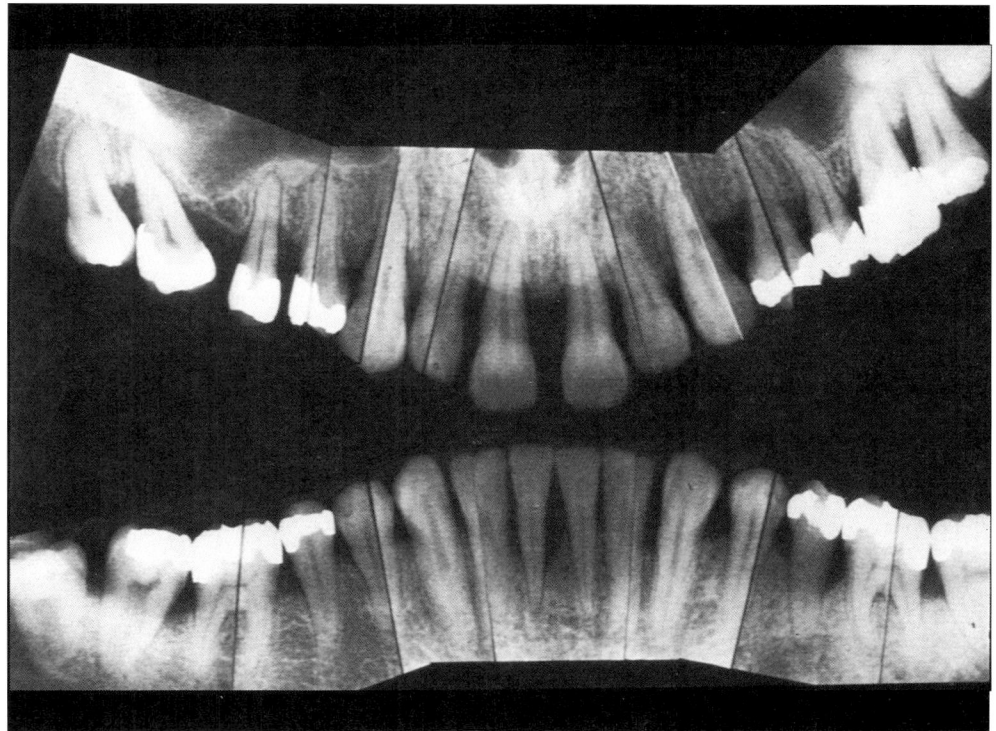

Fig 210 A young adult previously diagnosed with localized aggressive periodontitis, which has advanced to a more generalized form.

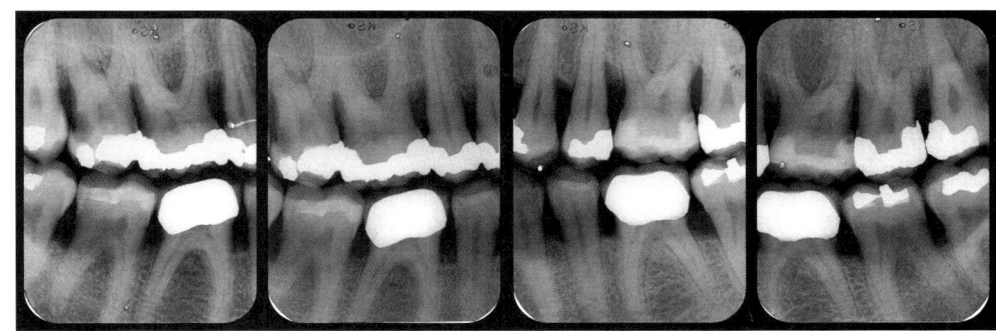

on the earliest erupting teeth (first molars and central and lateral incisors), there is no further spread of disease in the dentition. On the other hand, patients diagnosed with GEOP are frequently seronegative for *A actinomycetemcomitans*. A high IgG2 response against *A actinomycetemcomitans* has therefore been considered a protective mechanism against widespread EOP.

In addition, Lindskog and Blomlöf (1983) showed that first molars extracted because of a diagnosis of advanced LEOP exhibited multiple loci of cementum hypoplasia (Fig 212; see also Figs 170 and 171 in chapter 3). Adriaens et al (1988b) showed that bacteria could migrate into the root canal via the tubules of radicular dentin exposed by hypoplasia or aggressive scaling and root planing (see Figs 36a and 36b in chapter 1). Ehnevid (1995) showed that in teeth with infected root canals, bacteria and their products could migrate via the dentinal tubules to areas of cementum hypoplasia on the root surface and initiate localized periodontitis. Cementum hypoplasia is an impor-

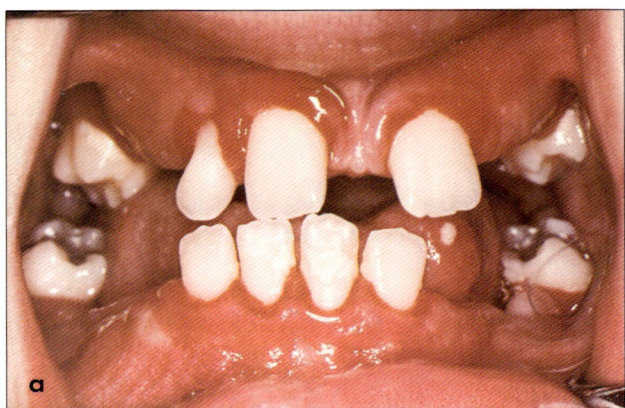

Figs 211a and 211b An 8-year-old patient with leukemia diagnosed with aggressive generalized early-onset periodontitis.

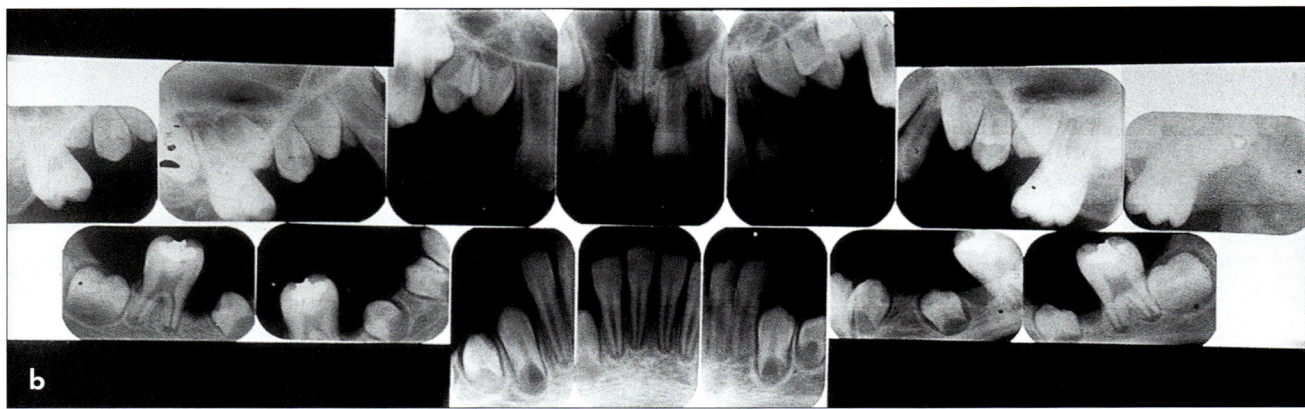

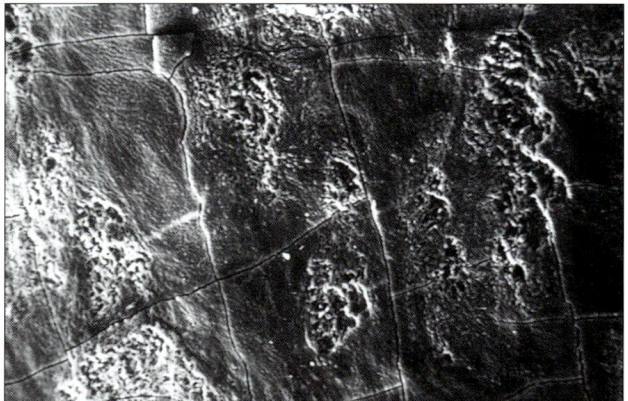

Fig 212 Cementum hypopolasia on a tooth extracted because of a diagnosis of advanced localized early-onset periodontitis (original magnification ×150). (From Lindskog and Blomlöf, 1983. Reprinted with permission.)

tant plaque retentive factor and may also facilitate lateral migration of the biofilm. Because the root cementum of the first molars and the central and lateral incisors develops at the same time, there is speculation that the prevalence of what was termed LEOP might be influenced indirectly by cementum hypoplasia, induced, for example, by overexposure of the cementoblasts to fluoride, analogous to its effect on ameloblasts in inducing enamel fluorosis (for details on the role of local risk factors see chapter 3).

Diagnoses of both GEOP and rapidly progressive periodontitis frequently have been associated with infection by *Porphyromonas gingivalis, Bacteroides forsythus,* and *A actinomycetemcomitans.* All these bacteria are gram-negative, but only *P gingivalis* and *B forsythus* are strictly anaerobic.

A relationship between bacterial counts of *A actinomycetemcomitans, P gingivalis,* and *B forsythus* and clinical response to treatment has been documented. Refractory lesions often contain elevated proportions of *A actinomycetemcomitans, P gingivalis,* and *B forsythus.* High local and systemic immune responses to *P gingivalis* have been demonstrated in patients diagnosed with GEOP.

In both types of the disease formerly referred to as EOP, although the periodontal pocket and the connective tissue contain considerably increased numbers of PMNLs, the chemotaxis, phagocytosis, and killing potential are impaired. This may be attributable to a combination of genetics and leukotoxins from *A actinomycetemcomitans,* particularly in patients diagnosed with LEOP. As in individuals with diabetes, endogenous matrix metalloproteinases (MMPs) from PMNLs will be released into the connective tissue, and periopathogens such as *A actinomycetemcomitans* and *P gingivalis* may invade the pocket epithelium and the connective tissue.

The local inflammatory response is characterized by high levels of not only prostaglandin E_2 (PGE_2), but also the proinflammatory cytokines interleukin-1 (IL-1) and tumor necrosis factor-α (TNF-α) in both gingival crevicular fluid and the connective tissue. In addition, local helper T-lymphocyte cells seem to be depressed in relation to suppressor T-cells. Patients diagnosed with GEOP tend not only to be seronegative against *A actinomycetemcomitans* but also to exhibit very low levels of serum antibodies against *P gingivalis,* and the antibodies have very low attachment strength (avidity) to the pathogens. In other words, patients diagnosed with GEOP exhibit impaired nonspecific (PMNLs) and specific (antibodies and helper T cells) host response against the most virulent periopathogens (*A actinomycetemcomitans* and *P gingivalis*). Unless optimal gingival plaque control is established from an early age (1 to 6 years), by the time the patient is a young adult, there will be advanced loss of periodontal support throughout the dentition (see Figs 209 and 210). In patients with severe immunodeficiency, what was known as GEOP will develop much more rapidly (see Figs 211a and 211b).

In the 1989 and 1993 classifications it was logically assumed that the above-mentioned forms of periodontal diseases had an early onset because they affected young people. However, many problems arose because of this classification:

- It was uncertain when the disease started and the first clinical signs of periodontal attachment loss appeared.
- There was considerable uncertainty about setting a correct upper limit for patients with so-called early-onset periodontitis.
- The relationship between different systemic diseases, specific microflora, genetics, and early-onset periodontitis, as opposed to adult periodonititis, was uncertain.
- The difference in progression rate between early-onset periodontitis and rapidly progressive adult periodontitis was uncertain.
- The difference in pattern of affected teeth (extent) between early-onset periodontitis and adult periodontitis was uncertain.

As a consequence of the above problems, classification terminologies that were age-dependent or required knowledge of rates of progression were discarded in the new classification system. Accordingly, highly destructive forms of periodontitis formerly considered under the term of "early-onset periodontitis," as well as the rapidly progressive forms of periodonititis in adults, were renamed using the term "aggressive periodontitis." In general, patients who meet the clinical criteria for LEOP or GEOP are now said to have "localized aggressive periodontitis" or "generalized aggressive periodontitis" respectively. So-called prepubertal GEOP related to systemic diseases is now placed under the heading of "periodontitis as a manifestation of systemic diseases" in this new classification.

It is pointed out in the new classification system that "aggressive periodontitis" is a specific type of periodontitis with clearly identifiable clinical and laboratory findings that make it sufficiently different from "chronic periodontitis" to warrant a separate classification. The common features of localized and generalized forms of aggressive peridontitis are:

- Aside from the presence of periodontitis, patients are healthy.
- Rapid attachment loss and bone destruction.
- Familiar aggregation.

Secondary features that are generally, but not universally, present are:

- Amounts of microbial deposits are inconsistent with the severity of periodontal tissue destruction.
- Elevated proportions of *A actinomycetemcomitans* and, in some populations, *P gingivalis*.
- Phagocyte abnormalities.
- Hyper-responsive macrophage phenotype, including elevated levels of PGE_2 and IL-1β.
- Progression of attachment loss and bone loss may be self-arresting.

Not all characteristics must be present to assign a diagnosis or classify the disease. The diagnosis may be based on clinical, radiographic, and historical data. If possible it should be supplemented with laboratory tests (eg, DNA-DNA checkerboard oral microbiology tests, genetic tests, gingival crevicular fluid tests).

There are enough specific features to allow subclassification of aggressive periodontitis into localized and generalized forms. Thus, in addition to the features common to all forms of aggressive periodontitis, the following specific features are identified:

- Localized aggressive periodontitis
  —Circumpubertal onset.
  —Robust serum antibody (particularly IgG_2) response to infecting agents (particularly *A actinomycetemcomitans*).
  —Localized first molar or incisor presentation with interproximal attachment loss on at least two permanent teeth, one of which is a first molar, and involving no more than two teeth other than first molars and incisors.
- Generalized aggressive periodontitis
  —Usually affects persons younger than 30 years, but patients may be older.
  —Poor serum antibody response to infecting agents (particularly *A actinomycetemcomitans*).
  —Pronounced episodic nature of the destruction of attachment and alveolar bone.
  —Generalized interproximal attachment loss attacking at least three permanent teeth other than first molars and incisors.

For details on aggressive periodontitis, see Tonetti and Mombelli (1999).

Periodontitis as a manifestation of systemic diseases

In the 1989 classification, one of the disease categories was "periodontitis associated with systemic disease." This category has been retained in the new classification because it is clear that destructive periodontal disease can be a manifestation of certain systemic dieases. Box 14 presents a list of systemic diseases in which periodontitis is a frequent manifestation. However, it should be observed that diabetes mellitus is not on the list. That is because uncontrolled diabetes can be a modifing risk factor of all forms of periodonititis, chronic as well as aggressive, but there are insufficient data to conclude that there is a specific diabetes melitus–associated form of periodontitis. For more detailed information on this topic see chapter 3 and Kinane (1999).

Necrotizing periodontal diseases

The acute and most severe forms of periodontal disease are necrotizing ulcerative gingivitis

(NUG) and necrotizing ulcerative periodontitis (NUP). The necrotizing diseases run an acute phase and are therefore sometimes called *acute necrotizing ulcerative gingivitis* (ANUG) and *acute necrotizing ulcerative periodontitis* (ANUP). However, there is no clear distinction between the two conditions: interproximally, not only is the free gingival papilla necrotized (Fig 213), but also the supra-alveolar attachment is destroyed, often resulting in an absence of papilla after healing. Therefore, ANUG and ANUP may be regarded as a single entity, *necrotizing ulcerative periodontitis*.

In Scandinavia, the prevalence is extremely low—only about 0.001%. In more than 40 years of practice, and with a specialty in periodontology, the author has personally seen only three cases. One of these is seen in Fig 213. However, in some developing countries, the prevalence may be as high as about 10%, and under the prevailing conditions—malnutrition, very poor oral hygiene, and almost total absence of dental care—NUP may progress to necrotizing stomatitis (NS) and the far more serious cancrum oris, also termed *noma*.

The microflora associated with NUP are completely dominated by a few gram-negative anaerobic microorganisms: *Treponema* species, *Selenomonas* species, *Fusobacterium* species, and *Prevotella intermedia*. Superinfection with *Treponema* species and *P intermedia* is indicated by very high antibody response against these microorganisms. Particularly *P intermedia* is considered to be the "key" etiologic factor in the necrotic lesion. However, spirochetes, for example, penetrate not only the epithelium but also the connective tissue.

Several observations indicate that the effects of endotoxins are more pronounced in NUP than in chronic gingivitis and periodontitis. Close to the connective tissue, the massive concentrations of gram-negative bacteria liberate large amounts of endotoxins. These can cause tissue destruction both directly, through a toxic effect, and indirectly, by activating and modifying the inflammatory and immune response, leading in turn to further tissue destruction.

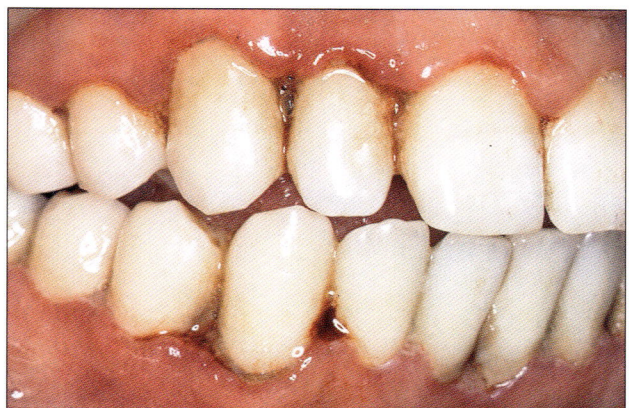

Fig 213 Necrotized free gingival papilla in a patient with necrotizing ulcerative periodontitis.

Although total leukocyte counts are similar in patients with NUP and control subjects, patients with NUP exhibit depressed PMNL chemotaxis and phagocytosis and reduced mitogen-induced proliferation of peripheral blood lymphocytes. Systemic diseases that impair immunity predispose to NUP, such as infection with HIV and other leukocyte disorders, including leukemia. Infection with HIV attacks the T helper cells of the body, causing a drastic change in the T helper (CD4$^+$)–T suppressor (CD8$^+$) ratio and severe impairment of host resistance to infection. Depleted peripheral T helper cell counts correlate closely with the occurrence of NUP, as shown in HIV-seropositive soldiers (Steidley et al, 1992). Malnutrition may also result in a reduced ratio of T helper–T suppressor cells (Enwonwu, 1972, 1985, 1994). In combination with a very high prevalence of HIV-seropositivity and poor oral hygiene, malnutrition is a major factor underlying the very high prevalence of NUP, NS, and noma among children and young adults in African countries. A history of previous NUP, sleep deprivation, extreme stress, and high alcohol and tobacco consumption, in combination with poor oral hygiene, further increases the risk for NUP (Horning and Cohen, 1995).

In the new classification, NUG and NUP are collectively referred to as "necrotizing periodontal diseases" with the subcategories NUG and

NUP. The definitions of these two subcategories follow.

Necrotizing ulcerative gingivitis. NUG is an infection characterized by gingival necrosis presenting as "punched out" papillae, with gingival bleeding and pain. Fetid breath and pseudomembrane formation may be secondary diagnosis features. Fusiform bacteria, *P intermedia,* and spirochetes have been associated with the gingival lesions. Predisposing factors may include emotional stress, poor diet, cigarette smoking, and HIV infection.

Necrotizing ulcerative periodontitis. NUP is an infection characterized by necrosis of gingival tissues, periodontal ligament, and alveolar bone. These lesions are most commonly observed in individuals with systemic conditions including, but not limited to, HIV infection, severe malnutrition, and immunosuppression. For details on this topic see chapters 1 and 2, Novak (1999), and Rowland (1999).

Abscesses of the periodontium

A periodontal abscess is a localized purulent infection of periodontal tissues and can be a common clinical finding among patients with moderate to advanced periodontitis. The microorganisms in periodontal abscesses are similar to bacteria detected in deep periodontal pockets—predominantly gram-negative anaerobic rods. Occlusion of the orifice of a deep periodontal pocket, systemic use of antibiotics in the absence of subgingival mechanical removal of the biofilms, and poorly controlled diabetes are common risk factors for development of the acute abcess. Abscesses of the periodontium may be associated with various combinations of the following clinical features: pain, swelling, color change, tooth mobility, fever, lymphadenopathy, and radiolucency of the affected alveolar bone. The lesions can be of short or long duration. Abscesses of the periodontium are classified as gingival abscesses, periodontal abscesses, or pericoronal abscesses, according to the following definitions:

- Gingival abscess: A localized purulent infection that involves the marginal gingiva or interdental papilla
- Periodontal abscess: A localized purulent infection within the tissues adjacent to the periodontal pocket that may lead to the destruction of periodontal ligament and alveolar bone
- Pericoronal abscess: A localized purulent infection within the tissue surrounding the crown of a partially erupted tooth (usually a third molar)

For details on abscesses of the periodontium see Meng (1999).

Periodontitis associated with endodontic lesions

Infected root canals may cause localized periodontal lesions via accessory root canals (particularly in furcation areas), apical foramina, exposed dentinal tubules as an effect of aggressive scaling, or cementum hypoplasia (Ehnevid 1995). The pulp may also be infected by microflora of infected periodontal pockets via exposed dentinal tubules (Adriaens et al, 1988b) as discussed earlier. In the new classification "combined periodontal-endodontic lesions," it is proposed either that the periodontal or endodontic lesion may be the cause or the result of the other, or that both may develop independently. For details on this topic see chapter 3 and Meng (1999).

Developmental or acquired deformities and conditions

Although the deformities and conditions listed in Box 14 are not separate diseases, they are important modifiers of the susceptibility to periodontal

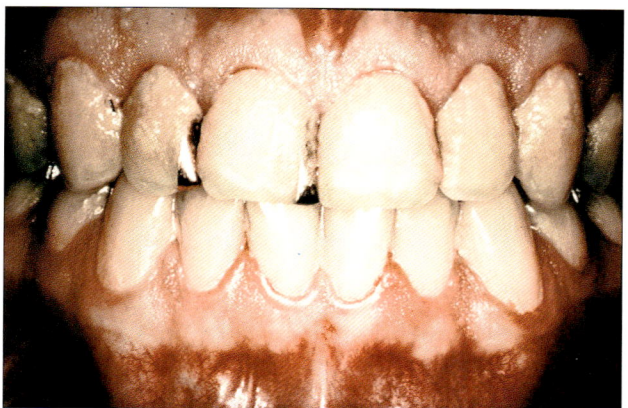

Fig 214 Plaque accumulation in a subject in an experimental gingivitis study. Note the relationship between the plaque and inflammation of the gingival margin. (From Löe et al, 1965. Reprinted with permission.)

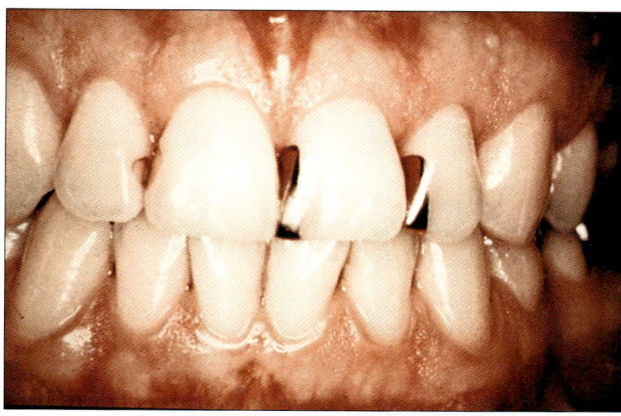

Fig 215 Resolution of the gingival inflammation shown in Fig 214, within 1 week of resumption of adequate oral hygiene. (From Löe et al, 1965. Reprinted with permission.)

disease and can dramatically influence the outcome of treatment. In addition, these conditions have been given a place in the new classification because periodontists are routinely treating many of them. For details on these topics see chapter 3, Blieden (1999), Hallmon (1999), and Prato (1999).

PATHOGENESIS OF PERIODONTAL DISEASES AT THE CLINICAL AND CELLULAR LEVELS

Experimental gingivitis

In 1965, Löe and associates demonstrated that in students with clinically healthy gingivae, clinical symptoms of gingivitis developed within 2 to 3 weeks if dental plaque was allowed to accumulate freely. Figure 214, a view of a subject in this classic study, shows the accumulated plaque and the consequent inflamed gingival margin, particularly at maxillary sites. Once adequate toothcleaning was resumed, the gingival inflammation subsided within a week (Fig 215).

The thickness of the gingival plaque gradually increased during the 3-week experimental period (Fig 216). For the first few days, this plaque was composed of gram-positive cocci and rods, representing the indigenous microflora of the tooth surface. After 4 to 5 days, filamentous organisms and gram-negative cocci as well as rods "infected" the gingival plaque. Gradually, nonattaching spirochetes appeared in the gingival sulcus, while the assortment of microorganisms in the gingival biofilm increased continuously. As a consequence, the first clinical signs of gingivitis developed within about 2 to 3 weeks. When the accumulated plaque was mechanically removed and daily oral hygiene was reestablished, the gingivae healed within about 1 week.

These findings have since been confirmed in many human and animal studies. Egelberg (1964) demonstrated subclinical symptoms of gingival inflammation, in the form of an exudate from the gingival sulcus, as early as 4 days after free plaque accumulation (Fig 217).

Animal experiments (Lindhe and Rylander, 1975), especially in dogs and monkeys, have also confirmed that undisturbed plaque accumulation results in gingival inflammation (Figs 218 and 219). Long-term experimental studies in dogs have shown that, at most sites, plaque-induced

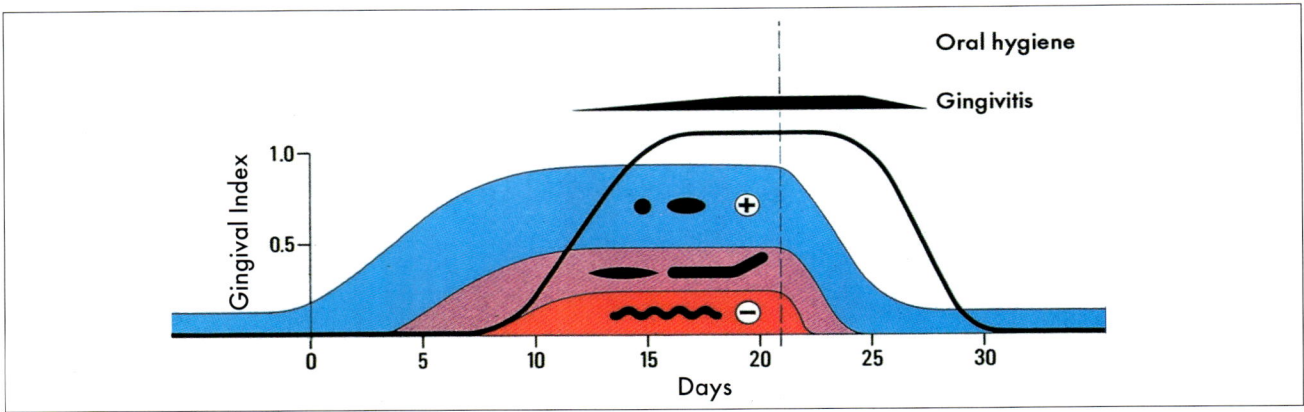

Fig 216 Increase in gingival plaque over the 3-week experimental period. For the first few days, this plaque is composed of gram-positive (+) cocci and rods, the indigenous microflora of the tooth. After 4 to 5 days, filamentous organisms and gram-negative (–) cocci and rods "infect" the plaque. Gradually, nonattaching spirochetes appear in the sulcus, while the assortment of microorganisms in the gingival biofilm increases continuously. As a consequence, the first clinical signs of gingivitis developed within 2 to 3 weeks. However, the gingiva healed when mechanical gingival plaque control was reestablished. (Modified from Löe et al, 1965. Reprinted with permission.)

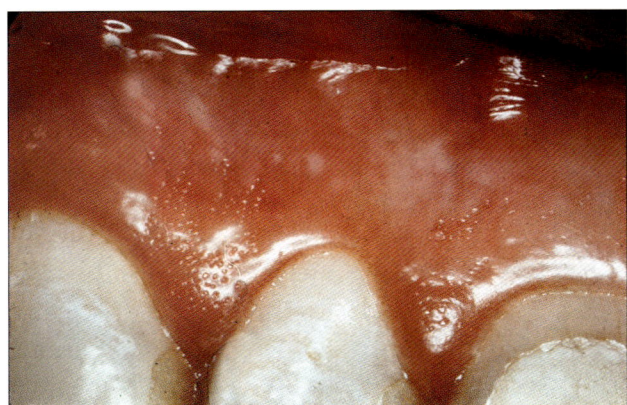

Fig 217 Exudate from the gingival sulcus, appearing 4 days after free plaque accumulation. (From Egelberg, 1964. Reprinted with permission.)

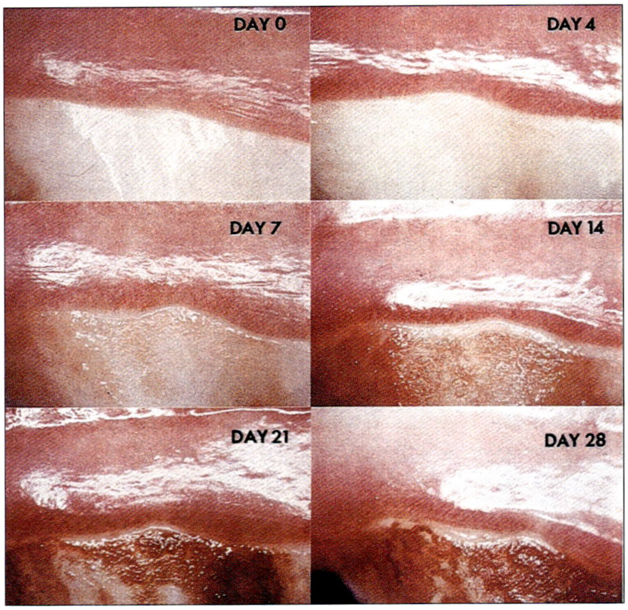

Fig 218 Gradual change in gingival status as plaque accumulates in a beagle, from healthy gingivae, associated with a clean tooth surface, to increasing severity of gingival inflammation after 4, 7, 14, 21, and 28 days. (From Lindhe and Rylander, 1975. Reprinted with permission.)

gingival inflammation remains unaltered as long as the gingival plaque remains; at some sites, however, gingivitis progresses to destructive periodontal disease with loss of connective tissue attachment and alveolar bone (Lindhe et al, 1975; Saxe et al, 1967).

Fig 219 *(left)* Histologic cross section of the healthy free gingivae at day 0. *(right)* Swollen and inflamed gingiva at day 28 (PAS and toluidine blue, original magnification ×200). (From Lindhe and Rylander, 1975. Reprinted with permission.)

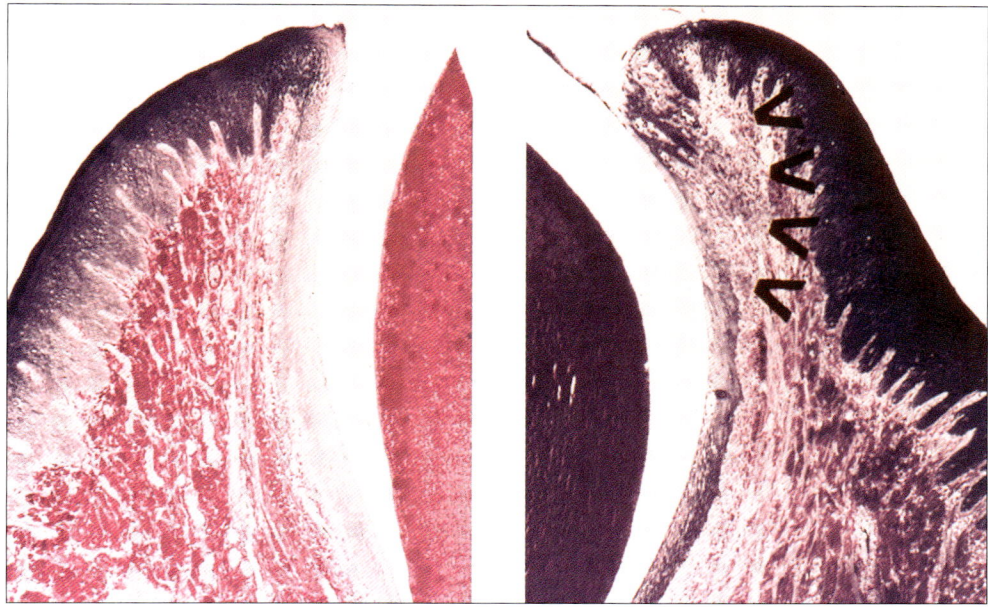

Histologic development of the periodontal lesion

The pathogenesis of human periodontitis was first documented in detail by Page and Schroeder in 1976 in an article that became a citation classic. Although lacking in detail, the general principles and the overall conclusions are still valid today. On the basis of the available histopathologic evidence, four phases of lesion progression were described: initial, early, established, and advanced. The initial and early phases were thought to reflect the histopathology of clinically "acute" or early stages of gingivitis, while the established lesion reflected the histopathology of "chronic" gingivitis. Progression of gingivitis to periodontitis was reflected in the histopathology of the advanced lesion. The evidence on which these descriptions were based was the prevailing information, originating mainly in animal biopsy material (Lindhe and Rylander, 1975) and some human adolescent samples.

It is virtually impossible to obtain pristine or noninfiltrated, histologically healthy gingival samples from humans. Nonhuman experiments are therefore the major source of material for the following illustrated summary (Figs 220 to 224) of lesion progression: the temporal, histopathologic sequences from healthy gingiva to an advanced, destructive lesion (periodontitis) (Page and Schroeder, 1976).

Histologic features of healthy gingivae (Fig 220) are presented in Box 15.

The initial lesion (Fig 221) occurs within 2 to 4 days of free plaque accumulation and the early lesion (Fig 222) within 4 to 14 days. Both lesions represent relatively acute stages of gingivitis and

---

Box 15 Histologic characteristics of healthy gingiva

- Normal junctional epithelium
- Few phagocytosing polymorphonuclear cells from the subepithelial vasculature in the junctional epithelium
- Minimal exudates from the sulcus
- Normal fibroblasts, connective tissue, collagen fibers, and alveolar bone

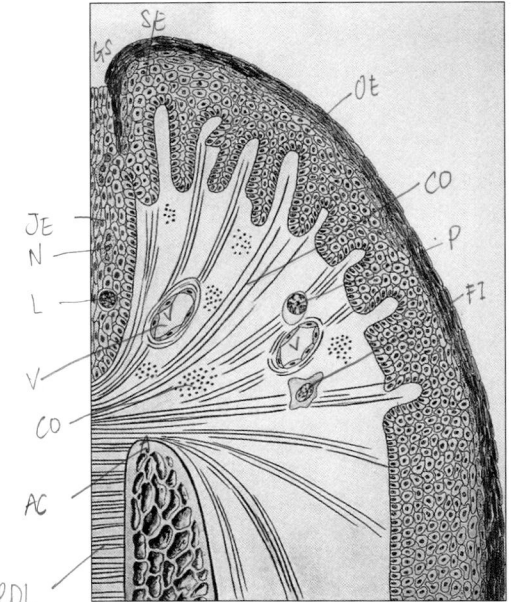

Fig 220 Healthy gingiva. (From Page and Schroeder, 1976. Reprinted with permission.)

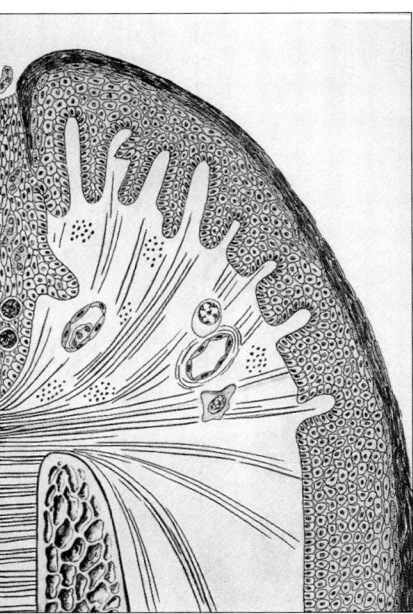

Fig 221 Initial gingival lesion. (From Page and Schroeder, 1976. Reprinted with permission.)

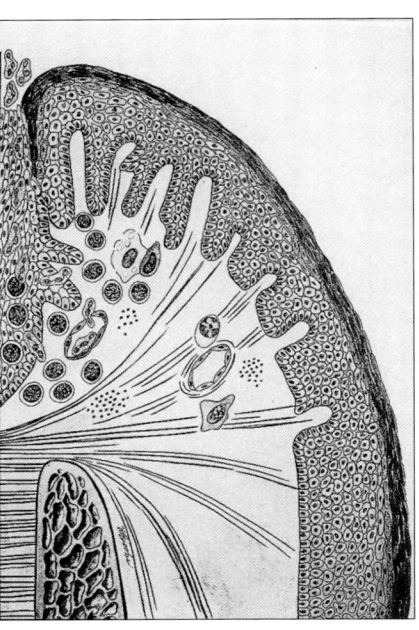

Fig 222 Early gingival lesion. (From Page and Schroeder, 1976. Reprinted with permission.)

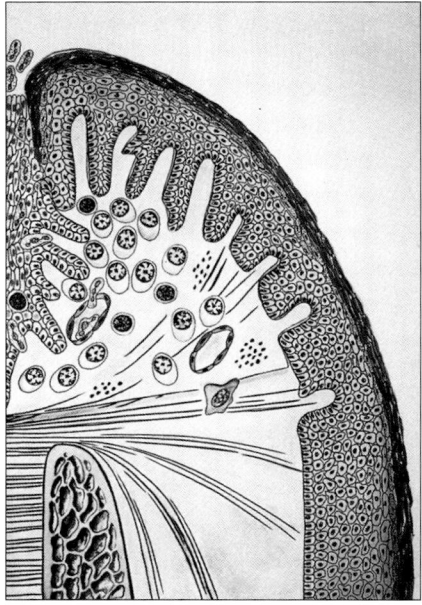

Fig 223 Established lesion (manifest gingivitis). (From Page and Schroeder, 1976. Reprinted with permission.)

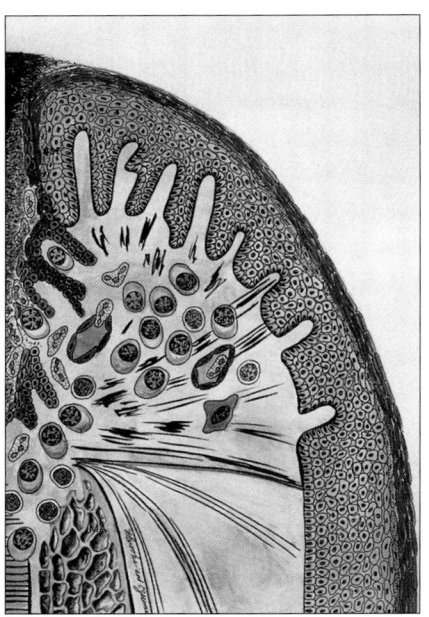

Fig 224 Progressive and destructive lesion (periodontitis). (From Page and Schroeder, 1976. Reprinted with permission.)

are the histologic precursors of the established lesion in adults (Box 16). In children, however, the "early lesion" may persist for prolonged periods.

The established lesion (Fig 223) often develops within 2 to 3 weeks of free plaque accumulation but may take months to develop. In adults, this stage may persist unchanged for years, sometimes for decades (Box 17). Adult gingivitis appears to be less the result of infection by specific microorganisms than of plaque quantity and plaque products.

For periodontitis to develop, periopathogens are an essential component of the gingival biofilm (for details see chapter 1); however, periopathogens alone are insufficient to cause destructive lesions. Progression from gingivitis to periodontitis is due to enhanced pathogenic potential of the gingival microflora and the interplay between altered host response and external modifying factors such as tobacco habits, medication, and so on, whereby the latter may outweigh the bacteria as determinants of the onset and the clinical severity of periodontitis (for details see chapters 2 and 3).

The histologic features of progressive and destructive lesions (periodontitis) (Fig 224) are listed in Box 18.

The histologic and clinical differences between gingivitis and periodontitis are summarized in Box 19.

Unique aspects of periodontal infections

As with other infectious diseases, the clinical outcome of periodontal diseases is determined by the severity of the bacterial challenge and the resistance of the host (Fig 225). However, the periodontal diseases are in some respects unique, mainly because of the anatomy: A mineralized structure, the tooth, passes through the integument, so that part of it is exposed to the external environment, the oral cavity, while part remains within the connective tissues. The tooth provides

---

Box 16 Histologic characteristics of initial and early lesions

- Increasing amounts of gingival plaque, dominated by facultatively anaerobic gram-positive cocci and rods
- Initial alteration and lateral proliferation of the junctional epithelium in the coronal region
- Increasing vasculitis and exudation of serum proteins
- Increasing numbers of migrating PMNLs, representing the nonspecific first line of defense
- Accumulation of lymphoid cells and monocytes and macrophages in the connective tissue but very few plasma cells
- Cystopathic alterations of fibroblasts
- Collagen loss in infiltrated connective tissue areas
- Vascular proliferation
- Normal alveolar bone

Box 17 Histologic characteristics of established lesions (manifest gingivitis)

- Increasing amounts of gingival plaque (dominated supragingivally by gram-positive facultatively anaerobic cocci and rods and subgingivally by gram-negative anaerobic rods)
- Continuing alteration and proliferation of junctional epithelium
- Deepening of the sulcus with the formation of a gingival pocket or pseudopocket
- Increase in size of the infiltrated connective tissue
- Continued migration of PMNLs and some monocytes and macrophages
- Acute inflammatory alterations: predominance of plasma cells and T lymphocytes accumulated in the infiltrated connective tissue, representing the specific second line of defense
- Increased vascular proliferation and vasculitis
- Increased loss of collagen
- Severe fibroblast injury
- Normal alveolar bone

Box 18 Histologic characteristics of progressive lesions

- Adherent gingival plaque (biofilm) supragingivally as well as subgingivally: predominantly gram-positive facultative anaerobic cocci and rods supragingivally and gram-positive and particularly gram-negative anaerobic rods subgingivally

- Nonadherent, anaerobic, motile or semimotile gram-negative microflora in the deeper part of the pocket

- Apical proliferation of pocket epithelium, true pocket formation, and ulceration of pocket epithelium

- Acute inflammatory alterations, as in gingivitis

- Increased connective tissue infiltrate

- Predominance of plasma cells (producing the specific antibody response) followed by lymphocytes in the connective tissue infiltrate

- Expansion of the inflammatory and immunopathologic reactions

- Increased exudation, often suppurative

- Further collagen loss in the infiltrated tissues; fibrosis in peripheral regions

- Destruction of the most coronal part of the periodontal ligament (clinical probing attachment loss)

- Resorption of alveolar bone next to the infiltrated connective tissue lesion (alveolar bone loss)

- Periods of quiescence and exacerbation

Box 19 Histologic and clinical characteristics of periodontitis in contrast to gingivitis

- Bone resorption (corresponding to radiographic evidence from standardized, digitized, or computer-aided radiographs)

- Apical proliferation and ulceration of the junctional and pocket epithelium

- Progressive loss of connective tissue attachment, corresponding to results of clinical evaluation (measurement of the distance from the cementoenamel junction to the base of the pocket with a manual or digital probe)

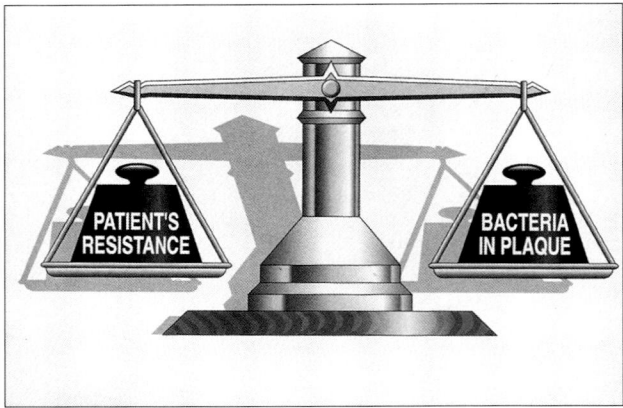

Fig 225 Factors affecting the clinical outcome of periodontal diseases. (Courtesy of B. Klinge.)

a "solid" surface for the colonization of diverse bacterial species.

Bacteria may attach to the tooth itself, to the epithelial surfaces of the gingiva or periodontal pocket, to underlying connective tissues (if exposed), and to other bacteria attached to these surfaces. In contrast to the outer surface of most parts of the body, the tooth has a no-shedding surface, which facilitates microbial colonization (accumulation). Microorganisms colonize a relatively stable surface, the tooth, in immediate proximity to the soft tissues of the periodontium, posing a potential threat to those tissues and, indeed, to the host itself. It is a tribute to the unique "seal" provided by the host and the nature of most of the colonizing organisms that causes periodontitis, but is relatively uncommon in systemic infections.

The presence of a tooth increases the complexity of the host-parasite relationship in a number of ways. The bacteria colonizing the tooth are by and large outside the body, where they are less able to be controlled by the potent mechanisms that operate within the tissues. The environment within a plaque (biofilm) with numerous microenvironments and a primitive circulatory system through which wastes are eliminated and nutrition provided may be conducive to microbial survival but is inaccessible to the host defense mechanisms (phagocytosing PMNLs) that seek out and destroy microorganisms (see Fig 39 in chapter 1). Factors such as pH, redox potential, and proteolytic enzymes can affect the performance of host defense mechanisms.

In addition, the tooth provides minute loci in which microorganisms can hide, persist at low levels during treatment, and then reemerge to cause further problems. Bacteria in the margins of restorations, in dentinal tubules exposed by aggressive scaling and root planing, in flaws in the tooth, or in areas demineralized by bacteria are not readily accessible to the much larger host cells (for details see chapter 3). There are similar obstacles to the function of noncellular host factors: diffusion barriers, lytic enzymes, and absorption by the mineral structure of the tooth. Organisms in the tooth cannot be reached by mechanical debridement, other than by vigorous removal of tooth substance. Chemotherapeutic agents are also ineffective in accessing such microenvironments and in penetrating thick plaque (biofilms). In particular, antimicrobial agents that require the bacteria to multiply would be adversely affected, because it is suspected that the rate of growth is low.

Altogether, infections of the tooth and its supporting structures present a formidable challenge to both the host and the clinician. The unique anatomic features of this "organ system" must be remembered during attempts to unravel the etiology and pathogenesis of periodontal diseases and to plan strategies for prevention or control. Periodontal diseases (periodontitis) are also different from other infectious diseases in that they leave a record of the disease on the periodontium, expressed as alveolar bone loss and/or loss of periodontal attachment.

This environment offers the potential for untreated periodontal diseases to progress unchecked in disease-susceptible individuals, until the teeth are lost. However, the process is not linear, and the rate of progression varies in different individuals and at different sites. These facts are exemplified by the case of the 21-year-old woman with unstable type 1 diabetes and almost complete loss of alveolar bone (see Figs 154 and 155 in chapter 3). In sharp contrast is an 80-year-old man (Fig 156 in chapter 3) who, despite massive plaque accumulation and total absence of dental care, has no missing teeth, almost no loss of periodontal attachment, and very vital and responsive gingival tissue. In this particular case, the internal (host) factors clearly outweigh the extreme bacterial challenge. However, it should be noted that the above two cases are extreme, with oral hygiene and dental care standards far below the Swedish norm, even 40 years ago. In contrast, most other infections are eliminated by the host response within a relatively short period of time, because the nonspecific defense, represented by the PMNLs, and the specific defense, represented by T lymphocytes and antibodies produced by plasma cells, generally have ready access to the pathogenic bacteria.

PATHOGENESIS OF PERIODONTAL DISEASES AT THE CELLULAR AND MOLECULAR LEVELS

Since the classic report by Page and Schroeder (1976) on the pathogenesis of gingival and periodontal lesions at the cellular level, much has been added to the profession's knowledge of the etiology, pathogenesis, and modifying factors at the molecular and the cellular levels.

The paradigm of the pathogenesis of periodontitis is shifting. Periodontitis is a family of related diseases that differ in etiology, natural history, disease progression, and response to therapy, but have a common underlying chain of events as discussed earlier in the chapter. For example, the histopathologic and ultrastructural features and pathways of tissue destruction as well as healing and regeneration are very similar, if not identical, in all forms of periodontitis. The same basic pathologic mechanisms underlie all forms of bacterially induced periodontitis. These common events are influenced by disease modifiers,

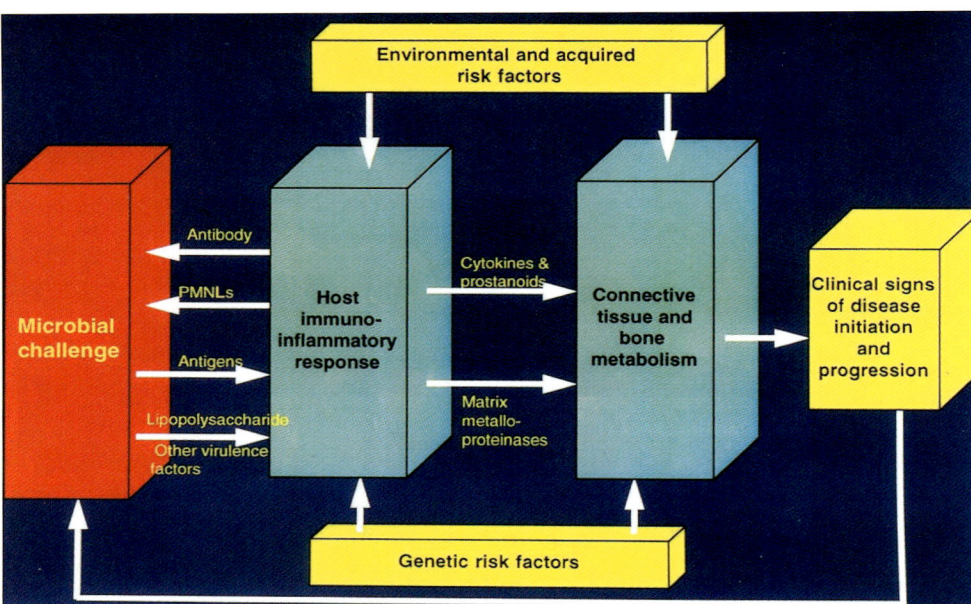

Fig 226 Current understanding of the pathogenesis of periodontal diseases: the microbial challenge and the host response, influenced by genetic and environmental modifying factors. PMNLs = Polymorphonuclear leukocytes. (From Page and Kornman, 1997. Reprinted with permission.)

both genetic and environmental, which may differ from one stage and form of disease to another. The resultant clinical features reflect the complex interplay of these events and modifiers and the microbial challenge.

During the 1970s and 1980s, great progress was made in elucidating the infectious nature of human periodontitis; recently it has emerged that, although bacteria are essential, their presence alone is insufficient for the onset of disease (for review see Offenbacher, 1996; Page and Kornman, 1997). Internal risk factors, such as impaired host defenses, and external risk factors, such as tobacco smoking, may even outweigh the bacteria as determinants of disease onset and clinical severity. These observations have led to major changes in ideas and concepts about the pathogenesis, prevention, and treatment of periodontal diseases.

The periopathogens tend to cause tissue destruction only indirectly, by activating various components of the host defense systems: It is enigmatic that activation of the host systems that provide protection and defense virtually always results in some degree of destruction.

The destruction may be greater if specific aspects of the host defense mechanisms within the local tissue are more active. This seems to be due, at least in part, to hyperresponsive host factors, both intrinsic (genetic) and induced (such as smoking), or to increased bacterial challenge within the tissues, as a result of compromised bacterial control mechanisms at the gingival sulcus. Most of the recent knowledge on the pathogenesis of periodontal disease involves the detailed molecular and cellular mechanisms regulating (1) the magnitude and balance of the host response within the tissues and (2) the quality of polymorphonuclear leukocytes (PNMLs) and antibody activity that reaches the gingival sulcus (for reviews see Kinane and Lindhe, 1997; Kornman et al, 1997b; Page et al, 1997).

Since the work by Page and Schroeder in 1976, the major development in this field has been the elucidation of the pathways through which antigens and various other virulence factors, and in some cases invading bacteria, activate host cells and systems in such a way that tissue destruction ensues, and of the pathways through which the extracellular matrix components of the gingiva and periodontal ligament are destroyed and alveolar bone is resorbed (for reviews see Darveau et al, 1997; Gemmell et al, 1997; Schwartz et al, 1997). Current understanding, although still incomplete, is now sufficient for the development and application of new diagnostic techniques and new preventive and treatment procedures targeted at blocking or altering these pathways.

Figure 226 illustrates current understanding of the pathogenesis of the human periodontal diseases: the microbial challenge, comprising antigens and various other virulence factors, and in some cases invading bacteria, and the host response, comprising an immediate inflammatory and immune response (the nonspecific first line of defense by the PMNLs, specific antibodies, etc). The host response also results in production of cytokines, prostanoids, other inflammatory mediators such as the kinins, complement activation products, and matrix metalloproteinases (MMPs), which perpetuate the response and mediate connective tissue and bone destruction. All these events are influenced by disease modifiers, both genetic and environmental. The resultant clinical features represent the final outcome of these events. The severity and rate of progression of disease feed back to influence the nature and magnitude of the microbial challenge by, for example, influencing the pH and availability of oxygen and various nutrients in the periodontal pocket. These events will be discussed in more detail later in this chapter.

Initial and acute phases of gingival inflammation

At the histologic level, perfectly healthy human gingiva—so-called pristine gingiva—does not exist, because the gingiva is always exposed to some bacterial challenge in the gingival crevice. The severity of this challenge may vary from clinically undetectable numbers of bacteria or colonies to gingival plaque (biofilm) and is strongly related to the quality and frequency of oral hygiene practices. Clinically healthy human gingiva therefore always exhibits histologic evidence of host response. The mildest form (see Fig 220) represents the first line of nonspecific defense: migration of PMNLs, through intact junctional epithelium, to phagocytose and "kill" the bacteria in the gingival crevice.

There are, however, several mechanisms in the vicinity of the teeth to fend off microbial infection and prevent the development of periodontitis. There is strong evidence that, in some individuals and under certain conditions, periodontal pathogens may be present, but clinical manifestations of disease do not develop. The intact epithelial barrier of the gingival, sulcular, and junctional epithelia normally prevents bacterial invasion of the periodontal tissues and is effective against penetration by bacterial products and components. Salivary secretions continuously flush the oral cavity and supply agglutinins and specific antibodies that can aggregate and kill bacteria, greatly influencing the species and numbers that can survive in the oral cavity. The gingival crevicular fluid (GCF) continuously flushes the sulcus or pocket and delivers all the components of blood serum, including complement proteins and specific antibodies, which bathe the bacteria of the subgingival flora. In inflamed gingiva, the amount of GCF per site is estimated to about 20 µL. A large population of B lymphocyte cells and plasma cells accumulate in the wall of the sulcus or pocket, producing antibodies that may be specific for antigens of challenging bacteria and may tag them for phagocytosis and killing.

High turnover of both the epithelium and the components of the extracellular matrix permits rapid replacement of cells and tissue components damaged by the microbial challenge. The turnover of the junctional epithelial cells is only 2 to 6 days, compared to a turnover of about 2 weeks for the oral epithelial cells. The normal gingival connective tissue consists of highly organized collagen fibers, proteoglycans, and serum-derived components, such as albumin. Some elastin fibers may also be present. Resident fibroblasts are uniformly distributed and a few macrophages and

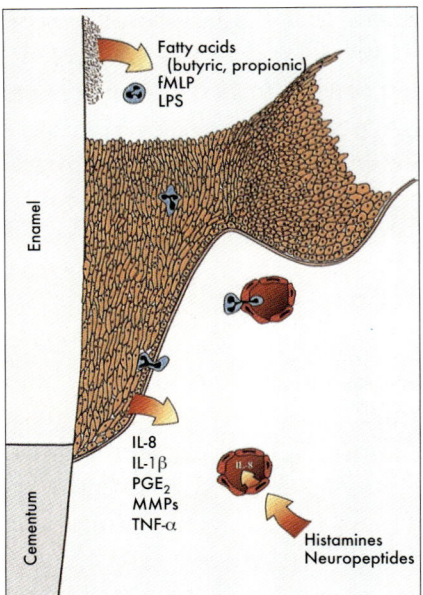

Fig 227 Schematic illustration of epithelial and vascular response to early gingival plaque accumulation. Bacterially released metabolic products such as fatty acids, peptides, and LPSs activate junctional epithelial cells to release various inflammatory mediators including IL-8, IL-1β, TNF-α, MMPs, and PGE₂. The bacterial products and epithelial response activate histamine release from the perivascular mast cells, resulting in vasodilation. fMLP = N-formyl-methionyl-leucyl-phenylalanine. (From Kornman et al, 1997b. Reprinted with permission.)

scattered infiltrating leukocytes, especially plasma cells, may be observed, but there are no foci of inflammatory cells.

If the gingiva is healthy, the bacteria adjacent to the gingival margin usually comprise the species that are early colonizers of the tooth surface, mainly gram-positive, facultatively anaerobic streptococci and actinomyces.

Accumulated gingival plaque, however, releases large quantities of metabolites that may diffuse through the junctional epithelium. These may include fatty acids such as butyric and pro-

pionic acids, which are toxic to the tissues; peptides, which are potent chemoattractants for leukocytes; and the LPS of gram-negative bacteria. Several other products of periodontal bacteria have been shown to activate various host mechanisms, but their relative importance in the disease process is unknown. These and other proinflammatory mediators synthesized by the junctional epithelium, such as interleukins (IL-1 and IL-8), TNF-α, PGE₂, and MMPs, can traverse the junctional epithelium and enter the connective tissues. It is via this mechanism that gingival vessels become inflamed and a gradient of chemoattractant signals is established, to guide the emigrating PMNLs to the location of the microbial plaque (Fig 227).

Other bacterial components, such as LPS, can activate the endothelial cells, directly or indirectly, by inducing the production and release of inflammatory mediators from various cells in the connective tissue (eg, histamine from perivascular mast cells; prostaglandins and interleukins such as interleukin-1β; and MMPs from resident tissue macrophages, fibroblasts, or keratinocytes). LPS can also activate the complement cascade via the indirect pathway as well as induce the production of kinins, all of which can act on the blood vessels and their endothelial cells.

Role of junctional epithelia

In "clinically healthy" gingiva and in the earliest acute phase of gingival inflammation, the junctional epithelium is the first structure directly challenged by bacteria. The junctional epithelium is a unique structure, differing in many respects from all other intraoral and extraoral epithelia. It manifests a uniform interface with the underlying connective tissue without rete ridges and is roughly 15 to 18 cells thick at the sulcus base, tapering to 4 or 5 cells at the most apical termination (see Figs 220 and 227). Junctional epithelium consists of basal and suprabasal strata, although all the cells are morphologically very similar. Although stratified, the cells do not undergo maturation.

Basal cells, which produce the basal lamina at the interface between junctional epithelium and the connective tissue as well as at the interface with the tooth surface, have the capacity to synthesize DNA and divide. The sloughing surface is at the sulcus base. Cells along the tooth surface and near the base of the sulcus contain acid phosphatase–positive lysosomes and manifest evidence of phagocytosis of PMNL granules and bacteria.

The cells express intercellular adhesion molecule-1 (ICAM-1) on their surfaces, even under healthy noninflammatory conditions; ICAM-1 expression by keratinocytes can be upregulated by proinflammatory cytokines but not by LPS. IL-8 messenger RNA was recently found to be present in gingival tissue and was localized primarily to the junctional epithelium. This localization plays an important role in directing PMNLs to the area of the gingival sulcus.

MMPs capable of degrading the extracellular matrix of the periodontium also have been identified in the gingival epithelium. In addition, epithelial cells in general are known to produce a broad range of cytokines, including interleukin-1α (IL-1α), IL-1β, IL-3, IL-6, IL-7, IL-8, IL-10, IL-11, IL-12, granulocyte-macrophage colony-simulating factor, interferon β, TNF-α, and transforming growth factor-β. In animals, the junctional epithelium also has been shown to include an unusually dense network of nerve fibers. These types of fiber routinely form localized loops that extend from the epithelium to innervate the local blood vessels and activate the mast cells that are normally resident adjacent to small vessels. The mast cell activation initiated by the fibers extending from the junctional epithelium may be effector mechanisms involved in the early vascular response and cellular replication.

The cytokines produced by the responding epithelial cells are also known to activate adhesion molecules on endothelial cells and cytokine production by endothelial cells. As mentioned previously, the turnover of the junctional epithelium is unusually high (2 to 6 days). Compared to other oral epithelial cells, cells of the junctional epithelium have fewer than half the number of desmosomes and wide extracellular spaces: In mild inflammation, these spaces are further expanded and filled with fluid, which can serve as a diffusion medium through which PMNL migration occurs.

As with all epithelial surfaces, an increased bacterial load in the gingival sulcus increases the cellular turnover rate of the sulcular epithelium. Infiltrating cells occupy about 1% to 2% of the extracellular space in human junctional epithelium and form a gradient in which the greatest number of cells is found coronally. Independent of this gradient, and in the absence of inflammation, large numbers of leukocytes migrate through the junctional epithelium at the rate of about 30,000/min. These are predominately PMNLs but also include monocytes and lymphocytes.

Acute inflammatory phase

Further exposure to bacterial challenge along the gingival margin generates proinflammatory afferent stimuli within the junctional epithelium. Early in the local inflammatory response, activation of the subepithelial venules causes an increase in vascular permeability, the expression of leukocyte cell adhesion molecules, and the release of specific leukocyte-activating agents. The net effect is thought to be increased leakage of plasma components, including acute-phase proteins, into the GCF and leukocyte extravasation, leading to the formation of a perivascular connective tissue infiltrate.

In the presence of LPS from gram-negative gingival microflora or cytokines, including IL-1β or TNF-α, the endothelial cells of the microcirculation are activated: The vessels become inflamed, dilated, and engorged with blood, and the blood flow slows. The endothelial cell junctions part, and protein-rich fluid leaves the vessels at the site of the postcapillary venules and accumulates in the extracellular matrix, resulting in edema.

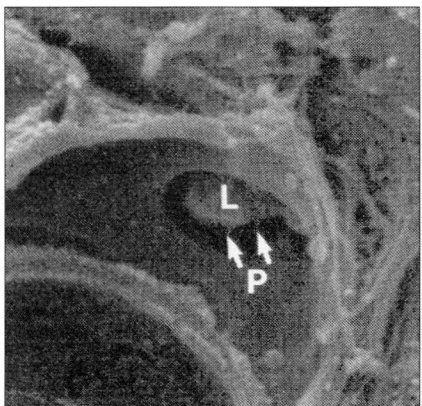

Fig 228 Polymorphonuclear leukocyte (L) migrating out from the vessel. P = Pseudopodium (original magnification ×6,000). (From Saglie et al, 1982c. Reprinted with permission.)

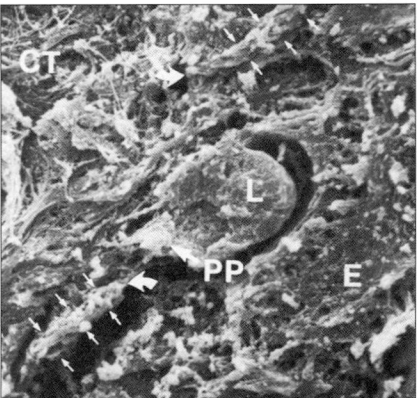

Fig 229 Polymorphonuclear leukocyte (L) with a polar pseudopodium (PP) penetrating the connective tissue (CT) and basement lamina and entering into the pocket epithelium (E). *Arrows* indicate migration of the polymorphonuclear leukocyte through the vessel wall (original magnification ×4,000). (From Saglie et al, 1982c. Reprinted with permission.)

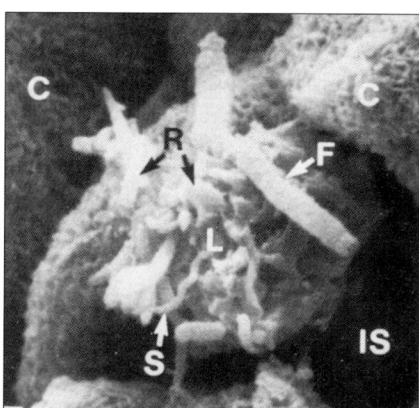

Fig 230 An aggressive competent polymorphonuclear leukocyte (L) entering the periodontal pocket through the intercellular space (IS) between epithelial cells (C), engulfing as many bacteria as possible, including rods (R), long rods (F), and spirochetes (S) (original magnification ×8,000). (From Saglie et al, 1982c. Reprinted with permission.)

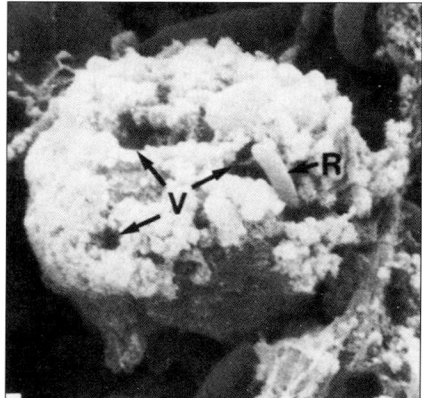

Fig 231 Long, rod-shaped bacterium (R) invaginated by a polymorphonuclear leukocyte. Three vacuoles (V) and "excrement" on the surface are evidence of previously phagocytosed bacteria and granular substance that could be lysosomal material (original magnification ×8,000). (From Saglie et al, 1982c. Reprinted with permission.)

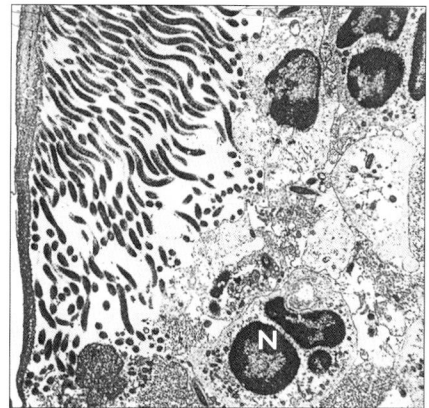 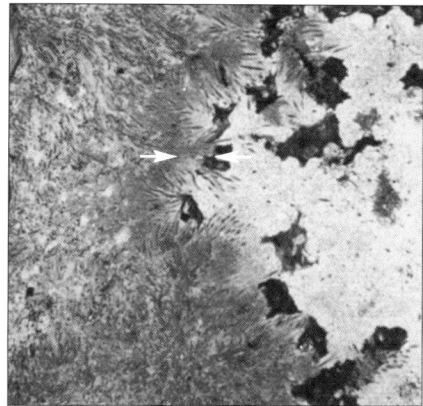 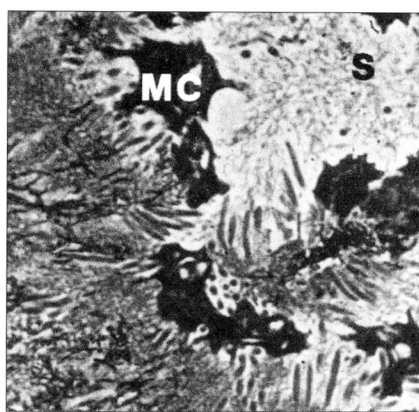

Fig 232 Polymorphonuclear leukocytes (N) acting as a barrier between the most apical subgingival microbial plaque biofilm and the gingival tissue (original magnification ×9,750). (From Theilade and Attström, 1985. Reprinted with permission.)

Figs 233 and 234 Aggressive polymorphonuclear leukocytes (black and irregularly shaped; MC) "tackling" and phagocytosing bacteria of the subgingival biofilm. Test-tube brush formations can be seen between the arrows in Fig 233 ([Fig 233] original magnification ×600; [Fig 234] original magnification ×2,000). (From Listgarten, 1976. Reprinted with permission.)

Role of polymorphonuclear leukocytes

As long ago as the late 1960s, Waerhaug, the founding father of modern periodontology, explained the important role of the phagocytosing PMNLs as the first line of nonspecific host defense in the pathogenesis of periodontal disease. Chemotactic antigens and other products are released from the gingival microflora, resulting in vasodilation and extravascular migration of PMNLs. Via attraction of chemotactic factors, the PMNLs are guided through the connective tissue and the junctional epithelium, to phagocytose and kill bacteria in the gingival sulcus.

As the first line of nonspecific defense against the subgingival microflora, preventing bacterial invasion of the tissue, the PMNLs have a major role. Many "aggressive," competent PMNLs, which migrate into the pocket, "guided" by chemotactic forces, are very beneficial (Saglie et al, 1982c) (Figs 228 and 229). An aggressive competent PMNL will engulf as many bacteria as possible, even long rods or spirochetes (Figs 230 and 231).

The PMNLs exit the inflamed vessels of the microcirculation and migrate along a gradient of chemoattractant through the connective tissues and the junctional epithelium, to form a barrier between the subgingival microbial plaque and the gingival tissue (Fig 232). Because these cells are still viable and capable of phagocytosis and killing bacteria, they prevent apical and lateral extension of the subgingival plaque biofilm (Figs 233 and 234).

Studies of host response in periodontal diseases have clearly identified the PMNL (neutrophil) as the key protective cell, which, under normal circumstances, limits the extent of damage by periopathogens. (For reviews see Dennison and Van Dyke, 1997; Hart et al, 1994. For details see chapter 3.) The PMNLs do not act alone, but as part of a neutrophil-antibody-complement axis that exerts a protective role against the gram-negative microorganisms that are the major pathogens of periodontal diseases.

As the predominant phagocyte in blood and inflamed tissues, and almost the exclusive form in the periodontal crevice and pocket, the PMNLs play a crucial role in the defense process against virulent bacteria. The association between defective PMNL function and advanced periodontal destruction has been demonstrated in both animals and humans (eg, in conditions such as cyclic neutropenia, leukocyte adhesion deficiency syndrome, and Chédiak-Higashi syndrome) (Hemmerle and Frank, 1991; Page et al, 1987; Waldrop et al, 1987). Defective PMNL function may also be induced by a number of drugs and smoking.

The most important evidence for the critical role of PMNLs in periodontal diseases comes from the identification of PMNL dysfunction in several forms of aggressive periodontitis. A large database supports the role of PNML abnormalities in localized aggressive periodontitis (for reviews see Dennison and Van Dyke, 1997; Hart et al, 1994).

Further evidence implicating the PNML as a major protective cell against oral bacterial pathogens is the observation that several periopathogenic bacteria have significant antiPMNL virulence factors. *P gingivalis* and *A actinomycetemcomitans* are leukoaggressive; ie, they produce toxins and other factors that either reduce PNML function or kill PNMLs. If the numbers of vital and aggressive phagocytosing PMNLs with sufficient versatility (lysosymal enzymes, etc) are inadequate in the gingival crevice or periodontal pocket, periopathic bacteria may invade the periodontal tissues during acute (active) phases of periodontitis (bursts or exacerbation), sometimes resulting in formation of a microabscess or macroabscess (Frank 1980; Saglie et al, 1982a, 1982b, 1985, 1986b, 1987, 1988a, 1988b) (see Figs 45 and 46 in chapter 1).

It has been shown that bacteria invade the pocket epithelium cells (Saglie, 1991). Experimentally, Madianos et al (1996) have shown that the well-known periopathogen *P gingivalis* may not only invade the epithelial cells but also multiply in the cells. Other studies have shown that, in cases of aggressive periodontitis, even mycoplasma (a macrovirus) can invade the connective tissue and attack lymphocytes as well as plasma cells (see Fig 49 in chapter 1). As early as 1978, Frank

and Voegel showed that direct bone resorption by bacteria was possible in advanced cases of human periodontitis (see Figs 47 and 48 in chapter 1).

Molecular regulation of leukocyte function

At the molecular level, there is good evidence that the movement of leukocytes from the vasculature to the tissues is regulated by different types of adhesion molecules expressed on endothelial cells and the leukocytes. The specificity of the adhesion molecules for leukocyte subpopulations determines which cells migrate into the tissue. The local immunoinflammatory response is determined by which cells are in the tissue and by the mediator signals that influence the behavior of the cells.

Entry of leukocytes into tissues is a tightly regulated process that has evolved to ensure optimal availability of inflammatory cells to injured tissues while avoiding unnecessary damage. Entry of leukocytes into the periodontium requires an increase in the "stickiness" of the leukocytes in response to bacterial LPSs and the intravascular release of proinflammatory agents, including the cytokine IL-8, by activated endothelial cells (Fig 235). This induces rolling of the leukocytes on the endoluminal aspect of the venules and increases the probability of specific interactions among vascular cell adhesion molecules and leukocyte integrins and thus the potential for inducing leukocyte extravasation by diapedesis into the extravascular spaces.

Specific differences in the resultant inflammatory infiltrate in various tissues indicate that this process is highly specific, enabling the selective enrichment of specific cell types. The selectivity of the process seems to be determined by the expression on the endothelial cells of specific adhesins, such as endothelial cell adhesion molecule-1 (ECAM-1) and vascular cell adhesion molecule-1 (VCAM-1): Specific leukocyte subpopulations carry complementary receptors to these adhesion. For example, ECAM-1 is thought to be important

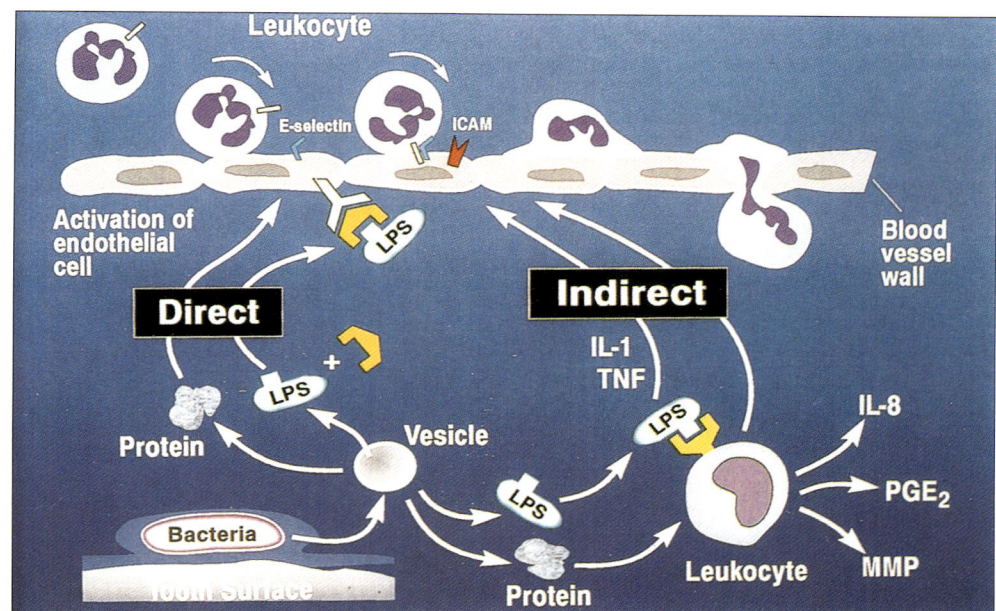

Fig 235 Schematic drawing showing how endothelial cells of the venules become activated by LPSs as well as proinflammatory cytokines IL-1β, IL-8, and TNF-α, thereby becoming induced to express E-selectin. Via expression of binding molecules to E-selectin, the PMNLs are slowing to a rolling motion along the endothelial surface. Leukocyte adhesion receptors form a tight binding with the intercellular adhesion molecule (ICAM), which is expressed by the endothelial cells, and initiate movement of the leukocyte between the endothelial cells into the extravascular compartment. (From Darveau et al, 1997. Reprinted with permission.)

for the extravasation of PMNLs and some lymphocytes. VCAM-1 is thought to be more specific for mononuclear leukocytes.

Following extravasation, the PMNLs (neutrophils) seem to gain access to the more coronal portion of the junctional epithelium and to migrate selectively through this multilayered epithelium to gain access to the bacterial flora. At least two mechanisms are considered important in the regulation of this transmigration following extravasation: (1) the expression of leukocyte adhesion molecules, such as ICAM-1, in epithelial cells and (2) a newly identified family of low–molecular weight cytokines with potent, mainly cell type–specific leukocyte chemotactic properties: the chemokines, and in particular the PMNL-selective IL-8 (Figs 236 and 237).

ICAM-1 and the cytokine IL-8 seem to be the most important chemokines (chemotactic fac-

tors) for the guidance of the PMNLs through the connective tissue and the junctional and pocket epithelium into the gingival crevice and periodontal pocket. Keratinocytes in junctional epithelium have been shown to express high levels of ICAM-1 and IL-8. The amount of ICAM-1 increases within the junctional epithelium in an apicocoronal direction: The superficial keratinocytes, possibly exposed to accumulation of bacterial plaque, express most of these molecules in the junctional epithelium. Expression of ICAM-1 in the gingival epithelium is limited to the junctional epithelium, the only epithelium associated with significant PMNL transmigration.

The biologic effects of IL-8 on PMNLs have been shown to be dose dependent: Lower concentrations stimulate cellular migration, and higher doses lead to activation of PMNL antibacterial mechanisms. Higher concentrations of IL-8 on the

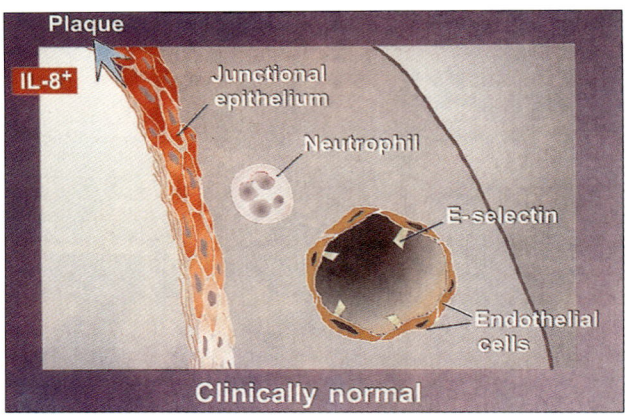

Fig 236 Exclusion of neutrophils (PMNLs) through the connective tissue and the junctional epithelium in clinically normal gingiva. Expression of E-selectin and ICAM from the endothelial cells facilitates the exit of neutrophils from the vasculature into the connective tissue. A gradient of IL-8 in a coronal direction attracts the neutrophils through the junctional epithelium to attack the bacteria in the gingival sulcus. (From Darveau et al, 1997. Reprinted with permission.)

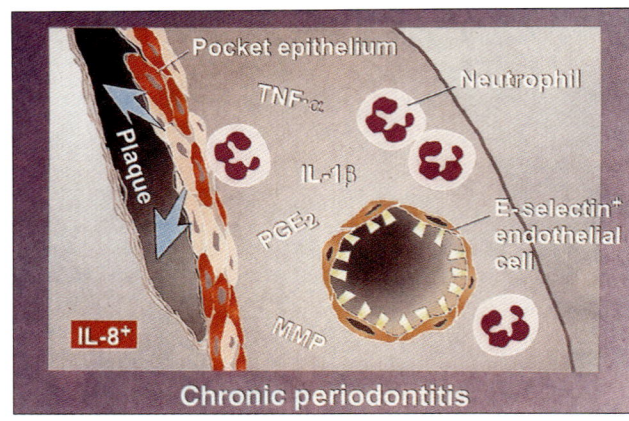

Fig 237 In chronic periodontitis, the molecular mediators of inflammation that are expressed in clinically healthy tissue are expressed at higher levels and new mediators are present. The gradient of IL-8 expression found in healthy tissue is disrupted and a pocket epithelium is formed. (From Darveau et al, 1997. Reprinted with permission.)

epithelial surface thus lead to activation of PMNLs (neutrophils). The exudate observed initially is predominated by PMNLs and has all of the manifestations of an acute inflammatory response.

The important functional role of the PMNL-dominated exudate cannot be overemphasized. In animal experiments, a large reduction in numbers of circulating PMNLs has been found to result in rapid invasion of the periodontal tissues by pathogenic bacteria (Hemmerle and Frank, 1991). However, suppression of lymphocytes does not enhance invasion. It also would be interesting to evaluate the quality of the PMNLs in the gingival exudate, for example, the proportion of cells that have degranulated (have used their weapons) (see Fig 231). It is paradoxical that the formation of the acute inflammatory exudate is accompanied by alterations in the perivascular connective tissue components, specifically destruction of collagen, which is probably attributable to release of a preformed collagenase or to activation of precollagenase stored in the connective tissue.

Most PMNLs recruited into the gingival tissues migrate into the sulcus, but the majority of the mononuclear cells (monocytes, macrophages, B lymphocytes, T lymphocytes, and plasma cells) persist in the perivascular connective tissue as components of the local inflammatory infiltrate (see Figs 222 and 223). The spatial demarcation of the area of leukocyte infiltration is attributed in part to specific chemokines, such as monocyte chemoattractant protein 1, produced within the inflammatory infiltrate.

As long as the standard of gingival plaque control is unchanged, the gingival infiltrate often remains constant over time. The complicated molecular regulation of the leukocytes as a reactive response to bacterial products during the acute gingival inflammatory phase is illustrated in Fig 238. After the initial macrophage activation and migration of PMNLs into the gingival crevice (see Fig 227), vascular leakage and activation of serum proteins, such as complements, begin to amplify the local inflammatory response, further enhancing endothelial cell activation. Additional leukocytes and monocytes are recruited, and activated macrophages produce many mediators of the immune and inflammatory responses, including IL-1β, interleukin-1 receptor antagonist (IL-1ra), IL-6, IL-10, IL-12, TNF-α, PGE₂, MMPs, interferon-γ (IFN-γ) and a series of chemotactic substances: monocyte chemoattractant protein, macrophage inflammatory protein, and regulated-on-activation normal T cell, expressed and secreted (RANTES).

Established gingival inflammation

After increased gingival plaque accumulation and long-term exposure (more than 2 to 3 weeks) to bacterial challenge, early acute gingival inflammation is followed by so-called established gingival inflammation. This is characterized at the cellular level by an accumulation of B lymphocytes, T lymphocytes, plasma cells, and macrophages in the inflamed gingival connective tissue. On the other hand, the number of fibroblasts is reduced. Destruction of the collagen fibers and the extracellular matrix also occurs, as does an increase in the volume of so-called infiltrate in which blood vessels proliferate.

While increasing numbers of PMNLs continue to migrate into the gingival crevice, directly phagocytozing and killing the bacteria, this first, nonspecific line of defense is now reinforced by mobilization of the specific host immune response, via antibodies produced by plasma cells, and the specific cell-mediated immune response by T cells. In addition, increasing numbers of macrophages participate in phagocytozing and killing the bacteria and removing "dead" PMNLs and toxic products of the bacteria.

Role of macrophages

As long ago as the late 1960s, Waerhaug described the macrophages as "scavengers," phagocytozing and "spy" or antigen-processing cells supporting

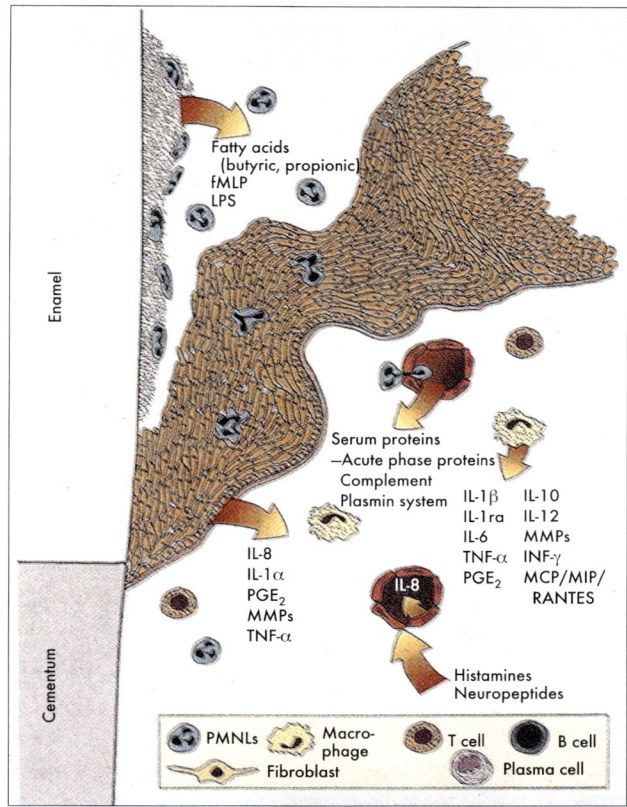

Fig 238 Molecular regulation of the polymorphonuclear leukocytes (PMNLs) as a reactive response to bacterial products during the acute gingival inflammatory phase. IL-1ra = Interleukin-1 receptor antagonist; IFN-γ = Interferon-γ; MCP/MIP/RANTES = Monocyte chemoattractant protein/macrophage inflammatory protein/regulated-on-activation normal T cell, expressed and secreted. (From Kornman et al, 1997b. Reprinted with permission.)

the development of a specific immune response (Figs 239 to 241).

Macrophages play a central role in mobilizing the host defense mechanisms against bacterial infection, because they are involved both in the initiation of responses as antigen-presenting cells and in the effector phase as inflammatory, tumoricidal, and microbicidal cells, in addition to their regulatory functions. After exposure to foreign microbes, macrophages develop an increased capacity to kill bacteria and secrete a number of immune mediators that stimulate antibacterial responses by other cells.

Figs 239 to 241 Development of a specific immune response. (Courtesy of J. Waerhaug.)

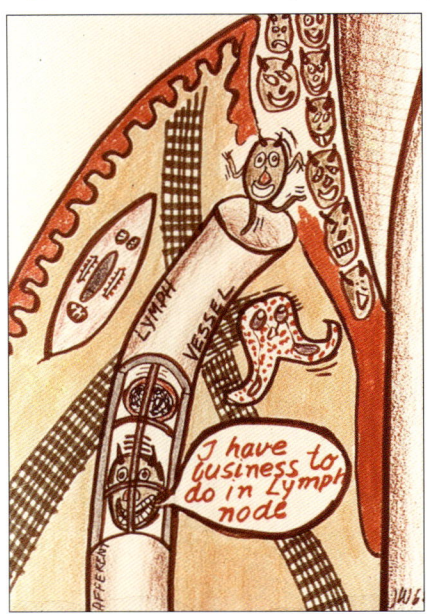

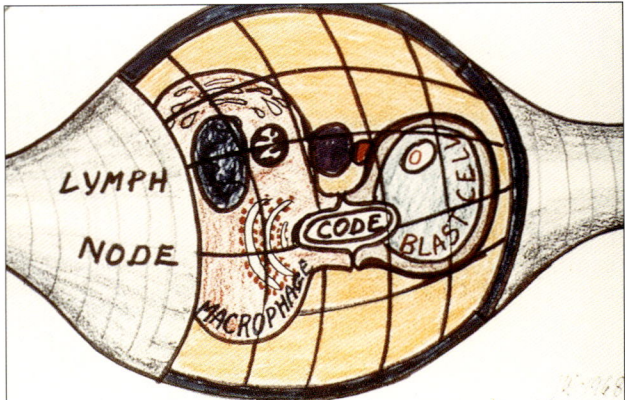

Fig 240 Macrophage bringing or processing bacteria and their antigens to B lymphocytes in the local lymph nodes.

Fig 239 Macrophage capturing and identifying bacteria and their antigens.

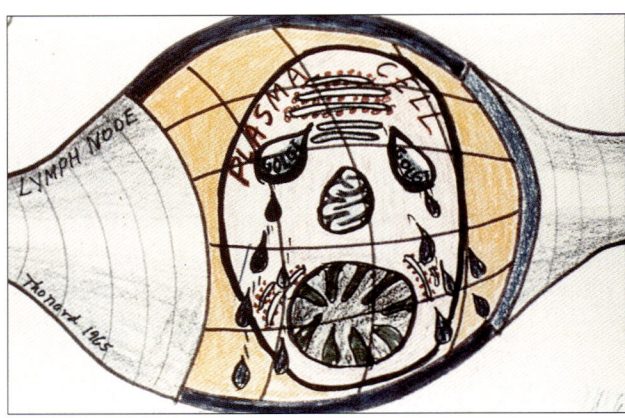

Fig 241 Stimulated B lymphocyte differentiating into a clone of plasma cells to produce specific antibodies.

Macrophages are scarce in healthy gingiva. Although they increase in the presence of gingivitis and periodontitis, density in the tissue is never pronounced, and they remain in low proportions relative to other cell types.

The macrophages originate from monocytes: After exposure to, for example, antigens, monocytes differentiate into macrophages. The functions of macrophages vary within and between the different tissue compartments.

Like the PMNLs, the macrophages are actively phagocytic cells, capable of ingesting and digesting exogenous antigens. In the first step in phagocytosis, macrophages are attracted by and move toward a variety of substances generated in an immune response; this process is called *chemotaxis.* The next step involves attachment of the antigen to the macrophage's cell membrane. Attachment induces membrane protrusions, called *pseudopodia,* to extend around the attachment material (Figs 242a and 242b).

The macrophages may also act as cleaning and "conditioning" cells on the root surface (Figs 243a and 243b). This effect of macrophages could be beneficial during healing after periodontal therapy, particularly regenerative therapy.

Other macrophages reside in the tissues, where they ingest foreign substances (antigens) and then present the antigens on the macrophage cell surface after "processing." The combination of the antigen with appropriate histocompatibility molecules enables T-lymphocyte recognition, stimulating the release of cytokines that amplify

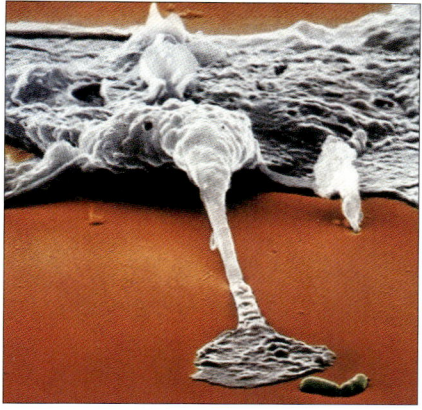

Fig 242a Macrophage approaching a bacterium (original magnification ×4,000). (Courtesy of L. Nilsson.)

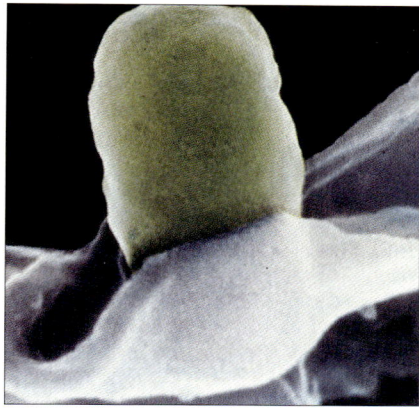

Fig 242b Bacterium captured by the macrophage for phagocytosis (original magnification ×25,000). (Courtesy of L. Nilsson.)

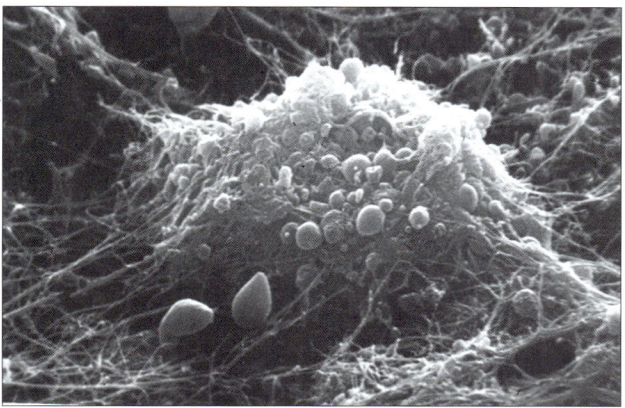

Fig 243a Macrophage attached to the root surface, which appears somewhat demineralized (original magnification ×4,000). (From Lindskog and Blomöf, 1992. Reprinted with permission.)

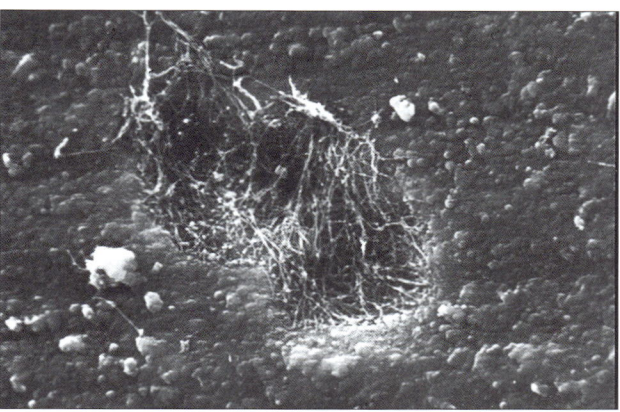

Fig 243b Exposure of a collagen network of fibers after removal of the macrophage (original magnification ×4,000). (From Lindskog and Blomöf, 1992. Reprinted with permission.)

the specific immune response: cell-mediate via T cells and humoral via antibody production by plasma cells.

In addition to processing antigens for activation of the specific immune system, macrophages within the tissues secrete a number of cytokines in response to antigens and other agents associated with microorganisms. These cytokines have several functions, including amplifying the specific immune system, inducing and amplifying inflammation, and stimulating tissue breakdown. Tissue breakdown can result either directly, from macrophage-secreted enzymes, or indirectly, from enzymes stimulated in cells such as fibroblasts (collagenase). In addition, the macrophage produces cytokines such as IL-1β and PGE$_2$, which can promote breakdown of bone by stimulating osteoclasts.

Molecular regulation of the immune inflammatory response

The events that constitute the pathogenesis of periodontitis are initiated, driven, and regulated by mediators of the inflammatory process. They are known to be major participants in acute and chronic inflammation, regardless of its location, and there is strong evidence for participation of these mediators in periodontitis. They are produced by activated resident gingival cells and infiltrating leukocytes and the complement cascade and kinin system in blood plasma. Macrophages (monocytes) from individuals susceptible to or suffering from severe periodontitis produce increased amounts of mediators, which are found in elevated concentrations in inflamed gingiva and in gingival crevicular fluid from diseased sites. These concentrations decrease following a positive response to therapy.

Role of cytokines

Cytokines are soluble proteins, secreted by cells; the cytokines act as messenger molecules transmitting signals to other cells. They have numerous actions, which include initiation and maintenance of immune and inflammatory responses and regulation of growth and differentiation of cells. The interleukins are important members of the cytokine group and are primarily involved in communication between leukocytes and other cells involved in both immune and inflammatory processes, such as epithelial and endothelial cells and fibroblasts. These molecules are released in small amounts and have a variety of actions on cells carrying the specific receptor for this cytokine. Cytokines are numerous; many have overlapping functions, and they are interlinked, forming an active network that controls the host response. Control of cytokine release and action is complex and involves inhibitors and receptors. Many cytokines are capable of acting on the cell that produced them so as to stimulate their own

production and the production of other cytokines.

IL-1 is a major mediator in periodontitis. Interleukin-1β comes mostly from activated macrophages and fibroblasts and IL-1α from keratinocytes of the junctional or pocket epithelium. Production is induced by LPSs and other bacterial components.

IL-1 upregulates complements and Fc receptors on PMNLs and monocytic cells as well as adhesion molecules on fibroblasts and leukocytes. It induces homing receptors for lymphoid cells in the extracellular matrix and induces osteoclast formation and bone resorption. It enhances production of itself, MMPs, and prostaglandins by macrophages, fibroblasts, and PMNLs. In addition, IL-1 upregulates major histocompatibility complex expression by B and T cells to facilitate their activation, clonal expansion, and immunoglobulin production. Recent studies by Kornman et al (1997a) have shown that adult subjects with genetically increased production of IL-1 are about four times more susceptible to severe periodontal diseases than are others. Other recent studies have shown that genetic polymorphism of IL-1 in combination with smoking seems to have a synergistic negative effect on tooth loss because of periodontitis (Axelsson et al, 2001; McGuire and Nunn, 1999) and alveolar bone loss (Axelsson et al, 2001). For details see chapter 3.

Among other things, IL-2, IL-3, IL-4, and IL-5 are all involved in lymphocyte clonal expansion, differentiation of B cells into antibody-producing plasma cells, and isotope switching. Interleukin-2 is produced by T cells and antigen-presenting cells and, in the presence of antigen, induces expression of clones of specific T cells and secretion of IL-3 and IL-4. Interleukin-4 regulates immunoglobulin G1 (IgG1) and immunoglobulin E (IgE) production and suppresses activated macrophages. Interleukin-6 is produced by macrophages, fibroblasts, lymphocytes, and endothelial cells. Production is induced by IL-1 and LPSs and suppressed by estrogens and progesterone.

As discussed earlier, IL-8 is the most important chemokine (chemoattractant) for the PMNLs. It is produced by LPS-activated macrophages, synovial cells, endothelium, and junctional epithelial cells. The primary target cells, PMNLs, have high-affinity receptors, which can become occupied at low concentrations of chemoattractant and cause the cells to undergo directed migration, and low-affinity receptors, which become occupied at high concentrations of chemoattractant and cause the cells to undergo a metabolic burst and to degranulate on arrival at the site of challenge.

Monocyte chemoattractant protein 1 is a potent attractant for monocytes. Monocyte chemoattractant protein 1–producing cells are commonly found in inflamed gingiva, and there is a good correlation between cells that produce IL-8 and monocyte chemoattractant protein 1 and the accumulation and location of PMNLs and macrophages in sites with gingivitis and periodontitis.

Transforming growth factor-β is produced by activated T cells. It is a chemoattractant for monocytes and suppresses their activation. Transforming growth factor-β induces production of immunoglobulin A (IgA) and IgG2b. Transforming growth factor-β is produced by macrophages and serves as a mitogen for fibroblasts, epithelial cells, and endothelial cells. In contrast, IFN-γ recruits and activates macrophages to target, among other things, virally infected cells for killing.

Role of prostaglandins

Prostaglandins are arachidonic acid derivatives that are important mediators of inflammation. The proinflammatory cytokines are capable of stimulating macrophages and other cells to produce copious amounts of prostaglandins, particularly PGE_2, which are potent vasodilators and inducers of cytokine production by various cells. PGE_2 acts on fibroblasts and osteoclasts, together with cytokines, to induce production of MMP, which is relevant to tissue turnover and the periodontal destructive process. Many studies of the association of PGE_2 with periodontal disease have indicated that its concentration in gingival crevicular fluid increases in the presence of periodontitis and is very high during periods of disease progression (Offenbacher et al, 1993).

Role of matrix metalloproteinases

The MMPs comprise a large family of Zn++ dependent enzymes produced by macrophages, fibroblasts, PMNLs, and keratinocytes activated by LPSs or cytokines. These enzymes are currently designated as *MMP 1* through *MMP 17*, and the list is still growing. They fall into classes including collagenases, gelatinases, stromelysins, matrilysins, metalloelastase, and membrane-bound MMPs. Collectively, MMPs can digest all of the components of the extracellular matrix.

Production of these enzymes is tightly controlled, complex, and not well understood. Transcription is upregulated by IL-1 and transforming growth factor-α. With some exceptions, transcription is downregulated by transforming growth factor-β and IFN-γ. MMP activity is suppressed by tissue inhibitors of metalloproteinases, which are also produced by macrophages.

The rate of periodontal tissue destruction is strongly related to the interplay among endogenic MMPs, endogenic tissue inhibitors of metalloproteinases (TIMPs), exogenic enzymes, and MMP-stimulating products from the periopathogenic microflora.

In patients with genetic overproduction of MMPs and genetic underproduction of TIMPs, breakdown of the periodontal tissue will be more rapid than it will be in average patients harboring similar quantities of periopathogenic microflora. Therefore, research is in progress to develop pharmaceutical TIMPs for treatment of such high-risk patients. Of the drugs currently available, doxycycline, in low doses, seems to inhibit MMP activity.

Role of serum proteins (kinin and complement systems)

Serum proteins, such as the kinin and complement systems, provide a mechanism for rapid expansion of the inflammatory response. Bradykinin enhances permeability and inflammation of vessels of the microcirculation.

The complement cascade comprises 30 heat-labile plasma proteins that autoassemble after initiation of inflammation, forming a series of enzymes that catalyze each subsequent step in turn. The net effect is to augment opsonization of bacteria by antibodies, to allow some antibodies to kill bacteria, to recruit phagocytes to the site of complement activation, and to attack the membranes of pathogens, creating pores in the cell and lysis. Complement is classically activated by an antigen-antibody complex, requiring an acquired humoral immune response. The alternative pathway is initiated by LPSs or other bacterial products, resulting in the direct cleavage of the third component of complement (C3), which initiates activation of the terminal proteins of the cascade.

Role of specific immune responses

The specific immune responses comprise two categories: the so-called humoral immune response, represented by specific antibodies produced by plasma cells, locally and systemically, and the cell-mediated immune response, represented by specific T lymphocytes.

The function of these two specific immune systems is regulated by a complicated interaction between different mediators at the molecular level, as discussed earlier. Despite the progress in this field during the last decade, many details have yet to be explained.

In the established gingival inflammatory lesion, the cell-mediated host response predominates from 2 weeks up to some months after initiation of the lesion. However, in the long-established gingival lesion, and particularly in the destructive periodontal lesion, antibody-producing plasma cells dominate.

Role of humoral immune response

Bacterial infection usually occurs in the following stages: attachment to host cells, proliferation of organisms, avoidance of phagocytes, and damage to host cells. Host cells (plasma cells) produce antibodies that react with bacterial components (antigens) involved in these stages.

Established gingival inflammation is caused and maintained by the gingival plaque (biofilm), which contains a great assortment of gram-positive and gram-negative facultatively anaerobic and anaerobic bacteria, ie, a mixed infection by bacteria of varying pathogenicity, which results in a great range of specific antibodies. Present at different levels in the gingival biofilm may be other, highly pathogenic bacteria, implicated in the etiology of the destructive periodontal lesions: At this stage, these pathogens are held in check by the powerful host response. Persistent challenge by such periopathogens and weakening of the immune response will eventually result in a destructive periodontal lesion.

Recent data indicate that *A actinomycetemcomitans, P gingivalis,* and *B forsythus* are responsible for the initiation and progression of periodontitis. The anaerobic *P gingivalis* occurs mainly in deep periodontal pockets, especially at active sites. The facultatively anaerobic *A actinomycetemcomitans* is found in pockets from patients with localized aggressive periodontitis found in children and adults. The anaerobic *B forsythus* seems to be related to disease activity in chronic periodontitis. There are a number of critical antigens, including fimbriae, capsular polysaccharide, hemagglutinin, LPS, enzymes, and other protein antigens from *P gingivalis,* and serotype-specific carbohydrate, LPS, leukotoxin, fimbriae, and other protein antigens from *A actinomycetemcomitans.* (For details on specific periopathogens, see chapter 1.)

As the bacterial challenge increases, the host tissues are protected by PMNL activity in the sulcus, facilitated by specific antibody, produced both systemically and in the local tissues. Circulating antibodies may be far greater in amount and importance than locally produced antibody. Specific antibody from the blood constitutes a major portion of the specific antibody in gingival crevicular fluid. The local antibody response is directed by the cytokine profile within the tissues and the presentation of antigens by specific antigen-presenting cells such as the macrophage. Large numbers of plasma cells accumulate in localized gingival tissues with chronic inflammation, and the host immune system, which produces specific immunoglobulins, is activated by periopathic bacteria and their products.

Studies throughout the 1970s established that enzyme-linked immunosorbent assay can detect and measure isotype-specific antibodies to a variety of antigens, including sonicated extracts of periopathogenic microorganisms, cell-surface components, and their extracellular products. Many studies using enzyme-linked immunosorbent assay have confirmed the association between periodontal disease activity or severity and elevated levels of serum antibodies to periopathogenic bacteria (for review see Ishikawa et al, 1997). However, the relationship between local antibody levels and disease status has not been investigated as extensively.

In general, saliva contributes to the maintenance of health in the oral environment. During salivation, the secretory form of salivary IgA is found in large quantities. Humoral immune responses at the mucosal level are mostly of the IgA isotype. Secretory IgA is an antibody that can traverse mucosal membranes and prevent the entry of infectious microorganisms. Immunoglobulin A consists of IgA1, the predominant subclass in serum, and IgA2, which predominates in the secretory form. Schenck et al (1993) reported that high levels of salivary IgA directed against bacteria in dental plaque, such as *A actinomycetemcomitans, P gingivalis,* and *Streptococcus mutans,* might protect against the development of gingivitis.

The relative amounts of specific serum IgG subclass isotypes produced during the antibody response depend on the nature of the antigen. Bacterial protein antigens induce mostly IgG1 antibodies in humans and low levels of IgG3 and IgG4. In contrast, the IgG2 subclass predominates in response to bacterial polysaccharide antigens and LPS. In general, antibodies against components of the bacterial cellular surface are beneficial to host defense. The four IgG subclass isotypes (IgG1, IgG2, IgG3, and IgG4) have various defensive features, including opsonic activity, complement activation, and toxin inactivation.

Systemic (serum) antibody has been shown to function in antibacterial immunity by a variety of mechanisms. These include the abilities to aggregate the bacteria, inhibit adherence and colonization, enhance phagocytosis, lyse the bacteria, and detoxify endotoxins and exotoxins. With respect to periodontal disease, these functions have been investigated mainly from two aspects: *(1)* studies attempting to substantiate the protective aspects of the antibody by relating the levels or presence of antibody activity to the severity of disease and *(2)* studies examining the ability of antibodies to inhibit colonization and toxic and other proposed virulence components of the bacteria.

The first stage in any infection involves adhesion of the microorganisms to a host tissue, directly or via some intermediary microorganisms. Local and systemic antibodies function in antibacterial immunity through participation in several mechanisms, such as microorganism aggregation and inhibition of adherence and colonization by microorganisms.

The next event in the pathogenesis of most bacterial infectious diseases is microbial invasion of host cells. After colonization of the periodontium by periopathic bacteria, some species of microorganism can in fact invade the tissues (see Figs 45 to 48 in chapter 1). Saglie et al (1982a, 1988a, 1988b) detected antigens from *A actinomycetemcomitans* in gingival tissue from patients with severe periodontitis. Many bacterial species can invade eukaryotic cells: It is believed that entry is gained by phagocytosis. It has also been shown that the death of macrophages induced by *A actinomycetemcomitans* infection occurs through apoptosis; to induce this mode of killing, the microorganisms must gain entry into the macrophage.

The efficacy of the immune host defense mechanism via the antibody response can be determined by measuring the avidity of the antigen-antibody interaction. *Avidity,* the net binding affinity between antibodies and antigens, is a useful tool with which to diagnose infectious diseases and B-cell tolerance in immune responses.

Furthermore, serum antibody enhances phagocytosis and lyses bacteria. Phagocytosis occurs when PMNLs, and to some degree macrophages, encounter the bacteria. Phagocytosis is greatly enhanced by coating of the bacteria with antibody and/or complement. These coating molecules (collectively called *opsonins*) facilitate binding and internalization via receptors on the cellular surface, including Fc receptors (receptors for the Fc fragment of IgG) and receptors for complement, specifically CR1 and CR3.

During phagocytosis, parts of the phagocyte membrane are projected outward to surround and internalize the bacterium, forming an intracellular vacuole, or phagosome. Typically, the phagosome fuses with lysosomes to become phagolysosomes, within which bacteria are killed and fragmented by a variety of toxic substances, antimicrobial agents, and enzymes. The granules within the PMNL responsible for microbial killing are the primary and secondary (specific) granules. This mechanism of killing is termed *intracellular killing* and results in sequestration of the enzymes responsible for bacterial cell death (see Figs 230 and 231).

Killing can also occur through release of the granules into the tissues in the vicinity of the invading bacteria. This killing, termed *extracellular killing,* can also destroy adjacent normal tissue and cells through the action of myeloperoxidases, hydrolases, proteases, elastases, and collagenases.

In this context, several investigators have demonstrated that optimal PMNL opsonization and killing of *P gingivalis* require *P gingivalis*–specific antibody. The alternative pathway of complement fixation is not particularly effective. Specifically, antibodies directed toward neutralizing the immunoglobulin and complement-cleaving enzymes of *P gingivalis* appear necessary to enable normal phagocytosis and killing by PMNLs. However, recent studies by Madianos et al (1997) have shown that *P gingivalis* invasion of oral epithelium inhibits PMNL transepithelial migration. Therefore, phagocytes will be reduced in the periodontal pocket in spite of IgG2 and complements.

Figure 244 illustrates the defensive functions of antibodies against *A actinomycetemcomitans*: *(1)* inhibition of adhesion and invasion; *(2)* complement activation; *(3)* neutralization of leukotoxin; and *(4)* opsonization and phagocytosis. Proteases produced by *A actinomycetemcomitans* cleave IgG, IgA, and immunoglobulin M (IgM).

Undoubtedly, the specific antibody response plays an important role in preventing infection and promotes recovery from periodontal diseases. In the last two decades, there has been intensive research into the humoral immune response of children and adults with localized aggressive periodontitis. Page et al (1993) reported that some patients respond by producing serum antibodies against periopathic bacteria during the periodontal infections, whereas others do not. It is hard to explain this phenomenon because of the complicated subgingival microflora and existence of numerous cross-reactive bacterial antigens in periodontal pockets. They speculated that, on subclinical infection with periopathogenic bacteria, subjects resistant to periodontitis may produce sufficient levels of high-avidity antibody to clear the bacteria (Page et al, 1993). On the other hand, under the same conditions, susceptible subjects may mount no humoral immune response or may produce antibodies of low avidity that do not have the capacity to prevent the onset of periodontitis. Under such conditions, clinical disease is initiated and able to progress.

It has also been shown that most, although not all, patients with aggressive and chronic peri-

Fig 244 Defensive functions of antibodies against *A actinomycetemcomitans*. (From Ishikawa et al, 1997. Reprinted with permission.)

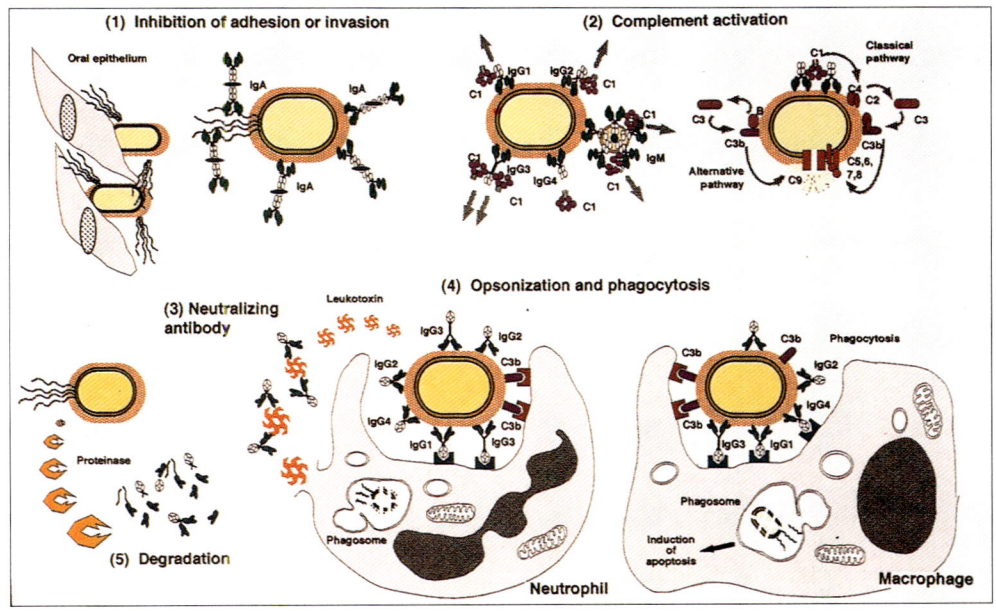

odontitis mount a systemic humoral immune response to antigens of the infecting bacteria. Remarkably high antibody titers are, however, often associated with low biologic activity, in terms of antibody avidity and capacity to opsonize and enhance phagocytosis and killing.

Role of cell-mediated immune response

The cell-mediated immune response is represented by the T lymphocytes and their products. The T cells originate from the thymus. In a naïve form, the cell-mediated immune response is initiated when antigens from the gingival plaque penetrate the junctional epithelium into the connective tissue. Antigen-presenting cells—particularly the macrophages, but also the Langerhans cells in the epithelium—process the antigen (see Figs 239 to 241) and alter it to an antigenic peptide form that is recognizable by the lymphocytes. The effect of antigenic stimulation is clonal expansion and differentiation on the T lymphocytes from naïve cells into memory or suppressor (cytotoxic) T cells. These T lymphocytes express either CD4 or CD8 molecules on their surface. The CD4+

and CD8+ T cells are referred to as *helper* and *suppressor (cytotoxic)* T cells, respectively. As CD4 binds class II major histocompatibility complex antigens, CD4+ T cells recognize the epitopes presented by these antigens. Whereas CD8 binds class I antigens, CD8+ T cells recognize those in the context of class I molecules.

The division of CD4+ T cells (helper T cells) into distinct subsets (T_H1 and T_H2), based on cytokine production, provided a new framework for studying immune responses to infectious diseases. The T_H1 cells produce IL-2 and IFN-γ and provide help for cell-mediated immunity and delayed-type hypersensitivity responses. The T_H2 cells secrete IL-4, IL-5, IL-6, and IL-10 and provide help for IgG, IgE, and IgA responses. A recently identified third type of T-cell clone (T_H0) produces IFN-γ, IL-2, IL-4, and IL-5. The effect of these cytokines has been discussed previously.

Evolution of the acquired (specific) immune system

The evolution of the immune system, from an innate to an acquired (specific) system, is illustrat-

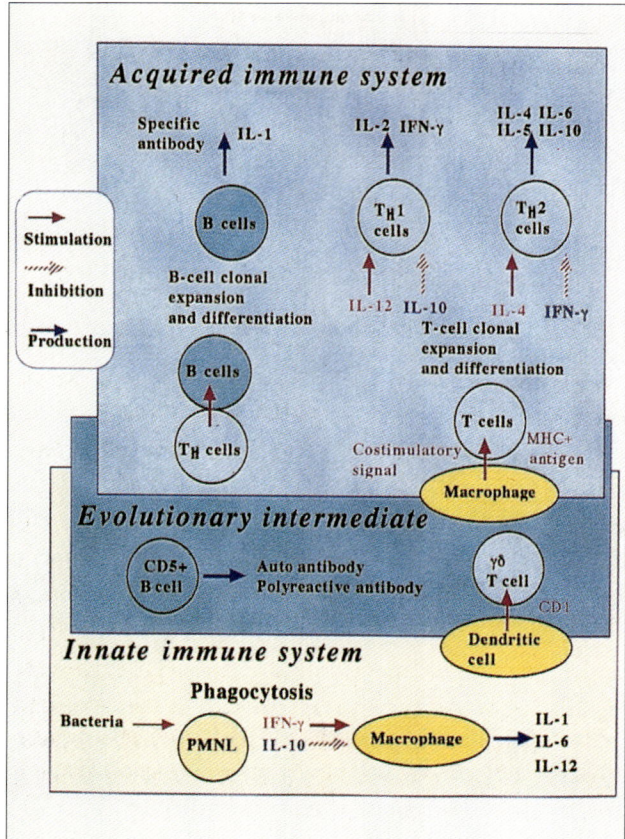

Fig 245 Evolution of the immune system. *(bottom)* In innate immune systems, antigens (bacteria) are recognized as non-self by phagocytic cells and eliminated by phagocytosis. This reaction is initiated by recognition and followed by elimination. *(middle)* The CD5+ B cells and γδ T cells are regarded as evolutionary intermediate cells. *(top)* The acquired immune system largely depends on innate immune systems. The T cells require costimulatory signals for clonal expansion and differentiation. Macrophages provide T cells with costimulatory signals during antigen presentation. In addition, macrophage-derived cytokines are important for T-cell differentiation into T_H1 and T_H2 cells. This reaction is initiated by recognition and followed by clonal expansion. MHC = Major histocompatibility complex. (From Ishikawa et al, 1997. Reprinted with permission.)

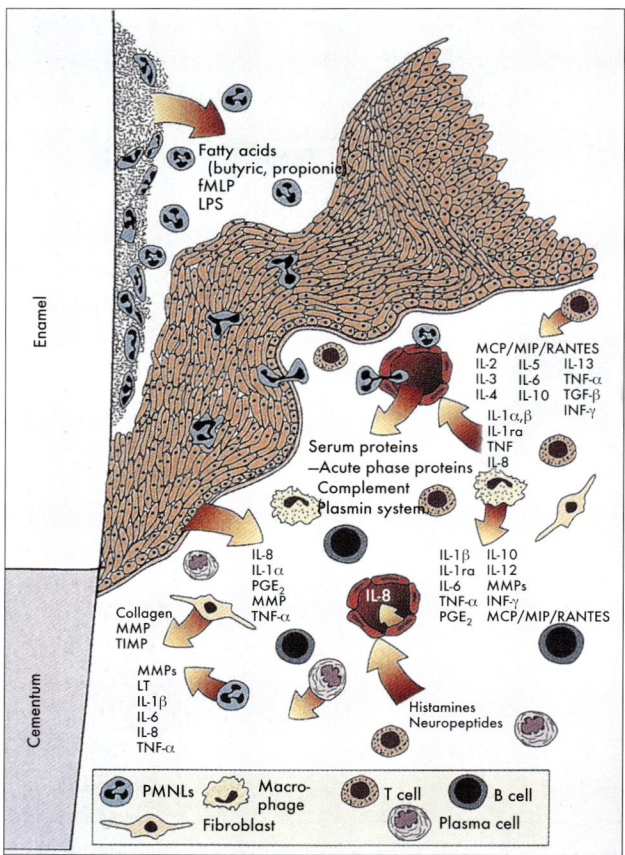

Fig 246 Cellular and molecular features of established gingival inflammation. TGF-β = Transforming growth factor-β; LT = Leukotrienes. (From Kornman et al, 1997b. Reprinted with permission.)

ed in Fig 245. The acquired system is layered on the innate system during evolution. In innate immune systems, antigens (bacteria) are recognized as nonself by phagocytic cells and eliminated by phagocytosis. The acquired immune system largely depends on innate immune systems. The T cells require costimulatory signals for clonal expansion and differentiation. Macrophages provide T cells with costimulatory signals during antigen presentation.

Cellular and molecular features of established gingival inflammation

Kornman et al (1997b) recently illustrated the complicated events at the cellular and molecular levels in established gingival inflammation (Fig 246). Unlike acute early inflammation (see Fig 238), in established inflammation the vascular exudate comprises mainly mononuclear cells. In addition to the macrophages and serum proteins, not only PMNLs, T cells, and B cells, but also plasma cells, become evident in the tissue. Activated T cells produce cytokines that help to shape the immune response, including IL-2, IL-3, IL-4, IL-5, IL-6, IL-10, IL-13, TNF-α, transforming growth factor-β, and IFN-γ. The T cells also produce a series of chemotactic substances: monocyte chemoattractant protein, macrophage inflammatory protein, and RANTES. Plasma cells become prominent in the tissues and produce immunoglobulins, such as IgG, and the cytokines IL-6 and TNF-α. Some of the PMNLs become activated in the tissue and produce IL-1α, IL-1β, IL-6, IL-8, TNF-α, leukotrienes, and MMPs. Fibroblasts produce collagen, MMPs, and tissue inhibitors of MMPs.

The destructive periodontal lesion

Today it is generally accepted that periodontitis represents a multifactorial family of diseases. Without bacterial challenge by a gingival biofilm containing periopathogens such as *P gingivalis, B forsythus,* and *A actinomycetemcomitans,* periodontitis, resulting in loss of periodontal support, will not occur. In other words the etiology of periodontal diseases is relatively well documented.

However, although a gingival biofilm containing periopathogens (mainly gram-negative anaerobic bacteria responsible for release of LPSs) is a prerequisite for the initiation and development of periodontitis, only a minority of individuals exposed to such a biofilm develop progressive periodontitis; however, probably all develop gingivitis. This may be exemplified by a recent study in a population of rural China, where oral care is minimal or nonexistent and the prevalence of most periodontal pathogens is about 90% to 95%. In fact, many or most subjects were infected, not with just a few of the species but with virtually all currently recognized pathogens. Nevertheless, the prevalence and severity of periodontal disease varied and were not substantially greater than in populations in industrialized countries (Papapanou et al, 1997a). This could partly be explained by the fact that only 2% of a Chinese population tested positive for genetic IL-1 polymorphism, compared to 30% to 40% of European and US populations (for details see chapter 3). That is because it has recently been estimated that external and internal modifying risk factors, such as smoking and polymorphism in the IL-1 gene family, together may identify more than 80% of adults susceptible to progressive destructive periodontitis, while periopathogens such as *P gingivalis* and *B forsythus* may identify fewer than 20% (Axelsson et al, 2001; Grossi et al, 1994; Kornman et al, 1997a; Kornman and di Giovine, 1998; McGuire and Nunn, 1999; Page et al, 1997).

These studies indicate that the role of other factors in predicting the development of destructive periodontitis has been underestimated: More attention should be paid to external and internal modifying risk factors, prognostic risk factors, and risk indicators (see chapters 2 to 4).

As discussed earlier, although there is consensus that periodontitis is preceded by gingivi-

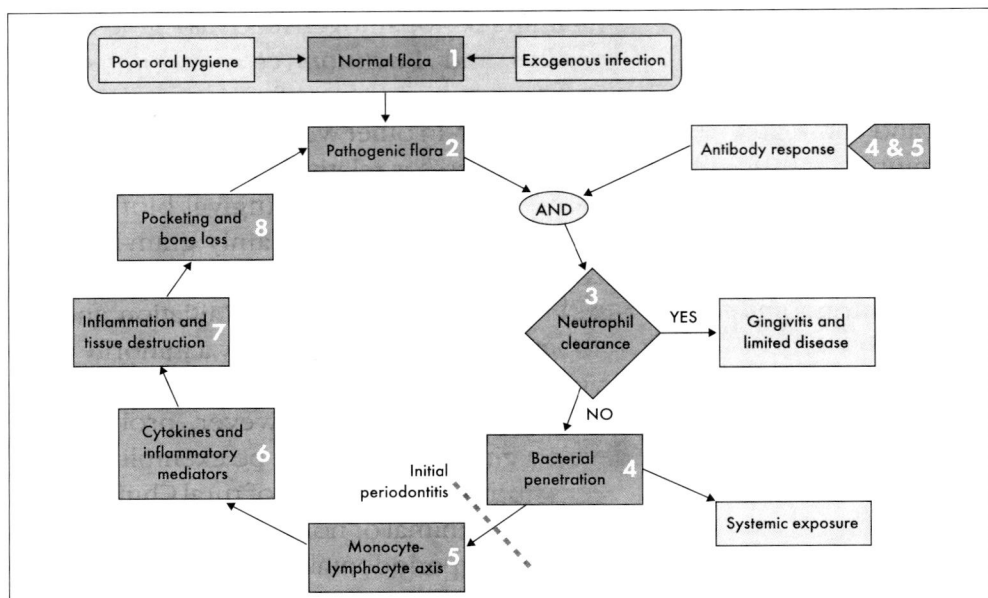

Fig 247 Critical pathway model for the pathogenesis of periodontitis demonstrating the overall sequence of events. (From Offenbacher, 1996. Reprinted with permission.)

tis, relatively few patients with gingivitis develop aggressive periodontitis. This is particularly obvious among children and young adults. In Scandinavia, which has high standards of oral hygiene and well-developed, school-based preventive programs, the prevalence of aggressive periodontitis in children is as low as 0.1% to 0.3% of the population. In countries without such resources, the prevalence of aggressive periodontitis in children is considerably higher. On this basis, populations may be broadly categorized as two subsets: patients with gingivitis and those with periodontitis.

Initiation and development of the destructive periodontal lesion

Recently Offenbacher (1996) illustrated the critical pathway model for the pathogenesis of periodontitis (Fig 247). In individuals with "normal" gingival microflora and fairly good gingival plaque control, the gingiva should remain clinically healthy. However if an individual with normal gingival microflora has poor oral hygiene, he or she will exhibit gingival inflammation (gingivi-

tis) at several sites. This results in increasing edema of the gingiva, the formation of pseudopockets, and increased release of gingival crevicular exudate (GCF) into the gingival sulcus. This environment favors the establishment of gram-negative anaerobic microflora in the gingival biofilm; ie, the individual will be more susceptible to exogenous infection by transmissible periopathogens such as *P gingivalis* and *A actinomycetemcomitans* as well as opportunistic endogenous infection by *B forsythus, P intermedia, Treponema denticola,* etc (Fig 247; 1). Individuals with gingival biofilm containing such periopathogens (Fig 247; 2) have the etiologic prerequisites for the development of periodontitis.

Despite this, only a minority of the adult population and very few young adults develop several destructive periodontal lesions because a competent nonspecific first line of defense is active in the gingival sulcus. The PMNLs (neutrophils) (Fig 247; 3) phagocytose and kill the bacteria and isolate the biofilm from the junctional epithelium, as described earlier. Supplementation by specific antibodies with good attachment strength to the bacteria and their antigens (Fig 247; 4 and 5) and complements (opsonins) further enhance the potential for the PMNLs to phagocytose and kill even the most virulent periopathogens (see Fig 244).

If this local cellular and humoral (antibodies produced by the plasma cells) immune response in the gingival sulcus is inadequate, periopathogens and their antigens (particularly LPS) will penetrate the junctional epithelium and the connective tissue (Fig 247; 4). This initiates not only a destructive periodontal lesion but also systemic exposure. There are several circumstances under which this occurs:

- It has been shown that LPSs from *P gingivalis* do not stimulate the production of E-selectin in human epithelial cells and also inhibit stimulation of E-selectin by other bacteria. In addition, *P gingivalis* or its LPSs inhibit monocyte chemotaxis, IL-8, and intercellular adhesion molecule expression in the endothelial cells, fibroblasts, and gingival epithelial cells. Increased numbers of *P gingivalis* in the apical part of the subgingival biofilm will therefore block the migration of phagocytosing PMNLs into this part of the gingival pocket (see Fig 72 in chapter 1).
- Periopathogens may also release different leukotoxins that may kill the PMNLs or limit their functions (for details see chapter 1).
- Genetic or acquired dysfunction of the PMNLs: There is strong evidence from the literature that patients with generalized PMNL defects, which impair clearance of bacteria, are at clear risk for periodontitis. Furthermore, certain individuals may exhibit abnormal PMNL clearance for only specific organisms, as is the case in patients with aggressive periodontitis. Systemically compromised patients, such as diabetics, experience transient PMNL impairment: Instead of migrating into the pocket, the PMNLs remain in the connective tissue and degranulate. It is also known that the PMNLs are impaired in smokers (for details see chapter 3).
- There is also reason to believe that certain bacterial challenges are capable of shifting the T-

cell and B-cell responses, resulting in less effective antibody function. Selected periodontal bacteria produce proteases that cleave the Fc regions of IgG or degrade the C3 component of the complement, thereby interfering with phagocytosing and killing. In addition, antibody avidity (attachment strength) to *P gingivalis* is higher in periodontally healthy individuals and patients with chronic periodontitis than in those with aggressive periodontitis and improves following therapy.

It is reasonable to expect these factors to substantially alter the protective balance within the sulcus. When the first line of defense (PMNLs) is overwhelmed and failing in the gingival pocket, there is an accompanying shift in the lymphocyte population, from T-cell– to plasma-cell–dominant. At this point, if the host can quickly mount an antibody response that is sufficiently protective, the bacteria are held in abeyance, and the disease is mild or "limited" (Fig 247; 4 and 5). However, if the antibody-neutrophil axis does not provide sufficient clearance, bacterial proliferation and deeper penetration of bacterial products and antigens ensue, resulting in recruitment and activation of the monocyte-lymphocyte axis (Fig 247; 5).

The host's immune response is determined largely by genes that regulate differences in the monocyte-macrophage (MØ)–T-cells response traits to different antigens, which in turn determine both the nature of the protective antibody response and the magnitude of the tissue-destructive, inflammatory response. The quality of the antibody response by resident plasma cells, and the regulatory effects of MØ–T-cell cytokines, secondarily result in differences in the functional responses of the PMNL to bacteria. Thus, it is reasonable to suggest that the interindividual differences in the severity of disease expression to a given infectious challenge are due largely to intrinsic differences in the MØ–T-cell response traits. In either event, LPS challenge to the monocyte-lymphocyte axis would result in the secretion of catabolic cytokines and inflammatory mediators, of which

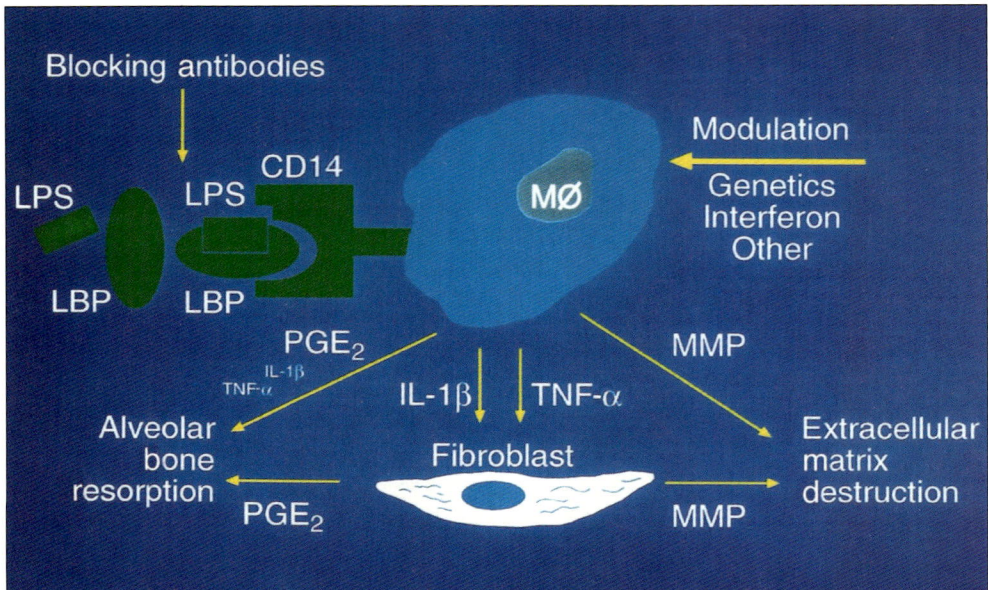

Fig 248 Role of monocytes/macrophages (MØ) in the development of destructive periodontal lesions. LBP = Lipid-binding proteins. (From Page et al, 1997. Reprinted with permission.)

PGE_2, IL-1α, IL-1β, TNF-α, and IL-6 would appear to dominate (Fig 247; 5 and 6).

Figure 248 by Page et al (1997) illustrates the central role of monocytes and macrophages in this phase of the development of destructive periodontal lesions. Macrophages activated by LPS produce IL-1β, TNF-α, MMPs, and PGE_2. Both IL-1β and TNF-α activate resident fibroblasts to produce PGE_2 and MMPs. Both activated cell types decrease the production of tissue inhibitors of MMPs, resulting in greatly increased relative levels of MMPs. This destroys components of the extracellular matrix, creating space for the enlarging inflammatory cell infiltrate. The microbial biofilm may extend apically and laterally. The epithelial cells activated by LPS can produce MMPs, which can destroy attached collagen fibers at the apical terminus of the junctional epithelium, allowing apical extension of the epithelium, formation of additional pocket epithelium, and deepening of the pocket. As this occurs, MMPs mediate clinical attachment loss and PGE_2 mediates resorption of the alveolar bone, and the gingival pocket progresses to become a periodontal pocket (see Fig 247; 6 to 8).

Interaction of periopathogens and host defenses

The events constituting the formation of gingival and subsequently periodontal pockets as presented may appear unidirectional. However, this is not the case: They are interactive, involving cross-communication between the microbial challenge and the host defenses called into play. At any given point, host defenses may contain the challenge and arrest or reverse progression, or the challenge may overwhelm the defenses and enhance progression; ie, there may be periods of exacerbation (bursts) and quiescence (burnouts).

A study by Goodson et al (1982) demonstrated the dynamic nature of periodontal disease, with characteristic periods of exacerbation and remission, as well as periods of inactivity. In untreated subjects with existing periodontal pockets, probing attachment loss was measured every month for a year: There was no significant changes in 83% of the diagnosed sites, significant further loss of attachment in 6%, and less loss of attachment in 11%.

Other studies have confirmed that sites with destructive periodontal activity may show no fur-

Fig 249 Critical pathway model showing the effect of mechanical debridement on the pathogenesis of periodontitis. (From Offenbacher, 1996. Reprinted with permission.)

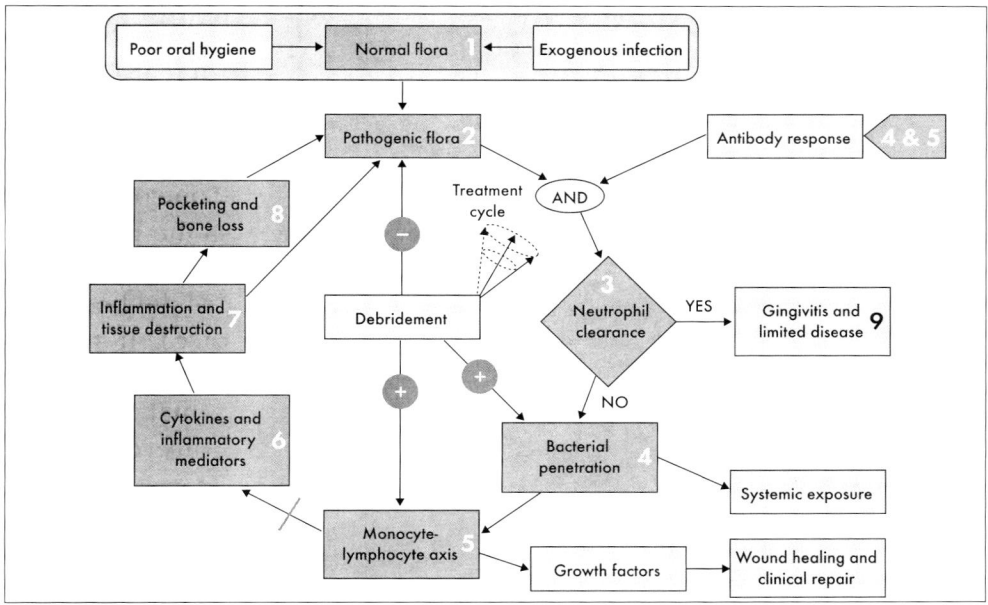

ther activity or subsequently undergo one or more exacerbations. Over a lifetime, there may be relatively short periods in which many sites undergo periodontal destruction, followed by prolonged periods of remission (Socransky et al, 1984).

Inflammation and pocketing both provide nutrients and an ideal environment for the continued growth and emergence of subgingival anaerobic bacteria. That is, more disease leads to deeper pockets, more inflammation, and an ecosystem that favors the overgrowth of pathogenic organisms. As these organisms overgrow, they present a chronic repeated challenge (see Fig 247; 2, 7, and 8). However, at this point, the antibody response has been reinforced (see Fig 247; 4 and 5): If it is sufficiently protective to enable PMNL clearance, then the disease will be limited as the infection is brought into homeostasis. With time, if the host becomes compromised so that either PMNL clearance or MØ–T-cell responses shift to a more inflammatory than protective balance, then the disease can exacerbate. Thus, in this critical pathway model of pathogenesis, a virulent flora and the evasion of PMNL clearance are prerequisites for initiation of disease, and the individual host response plays a determinant role in the severity of disease expression.

Subgingival debridement, mechanical removal of the subgingival biofilm, retards disease progression considerably: The procedure removes periopathogens within the biofilm that are inaccessible to PMNLs, macrophages, and antibodies as well as antimicrobial agents and antibiotics. However, debridement not only reduces the local bacterial burden but also results in a bacteremia, which serves to "boost" host immunity by enhancing local antibody opsonic potential. Removal of the microbial challenge, combined with blood clotting factors, initiates the change in monocytic phenotype, from a catabolic septic phenotype to an aseptic reparative phenotype, which now secretes growth factors to facilitate periodontal repair. Reduction of the microbial burden attenuates the inflammatory stimulus, reducing pocketing and inflammation, to suppress the reemergence of the flora (Fig 249). However, as described for patients with aggressive periodontitis and refractory cases, patients who do not show a clinically favorable response to debridement because of a MØ+ phenotype might experience persistent inflam-

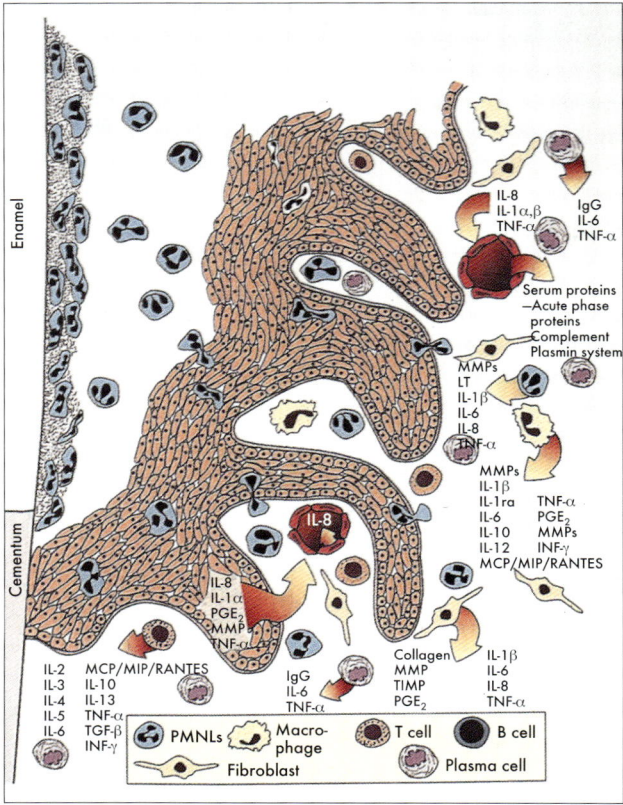

Fig 250 *Development of the initial destructive periodontal lesion. (From Kornman et al, 1997b. Reprinted with permission.)*

mation, fostering early reemergence of the pathogenic flora.

Figure 250 illustrates the complicated interplay, during development of the initial destructive periodontal lesion, among the subgingival biofilm that contains periopathogens, the PMNLs in the periodontal pocket, and the PMNLs, macrophages, T cells, B cells, plasma cells, fibroblasts, and their molecular regulation in the inflamed connective tissue. Compared to the established gingival inflammation lesion (see Fig 246), the initial destructive lesion demonstrates increased mononuclear cell activity in the tissues. The inflammatory mediator load in the tissues increases and includes contributions by the fibroblasts of IL-1β, IL-6, IL-8, PGE_2, and TNF-α, as well as collagen, MMPs, and tissue inhibitors of MMPs. Plasma cells are prominent.

FACTORS AFFECTING RATES OF PERIODONTAL DISEASE PROGRESSION

The net outcome of the infectious periodontal diseases is the relationship between the bacterial challenge of the gingival plaque (biofilm) and the power of the host's immune response (patient's resistance). If the bacterial challenge is not matched by the immune response, destruction of periodontal tissue will progress (Figs 251 and 252). However, as discussed earlier, the progression rate may vary considerably from time to time and among different individuals and sites.

Apart from the familiar clinical variables such as probing attachment loss, radiographs, and periodontal pocket temperature, the level of PGE_2 in the GCF is a very valuable indicator of ongoing destruction of periodontal tissues, particularly bone resorption (see Figs 248 and 252). The level of PGE_2 in GCF may be 10 to 15 times higher at sites of progressive periodontal destruction than it is at healthy sites.

Recent data suggest that the levels of PGE_2 in GCF are substantially higher in certain high-risk patients, such as those with aggressive refractory disease, aggressive periodontitis, or diabetes, than they are in other patients. In these patients, even clinically healthy sites (0- to 3-mm pockets; no inflammation) have higher levels of PGE_2 in GCF than do corresponding sites in patients with the more prevalent chronic periodontitis or with healthy sites. Thus, the interpretation of levels of PGE_2 in GCF in these high-risk patient categories should be considered in more detail.

It appears that the increased local PGE_2 response in GCF observed in these patients is coincident with an upregulated monocytic macrophage phenotype (MØ⁺). Thus, even low levels of endotoxin challenge within the periodontal pocket seem to induce high levels of PGE_2 secretion at these sites. Together with IL-1α and IL-1β and TNF-α, the osteoclasts will be overstimulated (see Figs 248 and 250); as a result, loss of alveolar bone will proceed more rapidly in these

Fig 251 Progression of periodontal destruction. (From Schwartz et al, 1997. Reprinted with permission.)

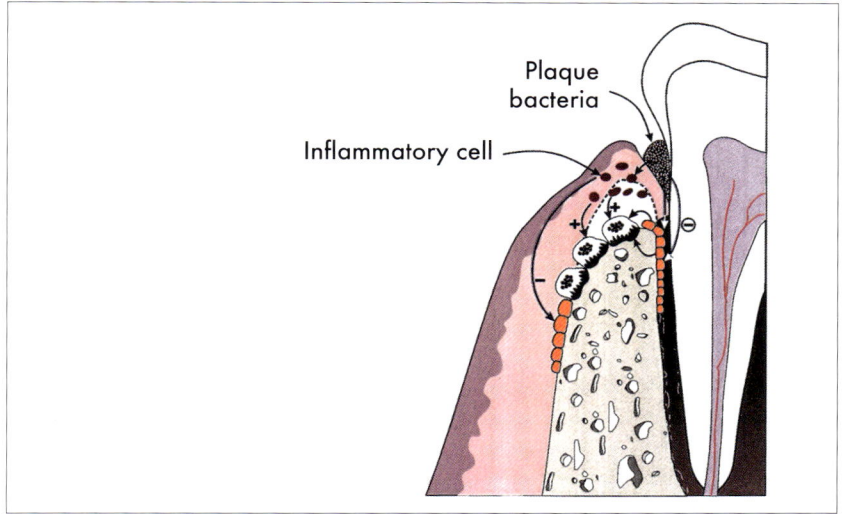

Fig 252 Bone remodeling during progressive periodontal disease. Local factors are released by inflammatory cells, osteoclasts, and osteoblasts, which inhibit osteoblasts and stimulate osteoclasts. BMP = Bone morphogenetic protein. (From Schwartz et al, 1997. Reprinted with permission.)

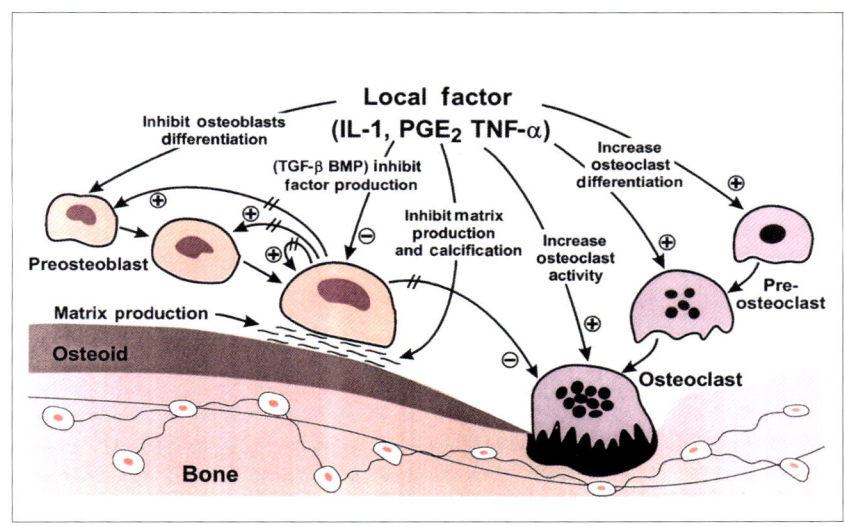

at-risk patients than in other patients with chronic periodontitis.

However, there are also other differences in immune response and bacterial challenge between these risk groups, as was discussed earlier.

Type 1 diabetes mellitus

In addition to overstimulated alveolar bone resorption, patients with type 1 diabetes mellitus ex-

hibit impaired PMNL function with respect to adhesion, chemotaxis, phagocytosis, and killing of the bacteria. This failing first line of defense in the periodontal pocket causes accumulation of PMNLs in the connective tissue and the release of many endogenous MMPs. However, the periodontal health of patients with well-controlled diabetes can be maintained after successful periodontal treatment, provided that the bacterial challenge is minimized by excellent gingival plaque control (Fig 253). As a contrast, see Figs 154 and 155 in chapter 3 (a 21-year-old woman

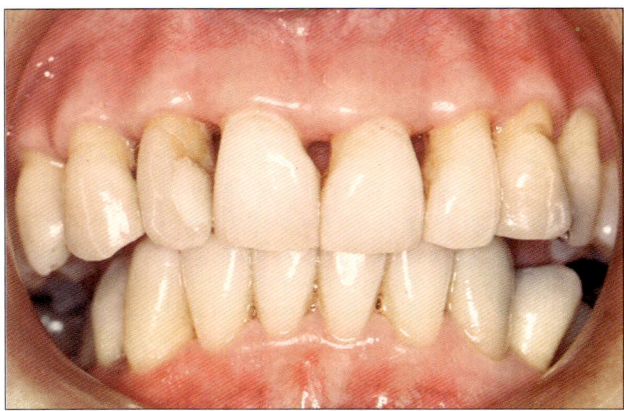

Fig 253 Forty-year-old man with type 1 diabetes mellitus. Results of successful periodontal treatment have been maintained by excellent plaque control.

with early-onset, poorly controlled type 1 diabetes; poor oral hygiene and dental care habits; and almost complete loss of periodontal support). For details on type 1 diabetes, see chapter 3.

ARREST AND CONTROL OF PERIODONTAL DISEASES

Today it is possible not only to control periodontal disease but also to regenerate lost periodontal support. However, from the point of view of cost effectiveness, materials and methods of choice for prevention and control of periodontal diseases must be based on comprehensive and accurate diagnosis, history taking, and risk prediction, as discussed in chapters 1 through 4 and 6. Fig 254 illustrates briefly the most important methods that could be used for successful prevention, treatment, and control of periodontal diseases.

Periodontal therapy and high-quality oral hygiene

Scaling and root planing (SCRP) followed by nonaggressive mechanical removal of newly formed subgingival biofilms and excellent gingival plaque control in the maintenance program are remarkably effective methods that have been the mainstay of periodontal therapy for almost 50 years. It is considered to be the gold standard against which all other forms of therapy are generally measured. SCRP and nonaggressive mechanical removal of the subgingival biofilm operate mostly at the microbial-host interface by enhancing host defense and reducing the microbial challenge as illustrated schematically in Fig 255. The procedure mechanically removes and disrupts the subgingival biofilms; the resulting bacteremia and spread of endotoxins such as LPSs may induce a humoral immune response. Moreover, specific antibodies entering the periodontal pocket can, together with complements, enhance PMNLs phagocytotis and destruction of the remaining disrupted subgingival bacteria.

Evidence from studies

More than 40 years ago, in a 5-year study, Lövdal et al (1961) showed that a maintenance program based on oral hygiene training and scaling two to four times per year reduced gingivitis and tooth loss. In 1973, Ramfjord et al reported the results of a 7-year study showing that periodontal attachment could be maintained in patients with advanced periodontal disease. After initial nonsurgical or surgical periodontal treatment, the patients had been recalled every third month for oral hygiene training, professional mechanical toothcleaning (PMTC), and subgingival scaling or debridement. Nonsurgical and surgical treatment were shown to be equally effective. Similar results were reported by Wennström et al (1986) in a 6-year longitudinal study in a selected group of patients with a history of aggressive periodontitis.

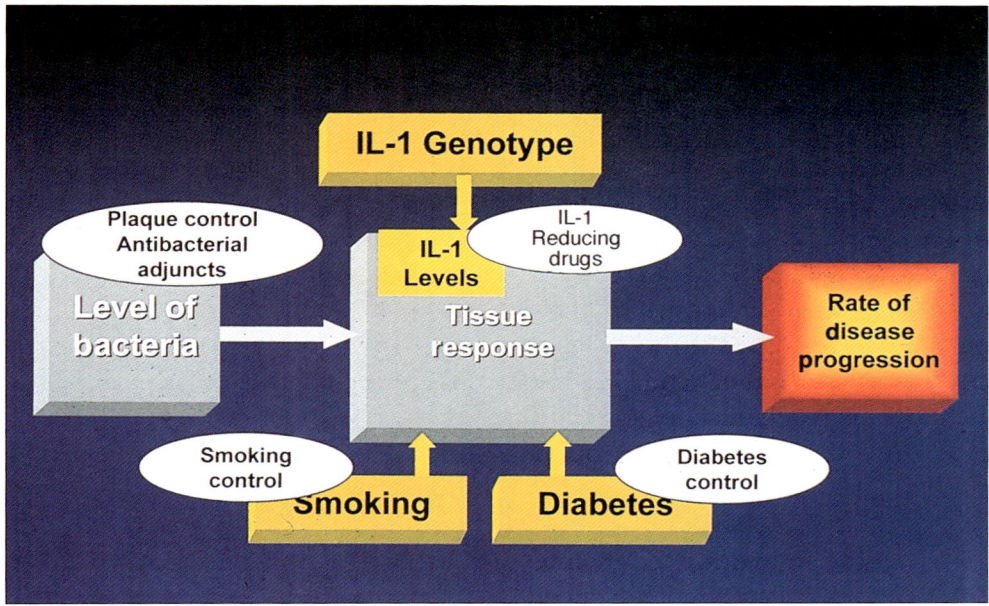

Fig 254 Schematic illustration of how periodontal diseases can be prevented and controlled related to comprehensive diagnosis, history taking, and risk prediction. (Courtesy of K. Kornman.)

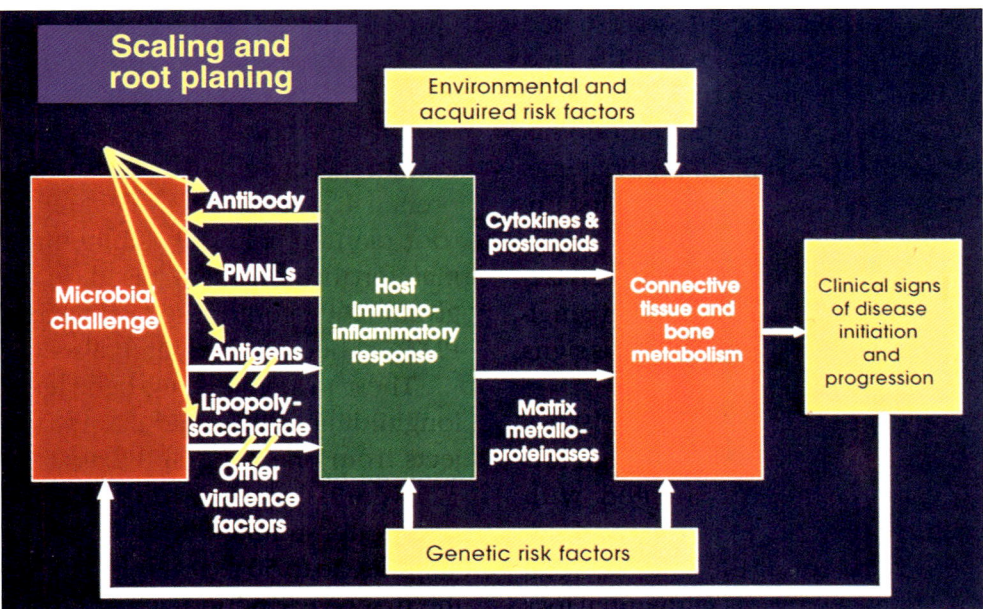

Fig 255 Schematic illustration showing how mechanical removal of subgingival biofilms by scaling and root planing and nonaggressive debridement is interfering in the pathogenesis of periodontal diseases by reducing the bacterial challenge and thereby enhancing the host defense. (From Page, 1999. Reprinted with permission.)

Frequent PMTC has also been successfully used in maintenance programs after initial non-surgical or surgical treatment of marginal periodontitis. In a 2-year study by Rosling et al (1976a), patients with a high prevalence of infrabony pockets were randomly allotted to a test or a control group. After initial open flap surgery, scaling, and root planing, the test group received PMTC every second week: On reexamination, about 95% of the infrabony pockets had healed and the gingival condition was excellent. In the matched control group without intensive mechanical plaque control, there was advanced recurrence of periodontal attachment loss.

Axelsson and Lindhe (1981b) also demonstrated the value of a carefully designed maintenance program following treatment of advanced periodontal disease. Seventy-seven patients were examined before treatment, 2 months after the last surgical procedure, and after 3 and 6 years. Two of three patients (52) were enrolled in a supervised maintenance program that included oral hygiene education, PMTC, and needs-related debridement every 2 months for the first 2 years and every 3 months for the last 4 years of the observation period. The remaining 25 patients resumed care with the referring dentist, who was informed of the importance of checking their oral hygiene, calculus formation, and gingival and periodontal conditions (nonrecall group). The recall patients were able to maintain proper oral hygiene and unaltered attachment levels. In the nonrecall group, plaque scores increased markedly from the baseline values, as did the number of inflamed gingival units. Concomitantly, there were obvious signs of recurrent periodontitis.

According to Lindhe and Nyman (1975), well-motivated patients who maintain high levels of oral hygiene can be managed with extended recall intervals, even in cases of advanced loss of attachment at the time of treatment. Seventy-five such patients with initial loss of alveolar bone amounting to half the length of the roots or more were treated and subsequently received PMTC, scaling, and oral hygiene instruction every 3 to 6 months. After 5 years, there was no radiographic evidence of further loss of alveolar bone.

In 1984, Badersten et al (1984b) demonstrated that, for single-rooted teeth, a single session of meticulous subgingival scaling and root planing was at least as effective as three sessions, even in patients with advanced periodontitis, provided that the patients were recalled for special oral hygiene training and PMTC at needs-related intervals.

Although so-called supragingival plaque control is considered to have little effect on the subgingival microflora of deep periodontal pockets, this may not apply to PMTC in moderately deep pockets (4 to 6 mm). A series of studies has shown that both probing depth and the total number of subgingival microflora gradually decreased in such pockets as a result of frequent PMTC without prior subgingival scaling. In addition, there was a shift from a periopathogenic to a less pathogenic microflora (for review, see Axelsson, 1994; Kieser, 1994). This may be attributable to the repeated removal of 2 to 3 mm subgingival plaque by PMTC, rather than the supragingival plaque control. In this way the edema of the gingival margin is eliminated and as a consequence the pocket depth and the anaerobic environment are reduced.

The most cost-effective rationale for treatment and control of periodontal diseases is initial, comprehensive, nonaggressive subgingival scaling, root planing, and debridement, followed by a maintenance program based on meticulous gingival plaque control: self-care, supplemented by PMTC at need-related intervals.

These principles have been tested in a 15-year longitudinal study in adults. Two groups of subjects from one geographic area were recruited; 375 were assigned to a test group and 180 to a control group, stratified into three age groups: 20 to 35 years, 36 to 50 years and 51 to 70 years. During the first 6-year period, the control patients were examined regularly once a year and given traditional dental care. The subjects in the test group underwent initial nonaggressive scaling, root planing, and debridement and were then recalled every 2 months for the first 2 years and once every third month for the following 4 years. They were individually educated in proper oral hygiene techniques, based on self-diagnosis. Professional mechanical toothcleaning, supplemented by debridement when necessary, was provided by a dental hygienist. Reexaminations were carried out toward the end of the third and sixth years of the study.

On average, the control group lost 1.2 mm of periodontal attachment per individual, while the test group lost none. Although there was no attachment loss in most of the subjects in the control group, there was serious deterioration in a few (Axelsson and Lindhe, 1978, 1981a). For ethical reasons, after the 6-year period, the control subjects were also offered needs-related prevention, and many accepted. For the following 9-year period, up to the 15-year reexamination, all test subjects received an individualized secondary preventive program, supervised by the same dental hygienist. To maximize cost effectiveness, not only the preventive measures, but also the recall intervals, were based strictly on individual needs: About 65% visited the dental hygienist only once a year, 30% twice a year, and 5% (the high-risk individuals) three to six times a year.

Over the 15-year period, only 0.23 teeth were lost per individual. These results could be extrapolated to infer that a 50-year-old subject enrolled in such a program would be more than 100 years old before losing another single tooth. During the same 15-year period, it is estimated that the Swedish adult population lost, on average, two to three teeth per individual.

The mean gain of probing periodontal attachment per individual, regardless of age, was 0.3 mm; this measurement was roughly the same in the 66 to 85 year olds as it was in the 36 to 50 year olds. It was estimated that the annual costs for dental care in the test group were only about 50% of the average annual costs for Swedish adult patients.

Case reports

The following case reports illustrate the long-term effect of the preventive program on tooth loss, loss of periodontal support, gingival health status, and standard of oral hygiene. At the baseline examination in 1972, all three subjects in cases 1 to 3 exhibited more than average loss of periodontal support for their age group.

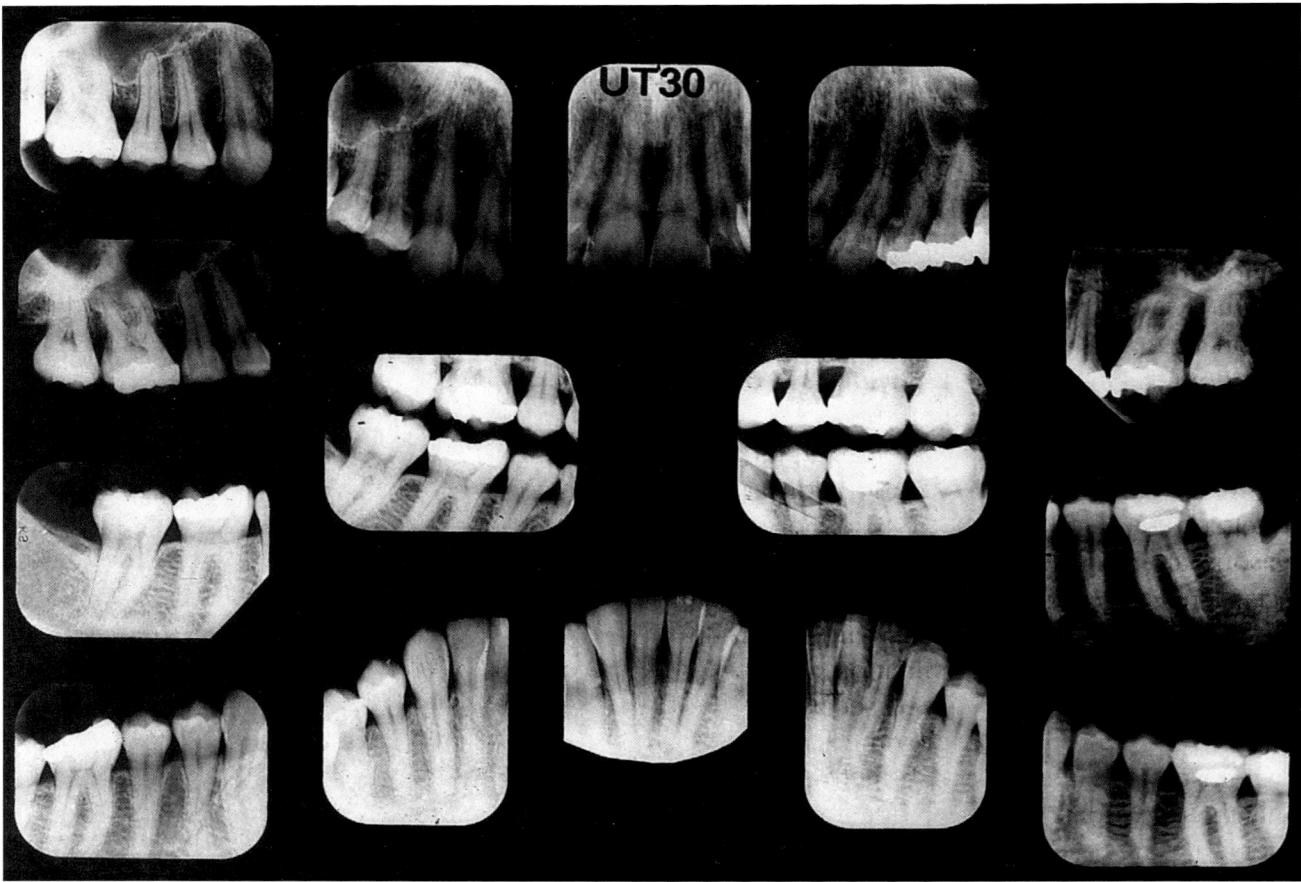

Fig 256 Complete-mouth radiographs of a 30-year-old woman in test group 1 (professional mechanical toothcleaning) at the baseline examination (1972). Aggressive periodontitis has resulted in loss of periodontal support around the maxillary first molars.

Case 1. A 30-year-old woman entered test group 1 in 1972 (Fig 256). As an effect of localized aggressive periodontitis, in 1972 the patient had more than average loss of periodontal support for her age around the maxillary first molars. During the following 15 years, no teeth were lost, there was no further loss of periodontal support, and no new caries lesions developed (Fig 257).

Figures 258 and 259 show the buccal gingival health status and level of oral hygiene at the 15-year reexamination (1987). On esthetic indications, many of the 25 to 30 amalgam restorations could have been replaced, for example with ceramic crowns, onlays, or inlays, but the patient chose to invest in preventive rather than restorative dentistry.

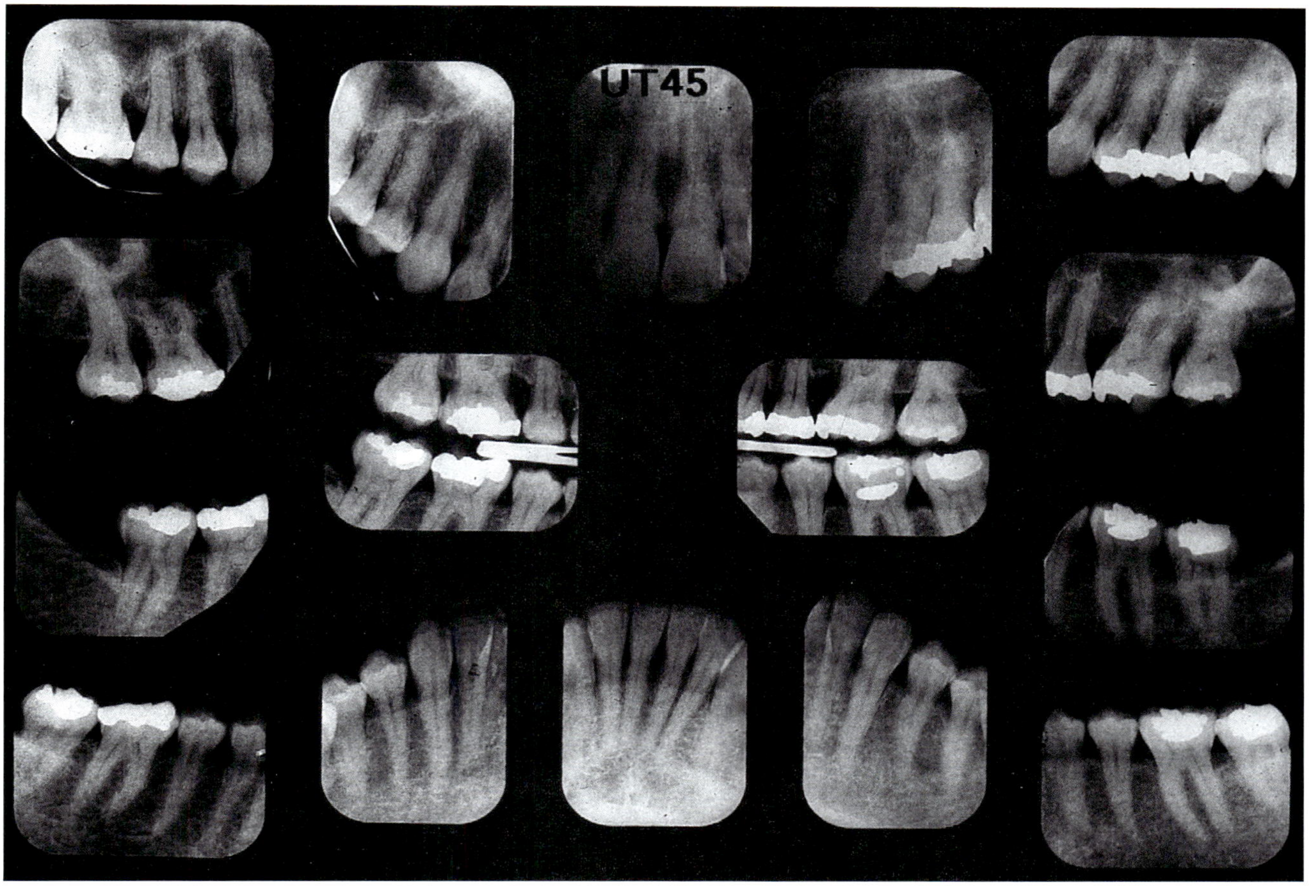

Fig 257 Complete-mouth radiographs of the patient in Fig 256, at the age of 45 years (1987). No teeth have been lost, there has been no further loss of periodontal support, and no new caries lesions have developed.

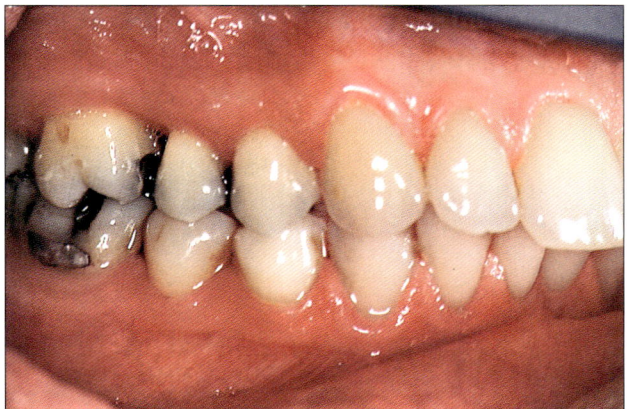 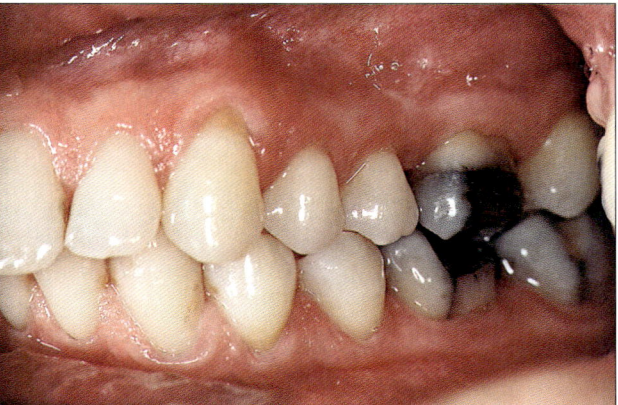

Figs 258 and 259 Buccal gingival health and oral hygiene status of the same patient at the 15-year reexamination (1987).

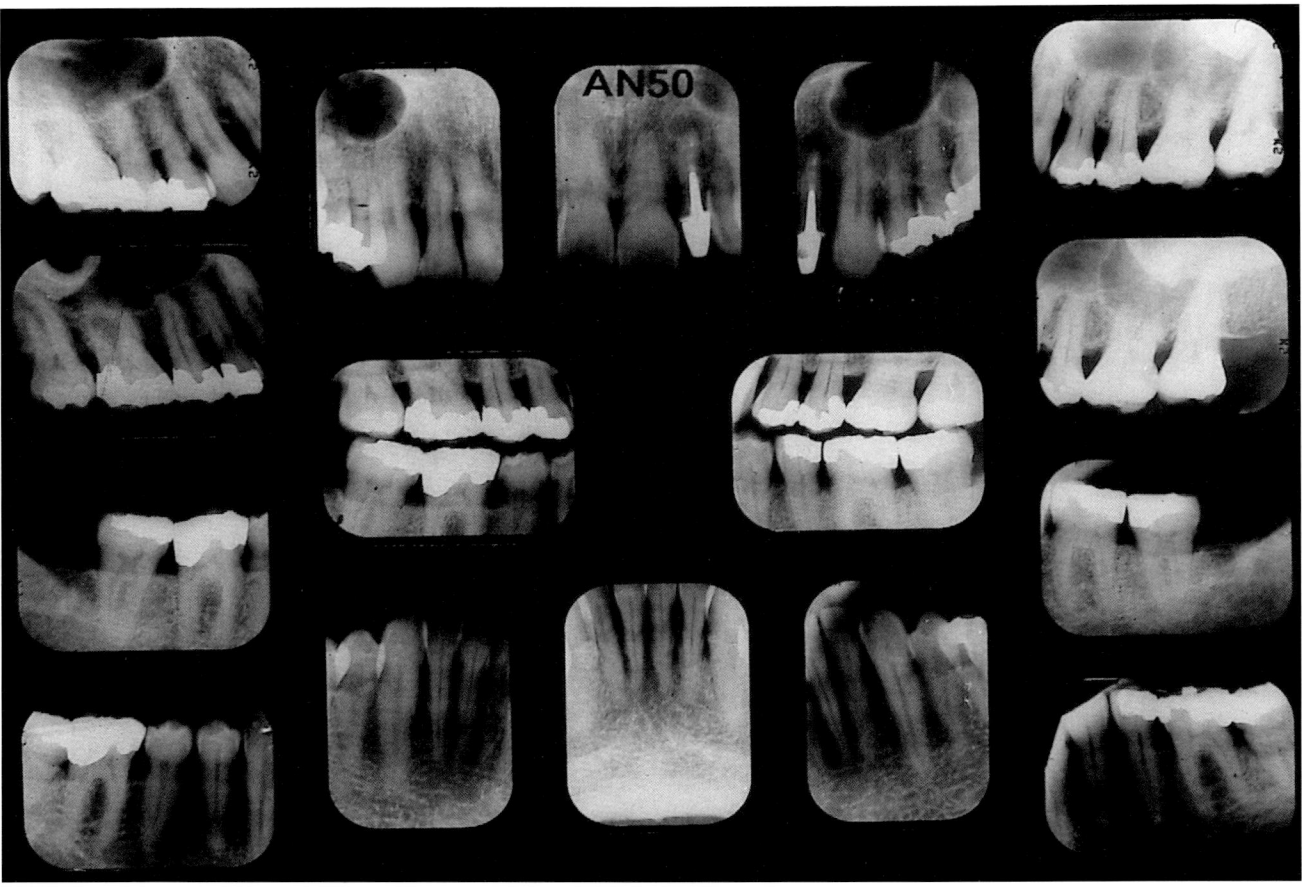

Fig 260 Complete-mouth radiographs of a 50-year-old man in test group 2 (professional mechanical toothcleaning) at the baseline examination (1972). He has greater-than-average probing attachment loss for his age, especially in the maxillary teeth.

Case 2. Complete-mouth radiographs from a 50-year-old man in test group 2 are shown at the baseline examination in 1972 (Fig 260) and at the 15-year reexamination in 1987 (Fig 261). In 1972, the patient exhibited greater than average probing attachment loss for his age, especially in the maxillary teeth. During the following 15 years, no teeth were lost, there was no further attachment loss, and no new caries lesions developed.

The buccal gingival health status and level of oral hygiene at the 15-year reexamination are shown in Figs 262 and 263.

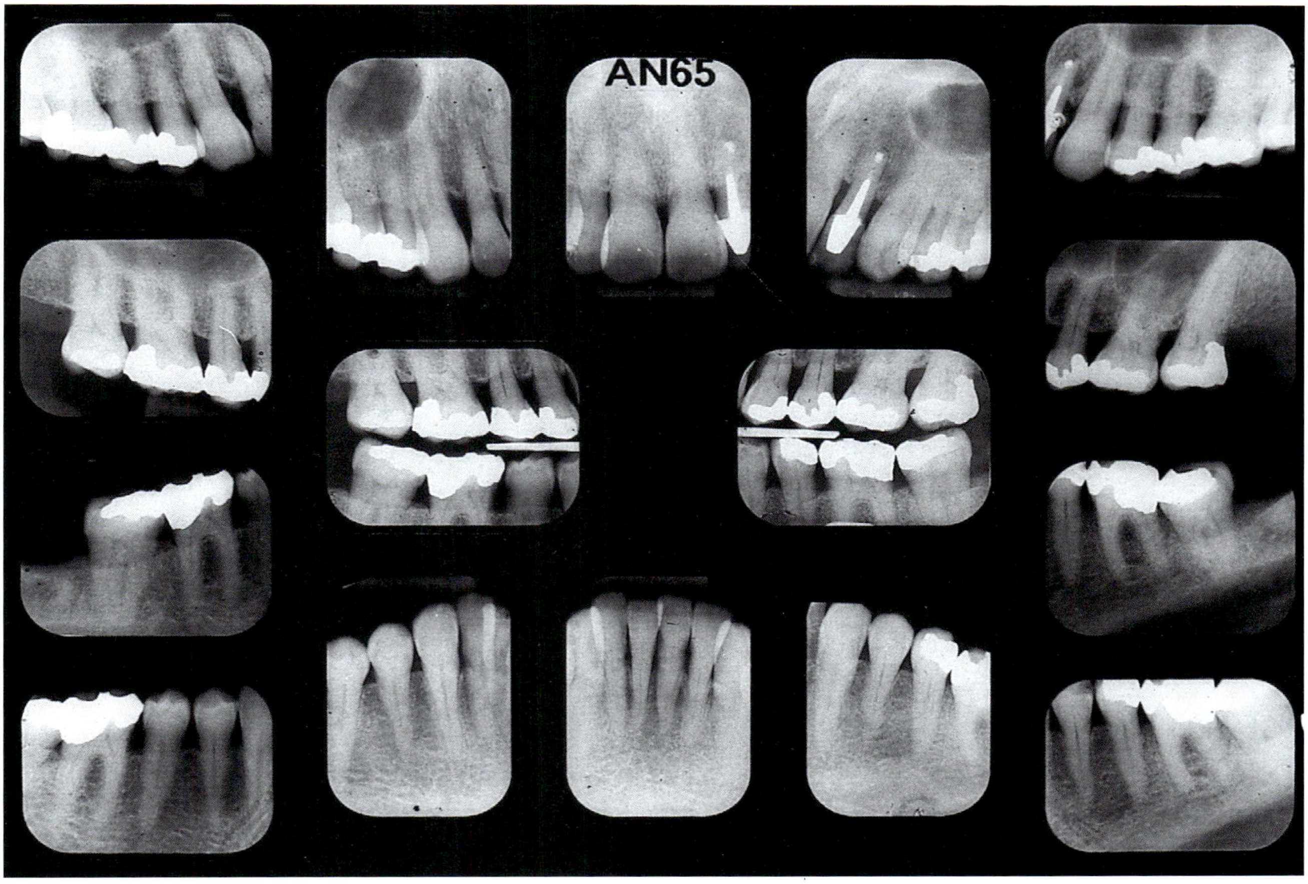

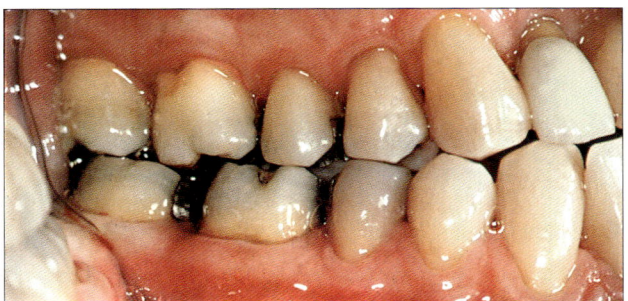

Fig 261 Complete-mouth radiographs of the patient in Fig 260, aged 65 years, at the 15-year reexamination (1987). No teeth have been lost, there has been no further loss of probing attachment level, and no new caries lesions have developed.

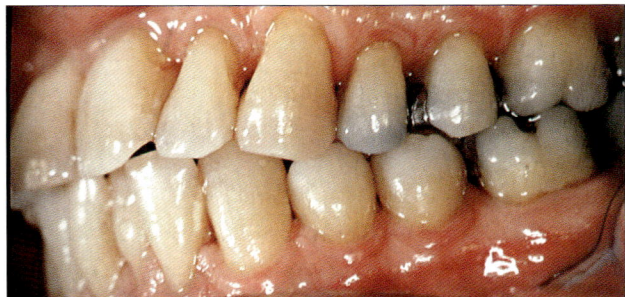

Figs 262 and 263 Buccal gingival health and oral hygiene status of the same patient at the 15-year reexamination (1987).

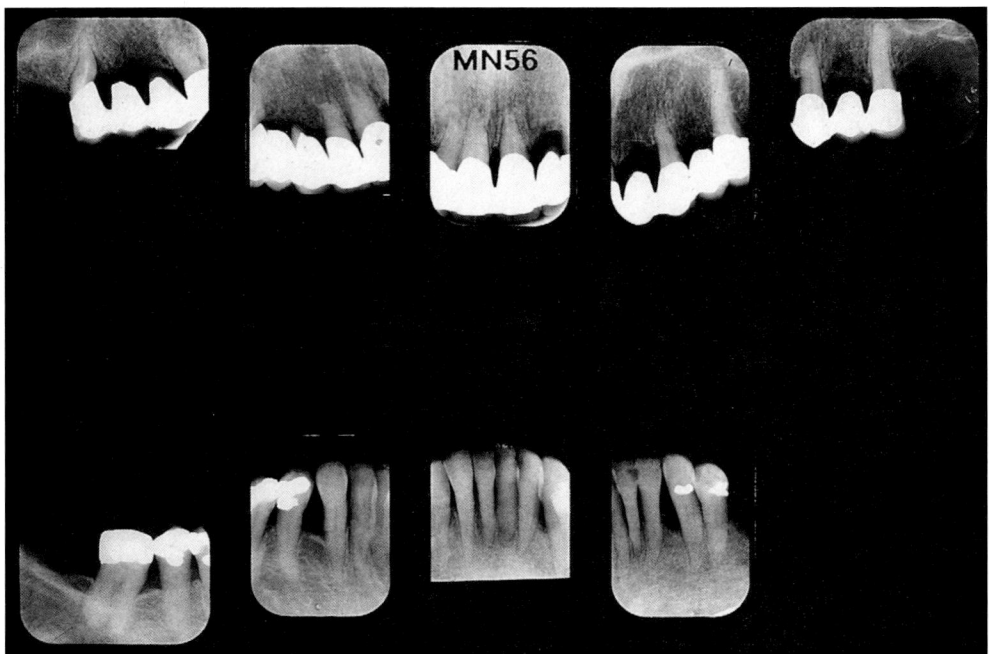

Fig 264a Complete-mouth radiographs of a 56-year-old woman in test group 3 (professional mechanical toothcleaning) at the baseline examination (1972). The number of remaining teeth and the amount of remaining periodontal support are below average for her age group.

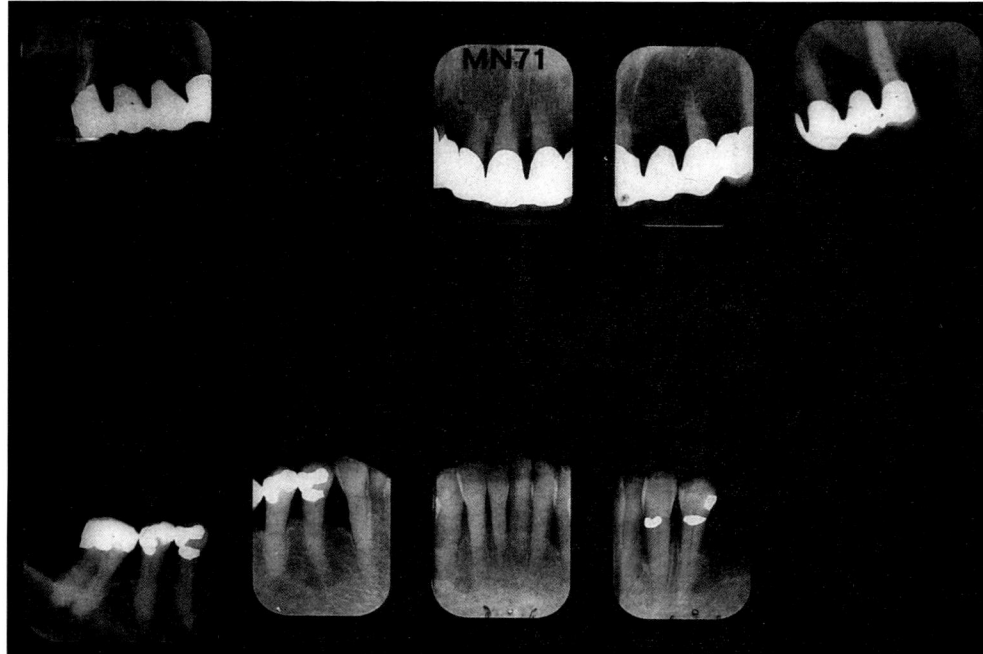

Fig 264b Complete-mouth radiographs of the patient in Fig 264a, aged 71 years, at the 15-year reexamination (1987). No additional teeth have been lost, no further loss of probing attachment level has been recorded, and no caries lesions have been detected. Compare the bone level on the mesial surface of the maxillary right second premolar (tooth 15) and the distal surface of the mandibular right canine (tooth 43) to that exhibited in 1972 (Fig 264a).

Case 3. Complete-mouth radiographs from a 56-year-old woman in test group 3 are shown at the baseline examination in 1972 (Fig 264a). Radiographs from the same patient, aged 71, are shown at the 15-year reexamination in 1987 (Fig 264b).

In 1972, the number of remaining teeth and remaining periodontal support were far below

Fig 265 Complete-mouth radiographs of the same patient, aged 77 years (1993).

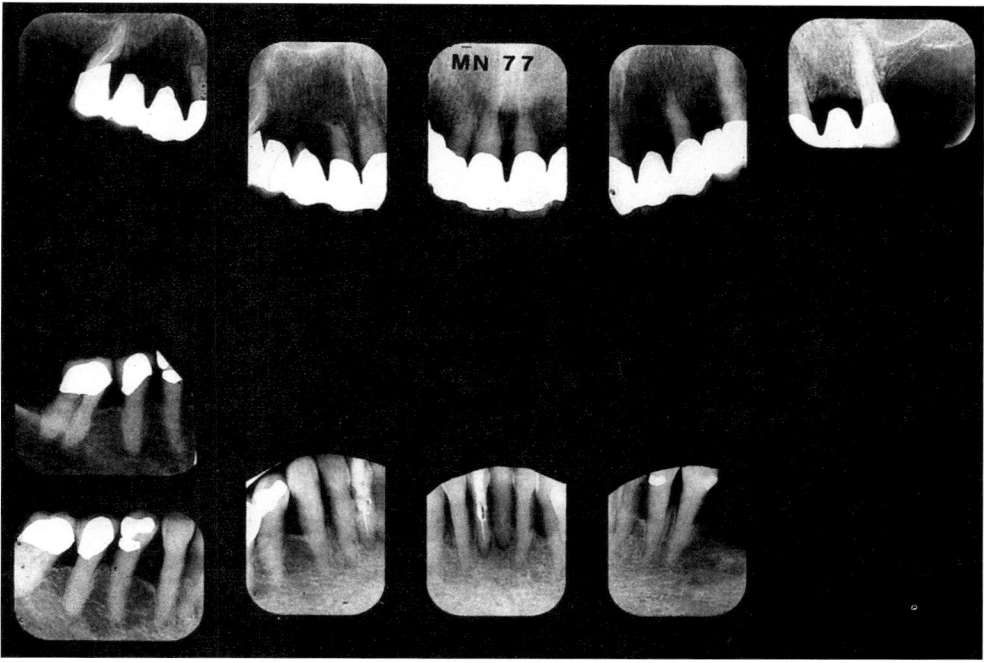

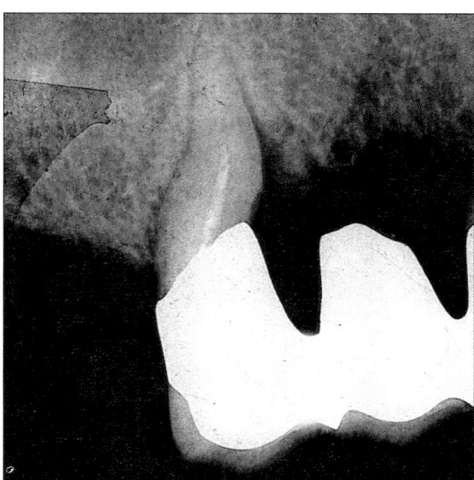

Fig 266 Radiograph of the maxillary right second premolar in 1972.

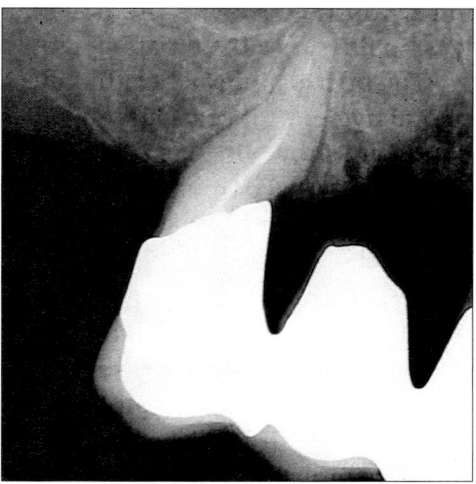

Fig 267 Radiograph of the maxillary right second premolar in 1993.

the average for 56 year olds. During the following 15 years, no teeth were lost, no further loss of attachment level was recorded, and no caries lesions were detected.

Complete-mouth radiographs from 1993 show the status at age 77 years (Fig 265). Figures 266 and 267 show details of the maxillary right second premolar in 1972 and 1993, respectively. De-

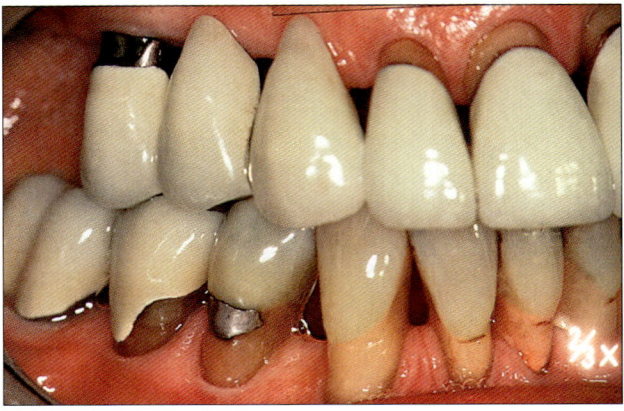 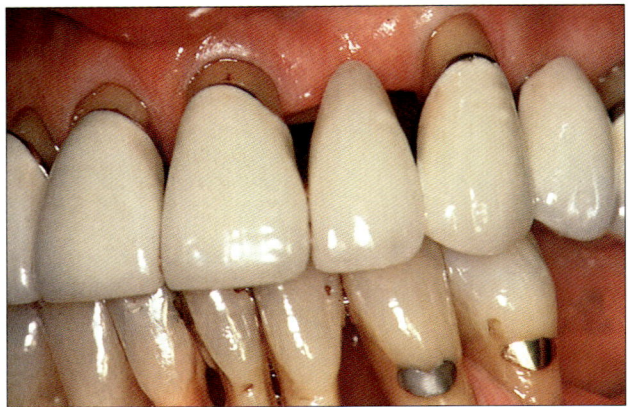

Figs 268 and 269 Buccal gingival health and oral hygiene status of the same patient, aged 76 years, at the 20-year reexamination. The maxillary fixed prosthesis, more than 20 years old, is still intact, without recurrent caries.

spite initially advanced loss of periodontal support and deep pockets, there was excellent healing around the second premolar, and the tooth was retained as a fixed partial denture abutment.

The buccal gingival health status and the level of oral hygiene 20 years after the baseline examination are shown in Figs 268 and 269. The maxillary fixed partial denture, more than 25 years old, is still intact and without recurrent caries.

Case 4. The long-term effect of excellent gingival plaque control is illustrated by further case documentation. The following case illustrates the effect of inadequate and excellent postoperative gingival plaque control in the same patient. Figure 270 shows complete-mouth radiographs of a 50-year-old man in 1969. While under the care of a general practitioner, he had undergone gingivectomy of all quadrants because of generalized pocketing of greater than 3 mm. He received no postoperative maintenance program for gingival plaque control. In addition, the patient developed polyarthritis, for which anti-inflammatory drugs were prescribed.

Three years later (1972), complete-mouth radiographs show dramatic postoperative loss of alveolar bone, particularly on the maxillary left anterior teeth (Nos. 21, 22, 23 [FDI tooth numbering system]) and the mandibular teeth (Nos. 44, 43,

42, 41, 31, 32, 33, 34) (Fig 271). In the absence of preoperative and postoperative gingival plaque control programs, periodontal surgery will accelerate loss of periodontal support.

In 1972, after detailed examination, followed by education in comprehensive self-care and self-diagnosis, he received an initial, thorough non-surgical scaling, root planing, debridement, and repeated PMTC. The effect of this initial treatment was evaluated after 1 month. A supplementary modified Widman flap surgery was then performed, from the maxillary right central incisor to the left second premolar; this was combined with apicoectomy and retrograde root filling of the left canine, which had a periapical lesion and a mesiopalatal marginal-apical communication. At the same session, the maxillary right second premolar was extracted because of root fracture and marginal-apical communication.

After a 2-month healing period, including excellent gingival plaque control by self-care (0.2% chlorhexidine mouthrinse twice a day for 2 weeks and mechanical cleaning) and PMTC once every 2 weeks, the maxillary lateral incisors and the four mandibular incisors were extracted and provisional fixed partial dentures were made. Three months later, maxillary and mandibular prostheses were made on the following abutments: teeth 13, 11, 21, 23, and 25 and teeth 44, 43, 33, and 34.

Fig 270 Complete-mouth radiographs of a 50-year-old man in 1969. The patient had undergone gingivectomy in all quadrants.

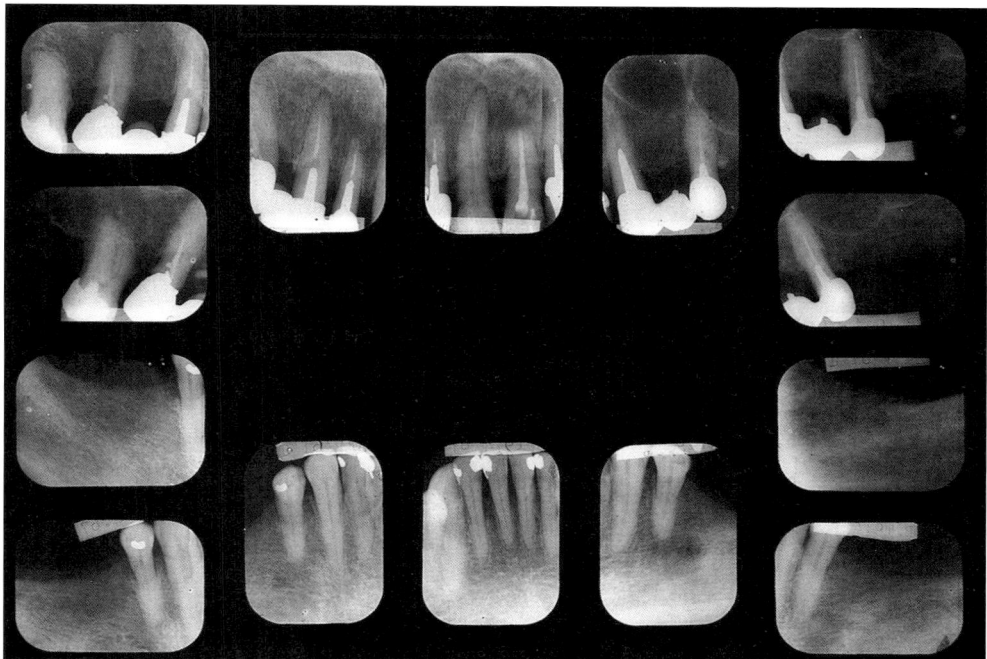

Fig 271 Same patient, exhibiting dramatic postoperative loss of alveolar bone, 3 years after surgery (1972). He had not been provided with any postoperative program to maintain plaque control.

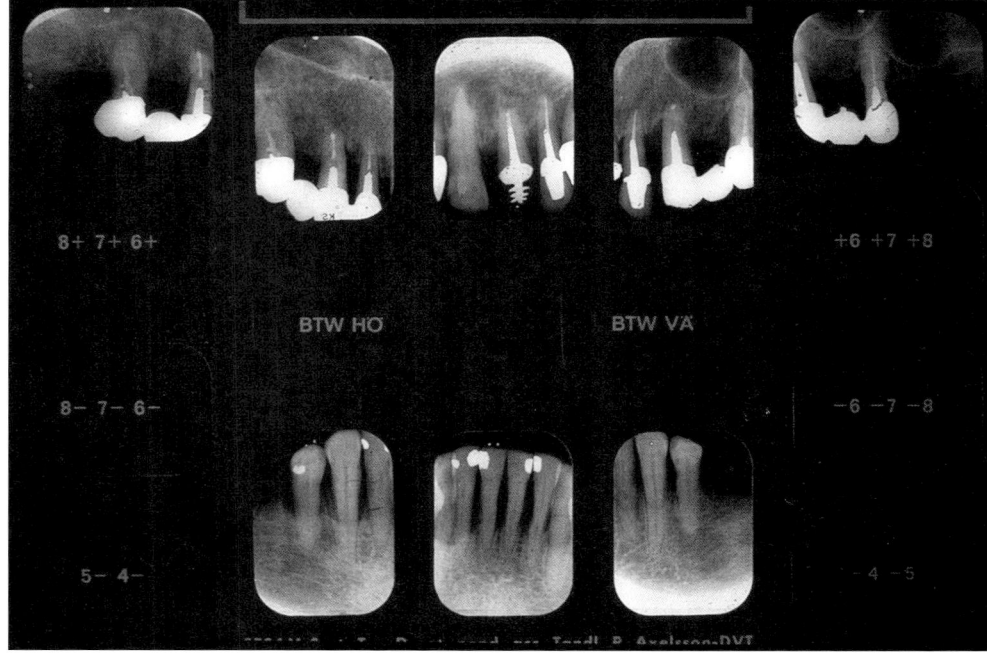

Figures 272a and 272b show complete-mouth radiographs after 13 (1985) and 23 (1995) years, respectively. Excellent gingival plaque control was achieved by a maintenance program comprising self-care supplemented by PMTC and debridement at needs-related intervals. No further teeth were lost, nor was there any further loss of periodontal support. Figures 272a and 272b show some gain of support, notably on the mesial surfaces of the maxillary left and right canines and

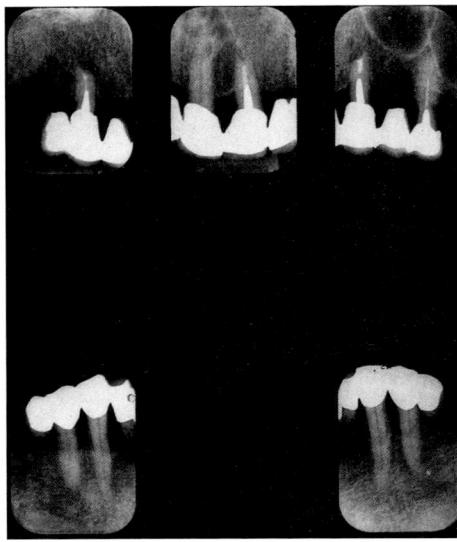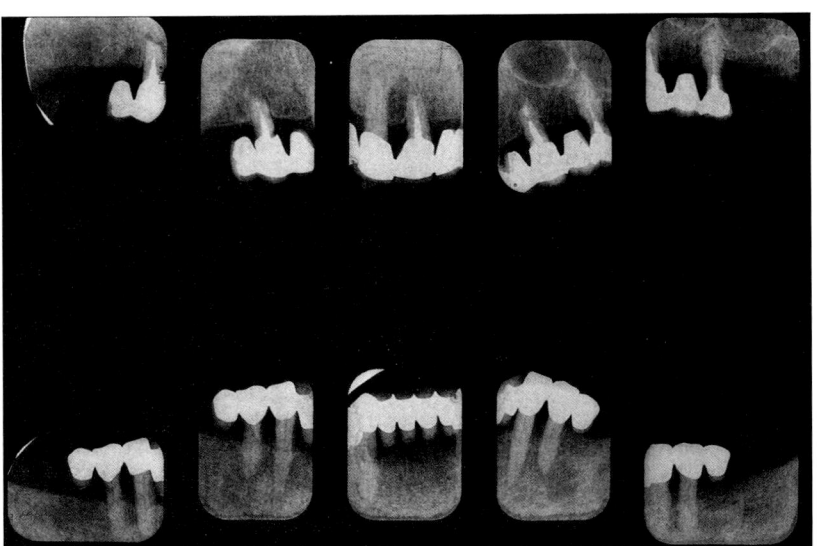

Fig 272a Same patient in 1985, 13 years after a second round of periodontal surgery and restoration of the dentition. This time, the patient was provided with a rigorous maintenance program to ensure excellent gingival plaque control.

Fig 272b Same patient in 1995. No further teeth have been lost, and there has been no further loss of periodontal support. In fact, some support has been gained, especially on the mesial surfaces of the maxillary left and right canines and the distal surface of the maxillary left central incisor. Intensive mechanical cleaning has resulted in some loss of tooth substance from the exposed roots, particularly from the maxillary abutment teeth.

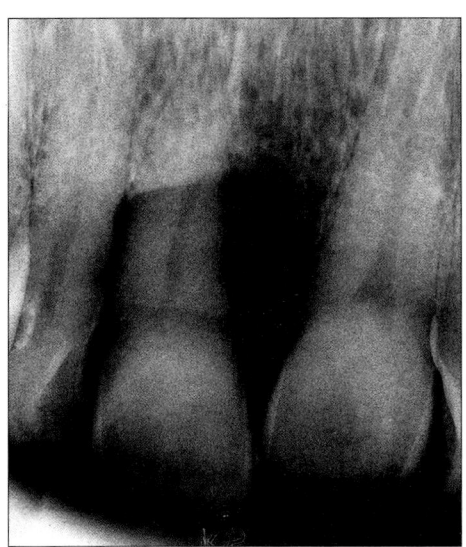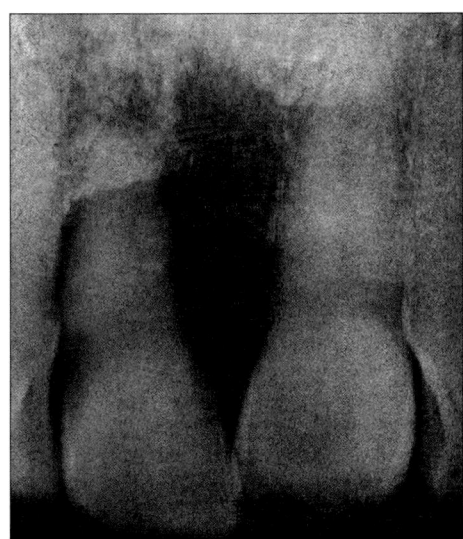

Fig 273a Advanced loss of bone support at the beginning of treatment in 1972.

Fig 273b Stable periodontal attachment level 22 years later (1994), maintained because of the patient's excellent plaque control.

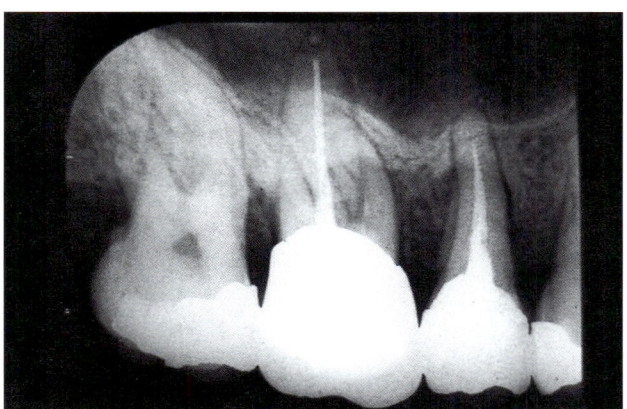

Fig 274 Advanced loss of alveolar bone around the maxillary right posterior teeth in a 40-year-old smoker.

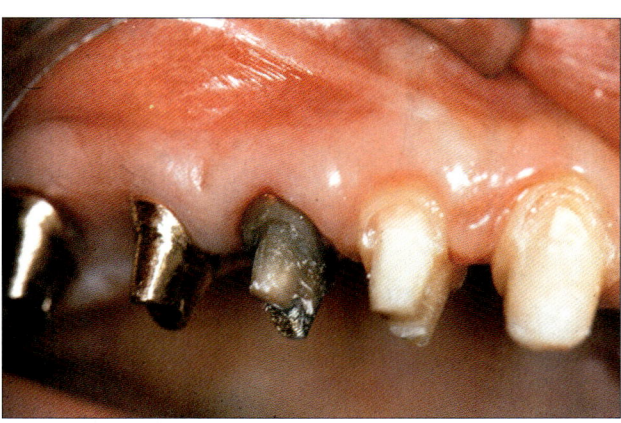

Fig 275 Cast gold post and cores with collars made for the mesiobuccal roots of the molars in the same patient.

the distal surface of the maxillary left central incisor. After 23 years of intensive mechanical cleaning by self-care, there has been some iatrogenic loss of tooth substance from the exposed roots, particularly the maxillary abutment teeth.

Case 5. Even teeth with very advanced loss of periodontal support may be maintained for many years after active periodontal therapy when a balance between etiologic factors and host response has been established by a needs-related maintenance program. Because excellent gingival plaque control habits, based on self-diagnosis, had been established in 1972, the probing attachment level on the maxillary right central incisor remained stable from 1972 to 1994 (Figs 273a and 273b). Over the last 20 years, the patient has been recalled only once or twice a year for supportive PMTC and debridement by a dental hygienist and has been reexamined by a dentist every second year.

Case 6. The radiograph in Fig 274, taken in 1975 in a 40-year-old female smoker, shows very advanced loss of alveolar bone around the maxillary right posterior teeth (Nos. 15, 16, 17). There was grade III furcation involvement on the mesial, buccal, and distal aspects of the first and second molars. After initial nonsurgical scaling, root plan-

ing, debridement, PMTC, and oral hygiene education based on self-diagnosis, the first and second molars were hemisectioned without flap surgery. The distobuccal and palatal roots of the molars were extracted after hemisection and endodontic treatment of the mesiobuccal roots.

The canine (tooth 13), premolars (teeth 14 and 15), and the mesiobuccal roots were prepared as abutments for a fixed partial denture. Cast gold posts and cores with collars were made for the mesiobuccal roots (Fig 275). Five "single-rooted" teeth in a "straight" row were used as abutments, which is favorable for hygiene. A shoulder was prepared mesiobuccally on the canine and the two premolars (Fig 275), and the porcelain abutted the shoulder directly (Fig 276). This allowed supragingival positioning of the margins of the prosthesis, facilitating gingival plaque control without compromising esthetics by a visible gold margin.

Figure 277 shows a radiograph taken 2 years after treatment (1977). Figure 278, taken 17 years after treatment (1992), shows even further improvement in alveolar bone support as an effect of a maintenance program based on excellent gingival plaque control by self-care, supplemented at needs-related intervals by PMTC.

Even in individuals with advanced forms of periodontal disease, further periodontal attachment loss can be prevented by long-term mainte-

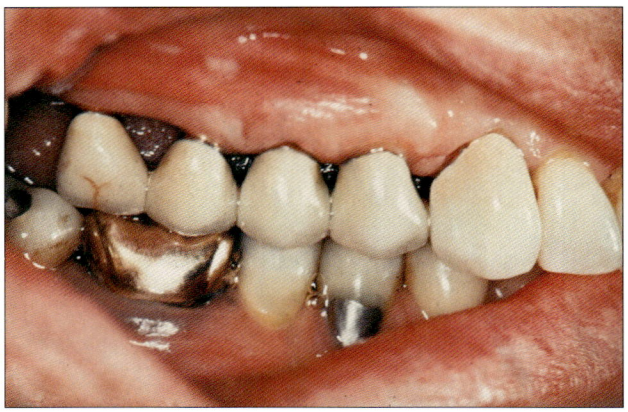

Fig 276 Permanent fixed partial denture in the same patient. The supragingival positioning of the margins of the prosthesis facilitates gingival plaque control.

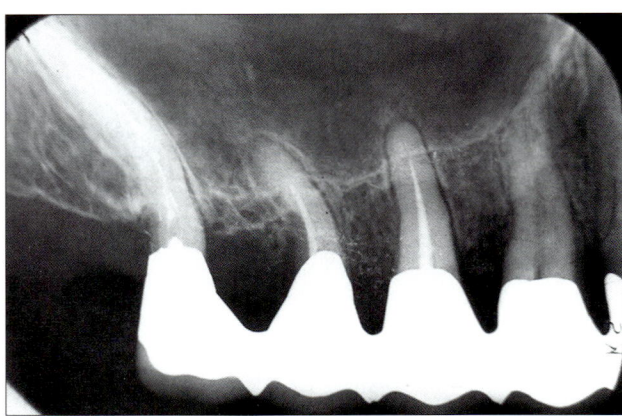

Fig 277 Radiograph taken in 1977, 2 years after treatment.

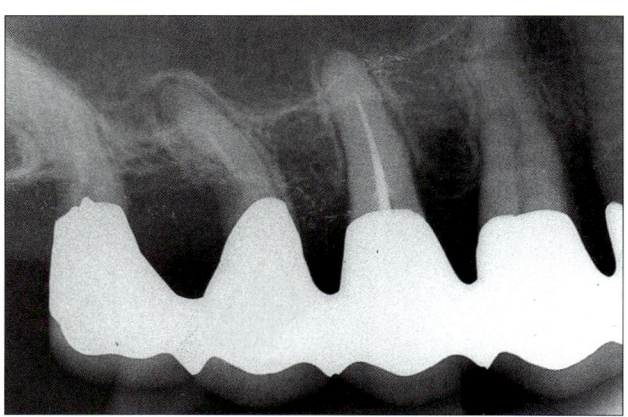

Fig 278 Radiograph taken in 1992, 17 years after treatment, revealing further improvement in alveolar bone support as a result of an effective maintenance program.

nance programs. These programs must be based on recognized methods for mechanical removal of gingival plaque by self-care, supplemented at needs-related intervals by PMTC and nonaggressive removal of subgingival biofilms by debridement. These methods are effective because they are causally directed, targeting the gingival plaque and the subgingival biofilm, which contains periopathogens inaccessible to the phagocytosing PMNLs, chemical plaque control agents, and antibiotics.

Mechanical removal of the gingival plaque and the subgingival biofilm facilitates accessibility for antibodies and complements to the remaining periopathogens and their toxic products. The phagocytosing and killing potential of PMNLs and macrophages are enhanced. In addition a "booster" effect from antigens into the connective tissue may be expected each time the gingival plaque and subgingival biofilm are removed, gradually improving the efficiency of the specific immune response, as discussed earlier (see Fig 255).

During the last few years, DNA probe techniques have been developed for comprehensive analysis of the subgingival periopathogenic microflora, facilitating detection of the most virulent periopathogens (*P gingivalis, A actinomycetemcomitans,* and *B forsythus*) in individuals susceptible to periodontitis (for details see chapter 1).

New knowledge about the pathogenesis of periodontal diseases, at not only the cellular but

Fig 279 Schematic illustration showing how antimicrobials, low-dose doxycycline hyclate (Periostat), alendronate, and NSAIDs may influence the pathogenesis of periodontal diseases. (From Page, 1999. Reprinted with permission.)

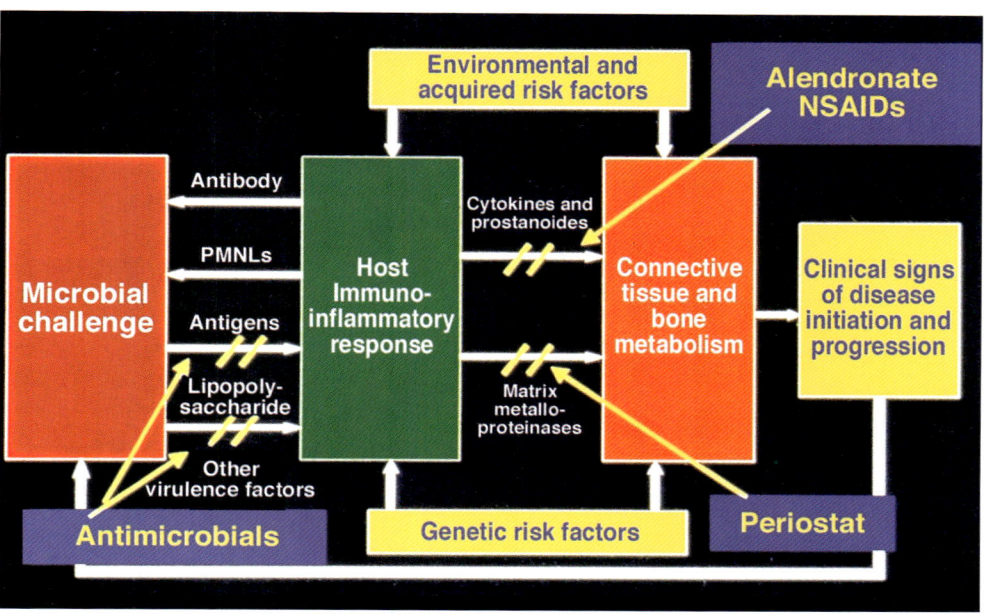

also the molecular level, has clarified the question of individual variations in susceptibility to periodontal diseases, on the basis of genetics, systemic diseases, and external modifying risk factors, such as smoking. New test methods and diagnostic tools have been developed to identify susceptible patients, which is important from a cost-effectiveness aspect. There are, for example, tests to identify genetic IL-1 polymorphism, methods for analysis of the gingival crevicular fluid PGE_2 levels, and measurement of periodontal pocket temperature as an indicator of active lesions. As mentioned earlier, IL-1 polymorphism and smoking may together identify more than 80% of susceptible patients (see chapters 2 to 4).

To supplement the highly effective mechanical methods for removal of gingival plaque and subgingival biofilms, new, efficient chemical plaque control agents and delivery systems have been developed. New principles for the use of antibiotics have been introduced, specifically restricting their use to susceptible patients in whom the periopathogens have been identified. In addition to their well-known antimicrobial effects, low doses of tetracycline antibiotics are effective chelators and inhibitors of MMPs. Low doses of

doxycycline hyclate (Periostat, CollaGenex, Newtown, PA) reduce destruction of collagenous connective tissue of gingiva and periodontal ligament by inhibiting MMP activity. Other new products include alendronate, a bisphosphorate, and nonsteroidal anti-inflammatory drugs (NSAIDs). Alendroin, taken orally, decreases alveolar bone resorption presumably by enhancing bone deposition. The NSAIDs used topically as an oral rinse or in toothpaste decrease alveolar bone loss by suppressing the production of prostaglandins. How these new drugs may interfere in the pathogenesis of periodontal diseases is schematically illustrated in Fig 279. Thus, application of current knowledge, materials, and methods should allow effective treatment and control of periodontal diseases, even in highly susceptible individuals.

Repair or regeneration of periodontal tissues

Not only repair (bone fill) of alveolar bone pockets, but also true regeneration of all components of the periodontal support (root cement, peri-

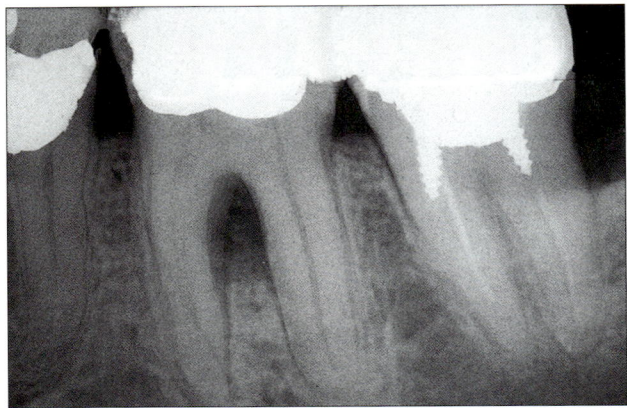

Fig 280 Advanced loss of alveolar bone in the furcation area of the mandibular left first molar (May 1990).

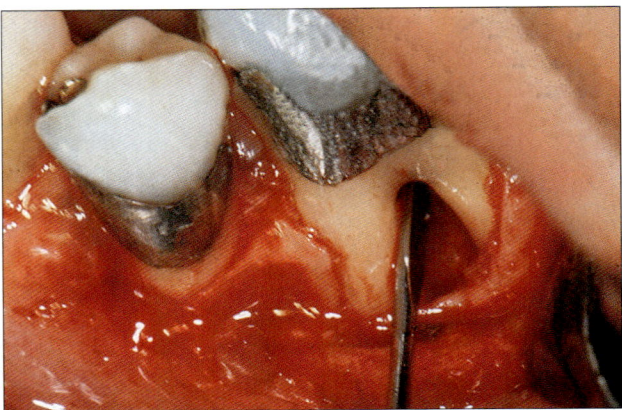

Fig 281 Extremely advanced furcation defect, visible during debridement and root planing with a PER-IO-TOR 4 reciprocating instrument.

odontal ligament, and alveolar bone) is possible today. The two most frequently used methods for regenerative therapy are so-called guided tissue regeneration by the use of barriers and matrix-guided regeneration using enamel matrix derivate (EMD) gel (Emdogain, Biora, Lund, Sweden).

Guided tissue regeneration

So-called guided tissue regeneration (GTR), based on original research by Nyman et al (1982a, 1982b, 1987), was introduced during the late 1980s. In principle, after open flap surgery and cleaning of the root surface, a nonresorbable or resorbable membrane (barrier) is inserted between the soft tissue flap and the root surface to maintain a space during the healing period. Today it is questioned whether arrest of the periodontal defect by GTR should be considered as true regeneration or as repair of the periodontal tissue (Araujo et al, 1999). More important is the long-term outcome of the treatment, exemplified by the following case.

Primary radiographs showed advanced loss of alveolar bone (more than 50%) in the furcation area of the mandibular left first molar (Fig 280). The initial buccal probing depth was 12 mm.

Grade II to III furcation involvement was diagnosed clinically on the buccal surface. Before surgery, the patient received oral hygiene education, PMTC, and nonsurgical periodontal treatment including scaling, debridement, and root planing. In response to treatment, the buccal probing depth decreased by 3 mm and the gingival margin healed.

The furcation area was exposed by open full-thickness flap surgery. The narrow dome of the deep furcation area was briefly scaled with a universal curette; this was followed by final nonaggressive scaling, debridement, and root planing with PER-IO-TOR 2 and 4 (Dentatus, Hägersten, Sweden) (Fig 281). The root surfaces were cleaned of debris and washed with sterile saline. Figure 281 shows the extremely advanced furcation defect during debridement and root planing. Only a partial, paper-thin lingual bony wall remained. At surgery, vertical probing attachment loss was 12 mm and horizontal attachment loss was 9 mm. Vertical probing depth was 9 mm; ie, there was 3 mm of gingival recession.

For regenerative therapy by GTR, a nonresorbable Gore-Tex expanded polytetrafluoroethylene membrane of single-tooth width was applied to the buccal surface in May 1990 (Fig 282). From 1 week before to 6 weeks after surgery,

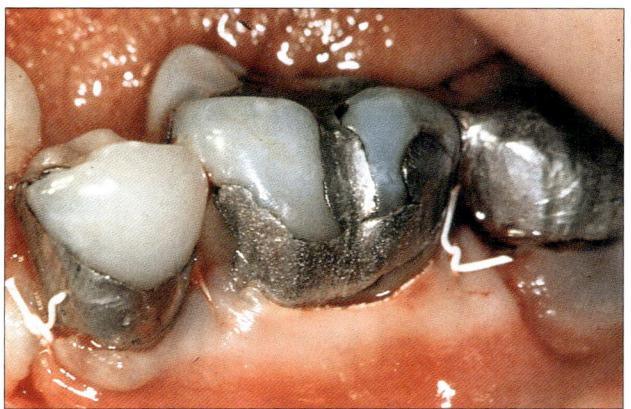

Fig 282 Replaced and sutured flap, which covers a nonresorbable expanded polytetrafluoroethylene barrier membrane.

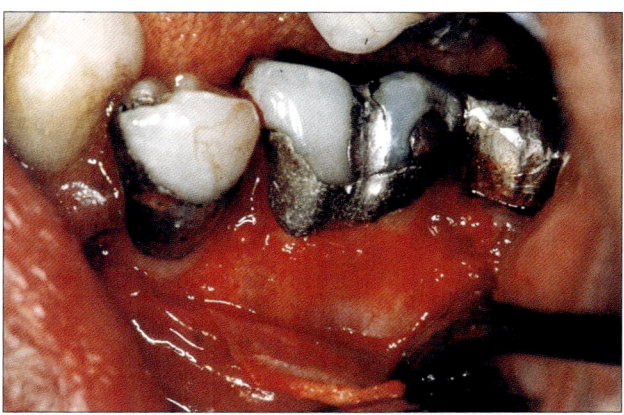

Fig 283 Furcation defect filled with noninflammatory, nonmineralized osteogenic tissue at membrane removal, 6 weeks after flap surgery.

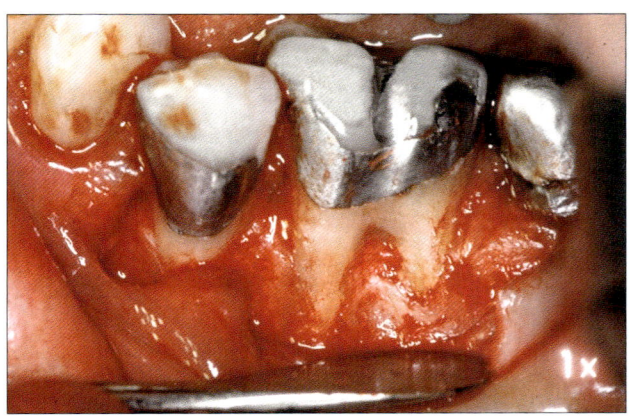

Fig 284 Complete bone regeneration of the formerly advanced furcation defect (May 1991).

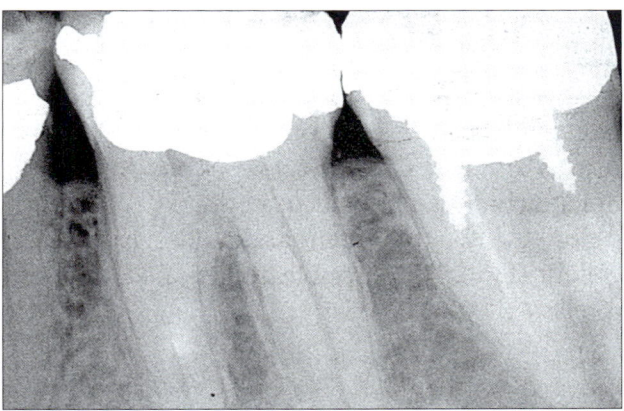

Fig 285 Total arrest of the advanced furcation defect and formation of a new periodontal ligament space around the furcation area (May 1991).

chemical plaque control was established by rinsing twice a day with 0.1% chlorhexidine solution. Six weeks after treatment, the barrier membrane was removed. The furcation defect was already filled with noninflammatory, nonmineralized osteogenic tissue (Fig 283).

For the first month after removal of the membrane, the patient was included in a weekly maintenance program including self-care education and PMTC; thereafter the patient returned once a month for the following 6 months. At the 1-year

reexamination (May 1991), the buccal probing depth was only 1 mm. The grateful patient then generously consented to direct inspection of the healing tissue by reentry surgery (Fig 284).

A radiograph (Fig 285) taken 1 year later (1991) shows total arrest of the extremely advanced furcation bone defect and the formation of a new periodontal ligament space all around the furcation area. Because of the maintenance program, based on excellent gingival plaque control, at the 8-year follow-up there was no deterio-

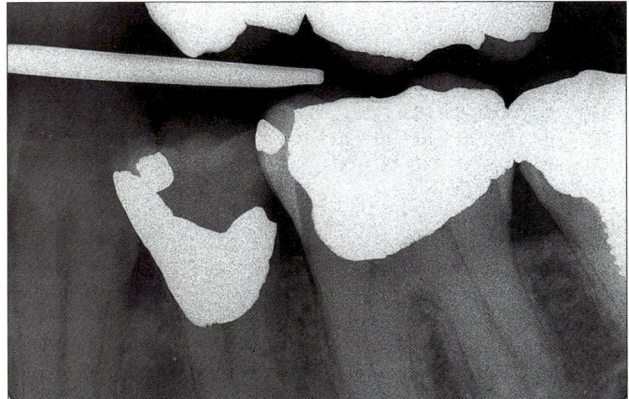

Fig 286 Radiograph in 1998 shows complete bone arrestment 8 years after the regenerative therapy.

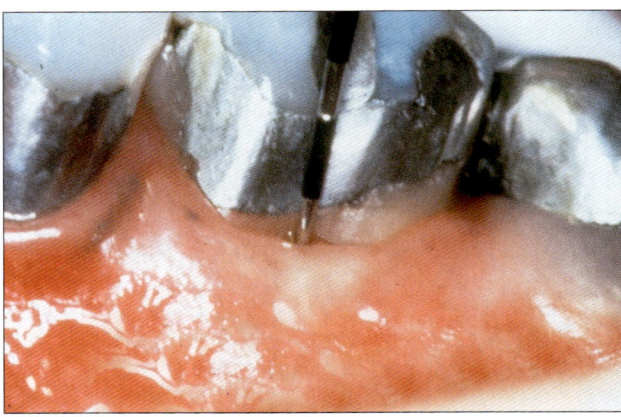

Fig 287 Probing depth of 1 mm at the 8-year follow-up. There has been no deterioration of the initial healing. Healthy gingiva and vertical and horizontal attachment gain of 9 mm has been maintained for 8 years.

ration in the initial healing. There was still complete bone arrestment in the furcation area according to the radiograph taken in 1998 (Fig 286). The probing pocket depth was still only 1 mm. After 1 and 8 years, vertical and horizontal probing attachment gain was more than 9 mm. In addition, the health of the marginal gingiva was excellent (Fig 287) (unpublished data, Heden and Axelsson, 1990, 1998).

Matrix-guided regeneration

An even more promising regenerative method is based on matrix-guided regenerative factors, using Emdogain gel. The product is based on the numerous observations of a link between the enamel matrix and cementum formation.

The EMD protein is extracted from the immediate layer between root cementum and root dentin. Figures 288a and 288b show histologic evaluation of periodontal regeneration with enamel matrix derivates in monkeys. The third molar of a young monkey was extracted and the enamel matrix was mechanically taken from the developing crown. The maxillary lateral incisor was gently extracted, and a cavity was made in the mesial surface of the root. The enamel matrix was

placed in the cavity, after which the incisor was immediately reimplanted. A similar extraction-reimplantation procedure was performed with the contralateral incisor, but no enamel matrix was placed in the cavity.

Eight weeks after the reimplantation, the monkey was sacrificed and the teeth with surrounding periodontal tissues were decalcified, sectioned, and examined in the light microscope. A layer of acellular cementum, firmly attached to the dentin, had been formed in the cavity where enamel matrix had been placed before the replantation (see Fig 288a). Complete regeneration of the periodontal ligament was achieved, with natural orientation of the principal fibers, their attachment in the newly formed root cementum surface, and regenerated alveolar bone. This is seldom achieved with GTR therapy. In the control tooth, where no enamel matrix was placed, fragments of acellular, poorly attached hard tissue had been formed in the cavity (see Fig 288b).

The following cases, which use the matrix-guided method, illustrate the results that can be achieved during a relatively short period of time (unpublished data, Axelsson, 1995 to 2002).

Before treatment, new patients undergo comprehensive history taking and clinical diagnosis, followed by education and training in self-

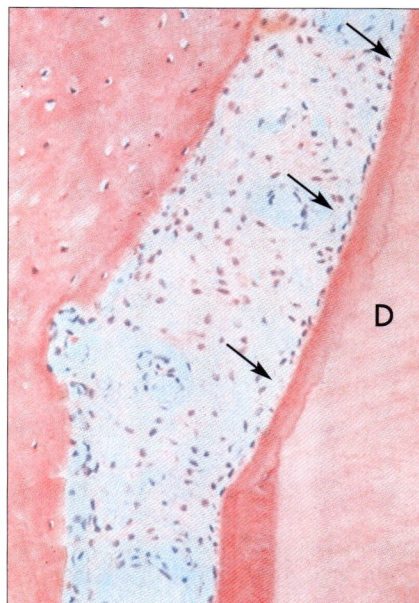

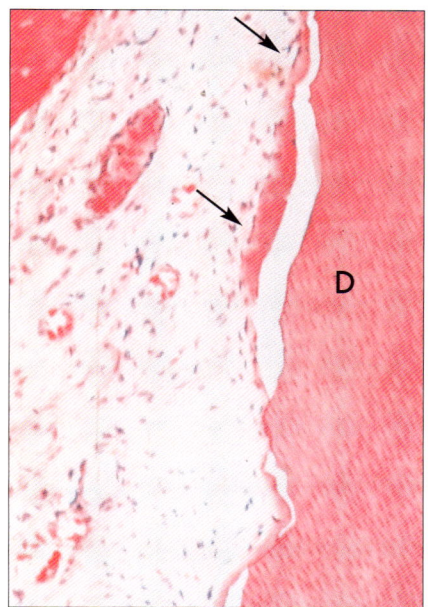

Fig 288a Histologic evaluation of periodontal regeneration with enamel matrix derivatives in monkeys. A layer of acellular cementum firmly attached to the dentin (D) has formed in the cavity *(arrows)*, where enamel matrix had been placed before reimplantation (H&E, original magnification ×1,500). (From Hammarström, 1997. Reprinted with permission.)

Fig 288b Histologic evaluation of periodontal regeneration in a control tooth, in which no enamel matrix was placed. Fragments of a cellular, poorly attached hard tissue *(arrows)* have formed in the cavity. D = Dentin (H&E, original magnification ×1,500). (From Hammarström, 1997. Reprinted with permission.)

diagnosis and self-care, to optimize daily gingival plaque control. To reduce the microbial challenge as much as possible, comprehensive nonaggressive scaling, root planing, and debridement, combined with bacteriocidic antimicrobial pocket irrigation (0.1% iodine solution), are followed by PMTC to eliminate the subgingival biofilm, nonattaching microflora, and calculus. So-called "full-mouth disinfection" is performed, including not only toothcleaning, but also tongue scraping and chemical plaque control (Axelsson et al, 1987; Quirynen et al, 1995).

The effect of this initial hygiene phase is evaluated by DNA probe analysis of the subgingival microflora. Antibiotics are not usually necessary but may be used restrictively in the most highly susceptible patients and patients with cardiovascular disease or diabetes and when there are persistently high counts of the most virulent pathogens: *P gingivalis, B forsythus,* and *A actinomycetemcomitans.* For patients with high counts of all three pathogens, amoxycillin (375 mg) with metronidazole (400 mg) is used 3 times/day for 10 days, starting 2 days preoperatively.

A final subgingival debridement combined with antimicrobial irrigation is carried out to remove remaining biofilms and to increase the accessibility of the antibiotics 2 days before surgery. The aim is to achieve an oral cavity and particularly preoperative lesions as free of infection as possible. As an effect of this intensive presurgical treatment, even the sites that will receive regenerative therapy are healed. Therefore, bleeding during surgery is signifcantly reduced, which optimizes both the accessability for the Emdogain gel and the oucome of therapy. If there is no *A actinomycetemcomitans* infection in the sites to be treated, only metronidazole should be used. Al-

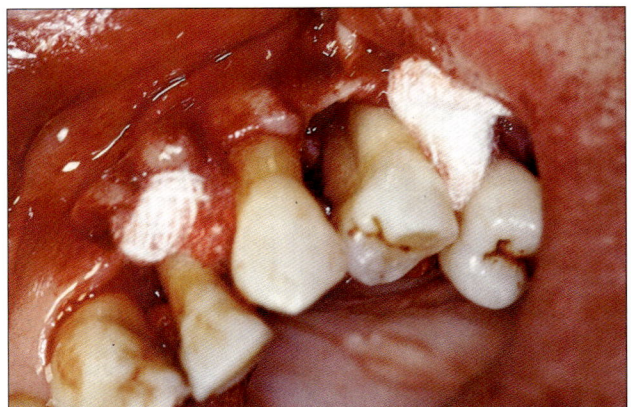

Fig 289a Intrabony defect after removal of granulation tissue mesial of the maxillary left first premolar (tooth 24).

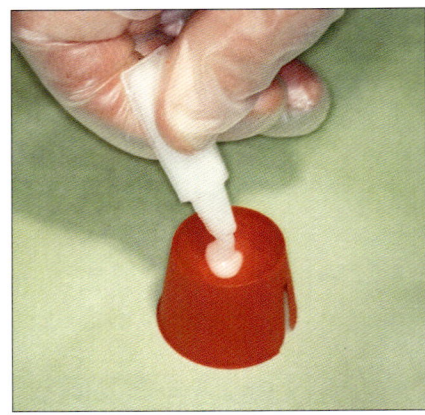

Fig 289b EDTA gel is pressed out from the original package.

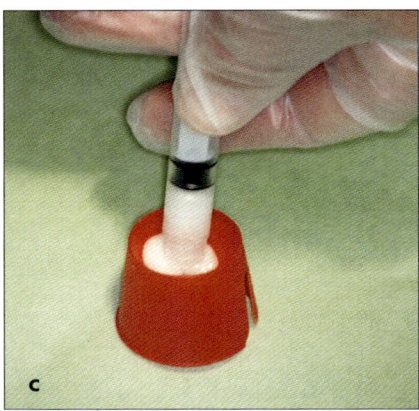

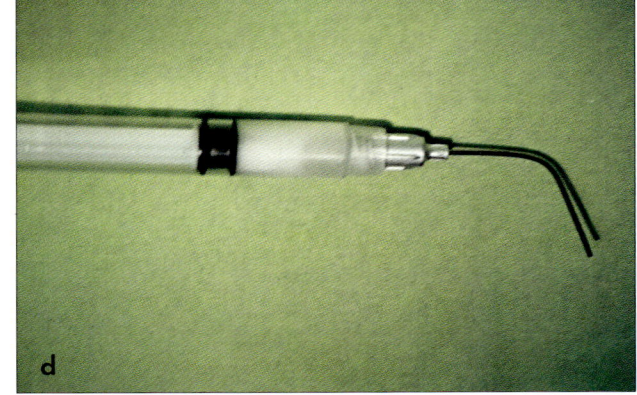

Figs 289c and 289d EDTA gel is placed into a syringe.

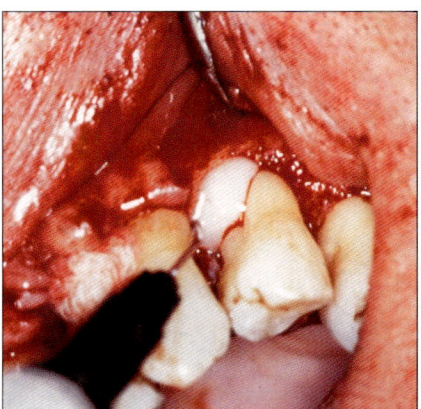

Fig 289e After naonaggressive mechanical cleaning of the root surface. The EDTA gel is applied with the syringe. After 2 minutes the gel is removed by generous irrigation with saline solution and the root surface is dried.

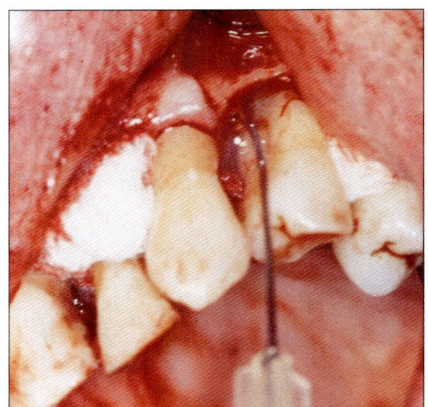

Fig 289f The Emdogain gel in a syringe is applied in the intrabony defect. Thereafter it was also applied on the roots of teeth 22, 23, and 25. Radiographs before and after treatment are shown in Figs 146 to 149 in chapter 3.

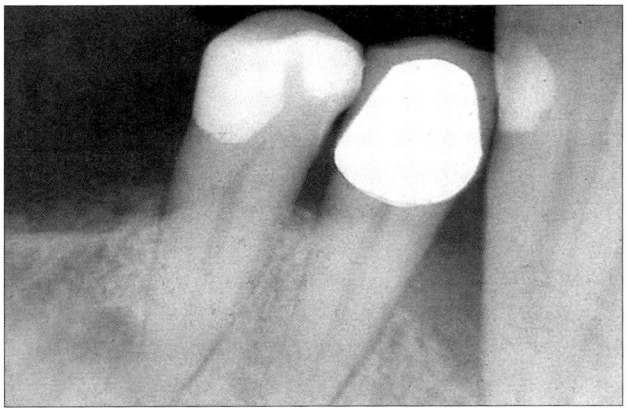

Fig 290 One- and two-wall defects along the distal surface of the mandibular right canine before treatment.

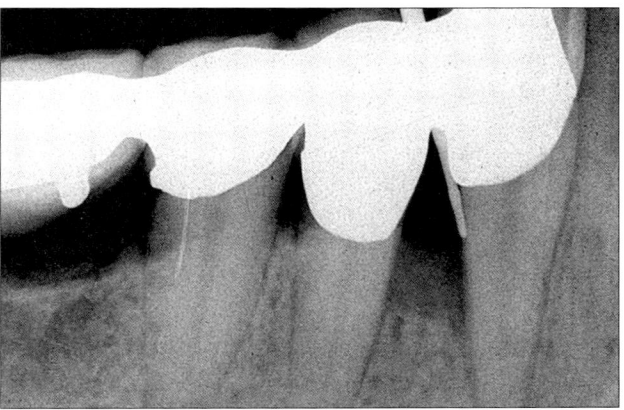

Fig 291 Considerable gain in periodontal support 11 months after treatment with matrix-guided material (Emdogain gel).

ternatively, the sites could be treated topically with tetracycline fibers or metronidazole or doxycycline gels during the week before treatment.

For self-care, the patient supplements mechanical plaque control and tongue scraping with a chlorhexidine mouthrinse (0.12%) used twice a day during the week before treatment and for 6 weeks after treatment. However, it should be noted that a toothpaste without anions, such as sodium lauryl sulphate and monofluorophosphate, must be used to avoid inactivation of the cationic chlorhexidine. The patient refrains from interdental mechanical toothcleaning near the wound for the first 4 weeks of healing. However, a special "extra extra soft" toothbrush may be used with caution around the treated teeth from 2 to 3 days after surgery.

Surgical access to the site is gained by a tailored miniflap. After removal of granulation tissue in order to optimize accessability and reduce bleeding (Fig 289a), supplementary mechanical cleaning of the visible root surface by nonaggressive debridement is performed. Thereafter the root surface is chemically cleaned and conditioned with an ethylenediaminetetraacetic acid (EDTA) gel (Figs 289a to 289e), irrigated with

saline solution, and dried before application of the Emdogain gel via a syringe (Fig 289f). Two to six teeth can be treated at the same visit with one package of gel. After 2 weeks, the sutures are removed. The professional part of the maintenance program, based on meticulous gingival plaque control, starts after 4 weeks, with three PMTCs, once every 2 weeks, and then monthly for the following 5 months. The first reexamination, including radiographs, is normally scheduled for 6 months.

Case 1. Figure 290 shows a deep, combined one- and two-wall defect on the distal aspect of the mandibular right canine (tooth 43) in a 42-year-old woman, a heavy smoker for about 20 years (30 pack years). After 1 year, a probing attachment gain of 6 mm had been achieved, as well as considerable bone regeneration (Fig 291). Typical for this kind of regenerative therapy is that the attachment gain occurs during the first few months postoperatively, but bone mineralization may continue for some years. At the same visit, the maxillary right first and second premolars (teeth 14 and 15) and the palatal root of the maxillary right first molar (tooth 16) were also treated with the

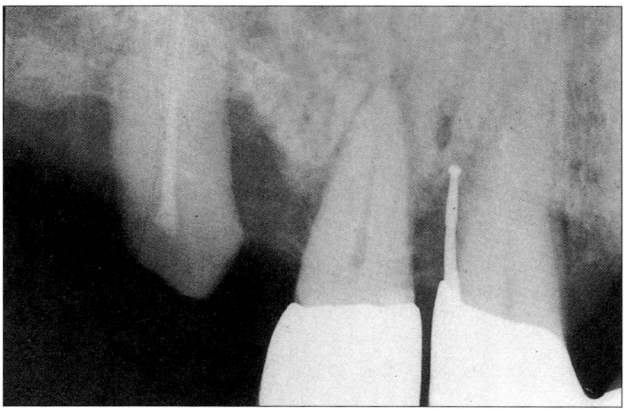

Fig 292 Advanced one- and two-wall bony defects mesial of the palatal root of the maxillary right first molar (tooth 16) before treatment. A thin buccal bone wall remained on the premolars (teeth 14 and 15).

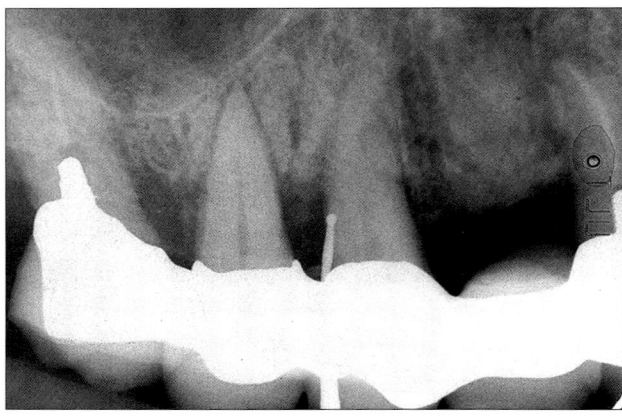

Fig 293 Result 1 year after treatment with matrix-guided material. Observe the complete arrestment of the mesial bone defect of the first molar and the considerable increase in bone around the premolars.

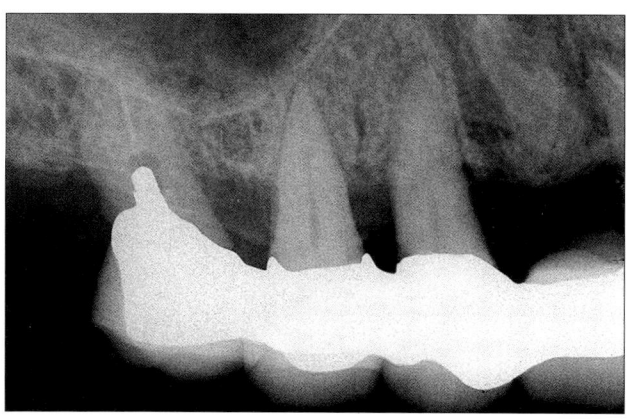

Fig 294 The result was still maintained almost 6 years after regenerative therapy.

same regenerative therapy because of a deep one- and two-wall bone defect mesial of the first molar (tooth 16) and palatal one-wall bone defects at the premolars (teeth 14 and 15) (Fig 292). The molar was recently hemisectioned because of furcation involvement degree 3 mesially and distally. The patient was motivated to stop smoking after treatment.

Figure 293 shows the arrested result, particularly at the mesial surface of the palatal root of the first molar (tooth 16) after 1 year. This result was still well maintained almost 6 years after treatment

(Fig 294). There was even a considerable gain of periodontal support around the premolars.

Case 2. A 45-year-old nonsmoking male patient presented with a combined one- and two-wall periodontal defect on the distal surface of the maxillary left first premolar (tooth 24) (Fig 295). Figure 296 shows healing after only 6 months. The inserted probe clearly shows the considerable probing attachment gain, and new bone has formed up to the horizontal crest. The mesiobuccal root of the second molar was hemisectioned because of

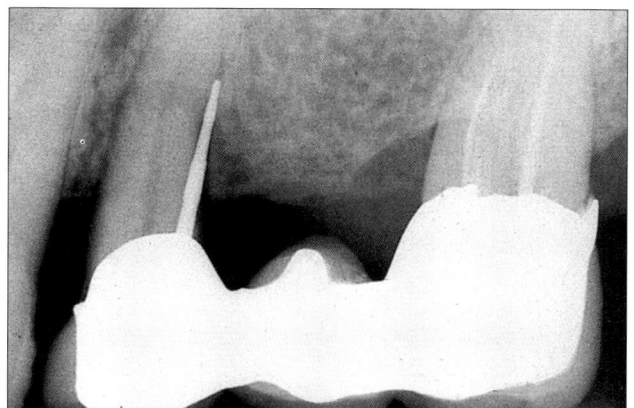

Fig 295 One- and two-wall alveolar bony defect on the distal surface of the maxillary left first premolar (tooth 24) before treatment.

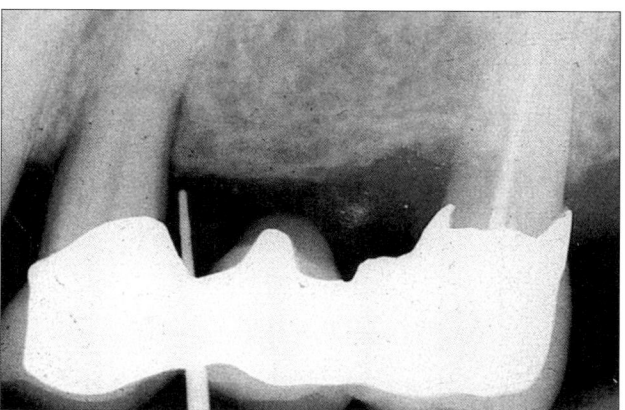

Fig 296 Result 6 months after regenerative therapy.

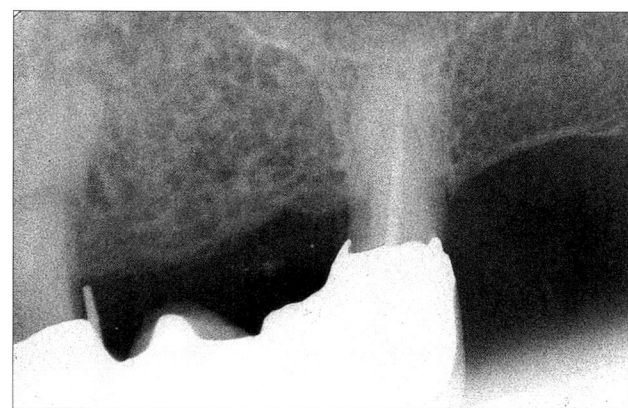

Fig 297 Well-maintained result almost 5 years after treatment.

grade III furcation involvement. (The distobuccal root had already been removed.) This result was still well maintained almost 5 years later (Fig 297).

Case 3. A 68-year-old man, a former smoker (more than 20 cigarettes a day for more than 40 years or 50 pack years), had an apical-marginal communication on the mesial and buccal surfaces of the maxillary left first premolar (tooth 24) (Fig 298). Because the tooth was the posterior abutment of a four-unit bridge, hemisection of the buccal root was planned after explorative flap surgery. How-

ever, after hemisection, the entire buccal surface of the lingual root was visible up to the apex (Fig 299). The gutta-percha root filling material was visible through the thin buccal root wall. As a last resort, the buccal root surface was nonaggressively mechanically cleaned and then chemically cleaned and surface conditioned with EDTA gel, before application of the Emdogain gel and resuturing of the flap. Considerable regeneration of alveolar bone around the apex and the mesial aspect of the lingual root was found only 4 months postoperatively (Fig 300). Figure 301, taken after 1.5 years, shows

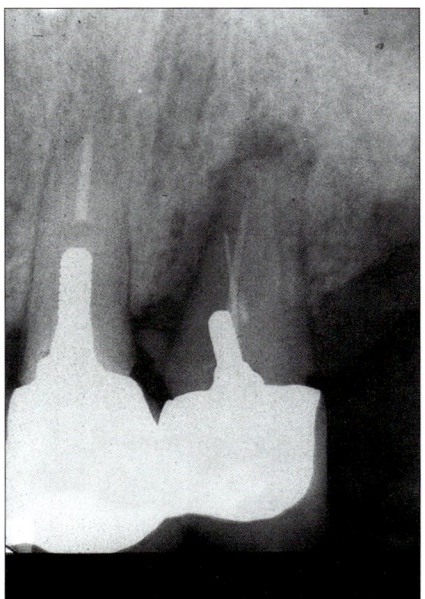

Fig 298 Apical-marginal communication on the mesial and buccal surfaces of the maxillary left first premolar in a 68-year-old former smoker.

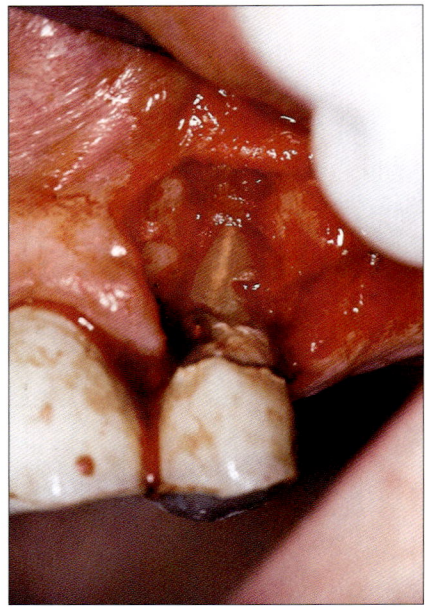

Fig 299 Hemisection of the buccal root in the same patient. The buccal surface of the lingual root is visible to the apex. Gutta-percha filling is visible through the thin buccal root wall.

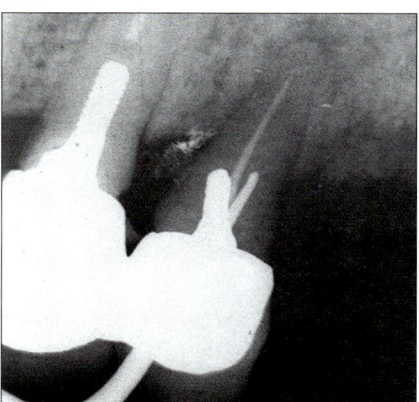

Fig 300 Regeneration of alveolar bone around the apex and the mesial aspect of the lingual root only 4 months after surgery.

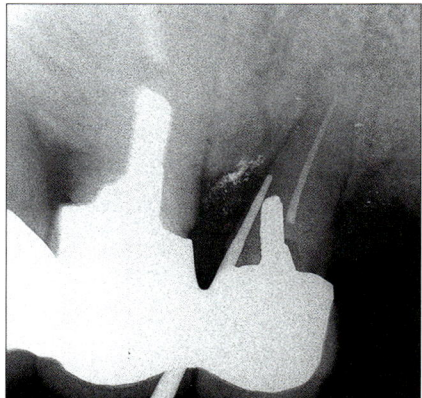

Fig 301 Probing attachment level on the mesial surfaces, 18 months after surgery. The attachment level is indicated by a periodontal probe placed in the base of the pocket. On the buccal surface, the probing depth is only 1 mm and the margin of the gingiva is located at the exposed tip of the post.

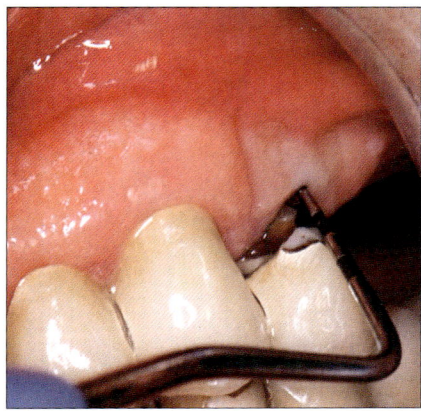

Fig 302 The buccal gingiva had healed and the pocket depth was only 1 mm 18 months after therapy.

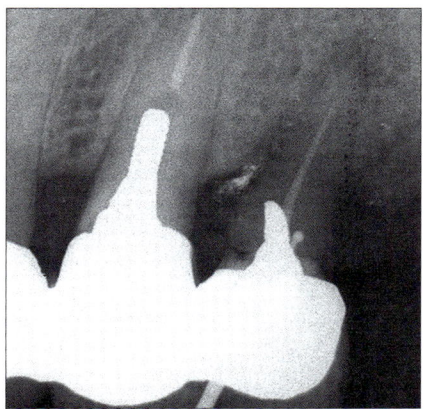

Fig 303 Almost 3.5 years after therapy, the initial result was still well maintained.

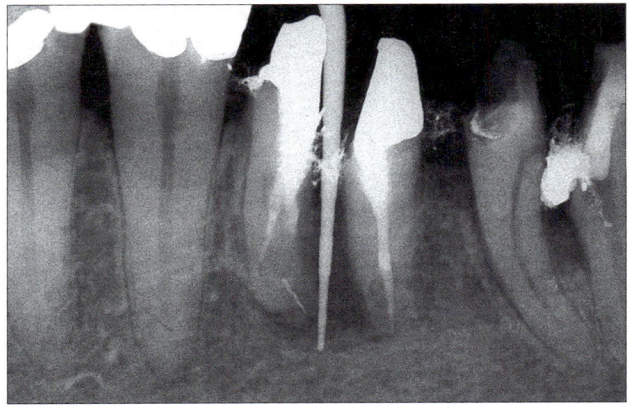

Fig 304 Very advanced loss of periodontal support and "through-and-through" furcation involvement of the mandibular left first and second molars. The inserted periodontal probe reaches the apical area after hemisection of the roots.

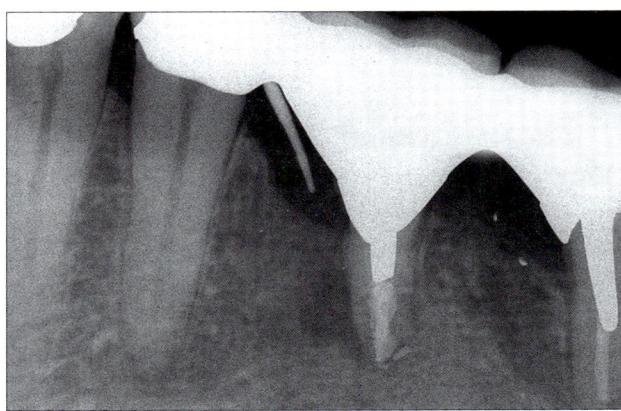

Fig 305 One year after regenerative therapy, most of the original alveolar bone level had been regenerated along the mesial surfaces of the distal roots, as shown by the inserted periodontal probe.

the probing attachment level on the mesial surfaces in relation to a periodontal probe inserted to the base of the pocket. On the buccal surface, the probing depth was only 1 mm, and the margin of the gingiva was located at the exposed tip of the post (Fig 302). Almost 3.5 years after therapy the tooth was still well maintained according to the radiograph with inserted probe on the buccal surface to the bottom of the pocket (Fig 303).

Case 4. A 58-year-old, nonsmoking man with generalized aggressive periodontitis had several severely diseased teeth, including the mandibular left first and second molars (teeth 36 and 37) with furcation involvement grade III ("through-and-through") (Fig 304). After hemisection and extraction of the mesial roots, regenerative therapy with Emdogain was carried out around the distal roots. Because a dramatic gain of periodontal sup-

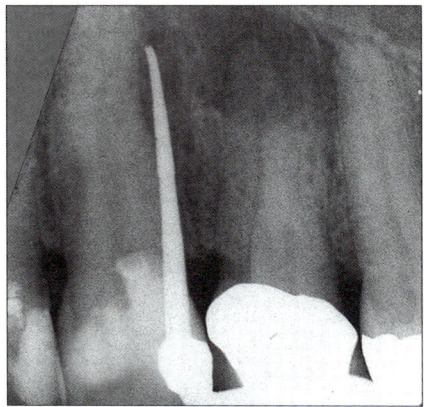

Fig 306 Radiograph showing the inserted periodontal probe almost to the apex along the distal surface of the maxillary left canine before regenerative therapy.

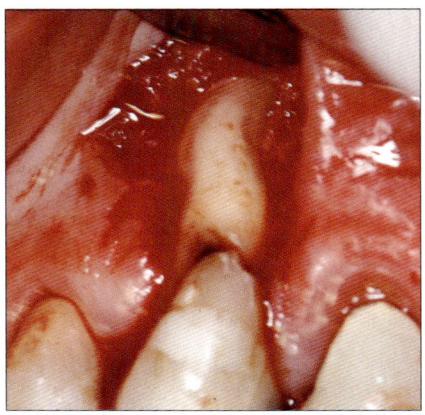

Fig 307 Mini flap surgery shows the exposed buccal and distal root surfaces almost to apex.

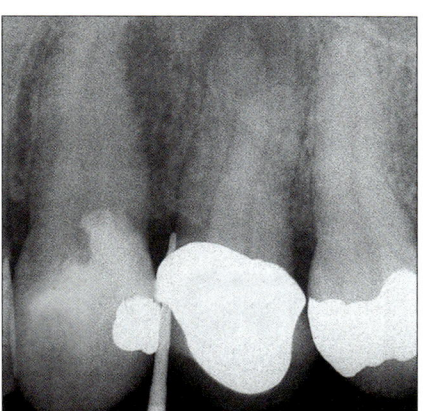

Fig 308 Three months afer regenerative therapy.

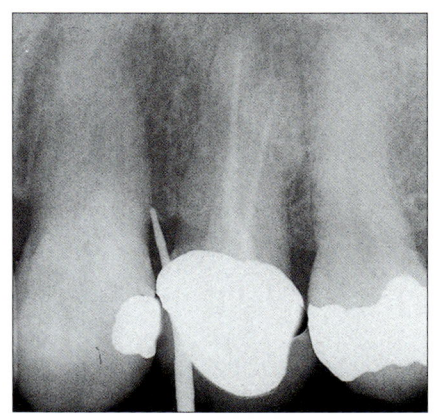

Fig 309 Two years after regenerative therapy.

port was achieved at the 6-month reexamination, the distal roots of the two molars were used as abutments for a fixed prosthodontic reconstruction. Figure 305 shows the result 1 year after regenerative therapy.

Case 5. A 65-year-old, nonsmoking woman had close to a marginal-apical communication at the buccal and distal surfaces of the maxillary left canine (Fig 306). Figure 307 shows the exposed root close to the apex during mini flap surgery. Three

months after regenerative therapy, alveolar bone regeneration had been achieved to 3 mm from the cementoenamel junction (CEJ) along the distal surface (Fig 308) and the pocket depth was only 1 mm buccally and 2 mm distally. Two years later, the initial result was maintained and healing at the apical periodontitis of the first premolar was ongoing after endodontic therapy (Fig 309).

Case 6. A 63-year-old, nonsmoking woman had a marginal-apical communication along the mesio-

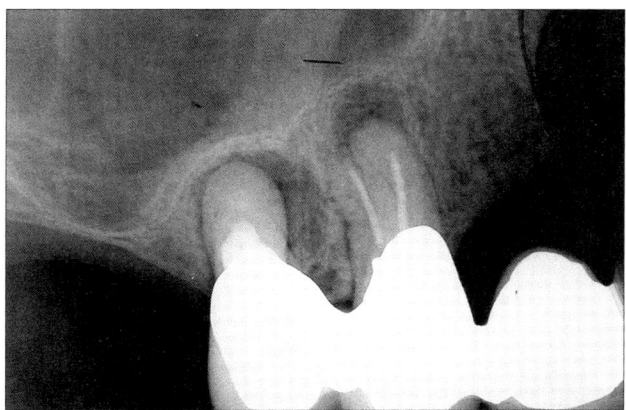

Fig 310 Marginal-apical loss of alveolar bone along the mesial surface of the maxillary second premolar and apical lesion on the first premolar.

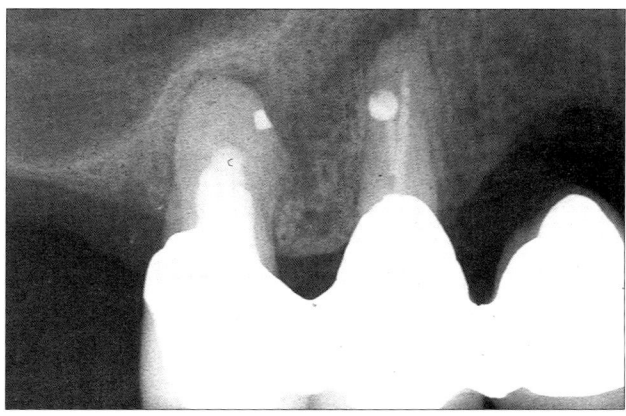

Fig 311 Complete regeneration of alveolar bone 3 months after retrograde root fillings and regenerative therapy.

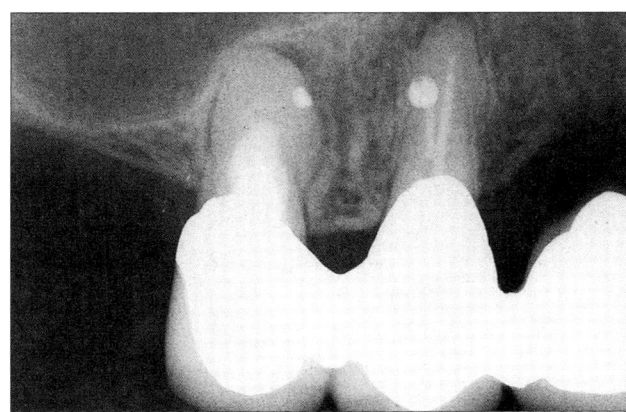

Fig 312 Results 3 years after therapy.

buccal surface of the maxillary right second premolar (tooth 15) and apical periodontitis on the first premolar (tooth 14) (Fig 310). During open flap surgery a perforation or accessory root canal less than 1 mm in diameter was discovered. After retrograde root fillings with Ketac (Espe, Seefeld, Germany) silver glass-ionomer material and comprehensive mechanical cleaning and chemical conditioning with EDTA gel, regenerative treatment with Emdogain was performed along the mesiobuccal surface, around the apex of the sec-

ond premolar, and apically of the first premolar. Three months after therapy, complete regeneration of alveolar bone was achieved (Fig 311). Figure 312 shows the result 3 years after therapy.

The short- and long-term effect of regenerative therapy with enamel matrix-guided technique in four more cases with advanced loss of periodontal support are shown in Figs 90 to 101 in chapter 1 and Figs 142 to 149 in chapter 3.

The arrest of lesions achieved in these cases represents the net effect of a series of important steps:

- Comprehensive history taking and diagnosis, intensive elimination of the subgingival biofilm and infection, and the establishment of excellent gingival plaque control and full-mouth disinfection before surgery.
- Tailored, mini flap surgery; nonaggressive supplementary mechanical cleaning of the visible exposed root surfaces; chemical cleaning and conditioning of the root surface with EDTA solution or gel; and the regenerative potential of the enamel matrix derivative proteins in the Emdogain gel.
- Excellent gingival plaque control during the healing phase and during the following maintenance program. This is the key to long-term success.
- Cessation of smoking in smokers after treatment. Supplementary treatment with antibiotics was based on analyses of the subgingival microflora, periodontal susceptability, and general health conditions.

Materials and methods for prevention, control, and nonagressive treatment of periodontal diseases, as well as regenerative therapy, will be more comprehensively discussed in volumes 4 and 5 of this 5-volume series.

Conclusions

Classification

The periodontal diseases range in severity from infection and inflammation localized to the free gingiva, traditionally termed *gingivitis,* to rapidly progressive destruction of the periodontal support, *aggressive periodontitis,* which often terminates in tooth loss. Based on histologic findings at the cellular level, gingival and periodontal lesions may be described as initial or acute gingival lesions, established inflamed gingival lesions, or destructive periodontal lesions. The First European

Workshop on Periodontology, held in 1993, proposed the following classification of marginal periodontitis, based on the age of the patient, the pattern of periodontal attachment loss, and the incidence (progression rate) of periodontal disease:

- Early-onset periodontitis (EOP), which may be subdivided into localized and generalized forms (LEOP and GEOP)
- Necrotizing periodontitis (NP)
- Adult periodontitis (AP)

In 1999 a new and more comprehensive classification system for periodontal diseases and conditions was introduced at the international workshop arranged by the American Academy of Periodontology (see Box 14). The most important changes compared to earlier classifications were:

1. Introduction of a new section for gingival diseases and lesions that are either plaque-induced or not primarily associated with dental plaque.
2. "Adult periodontitis" was replaced with "chronic periodontitis," which may be classified as either localied or generalized.
3. "Early-onset periodontitis" was replaced with "aggressive periodontitis," which has two subclasses: localized or generalized.
4. A new section for "periodontitis as a manifestation of systemic diseases" was introduced.
5. "Necrotizing ulcerative periodontitis" was replaced with "necrotizing periodontal diseases," which was subclassified as "necrotizing ulcerative gingivitis" (NUG) and "necrotizing ulcerative periodontitis" (NUP).
6. New sections were introduced for "abscesses of the periodontium," "periodontitis associated with endodontic lesions," and "development of acquired deformities and conditions."

This most recent classification system is used in this volume.

Pathogenesis at the clinical level

The periodontal diseases represent a family of chronic and occasionally acute inflammatory infectious diseases, caused, like other infectious diseases, by pathogenic bacteria. However, unlike other infectious diseases, periodontal diseases are caused by different types of bacteria growing in the form of plaque at the gingival margin, and in a well-organized subgingival biofilm, from which bacteria may invade not only the junctional and pocket epithelium, but also the connective tissue. At the American Academy of Periodontology Workshop in 1996, five species of bacteria were acknowledged as particularly virulent, and responsible for both direct and indirect destruction of the periodontal tissues: *P gingivalis, B forsythus, A actinomycetemcomitans, P intermedia,* and *T denticola* (American Academy of Periodontology, 1996c).

As long as the periopathogens grow in the biofilms of the gingival and subgingival plaque, they are inaccessible to and protected from the first line of host defense, the phagocytosing PMNLs (neutrophils) as well as from chemical plaque control agents and antibiotics. To improve accessibility, the gingival plaque and the subgingival biofilm must be disrupted and mechanically removed. This explains the successful outcome of treatment and maintenance programs based on mechanical removal of supragingival and subgingival plaque (biofilms) by daily self-care, supplemented with repeated subgingival debridement, and professional mechanical toothcleaning.

Teeth that are kept meticulously clean will not decay, nor will gingivitis or periodontitis develop in the supporting periodontal tissues. However, as in other infectious diseases, the outcome of the bacterial challenge is always related to the host response. As shown by Löe et al (1965) almost everybody who refrains from oral hygiene for 2 to 3 weeks develops several sites with inflamed gingivae (gingivitis). Within a week of resumption of excellent gingival plaque control, the inflammation subsides.

There is general agreement that periodontitis is preceded by gingivitis, but only a few individuals or sites with gingivitis progress to destructive periodontitis. Recent studies have shown that screening for subjects potentially susceptible to progressive periodontitis on the basis of the occurrence of known periopathogens in periodontal pockets will disclose only about 20% of cases; more than 80% are identified when selection is based on smoking (external risk factor) combined with the occurrence of polymorphic IL-1 genes (internal, genetic risk factor). On the basis of comprehensive history taking and diagnosis, the absolute majority of patients can be categorized as low-risk (gingivitis) and a small minority can be labeled as periodontitis risk patients. The individual risk profile should be evaluated and a needs-related maintenance program should be established.

Pathogenesis at the cellular and molecular levels

The classic research by Page and Schroeder (1976), using histologic findings to classify initial, early, established, and destructive gingival and periodontal lesions is still valid at the cellular level. However, in recent years, much has been added to the knowledge of the pathogenesis of the periodontal diseases, not only at the cellular, but also at the molecular and genetic levels, offering new potential for prediction of risk and for treatment and control of the periodontal diseases. Much of this field remains to be explored. Some of the molecular mediators from the bacteria and host cells, which are responsible for periodontal tissue destruction, have been identified, and there is new but incomplete knowledge about the genetic interaction regarding molecular immunoregulating mediators of destruction and of healing in the periodontal tissues.

Of utmost importance is the nonspecific first line of defense in the gingival sulcus or periodontal pocket, by numerous vital and aggressive PMNLs, which phagocytose and kill accessible bacteria and wall off the subgingival biofilm from direct contact with the junctional and pocket epithelium. If this first line of defense is weak, periopathogens may invade the periodontal tissues. Available data show that the efficacy of this first line of host response in the acute phase of gingival inflammation is critical in protecting the periodontal tissues from the pathologic sequelae of bacterial colonization and invasion.

Normal, efficient PMNL function may explain why most adults and almost all children can be regarded as "gingivitis patients." On the other hand, it has long been recognized that abnormalities of PMNL function adversely affect periodontal health. Constitutive defects in PMNL function or number are expressed as severe inflammation of the periodontium, loss of alveolar bone, and destruction of the supporting connective tissue. Among others, smokers and individuals with type 1 diabetes may exhibit impaired PMNL function.

As the understanding of host defense has improved, knowledge of other components involved in PMNL function has grown. It is now apparent that the bacteria associated with periodontal disease elicit predominantly IgG2 antibodies and that bacteria opsonized with this antibody are most effectively phagocytosed by PMNLs of the high-responder, FcγRIIA, allotype. Future studies should determine whether low titers of antigen-specific IgG2 antibody and/or PMNLs of the low-responder, FcRIIA, allotype are risk factors for periodontal disease development or progression.

An important conceptual advance has been the realization that, to avoid phagocytic cells, bacteria use a number of strategies, including molecular mimicry, direct destruction of phagocytic signals, and direct alteration of the phagocyte itself. As knowledge in this area advances, intervention at the molecular level is the goal.

The established gingival lesion is characterized by continuous emigration of PMNLs into the gingival crevice, guided by chemoattractants such as interleukin-8 in the junctional epithelium and bacterial products. Gingival crevicular fluid from gingival lesions contains high levels of PMNLs and their degranulation products. The connective tissue infiltrate is dominated by B lymphocytes, T lymphocytes, monocytes and macrophages, and relatively few plasma cells and fibroblasts.

The destructive periodontal lesion is dominated by plasma cells, which produce large quantities of specific antibodies against the subgingival periopathogens and their antigens. The periodontal tissues are continuously exposed to specific bacterial components, particularly LPSs from the subgingival gram-negative periopathogens, that alter and mediate many local cell functions. Particularly macrophages, but also T cells, are stimulated by LPSs to produce selective subsets of cytokines (particularly IL-1β and TNF-α), PGE$_2$, and MMPs. Both IL-1β and TNF-α may stimulate local fibroblasts to produce PGE$_2$ and MMPs. MMPs result in destruction of the extracellular matrix in the connective tissue, while PGE$_2$ particularly but also IL-1β and TNF-α may mediate alveolar bone resorption by stimulation of the osteoclasts. Thus elevated and high levels of LPS, PGE$_2$, IL-1β, TNF-α, and MMPs indicate tissue inflammation that may be associated with active periodontal destruction. Particularly high levels of PGE$_2$ in the gingival crevicular fluid may be associated with severe periodontitis.

Removal of the subgingival biofilm and establishment of excellent gingival plaque control will result in the elimination of or marked reduction in LPSs and thereby lead to reduced levels of PGE$_2$, IL-1β, TNF-α, and MMPs.

Arrest and control of periodontal diseases

Based on current knowledge, the strategy for prevention, control, and arrest of periodontal diseases should be:

- Introduction of regular toothcleaning by the parents, from the time the child reaches the age of 1 year.
- Establishment of needs-related oral hygiene habits in schoolchildren.

- School-based preventive programs against smoking, from the age of 12 years.
- Identification, as early as possible (prepuberty), of individuals susceptible to aggressive periodontitis, localized and generalized, by regular clinical examination; determination of smoking status; and possibly genetic screening for the IL-1 polymorphic gene family (such a test is already available), FCγRIIa phagocyte receptor affinity, and the capacity to mount an effective IgG$_2$ humoral immune response.

Once identified, young high-risk individuals should be examined regularly, using DNA probes to identify the exogenous periopathogens *A actinomycetemcomitans* and *P gingivalis* and the opportunistic endogenous periopathogens *B forsythus, P intermedia,* and *T denticola.* Whenever an infection is discovered, it should be eliminated by an initial combination of mechanical cleaning and chemotherapy by "completemouth" disinfection. This should be followed by a needs-related maintenance program, based on excellent gingival plaque control and regular clinical and DNA probe examinations.

Young adults and adults may be broadly selected into two groups: one large main group of healthy individuals and persons with gingivitis and a minor group of individuals with periodontitis subjects. In the minor group of subjects susceptible to periodontal disease, individual periodontal risk profiles should be evaluated, using comprehensive history taking; clinical examination (periodontal attachment loss, treatment needs, periodontal pocket temperature, gingival crevicular fluid analyses, etc); assessment of the standard of oral hygiene; measurement of plaque formation rate; DNA probe analyses of the subgingival microflora; and evaluation of external and internal modifying risk indicators, risk factors, and prognostic risk factors. Based on the risk profile evaluation, the basic strategy should be individualized treatment to eliminate infection by periopathogens and to reduce modifying risk indicators, risk factors, and prognostic risk factors as much as possible (par-ticularly smoking). As a consequence, the periodontal tissues will heal.

Initial healing will be maintained by an individualized maintenance program, based on the establishment of excellent gingival plaque control by self-care, supplemented by needs-related professional mechanical toothcleaning and nonaggressive subgingival debridement. The effect of the maintenance program will be evaluated at needs-related intervals. Use of antibiotics (topical or systemic) should be restricted to extremely high-risk patients with refractory aggressive periodontitis, and only after mechanical removal of the subgingival biofilms and identification of pathogens by DNA probe evaluation.

In the near future, specific methods to stimulate cytokines that suppress the immunoinflammatory response and tissue inhibitors of metalloproteinases will be used in combination with optimal reduction of the bacterial challenge in selected high-risk patients. Promising initial results with nonsteroidal anti-inflammatory drugs for slowing bone resorption and with chemically modified tetracycline (doxycycline) for reducing extracellular destruction have also been confirmed. Also promising are the results of a recent 3-year longitudinal study of the use of toothpaste with triclosan in selected patients with periodontitis (Rosling et al, 1997a, 1997b). Triclosan has antiplaque as well as anti-inflammatory properties.

Repair and regeneration of periodontal tissues is already a reality. So-called guided tissue regeneration by use of barriers was introduced in the late 1980s. The most promising method to date is the use of enamel matrix derivatives (Emdogain gel). Other combinations of biomaterials may be expected in the near future. (For reviews on the pathogenesis of the periodontal diseases, see Darveau et al, 1997; Dennison and Van Dyke, 1997; Ebersole and Taubman, 1994; Gemmell et al, 1997; Hart and Kornman, 1997; Holmstrup and Westergaard, 1997; Ishikawa et al, 1997; Kinane and Lindhe, 1997; Kornman et al, 1997b; Offenbacher, 1996; Page and Kornman, 1997; Page et al, 1997; Reynolds and Meikle, 1997; Salvi et al, 1997a; Schwartz et al, 1997; Tonetti, 1994; Tonetti and Mombelli, 1997.)

CHAPTER 6

DIAGNOSIS
OF PERIODONTAL DISEASES

The population can broadly be divided into two groups, on the basis of susceptibility to either gingivitis or periodontitis. However, there is no clear distinction between the two. Very few children or young adults exhibit aggressive periodontitis. In Scandinavia, the prevalence of aggressive periodontitis in these age groups is only about 0.1% of the population. There is general agreement that periodontitis (destruction of the periodontal support) is always preceded by gingivitis. However, in populations where high standards of gingival plaque control are established at an early age, only a minority of individuals will in adulthood develop destructive periodontal lesions (chronic periodontitis). An absolute minority exhibit aggressive periodontitis.

There is also general agreement that the prevalence of gingivitis is strongly correlated to the standard of oral hygiene (amount of gingival plaque) at the individual as well as at the site level. Some decades ago, when standards of oral hygiene were poor and the dental care resources available were inadequate almost worldwide, the prevalence of gingivitis was very high, even among children and young adults. These conditions still pertain to most of the world's population.

Persistently poor gingival plaque control results in a gradual increase in size of the inflamed and swollen gingiva, forming a so-called pseudo-pocket. This changes ecological conditions in favor of a gram-negative, anaerobic microflora, which forms a subgingival biofilm. Most periopathogens belong to this category of microflora.

With continual exposure to such a bacterial challenge, the individual subject or site will eventually develop periodontitis. The children most susceptible to periodontitis will develop generalized or localized aggressive periodontitis at an early age, while the most resistant will experience no destruction or limited destruction of periodontal support at a few sites during their lifetime. These facts explain why the prevalence of periodontitis is strictly age-related worldwide, representing the cumulative effect of all periods of exacerbation (incidence) and "burnouts." Clinically, the condition of the gingiva may be dichotomized into healthy or inflamed (gingivitis) on the basis of visible signs (swelling, redness, and altered surface texture) or bleeding on probing. The severity of gingivitis may also be classified by using different indices, eg, the Löe and Silness Gingival Index (GI).

There is a strong correlation between the volume of gingival crevicular fluid (GCF) and the severity of gingival inflammation, and the composition of GCF is different in gingivitis and periodontitis sites. At the surface level, there is a strong correlation between gingivitis and the amount and duration of gingival plaque. Evaluation of Plaque Index (PI) and Plaque Formation Rate Index (PFRI) are therefore essential for successful elimination of gingivitis and maintenance of healthy gingiva.

Clinical probing is the most commonly used method for assessing attachment loss (destruction of periodontal support) and probing depth, as well as pocket bleeding (treatment needs). Probing depth as well as attachment loss can be measured by manual probing or by more sophisticated, automated, computer-linked, pressure-sensitive periodontal probes.

Alveolar bone loss is still most frequently evaluated by conventional (vertical) bite-wing and complete-mouth radiographs. Panoramic radiographs may be used for screening. Recently, computer-aided digital subtraction radiography has been introduced. In contrast to conventional radiography, this method allows small changes in the mineral content of alveolar bone to be monitored over short periods of time (ie, months).

Over the last two decades, the Community Periodontal Index of Treatment Needs (CPITN), developed by the World Health Organization (WHO) and Fédération Dentaire Internationale, (FDI), has been applied at the individual and sextant levels in numerous national surveys of the epidemiology of periodontal diseases. This four-grade index considerably overestimates treatment need, not only at the individual and sextant levels, but also at the tooth level (the highest score per individual, sextant, or tooth is registered). In the individual patient, however, the CPITN may be useful at the surface level to evaluate treatment needs.

Probing attachment loss (PAL), periodontal probing depth, and alveolar bone loss provide retrospective information about destruction of periodontal support. Ongoing periodontal destruction at site level is disclosed by increased levels of prostaglandin E_2 (PGE$_2$), interleukins, and proteinases in the gingival crevicular fluid; suppuration; bleeding on probing; increased periodontal pocket temperature; and the occurrence of subgingival biofilms and specific periopathogens. To some extent, these variables are also predictors of further periodontal progression. Several methods are available for the detection of subgingival pathogens associated with periodontal diseases, including direct microscopy, microbial culture, and nucleic acid probe assays.

DIAGNOSIS OF CLINICALLY HEALTHY AND INFLAMED GINGIVA (GINGIVITIS)

Clinically healthy gingiva

The characteristics of clinically healthy gingiva are described in Box 20.

The thickness of the oral epithelium and thereby the color of the gingiva may vary, as a result of physical adaptation to variations of abrasiveness, shape and position of the teeth, the age of the individual, etc. In addition, the width of the so-called attached gingiva may vary considerably among individuals and different tooth surfaces exemplified in the following cases (Figs 313 to 317).

The connective tissue of the healthy free gingiva is covered by an outer oral epithelium, with an undulating border (rete pegs), and an inner junctional epithelium, with a straight border (Figs 318 to 321). The junctional epithelium is relatively thin, comprising 15 to 30 cells coronally and 5 to 10 cells apically, and has a rapid turnover (3 to 6 days) compared to the oral epithelium (14 to 20

Box 20 Characteristics of clinically health gingiva

- Pale pink color
- Stippled surface texture; resembling orange peel
- Thin marginal gingiva
- Free gingiva that is attached to the tooth surface
- On probing, a resilience resembling that of rubber

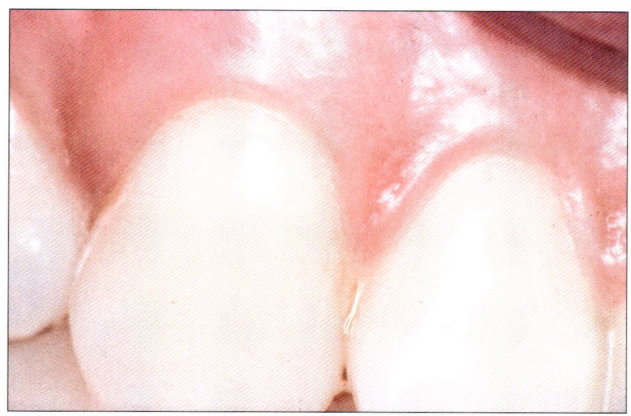 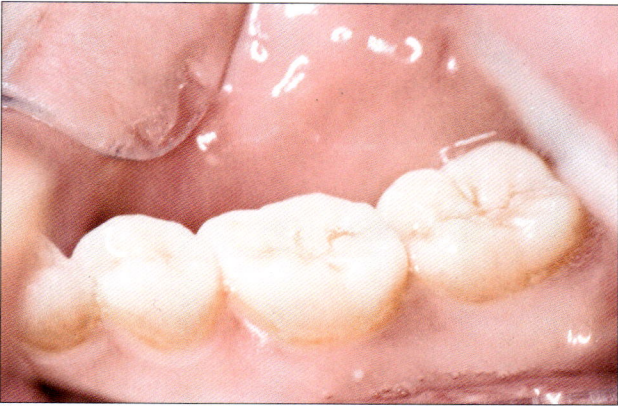

Figs 313 and 314 Clinically healthy gingiva in a 14-year-old girl. The oral epithelium is relatively thin.

Fig 315 Healthy gingiva in a young adult.

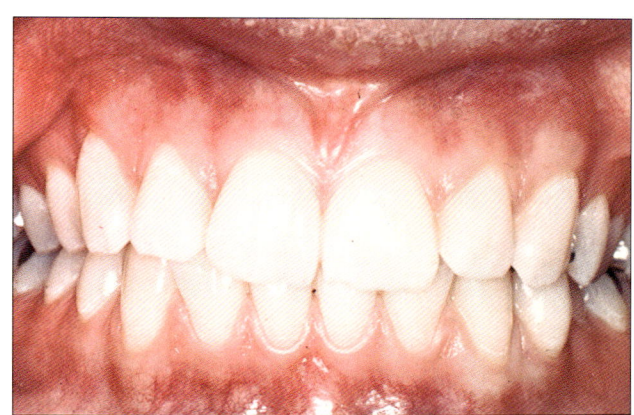

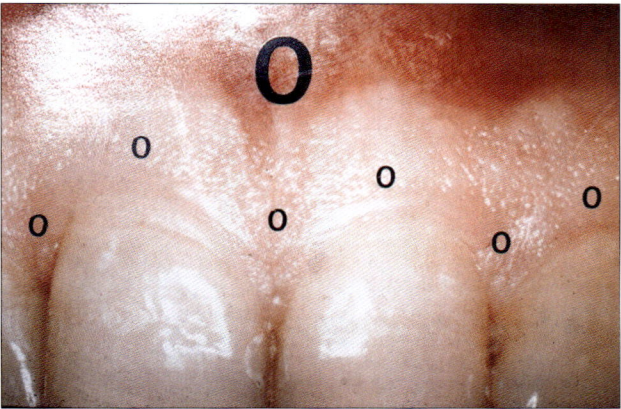 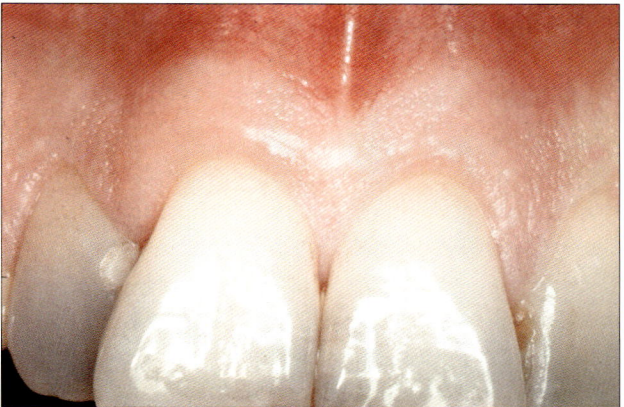

Figs 316 and 317 Healthy gingiva in two adults. These individuals have different tooth forms, but both exhibit very thick oral epithelium. The circles in Fig 316 mark thick, well-keratinized, healthy gingival margins.

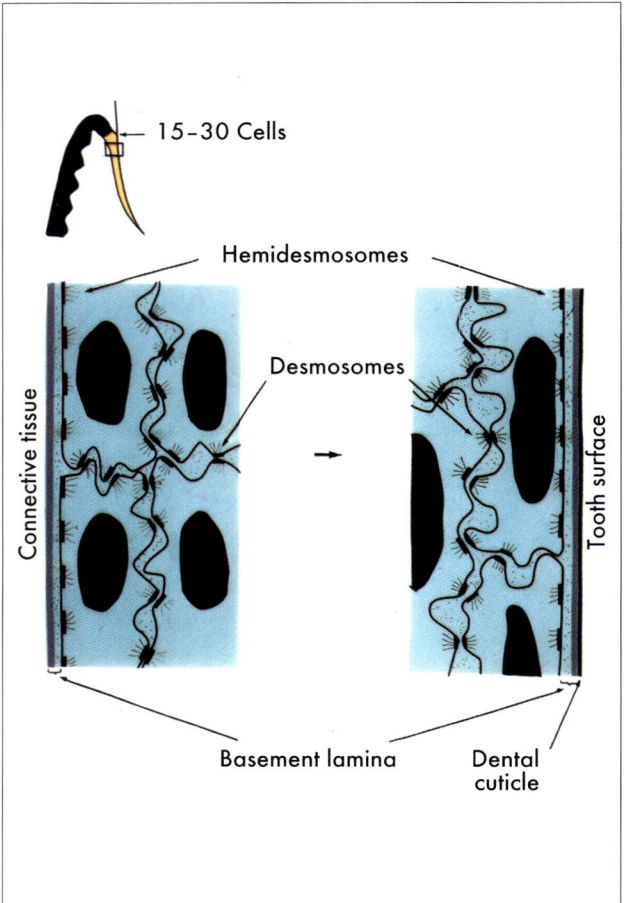

Fig 318 Cross section of the connective tissue of the healthy free gingiva. There is an oral epithelium, with an undulating border, and an inner junctional epithelium, with a straight border. The junctional epithelium cells are attached to the tooth surface and the basement lamina with hemidesmosomes and intercellularly with desmosomes.

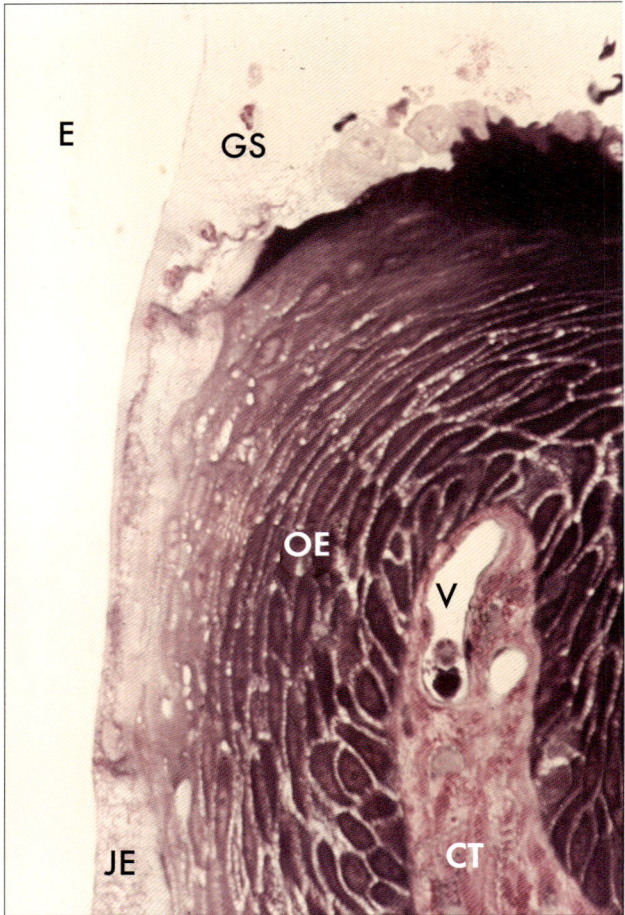

Fig 319 Histologic cross section of the gingival margin. The cells of the oral epithelium gradually become more flattened and dense toward the outer so-called stratum corneum, with semikeratinized cells. GS = Gingival sulcus; E = Tooth enamel; OE = Oral epithelium; JE = Junctional epithelium; CT = Connective tissue; V = Vessel (PAS and toludine blue, original magnification ×2,000).

days). The junctional epithelial cells are attached with equal strength to the tooth surface and the basement lamina against the connective tissue by hemidesmosomes and intercellularly by desmosomes (see Fig 318). Histologically, an intact junctional epithelium should therefore be regarded as a partial periodontal attachment.

The difference in histologic appearance reflects the different functions of the oral and the junctional epithelia. The densely packed and semikeratinized surface layer of the oral epithelium is impermeable to the oral microflora and their toxins and resistant to friction from food, etc (see Fig 321). The intact junctional epithelium is permeable to phagocytozing leukocytes, particularly polymorphonuclear leukocytes (PMNLs), but also macrophages, and attaches the free gingiva to the tooth surface (see Fig 320). However, long-term exposure to gingival plaque may also lead to some penetration of periopathogens through the junctional epithelium.

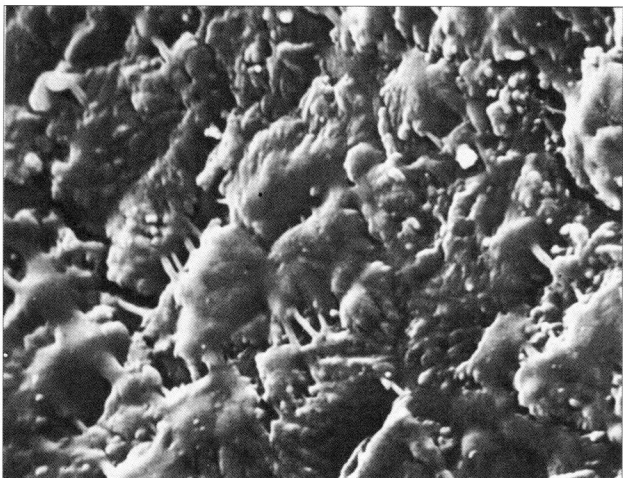

Fig 320 Scanning electron micrograph (SEM) of the outer surface of the junctional epithelium against the tooth surface. The cells of the junctional epithelium are loosely packed, are of the same shape, and have a wide intercellular matrix (original magnification ×2,000).

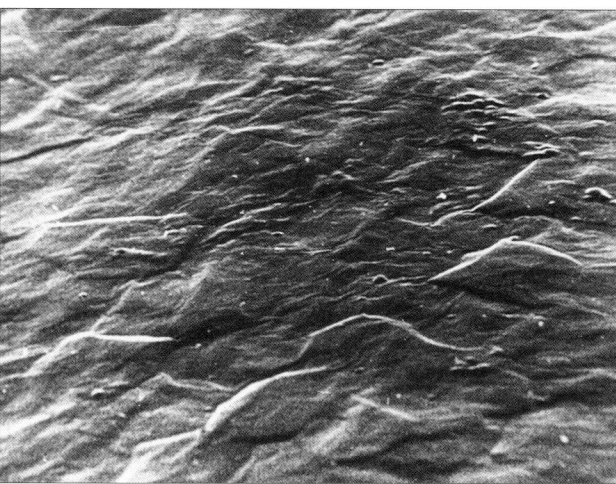

Fig 321 SEM of the outer surface of the oral epithelium. The epithelial cells are thin, flat, and densely packed in order to protect against transmission of bacteria, chemical agents, etc into the connective tissue (original magnification ×2,000).

Gingival inflammation (gingivitis)

Gingivitis represents the inflammatory response in the free gingiva to accumulation of gingival plaque. About 90% of the population will exhibit at least some inflamed sites. The lesion is usually confined to the gingival margin and may be local or general. Because there is a strong correlation between the amount and location of gingival plaque and the development of gingivitis, the most common sites are the areas that are difficult to keep clean, for example, the linguoapproximal surfaces of the mandibular posterior teeth (see Fig 207 in chapter 5).

The four cardinal signs of inflammation are redness (rubor), swelling (tumor), heat (calor), and pain (dolor). Inflamed periodontal tissues may also exhibit bleeding on probing, suppuration, gingival exudate, and ulceration. All cases of gingivitis or periodontitis must have one or more of these clinical signs of inflammation (Box 21). The presence of clinically detectable inflammation indicates that the periodontal tissues are not healthy.

A change in color is one of the most common clinical signs of gingival inflammation. Because of the increased vascularity at inflamed sites, the tissues usually exhibit various hues of red. An equally common sign of gingival inflammation is swelling or edema. Inflamed gingiva swells because fluid accumulates in the tissues as a result of increased vascular permeability at inflamed sites (Lindhe and Rylander, 1975). The primary clinical importance of gingival redness or swelling is to indicate that the tissues are diseased. However, as discussed earlier, this does not necessarily imply a greater risk of further attachment loss (that is, disease progression).

Box 21 Clinical signs of gingivitis
• Redness
• Swelling
• Bleeding on probing
• Exudate

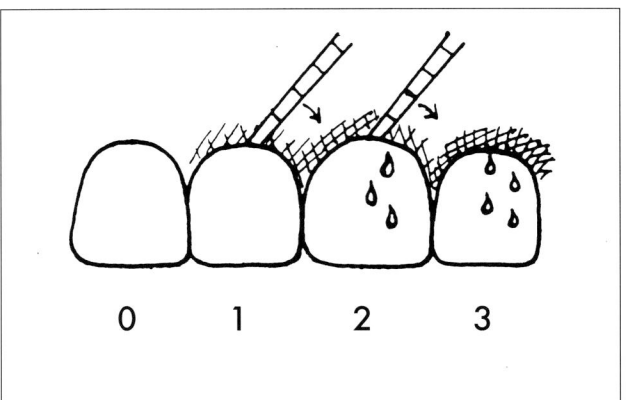

Fig 322 Löe and Silness Gingival Index (Löe and Silness, 1963). 0 = Normal gingiva, no inflammation, no discoloration, and no bleeding; 1 = Mild inflammation, slight color change, mild alteration of gingival surface, and no bleeding; 2 = Moderate inflammation, erythema, swelling, and bleeding on probing or pressure; 3 = Severe inflammation, severe erythema and swelling, tendency to spontaneous hemorrhage, and some ulceration.

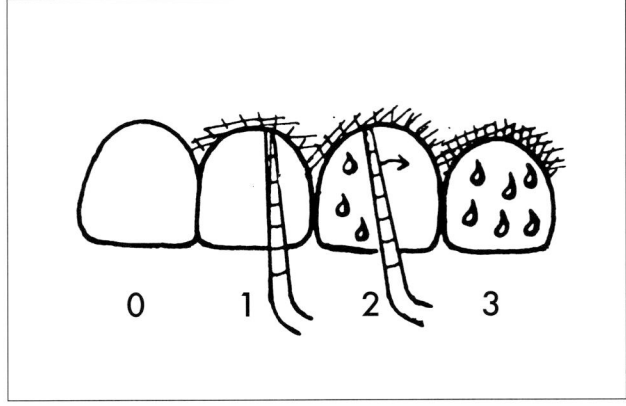

Fig 323 Löe's modification (Löe, 1967) of the Gingival Index. The technique changed from use of "pressure" to use of "probing."

Bleeding on probing is widely regarded as a relatively objective sign of gingival inflammation, because it is either present or absent, and is the basis of several indices used to assess the extent of gingival inflammation in clinical studies. Periodontal probes are usually the instruments of choice for eliciting bleeding, although wooden triangular toothpicks and dental floss have also been used for interdental diagnosis of gingivitis.

With some gingival assessment systems, such as the widely used Gingival Index by Löe and Silness (1963) (Fig 322), the probe is inserted just apical to the gingival margin and the tissues are gently stroked laterally with the edge of the instrument. Other bleeding indices specify that the probe be inserted to the base of the pocket (Fig 323). Comparison of the two methods of probe placement suggests that the results will differ. Angulation of probe insertion is another important variable influencing gingival bleeding responses. Because gingival bleeding can occur immediately or shortly after probing, some indices include a time factor for the appearance of bleeding. Finally, some indices call for qualitative assessments of the amount of gingival bleeding such as point bleeding with no flow along the gingival margin, bleeding with flow along the gingival margin, and copious bleeding with flow to the adjacent tooth (Figs 324a and 324b).

Although there is general agreement that bleeding on probing is a reliable sign of gingival inflammation, whether or not the tissues bleed depends on a variety of factors besides the extent of inflammation. For example, the percentage of sites with bleeding on probing increases significantly if patients brush their teeth before the examination. The prevalence of bleeding on probing is also increased by multiple sequential probe insertions at a single site. However, probably the most important variable (besides inflammation) affecting the prevalence of bleeding on probing is the pressure with which probes are inserted. The percentage of sites that bleed on probing is increased when greater insertion forces are used. In one such report, in patients with a reduced but healthy periodontium, bleeding on probing was more frequent with probing forces exceeding 0.25 N (Lang et al, 1991). It was suggested that high-

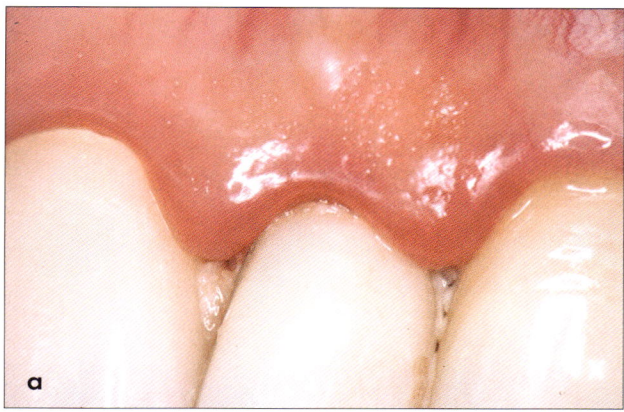 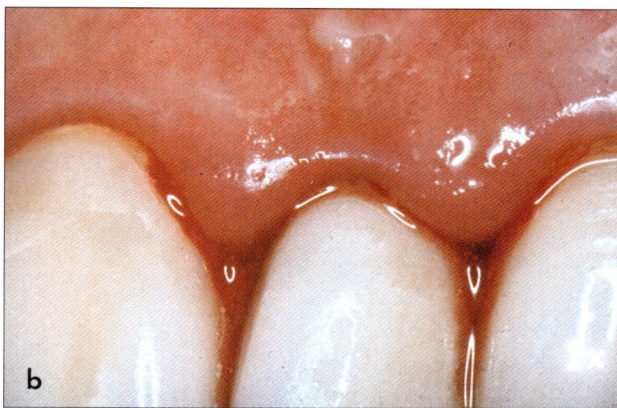

Figs 324a and 324b Interproximal sites with severe Gingival Index score 2.

er probing forces traumatize the tissues and induce bleeding, giving a false-positive result.

Gingivitis indices

Löe and Silness Gingival Index

Several indices have been designed for clinical assessment of gingivitis. The most frequently used index internationally, for epidemiologic and experimental studies, is the Gingival Index (GI) by Löe and Silness (1963), which scores gingival inflammation from 0 to 3 on the facial, lingual, mesial, and distal surfaces of all teeth (see Fig 322).

- Score 0 = Normal gingiva, no inflammation, no redness, and no bleeding
- Score 1 = Mild inflammation, slight color change, mild alteration of gingival surface, and no bleeding
- Score 2 = Moderate inflammation, erythema, swelling, and bleeding on probing or when pressure is applied.
- Score 3 = Severe inflammation, severe erythema and swelling, tendency toward spontaneous hemorrhage, and some ulceration

The GI was modified by Löe (1967), who changed the use of the probe from "pressure" to "probing" (see Fig 323).

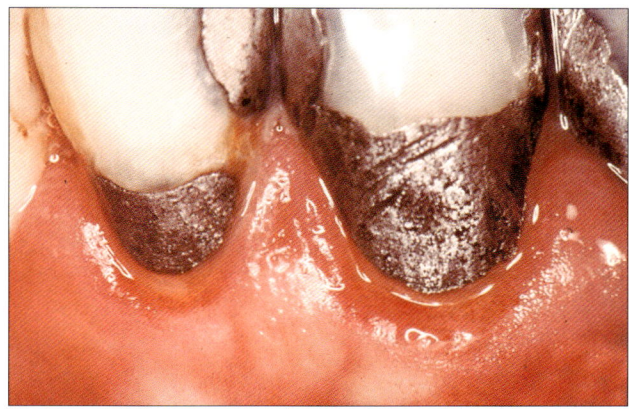

Fig 325 Two sites with different levels of Gingival Index score 1.

Figure 325 illustrates two buccal sites with different levels of GI score 1, while Figs 324a and 324b show two interproximal sites with severe score 2. Advanced forms of score 3 are shown in Figs 326 and 327 (extreme forms of hyperplastic gingival inflammation). Even such severe cases of gingivitis will heal rapidly following the establishment of meticulous gingival plaque control, debridement, and so on (Fig 328). In Scandinavia, GI scores of 3 are extremely rare because of the high standard of oral hygiene and regular dental care. In more than 40 years of practice, and with a specialty in periodontology, the author has seen

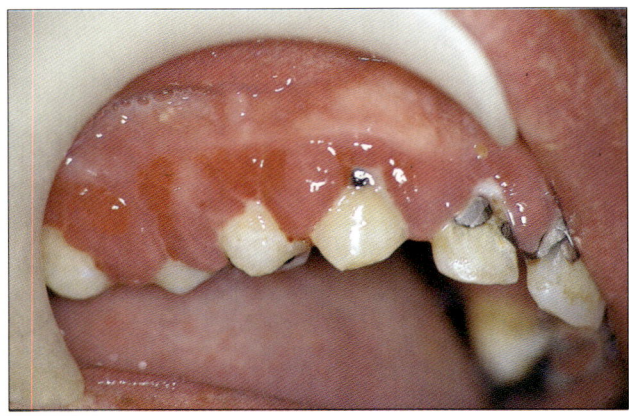
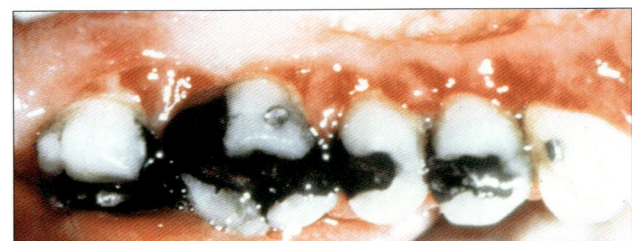

Figs 326 and 327 Advanced forms of Gingival Index score 3 (extreme forms of hyperplastic gingival inflammation).

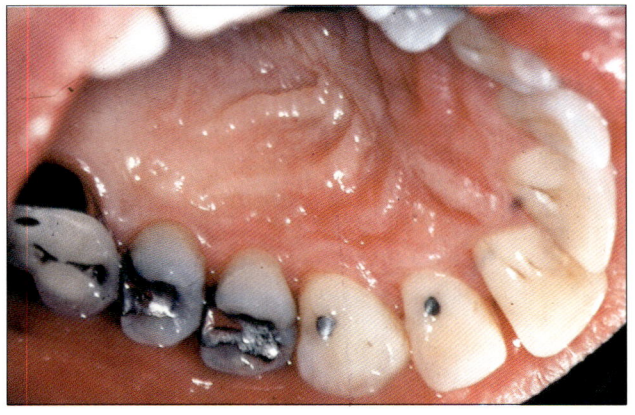

Fig 328 Gingiva in Fig 327, healed after debridement and establishment of meticulous plaque control.

only six cases, two of which are shown in Figs 326 to 328. See also the acute necrotizing ulcerative gingivitis case in chapter 5 (Fig 213).

Ainamo and Bay Gingival Bleeding Index

The Gingival Bleeding Index (GBI) by Ainamo and Bay (1975) is based on recordings from all four tooth surfaces of all teeth. Bleeding on probing is recorded as present (+) or absent (–). A minus (–) is the equivalent of GI scores 0 and 1, and a plus (+) is equal to GI scores 2 and 3. The

GBI is calculated as a percentage of affected sites (bleeding units). In adults, GBI is very useful for experimental studies and in practice on a routine basis in individual patients. In children, despite a high prevalence of GI score 1, scores 2 and 3 are very seldom recorded. Therefore, to avoid underestimation of the prevalence of gingivitis, in children, the Gingival Bleeding Index should be modified to include GI score 1 (Axelsson and Lindhe, 1974).

The patterns of dental plaque (PI), plaque formation rate (PFRI), and gingivitis (GI, GBI) vary from buccal to lingual and in maxillary and mandibular teeth. Six surfaces per tooth—mesiobuccal, buccal, distobuccal, mesiolingual, lingual, and distolingual—should therefore be recorded in experimental studies, in analytical epidemiology, and clinically in individual patients (Axelsson et al, unpublished data, 1990; Axelsson 1991, 1994).

Saxer and Mühlemann Papillary Bleeding Index

The Papillary Bleeding Index (PBI) by Saxer and Mühlemann (1975) is based on a 0 to 4 scale of bleeding 20 to 30 seconds after interproximal probing, from the buccal direction in the second and fourth quadrants and from the lingual direction in the first and third quadrants.

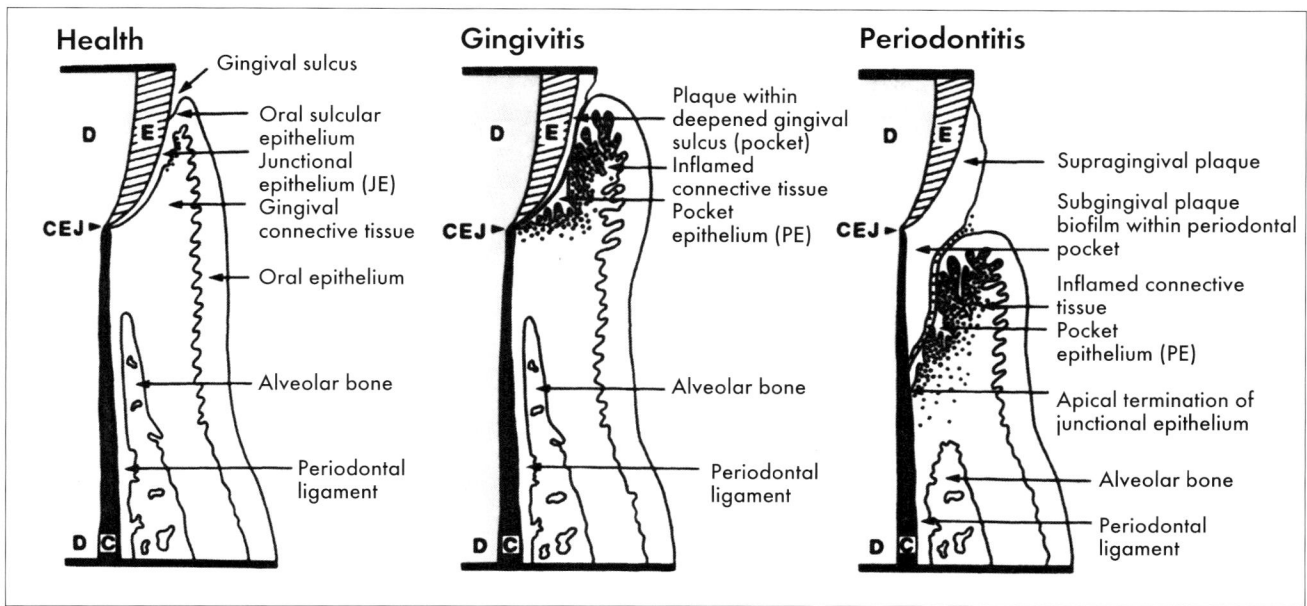

Fig 329 Cross sections of the periodontal tissues in good health and affected by gingivitis and periodontitis. D = Dentin; E = Enamel; C = Cementum. (From Armitage, 1995. Reprinted with permission.)

A simplified Papillary Bleeding Index was developed by Gjermo, based on the presence of papillary bleeding (+) after use of a triangular-pointed toothpick inserted from the buccal direction. This index is very useful for screening procedures and, in individual patients, for oral hygiene education based on self-diagnosis.

DIAGNOSIS OF PERIODONTAL ATTACHMENT LOSS

In contrast to assessment of healthy gingiva and gingival inflammation (gingivitis), examination for periodontitis must identify not only sites in the dentition with inflammatory alterations but also the extent of tissue breakdown at these sites. The main clinical signs of marginal periodontitis are loss of tooth-supporting tissues, attachment loss, and formation of suprabony and infrabony pockets.

In healthy gingiva and in inflamed gingiva (gingivitis with no past damage from periodontitis), the most apical epithelial cells against the tooth surface are located at the cementoenamel junction (CEJ) (Fig 329). Collagen fibers, representing the most coronal part of the periodontal attachment, are still attached to the root cementum, from the CEJ down to the alveolar crest (about 2 mm) (Fig 330). Thereafter, the collagen fibers of the periodontal ligament attach to the root cementum and to the alveolar bone (Fig 331). Deterioration from gingivitis to destructive periodontitis means that the most coronal collagen fibers attaching to the root cementum are lost, and the apical termination of the junctional epithelium proliferates apical to the CEJ and continuously follows the most coronal level of the attached collagen fibers. There is resorption of the alveolar bone crest, the periodontal pocket deepens, and subgingival plaque (biofilm) forms (see Fig 329). If gingival plaque control is inadequate and this subgingival biofilm is not mechanically removed, periodontitis generally progresses to ad-

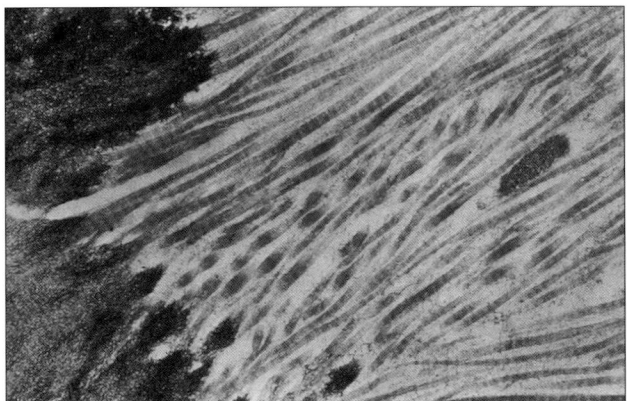

Fig 330 Histologic detail of collagen fibers inserted into the rough root cementum (original magnification ×25,000).

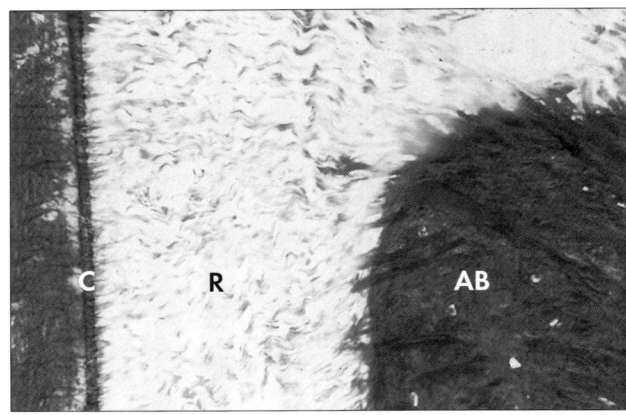

Fig 331 Histologic view of the collagen fibers of the periodontal ligament (R) attached to the root cementum (C, *left*) and the alveolar bone (AB, *right*) (original magnification ×160).

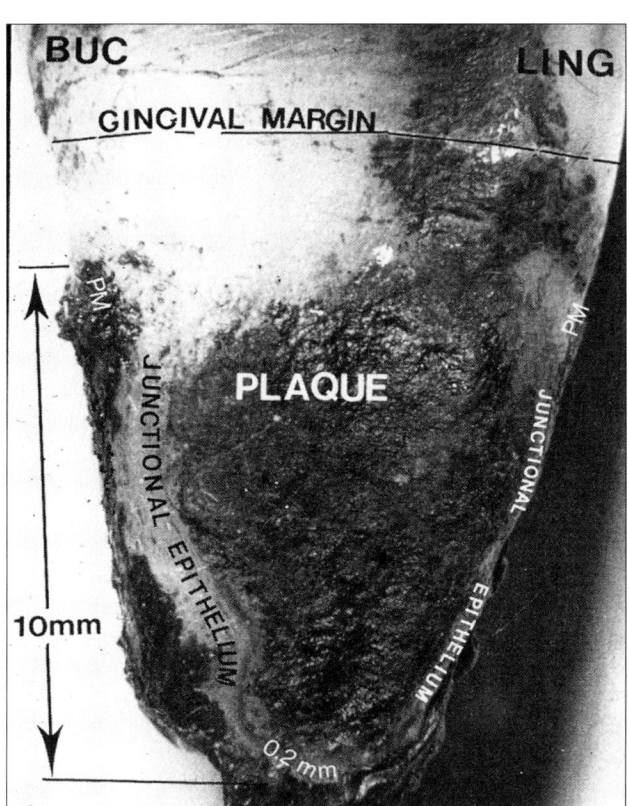

Fig 332 Autopsy material revealing the effect of subgingival plaque biofilm on tooth surfaces. Note the close relationship among the pattern of subgingival plaque, the junctional epithelium, and the remaining periodontal ligament. BUC = Buccal surface; LING = Lingual surface; PM = periodontal (membrane) ligament. (From Waerhaug, 1976. Reprinted with permission.)

vanced loss of periodontal support, but distribution in the dentition is haphazard. Isolated teeth and surfaces are affected (Fig 332).

Probing depth and loss of periodontal attachment

Clinical evaluation of periodontal tissue destruction may comprise a combination of visual detection of clinical signs of tissue destruction, assessment of probing depth and clinical attachment loss, and radiographic detection of bone loss. In current clinical practice, calibrated periodontal probes are used primarily to measure: *(1) probing depth,* or the distance from the gingival margin to the base of the probeable pocket, and *(2) clinical attachment loss,* or the distance from the CEJ to the base of the probeable pocket. In certain situations, a landmark other than the CEJ is used as a reference point from which attachment loss measurements are made, eg, the cervical margin of a restoration, the edge of a stent, or the occlusal surface of a tooth. Measurements made from these landmarks are referred to as *relative attachment loss.*

Measurements of probing depth are an essential part of any complete periodontal exami-

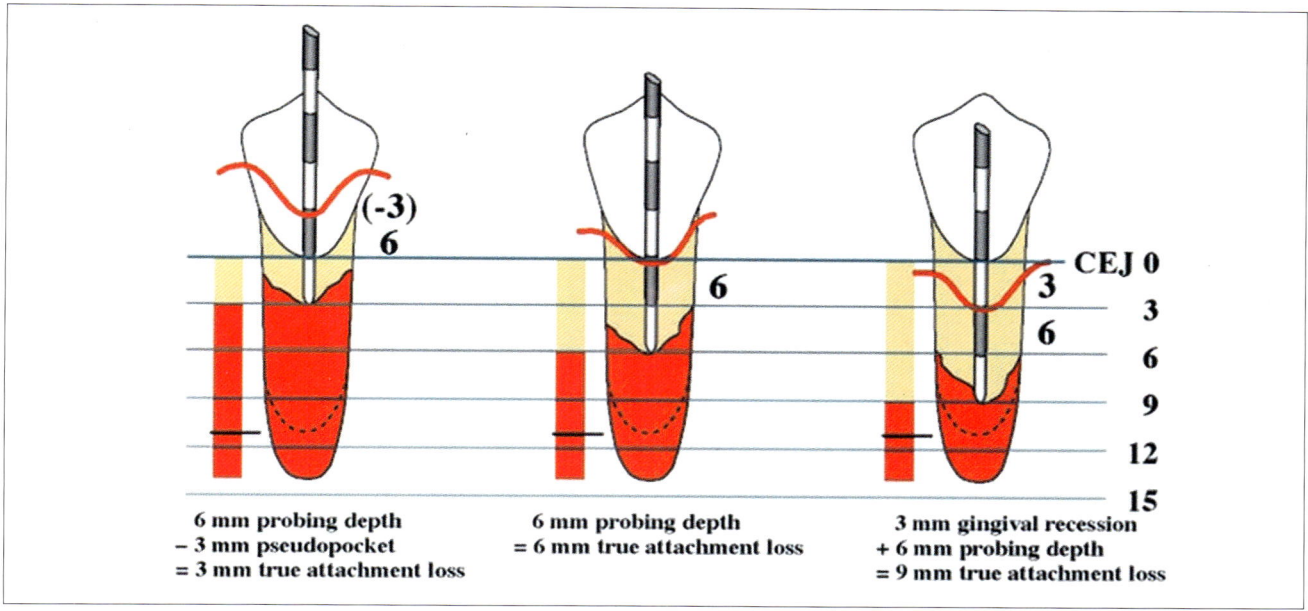

Fig 333 Relationship of probing depth to attachment loss. (Modified from Rateitschak et al, 1989. Reprinted with permission.)

nation and represent a clinically useful approximation of the depth of periodontal pockets. The primary clinical importance of periodontal pockets is that they are major habitats of putative periodontal pathogens. Deep pockets (greater than 5 mm) are particularly difficult for both the patient and therapist to clean, and their presence might increase the risk for progression of periodontitis.

However, probing depth does not disclose the "true" loss of periodontal attachment. Figure 333 shows three different clinical probing attachment levels (3, 6, and 9 mm) but the same probing depth (6 mm). Because of gingival recession and limited inflammation (edema) in the gingival margin, smokers in particular may have advanced PAL but limited probing depth. On the other hand, some drugs, systemic diseases, and hormonal changes may result in extremely hyperplastic gingiva, with formation of pseudopockets and relatively limited PAL. The absence of deep pockets is usually a good indicator of periodontal stability, while deepened pockets indicate periodontal instability.

Vertical probing attachment loss

In single-rooted teeth, loss of attachment occurs only vertically. In multirooted teeth, loss of attachment can also occur horizontally, indicating furcation involvement.

Manual probing

Vertical loss of attachment, the distance between the CEJ and the base of the pocket, can be measured manually with a millimeter-graded probe. When the CEJ is located subgingivally, loss of attachment is measured as shown in Figs 334 and 335. The probe is held with a light pencil grasp so it can be moved and directed with minimal force. The end of the probe is then placed against the enamel surface coronal to the margin of the gingiva, so that the angle formed by the working end of the probe and the long axis of the tooth crown is approximately 45 degrees. With slightly decreased probe-crown angle, the distance between

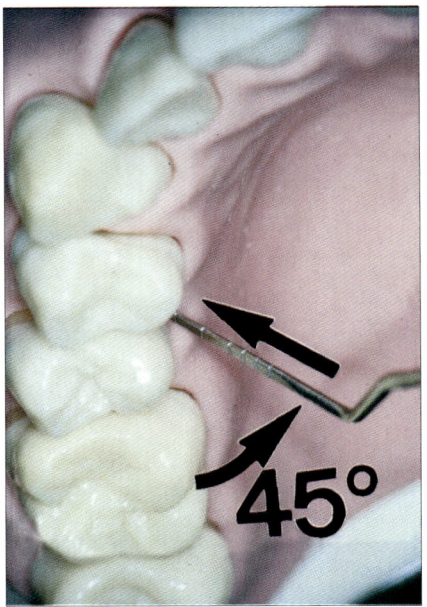

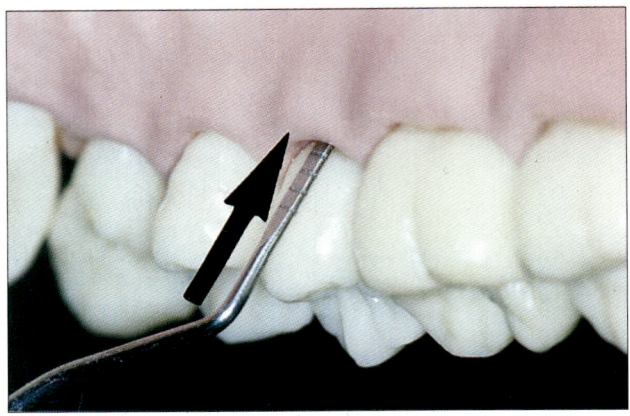

Figs 334 and 335 Measurement of loss of attachment. If the gingival margin is located coronally to the CEJ, the pocket depth is exceeding PAL.

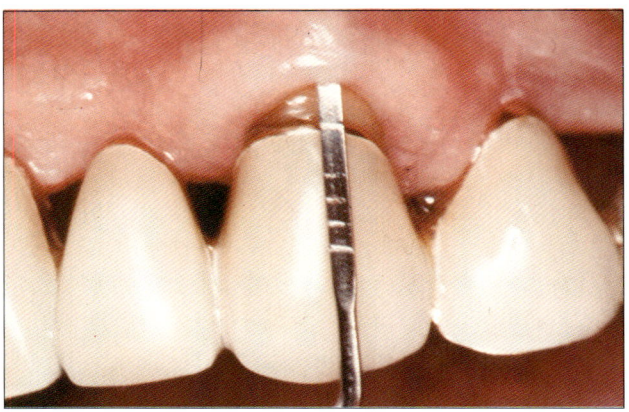

Fig 336 Measurement of attachment loss when the free gingival margin is located apical to the cementoenamel junction or crown margin. Attachment loss is measured directly from the visible cementoenamel junction to the bottom of the pocket.

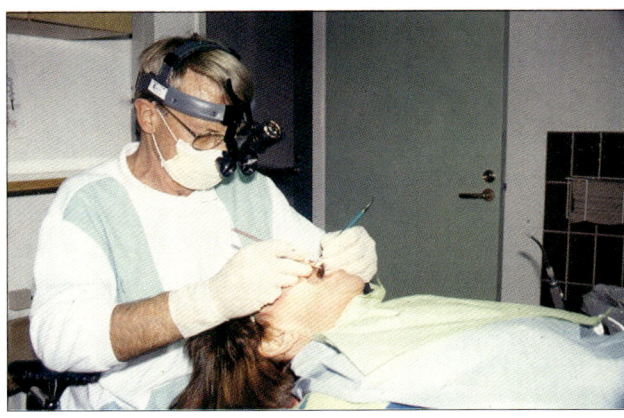

Fig 337 A combination of magnifying telescope (×3) and an extra zooming light improves visibility during the clinical examination.

the free gingival margin and the CEJ is measured. Then the distance between the gingival margin and the base of the pocket is measured (pocket depth). The difference between the two distances is the loss of periodontal attachment. In other words, PAL is 4 mm if the probing depth is 6 mm and the distance from the gingival margin to CEJ is 2 mm.

If the free gingival margin is apical to the CEJ or crown margin, attachment loss is measured directly from the visible CEJ to the bottom of the pocket (Fig 336). To improve visibility during the

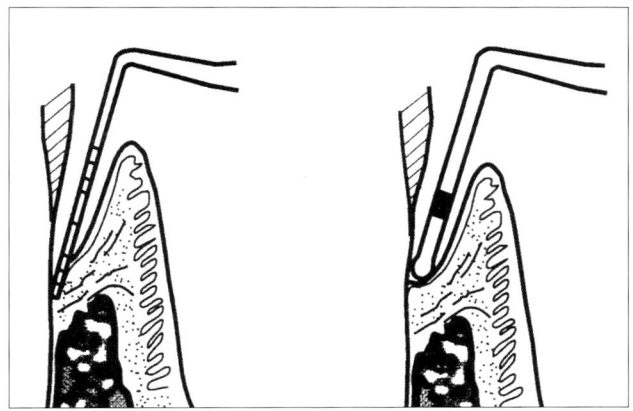

Fig 338 Effect of different sizes of periodontal probes on measurement of probing depth. (From Reddy, 1997. Reprinted with permission.)

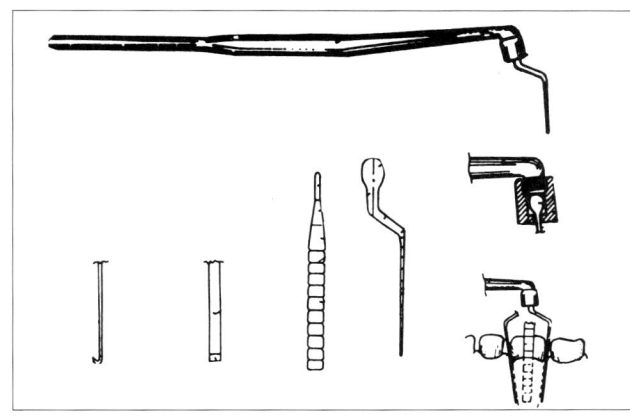

Fig 339 Use of a thin, blade-shaped probe to attain accurate measurement of probing depth. To access all sites, the probe must be rotated 360 degrees.

clinical examination, a combination of magnifying telescope (×3) and an extra zooming light (Orascoptic Direction 3 T, Orascoptic Research, Middleton, WI) are useful aids (Fig 337).

Variability in measurements using the vertical PAL method may be the result of several sources of inherent error, such as *(1)* the dimensions and shape of the periodontal probe; *(2)* the position of the probe and the reference point; *(3)* the coarseness of the measurement scale; *(4)* the probing force; and *(5)* the gingival tissue conditions.

Dimensions of the periodontal probe. It is obvious that different shapes and sizes of periodontal probes will yield different penetration depths into the periodontal tissues, even if all other variables are controlled (Fig 338). The use of probing instruments with standardized dimensions is therefore a prerequisite for repeated measurements of probing depth. Periodontal probes with a point diameter of 0.4 to 0.5 mm have been used successfully.

Most periodontal probes are circular in cross-section: A probe thin enough to reach the "true" attachment level under healthy conditions, with junctional epithelium and "resistant" connective tissue, will penetrate the less resistant, inflamed connective tissue in diseased pockets and overestimate loss by 0.5 to 1.0 mm. A thicker circular probe will not reach the true attachment level in healthy pockets. A thin, blade-shaped probe will give the most accurate result, but to access all the sites, it has to be able to be rotated 360 degrees (Axelsson, 1982) (Fig 339).

Positioning of the probe. Manual probing is subject to measurement error because of variations in the angulation and site of insertion of the probe and because of the difficulty in obtaining a fixed landmark as a reference point. The probe should be kept as parallel as possible to the long axis of the root. The tip should continuously follow the root surface, to prevent penetration of the pocket epithelium and connective tissue, resulting in underestimation of attachment loss (Figs 340 to 343).

Although the aim of probing depth is to identify the deepest part of the pocket at every site, PAL should be measured at the same, easily identifiable position at every examination, to enable changes to be monitored over time (Figs 344 and 345). The following principles are recommended to optimize reproducibility. The mesial surface is assessed mesiobucally and mesiolingually, and the higher value is registered as representing mesial loss of attachment. The distal surface is as-

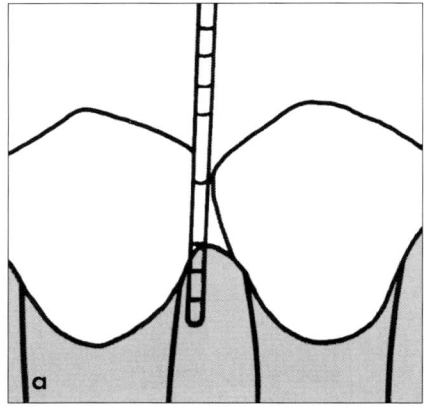 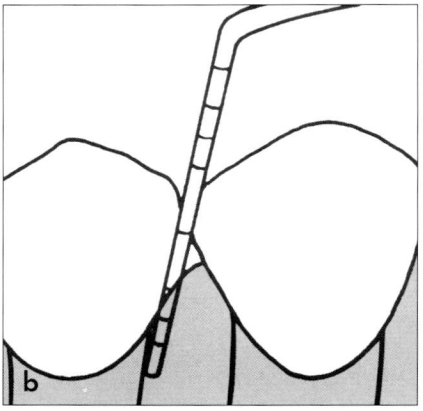

Fig 340a Underestimation of probing depth and PAL. (From Parr and Green, 1974. Reprinted with permission.)

Fig 340b Accurate probing depth and PAL attained by keeping the probe as parallel as possible to the long axis of the root. (From Parr and Green, 1974. Reprinted with permission.)

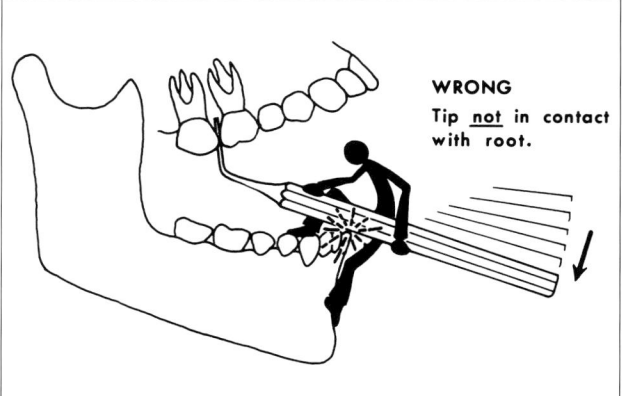

WRONG
Tip **not** in contact with root.

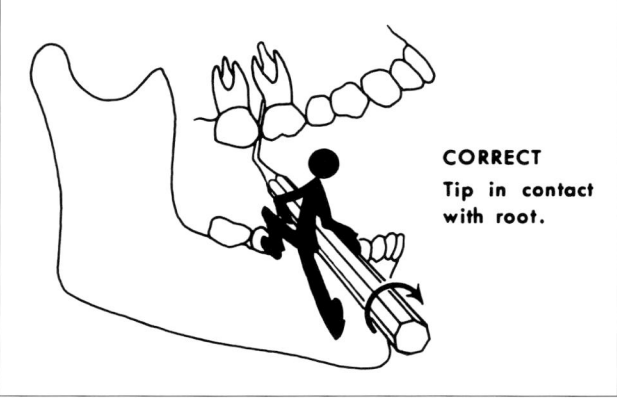

CORRECT
Tip **in** contact with root.

Fig 341 Incorrect placement of a periodontal probe for measurement of probing depth and PAL. (From Parr and Green, 1974. Reprinted with permission.)

Fig 342 Correct placement of a periodontal probe for measurement of probing depth and PAL. (From Parr and Green, 1974. Reprinted with permission.)

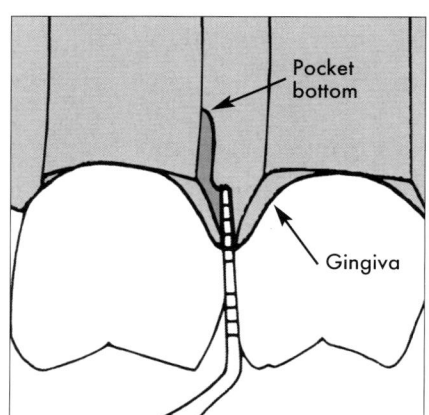

Pocket bottom

Gingiva

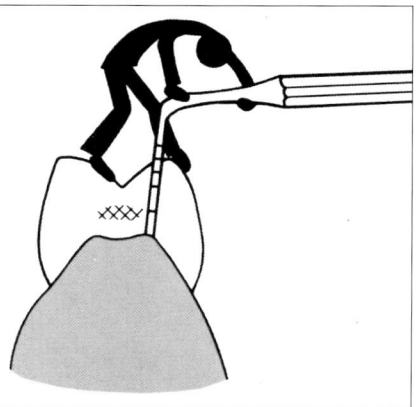 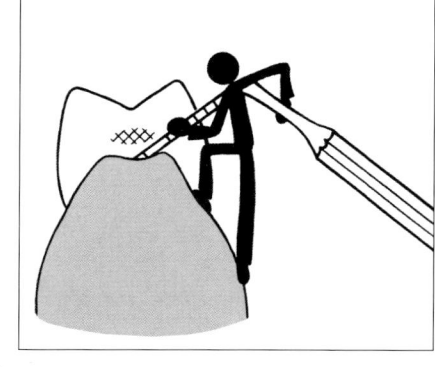

Fig 343 Incorrect placement of a periodontal probe, causing penetration of pocket epithelium and connective tissue and resulting in underestimation of probing depth and PAL. (From Parr and Green, 1974. Reprinted with permission.)

Figs 344 and 345 Effect of using different probe positioning during measurement of probing depth and PAL. Periodontal attachment loss should be measured at the same, easily identifiable position at every examination, to allow changes to be monitored over time. (From Parr and Green, 1974. Reprinted with permission.)

sessed only distobuccally. The buccal and lingual surfaces are measured at the most prominent part of the root surfaces. In multirooted teeth, the maxillary and mandibular molars, the highest buccal value is registered, as is the highest lingual value of the mandibular molars.

Coarseness of the measurement scale. Probing depth measurements are generally assessed to the nearest millimeter. For example, measurements of 2.0 to 2.5 mm are recorded as "2 mm," and measurements greater than 2.5 mm and up to 3.5 mm are recorded as "3 mm." Therefore, a recorded loss of attachment of 0.5 mm will include a high incidence of false-negative values. This, in turn, means that "true" disease progression may actually occur, but the intervals on the measurement scale are too coarse to disclose minor deterioration. Although commonly used periodontal probes, such as the WHO probes (LM Dental, Finland), are graded at 3.5 mm, followed by intervals of 2.0 mm, some of the new electric, pressure-controlled probes (eg, the Florida Probe, Florida Probe, Gainsville, FL) register PAL of 0.1 mm.

Probing force and gingival tissue conditions. In clinical application, periodontal probes used at clinically healthy sites, with what would be considered "gentle" (0.20- to 0.50-N) insertion forces, do not penetrate to the apical termination of the junctional epithelium. At sites treated for periodontitis, probes also fail to reach the apical termination of the junctional epithelium consistently. Furthermore, most studies of sites with untreated periodontitis indicate that probes tend to penetrate the tissues to a level apical to the apical termination of the junctional epithelium (Keagle et al, 1989). Apparently, the primary factor in resistance to probe insertion is the tone of the connective tissue adjacent to the pocket wall.

Based on the available data, it can be concluded that, at sites with periodontitis, the true levels of connective tissue attachment tend to be overestimated in pretreatment measurements of PAL and underestimated in posttreatment measurements (Robinson and Vitek, 1979). To ap-

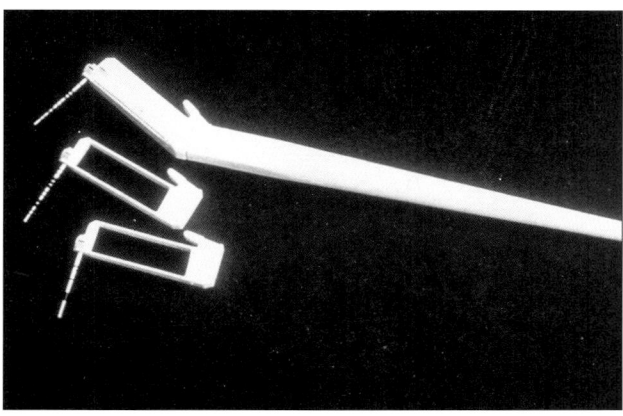

Fig 346 Hunter Probe, calibrated to insert the probe tip with a force of 20 g.

proximate true PAL more closely, the probing force would therefore need to be greater at healthy sites than at inflamed sites. However, it is also clear from data that, on average, the probeable discrepancy between pretreatment and posttreatment assessments of PAL is rarely more than 1 millimeter.

Automated probing

Because probing force is one of the major variables affecting the extent of probe penetration, several automated or controlled-force probes have recently been introduced. Most can be modified to deliver a range of insertion forces, some are computer linked to automatically record clinical measurements, and a few have resolutions of 0.1 to 0.5 mm.

The Hunter Probe (Vivadent, Liechtenstein) is a disposable device calibrated to insert the probe tip with a force of 20 g (Fig 346). The Foster-Miller Probe (Foster-Miller, Waltham, MA) is a controlled-force device capable of automatically recording the position of the CEJ. Of the other controlled-force probes, the Florida Probe is the most widely used. Comparative reproducibility data from many studies do not show major differences between conventional and controlled-force probes.

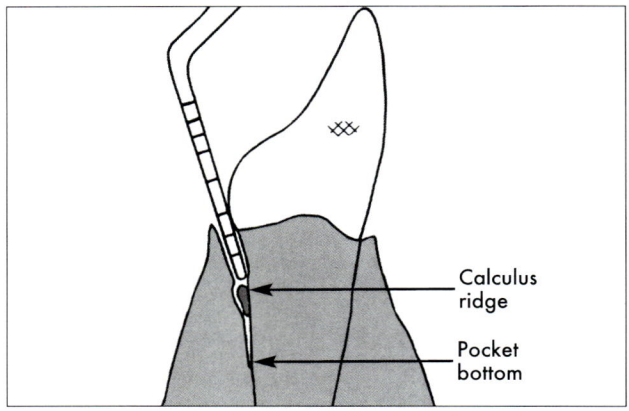

Fig 347 Pretreatment probing depth and PAL measurement. Calculus obstructs the probe, resulting in an inaccurate measurement. (From Parr and Green, 1974. Reprinted with permission.)

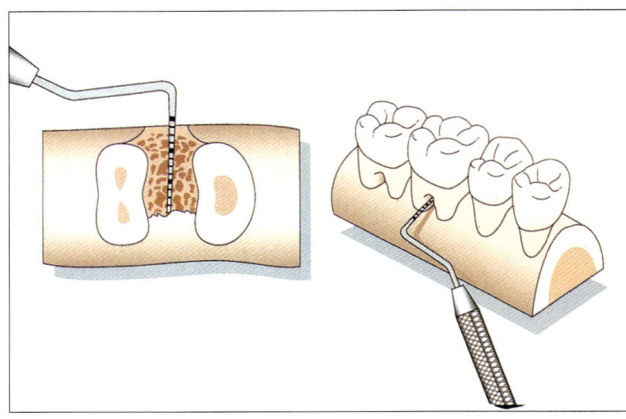

Fig 348 Advanced, grade II furcation involvement in a mandibular molar.

In a recent study, Reddy et al (1997) showed that both manual and controlled-force probes (Florida Probe) can provide measurement to within less than 1 mm of error.

The most important variable for evaluation of the long-term efficacy of therapy and maintenance programs is PAL. However, posttreatment evaluations are less subject to the confounding effects of measurement error than is pretreatment evaluation. Before treatment, the reference point (cementoenamel junction) may be obstructed by calculus (Fig 347) or by dental restorations, and the condition of the gingival tissues may readily allow the periodontal probe to penetrate the tissues, even when probe position and pressure are standardized. Initial periodontal therapy should minimize these biologic variables (tissue condition and the presence of calculus): For long-term clinical monitoring, periodontal reevaluation, following initial therapy and healing, should therefore be taken as the baseline. (For review on variables related to probing, see Garnick and Silverstein, 2000.)

Horizontal probing attachment loss (furcation involvement)

Progressive periodontal disease around two-rooted or multirooted teeth destroys the supporting structures of the furcation area. Because treatment is often complicated, precise identification of the presence and extent of periodontal tissue breakdown within the furcation area of each multirooted tooth is of importance for proper diagnosis and treatment planning. Three grades of furcation involvement may be classified.

- Grade I: Horizontal loss of supporting tissues not exceeding one third of the width of the tooth
- Grade II: Horizontal loss of supporting tissues exceeding one third of the width of the tooth but not encompassing the total width of the furcation area
- Grade III: Horizontal "through-and-through" destruction of the supporting tissues in the furcation

Figure 348 illustrates advanced furcation involvement (grade II—almost grade III) in a mandibular molar. Figure 349 shows cross sections of the roots of the maxillary and mandibular

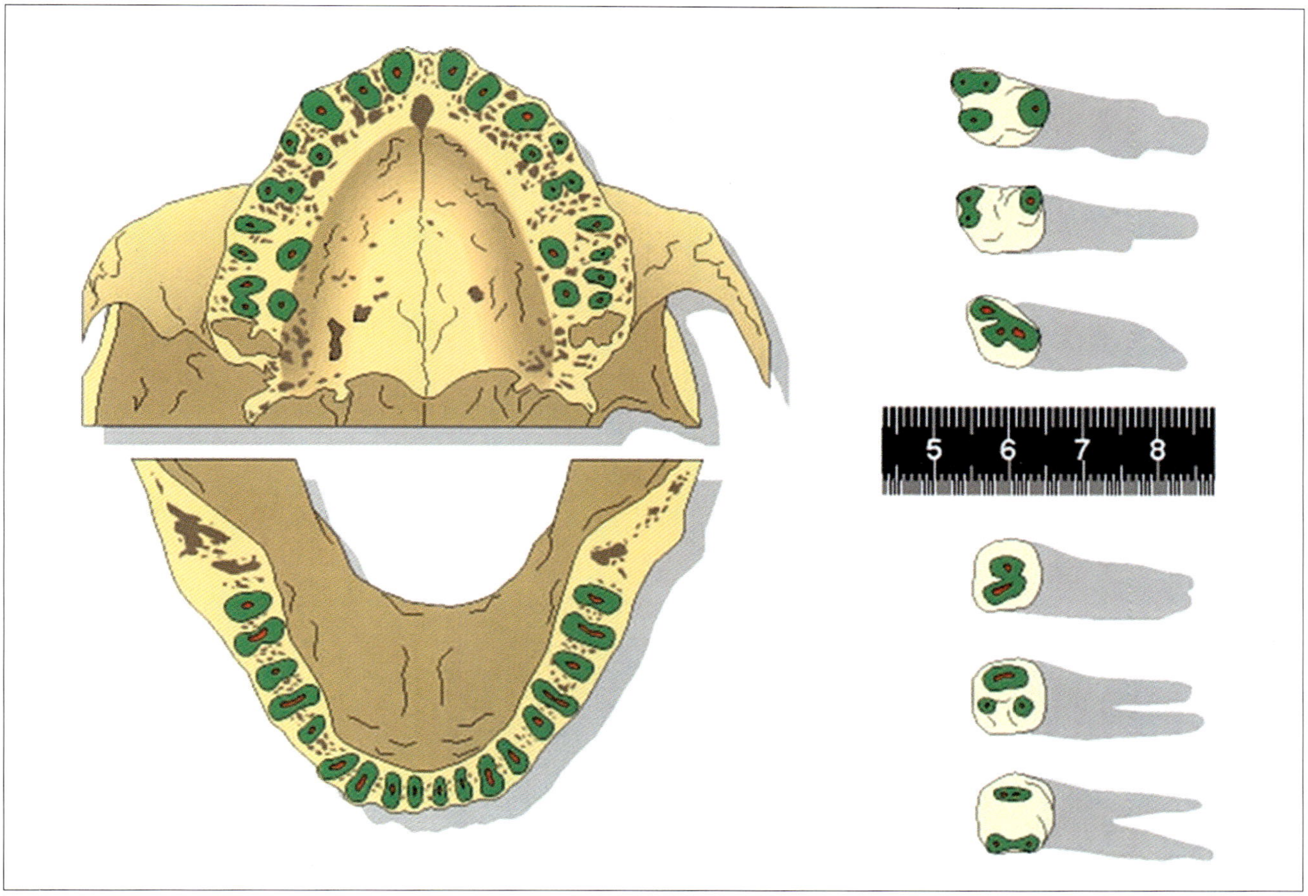

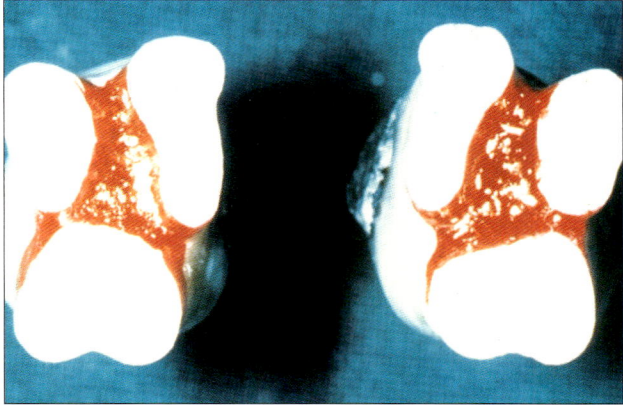

Fig 349 Cross sections of maxillary and mandibular teeth and variations in furcation topography on different teeth. (Modified from Rateitschak et al, 1989. Reprinted with permission.)

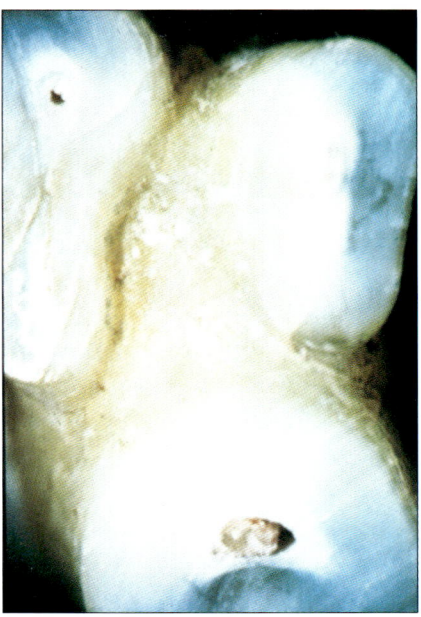

Figs 350 and 351 Cross section of the furcation regions of maxillary first molars.

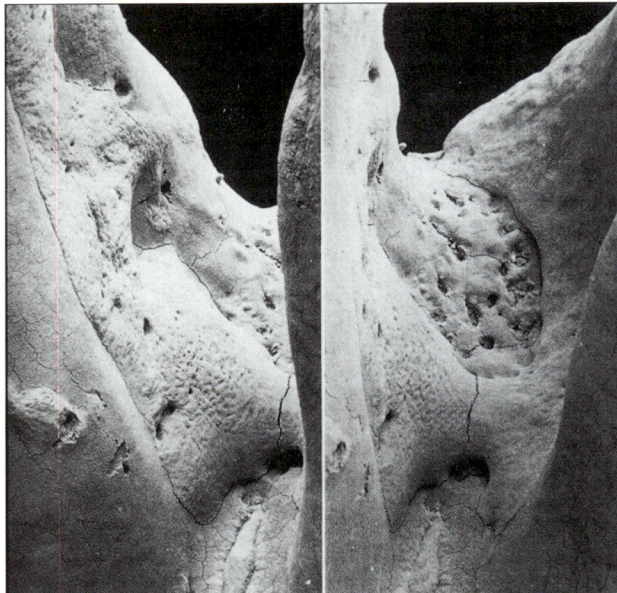

Fig 352 Detail of the furcation area. Perforations indicate accessory canals from the pulp, confirming the need to perform a pulp test for all teeth with furcation involvement.

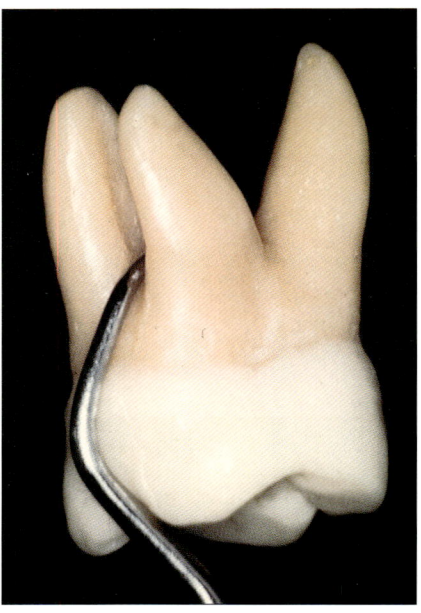 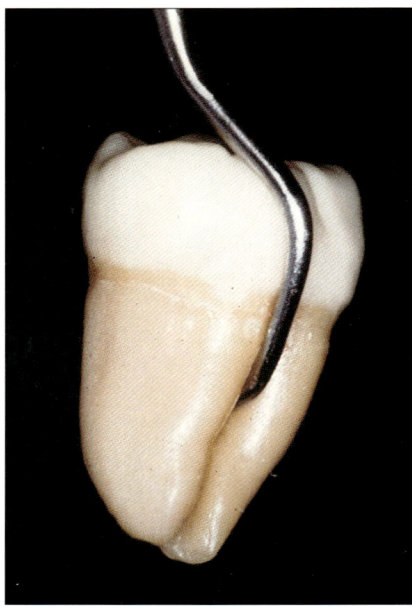

Figs 353 and 354 Double-ended Goldman-Fox No. 3 (Hu-Friedy, Chicago, IL), a long, slim curette, used for diagnosis of furcation involvement in maxillary and mandibular molars.

teeth and the possible variations of furcation involvement on different root surfaces.

Figures 350 and 351 show different cross sections of the furcation regions of the maxillary first molars. Because treatment of furcation involvement on the relatively inaccessible approximal surfaces of these teeth is complicated, gingival plaque control and early diagnosis of initial furcation involvement are of great importance. Figure 352 shows perforations indicating accessory canals from the coronal pulp, confirming the need to perform pulp tests for all teeth with furcation involvement.

For accurate diagnosis, a slim, curved instrument is necessary, eg, the double-ended curette, Goldman-Fox No. 3 (Figs 353 and 354). Specially

Fig 355 *(near right)* Mesial furcation involvement of the maxillary molar. This must be diagnosed in a mesiolingual-apical direction. MB = Mesiobuccal root; P = Palatal root; GF3 = Goldman-Fox No. 3 curette.

Fig 356 *(far right)* Distal furcation involvement of the maxillary molar. This must be diagnosed in a distobuccal-apical direction. DB = Distobuccal root; P = Palatal root.

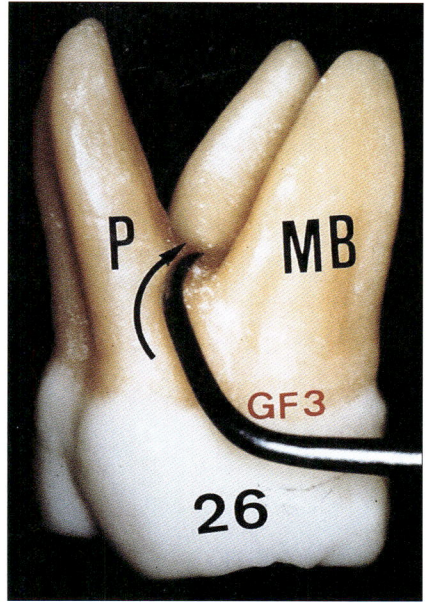

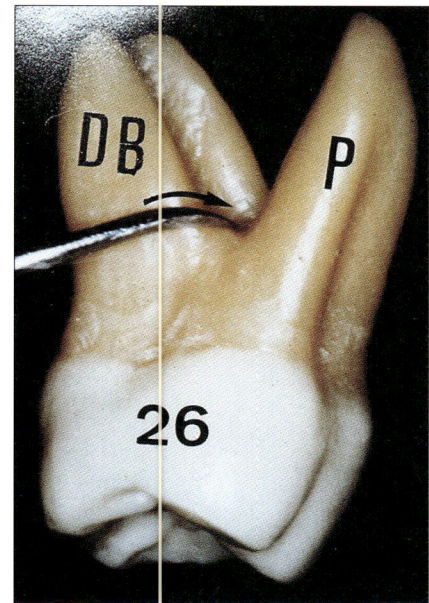

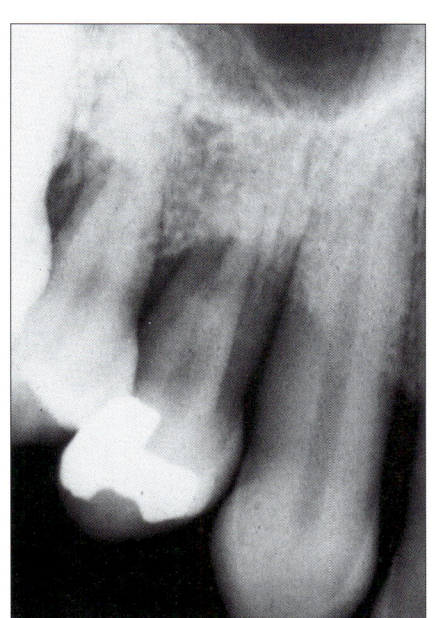

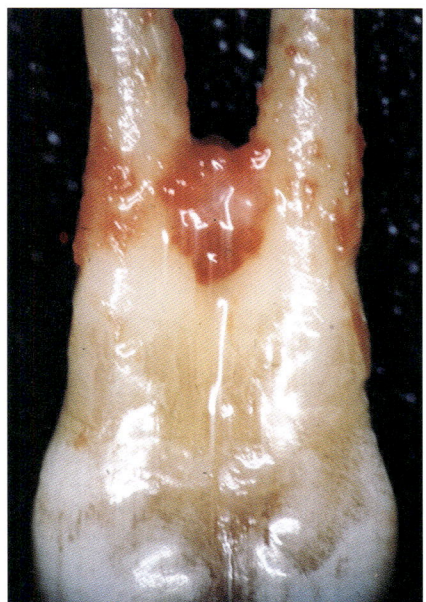

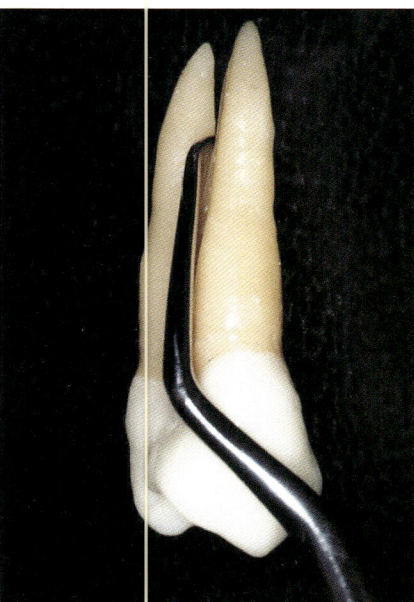

Fig 357 Eccentric radiograph of a maxillary first premolar for the diagnosis of furcation involvement. The level of the entrance of the furcation area should be compared with the most coronal margin of the alveolar bone. The obvious furcation involvement of the first premolar was finally confirmed by probing with a curette.

Fig 358 The maxillary first premolar in Fig 357 after extraction due to furcation involvement (grade III). Attached granulation tissue was shown in the furcation area.

Fig 359 Goldman-Fox No. 4, a thin curette with an elongated neck, used for diagnosis of furcation involvement in maxillary first premolars.

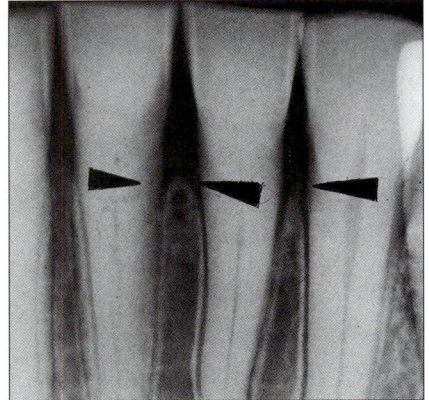

Fig 360 Radiograph revealing the height and configuration of the interproximal alveolar bone *(arrows)*.

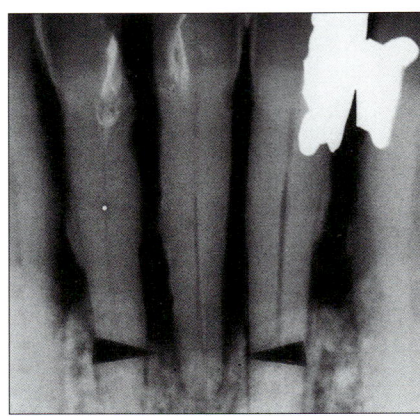

Fig 361 Radiograph revealing defects on the approximal root surfaces *(arrows)*.

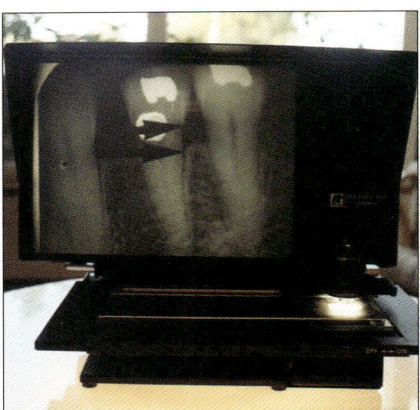

Fig 362 Use of a magnifying viewer to aid diagnosis of alveolar bone loss.

designed probes for diagnosis of furcation involvement are also available, eg, the flexible disposable tip of the TPS Probe (Vivadent) and the Furcation Probe (LM Dental). Clinical examination of furcations on the approximal tooth surfaces may be more difficult when neighboring teeth are present, especially if the teeth have broad approximal contact areas, as in maxillary molars. Furcations on the mesial surface of a maxillary molar should be probed from the mesiopalatal aspect (Fig 355) and those on the distal surface from the distobuccal aspect (Fig 356) in a slightly apical direction.

Eccentric radiographs should be used to detect furcation involvement, and the levels of the entrance of the furcation area should be compared with the most coronal margin of the alveolar bone. Thereafter, the diagnosis is verified by probing. In maxillary first premolars, this is particularly important for differentiating root grooves from furcation involvement between the buccal and lingual roots, because the entrance to the furcation is usually extremely apical (Figs 357 and 358). Such furcation involvement can be accessible to a thin curette (Goldman-Fox No. 4) with an elongated neck (Fig 359).

RADIOGRAPHIC DIAGNOSIS

Conventional radiographs

For detailed analysis of the alveolar bone, it is usual to take intraoral complete-mouth radiographs, supplemented with four vertical bitewing radiographs. A standardized technique is used, eg, film holders attached to the long cone. The radiographs provide information on the height and configuration of the interproximal alveolar bone (Fig 360) and disclose the presence of calculus and defects on the approximal root surfaces (Fig 361).

In experimental studies, measurement of interproximal alveolar bone loss is facilitated by the use of special films equipped with a millimeter grid, and a viewer with ×10 magnification (Fig 362). The normal threshold for no loss of alveolar bone is 1.5 to 2.0 mm from the CEJ to the most coronal level of the "intact" supporting bone. It is usually about 1.5 mm in children and young adults and 2.0 mm in adults and the elderly because of attrition and compensatory elongation. Thus, actual loss of alveolar bone is evaluated by measuring the distance from CEJ to the most coronal level of alveolar bone and subtracting 1.5 to 2.0 mm.

Fig 363 By combination of radiographs, probing depth, and attachment level data, different types of bony defects (three-, two-, and one-wall bony defects) may be diagnosed.

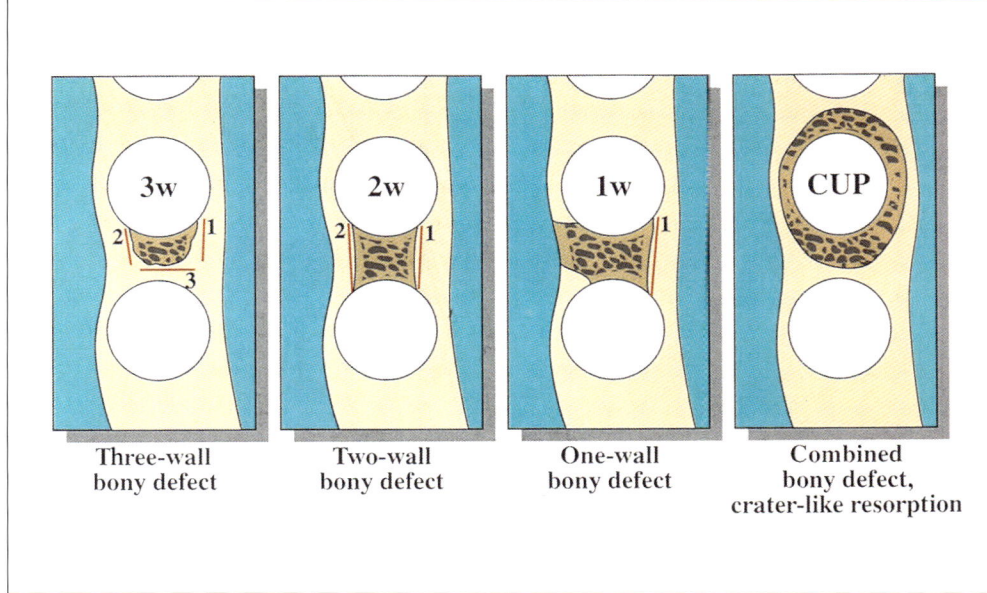

Three-wall bony defect

Two-wall bony defect

One-wall bony defect

Combined bony defect, crater-like resorption

Fig 364a An exposed infrabony pocket.

Fig 364b Placement of special millimeter-graded probe during radiography to aid analysis of the same infrabony pocket. In addition, a radiograph with a square millimeter grid was used.

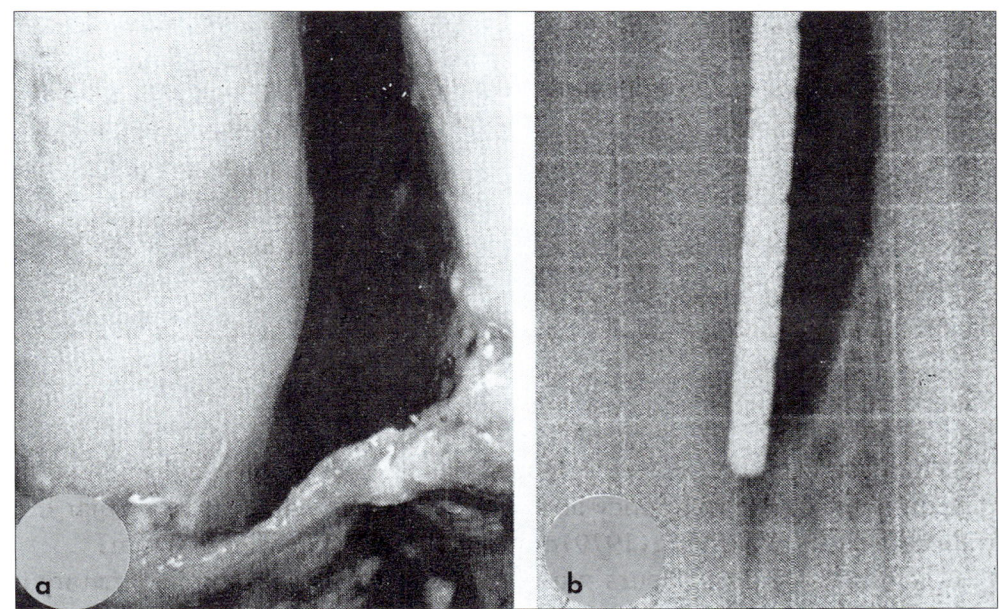

The outlines of the buccal and lingual crests of the alveolar bone tend to be obscured by overlying structures (bone tissue and teeth). Diagnosis of "horizontal" and "vertical" bone loss and different types of bone defects should therefore be based on a combination of radiographic analysis and detailed evaluation of probing depth and attachment level data (Fig 363). For detailed analysis of infrabony pockets, special millimeter-graded probes can be inserted into the pockets during radiography and the afore-mentioned film with a millimeter grid can be used (Figs 364a and 364b).

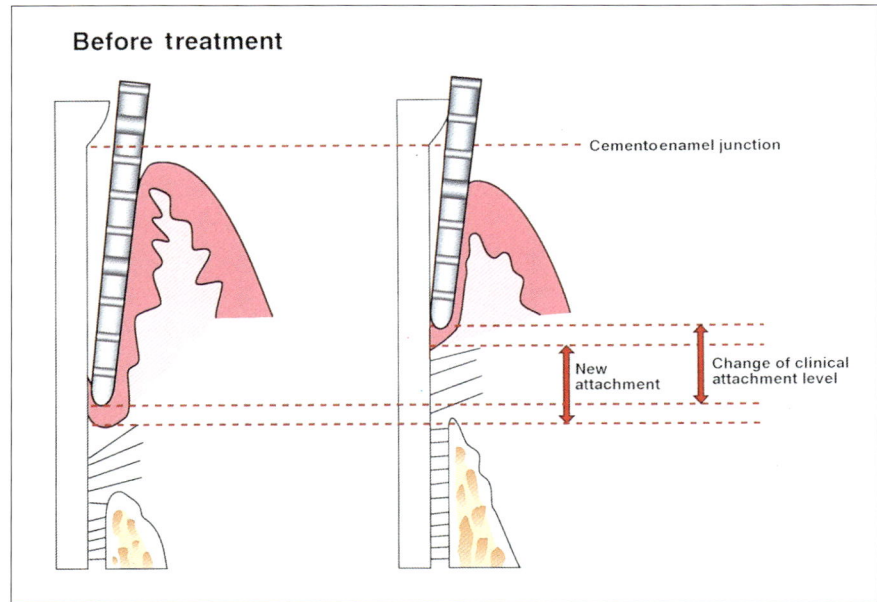

Before treatment

Cementoenamel junction

New attachment

Change of clinical attachment level

Figs 365 to 367 Monitoring the clinical outcome of regenerative therapy. *(Fig 365, left)* Analysis is aided by the placement of a periodontal probe to indicate periodontal attachment level during exposure of pretreatment and posttreatment radiographs. (Courtesy of K. Rateitschak.) *(Fig 366, below left)* Periodontal probe inserted mesially in a two-wall infrabony pocket of the second mandibular molar on the right side (tooth 47) before regenerative therapy with Emdogain (Biora, Lund, Sweden). *(Fig 367, below right)* The result after 13 months confirmed by radiograph and inserted probe.

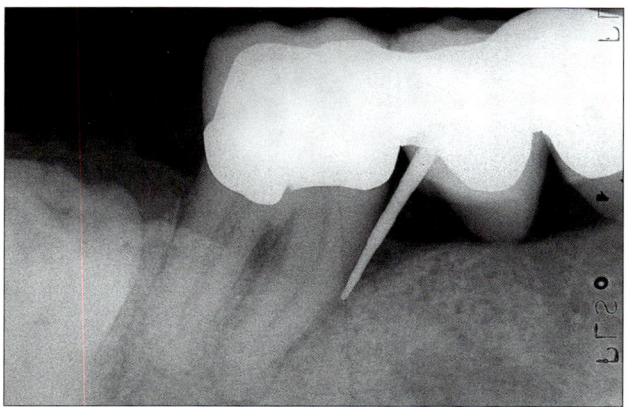
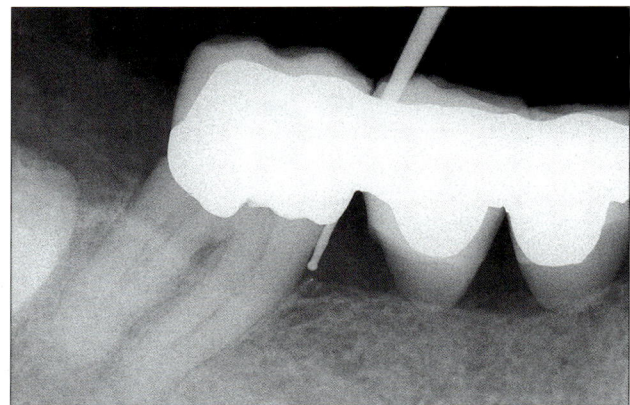

There has been considerable debate as to the determinants of the frequency and cause of infrabony lesions. Waerhaug (1979) demonstrated that bone resorption occurs when microbial plaque approaches to within 0.5 to 2.0 mm of the bone surface. Based on these and other observations, Page and Schroeder (1982) postulated a 2.5-mm range of influence of the subgingival plaque (biofilm) on alveolar bone loss. They stated that "when the bone surface has been resorbed to about 2.5 mm apical or lateral to the site of the bacteria, bone loss appears to cease and bone production takes over, until it equals or surpasses resorption." Therefore, infrabony lesions seldom develop on the buccal surfaces, where the alveolar bone is normally very thin (less than 3 mm).

The inflammatory infiltrate also plays a role: The closer the cells of the inflammatory infiltrate are to the bone, the more osteoclasts appear and the more bone is degraded (Schroeder and Lindhe, 1980). Tal (1984) provided data supporting this hypothesis by measuring infrabony lesions in 344 interproximal areas and 117 infrabony pockets in 84 patients. At interdental distances less than 2.6 mm, infrabony lesions were only rarely observed; they occurred on both adjacent teeth only at interdental distances greater than 3.1 mm.

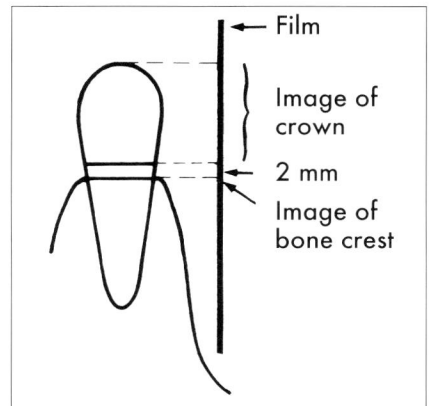

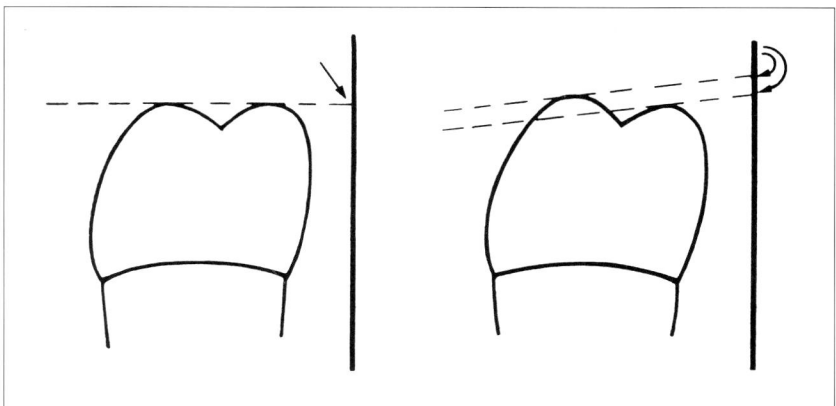

Fig 368 Correct positioning of film to attain an undistorted periapical radiograph. Dashed lines indicate direction of radiation (see also Figs 369 to 376). (From Parr and Green, 1974. Reprinted with permission.)

Fig 369 *(left)* Correct and *(right)* incorrect angulation of the X-ray beam for a periapical radiograph. If the angulation is correct, the buccal and lingual cusp tips appear to be at approximately the same level in the resulting radiograph. (From Parr and Green, 1974. Reprinted with permission.)

In order to arrive at a correct diagnosis with respect to the alveolar bone level, the presence of angular bony defects and interdental osseous craters, and so on, an additional method, called *sounding,* may be used. While the site is under local anesthesia, the periodontal probe is inserted into the pocket, the tip being forced through the supra-alveolar connective tissue to contact the bone, and the distance from the cemento-enamel junction to the bone is assessed in millimeters. A particularly useful technique for monitoring the clinical outcome of regenerative therapy is placement of a periodontal probe to indicate PAL as pretreatment and posttreatment radiographs are exposed (Figs 365 to 367; see also Figs 95 and 97 in chapter 1; Figs 142 and 145 to 149 in chapter 3; and Figs 295 to 297, 306, 308, and 309 in chapter 5).

Role of angulation

By their very nature, transmission radiographs are limited: They are two-dimensional representations of the three-dimensional alveolar bone, tooth, and soft tissue. This two-dimensional map-ping is highly subject to angulation error, incurred during positioning of the films and the X-ray tube head. The periapical view has been designed to minimize distortion of the bone-root relationship while the root apex is imaged (Fig 368). To achieve an accurate representation of the bone height along the root surface, the central ray must be perpendicular to the area of interest and the intraoral film. Periapical radiographs are subject to operator error, especially in the maxillary molar regions, and may present a distorted bone-tooth relationship, foreshortening, or elongation. The bone may even appear to cover the enamel of the teeth, increasing the risk of misdiagnosis.

The quality of the periapical radiograph may be evaluated by examining the cusp tips of the posterior teeth. Buccal and lingual cusp tips should appear at approximately the same level: When they appear at different levels, the cause is usually incorrect angulation of the film, which also distorts the apparent location of the bone height along the root surface (Fig 369). This is the underlying cause of the radiographic illusion of bone deposition or resorption, unrelated to any true change arising from therapy or disease progression (Figs 369 to 376).

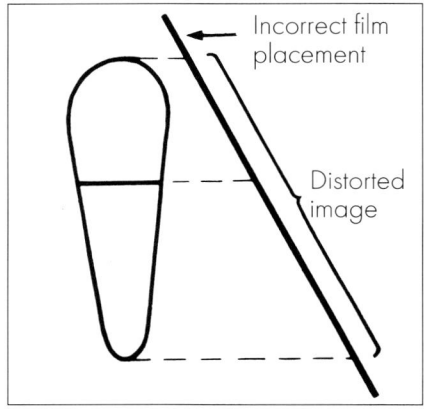

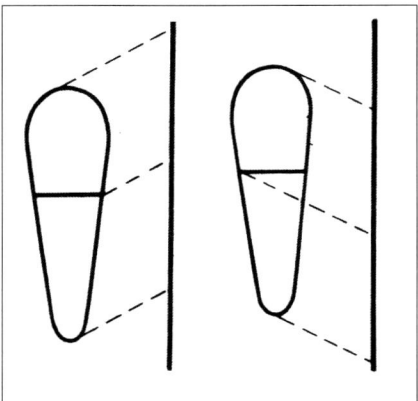

Fig 370 Incorrect angulation of the X-ray beam, which results in distortion of crown or root length in the radiograph. (From Parr and Green, 1974. Reprinted with permission.)

Figs 371 and 372 Incorrect vertical angulation of the X-ray beam, which results in distortion of bone height in the radiograph. (From Parr and Green, 1974. Reprinted with permission.)

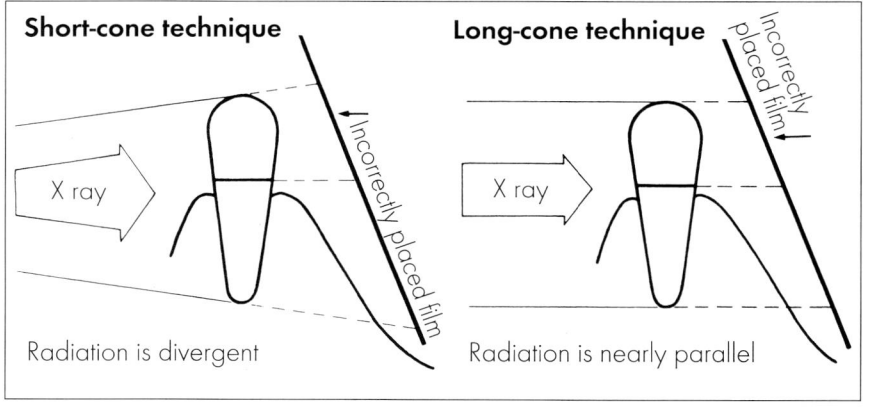

Fig 373 Effect of incorrect film placement on the results of short-cone and long-cone radiographs. (From Parr and Green, 1974. Reprinted with permission.)

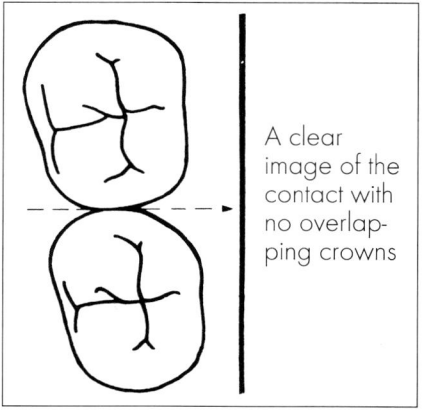

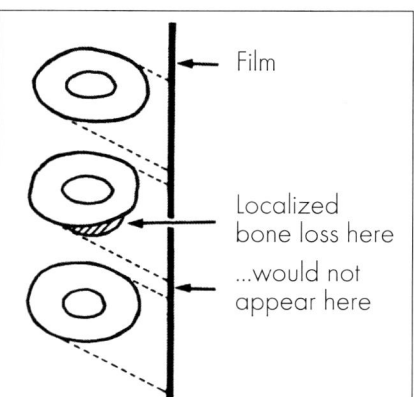

Fig 374 Correct horizontal angulation of the X-ray beam, which results in a clear image. (From Parr and Green, 1974. Reprinted with permission.)

Figs 375 and 376 Incorrect horizontal angulation of the X-ray beam, which results in obstruction of some details or overlapping of features. (From Parr and Green, 1974. Reprinted with permission.)

This source of distortion is readily minimized. First, a long cone should always be used. The relatively parallel rays minimize the distortion of the image that would result from divergence of the beam between the bone and teeth and the film. Second, commercially available paralleling positioning devices help to standardize the relationship among film, object, and X-ray source. Such devices reduce operator error and can aid in reducing radiation exposure by minimizing the need for retakes. A further benefit is enhancement of the diagnostic value of the radiograph, because the dentist has greater confidence in the validity of the relationship between the bone and the tooth root.

Other views are also useful for periodontal diagnosis: in fact, the bite-wing radiograph is often overlooked in periodontal diagnosis. Bite-wing radiographs are taken with the X-ray beam perpendicular to the bone and the tooth root, thus minimizing the distortion of the location of the bone height along the root. A disadvantage is the very restricted view of the osseous crest, which may preclude its application as a diagnostic aid, even in cases of periodontitis with only moderate bone loss.

Vertical, or standing, bite-wing radiographs are therefore recommended: The long axis of the film is placed vertically in the mouth, at either anterior or posterior sites. The resulting radiograph discloses considerably more bone and can be used to assess bone height in patients with moderate to severe bone loss (Figs 377 to 381). Compared with individual periapical radiographs, vertical bite-wing radiographs require a smaller radiation dose because several maxillary and mandibular teeth are included on one piece of film. The bone height is generally imaged very accurately along the root surface because of the ease of directing the X-ray beam perpendicular to the tooth, either by eye or with a specially designed vertical bite-wing positioning device.

Other limitations

Conventional radiographs are used not only in clinical practice, but also in most cross-sectional epidemiologic studies. Radiographs disclose the damage the disease has already caused to the supporting alveolar bone rather than current presence of the disease. Bone loss is usually assessed on intraoral radiographs. The interproximal bone is evaluated both quantitatively and qualitatively. The following features are recorded: the presence of an intact lamina dura, the width of the periodontal ligament space, the morphology of the bone crest ("even" or "angular") and the distance between the CEJ and the most coronal level of the "intact" alveolar bone. The last is the most common criterion, although it may be heavily influenced by projection geometry (see Figs 369 to 376). Bite-wing radiographic assessments have also been widely used in screening, particularly for localized aggressive periodontitis (Figs 382 and 383).

Conventional radiographic evaluation of periodontal status also has some important limitations, for example, the fact that there must be major loss of mineral mass (more than 50%) before it can be detected on a radiograph by the naked eye. In a study by Goodson et al (1984), standardized radiographs and repeated periodontal probing measurements were made on untreated subjects with destructive periodontal disease monitored for 1 year. Radiographs of selected sites were taken at 6 and 12 months and attachment levels were measured monthly. Significant PAL generally preceded radiographically detectable bone loss by 6 to 8 months.

At 4 mm PAL, subsequent bone loss would be predictive with a true-positive ratio of 60% and a false-positive ratio of 5%, indicating a high degree of predictive discrimination. In contrast, the potential for a true-positive ratio of bone loss on radiographs to predict PAL was 0%, and the false-positive ratio was 100%. For sites of active disease, PAL measurements changed by an average of 4.6 mm, while radiographic crestal bone height changed by 0.76 mm. These observations indicate that PAL precedes radiographic evidence of crestal alveolar bone loss during periods of periodontal disease activity. This study clearly demonstrated that radiation exposure and cost preclude the use

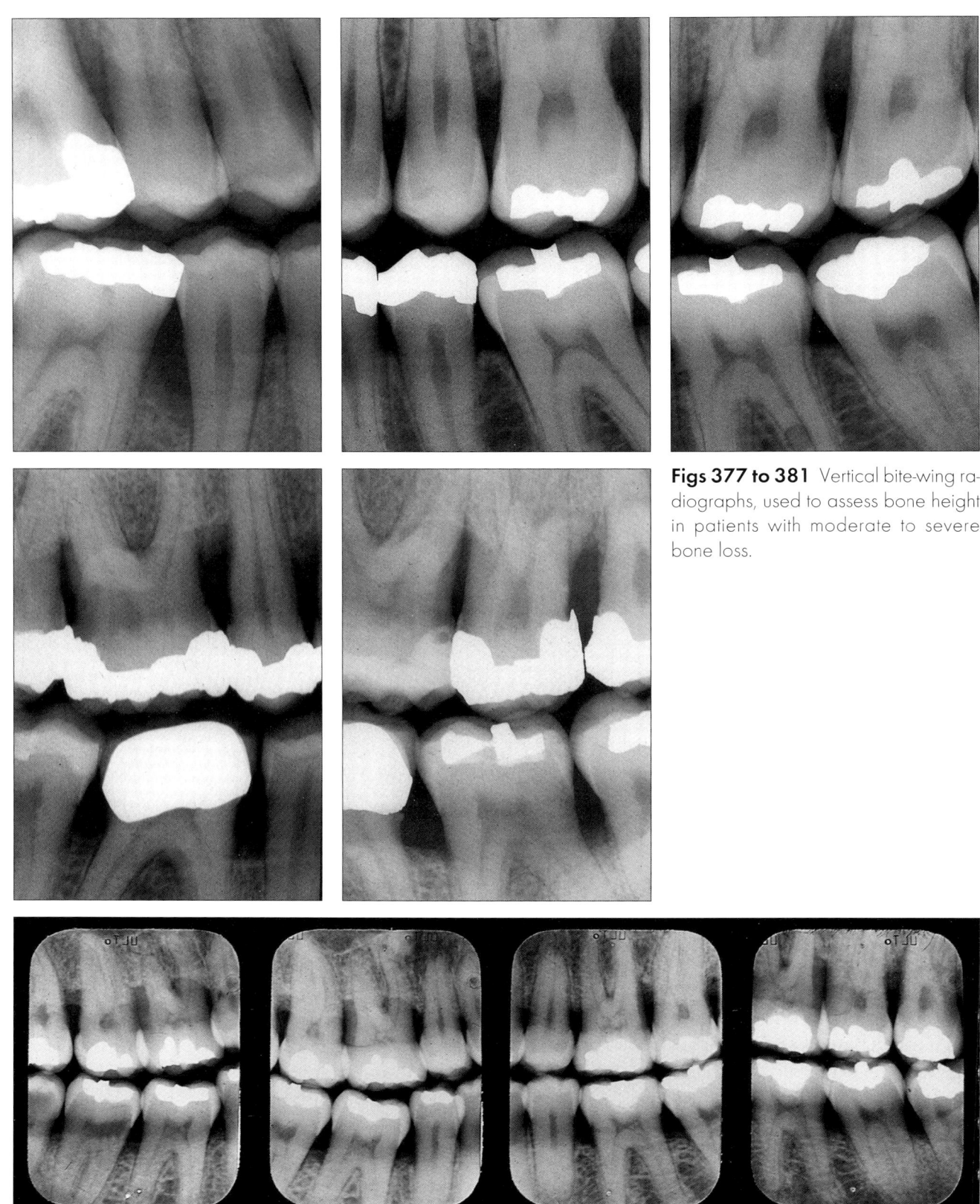

Figs 377 to 381 Vertical bite-wing radiographs, used to assess bone height in patients with moderate to severe bone loss.

Figs 382 and 383 Bite-wing radiographs, used to screen for cases of localized aggressive periodontitis.

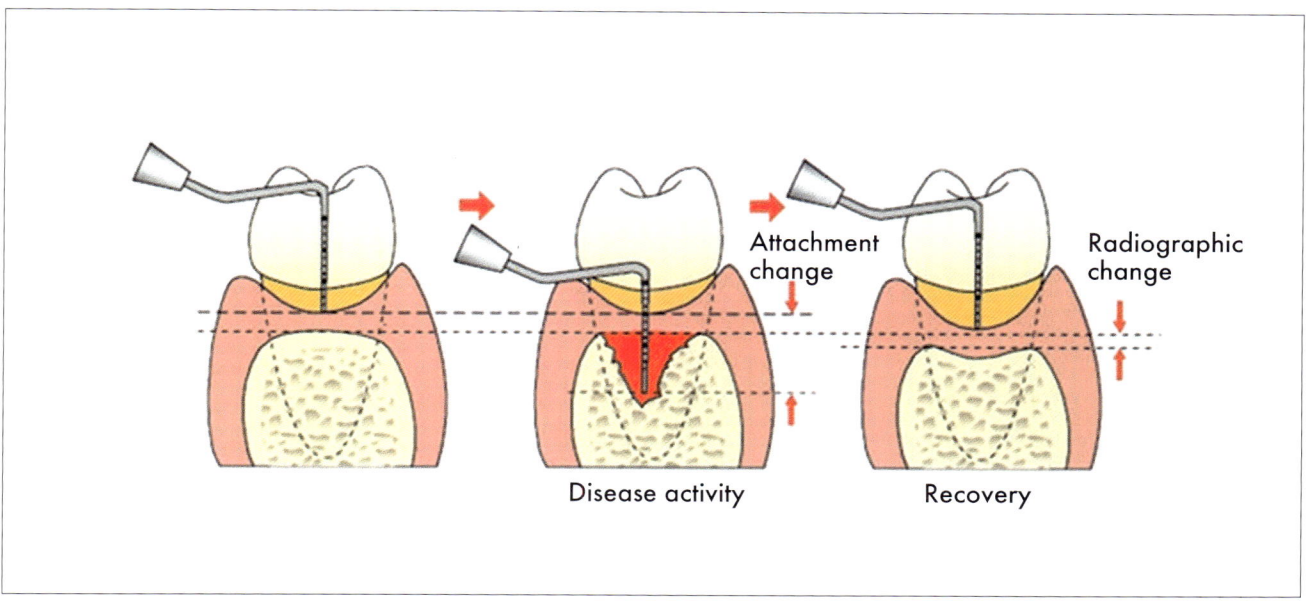

Fig 384 Relationship of probing attachment levels to radiographic change. (Modified from Goodson et al, 1984. Reprinted with permission.)

of complete-mouth radiographs for monitoring changes in periodontal support. (Goodson et al, 1984).

Figure 384 from the study illustrates possible attachment level and alveolar bone changes during a period of active destructive periodontal disease. The earliest phase results in medullary bone loss and an accompanying increase in probing attachment level. During this phase, radiographic evidence of bone loss is not apparent because the cortical bone height remains unchanged. At the end of the acute burst of active destructive disease, the probing attachment depth resumes a stable level, and the underlying bone undergoes remodeling. At that time, radiographic evidence of bone loss is detected, because of a decrease in the level of crestal alveolar bone, even though there has been repair of the approximal bone defect. This is due to the fact that the bone mass of the cortical bone was greater than that of the total spongiform bone, and the natural shape of the alveolar bone is being reestablished.

It has also been demonstrated that complete removal of medullary bone produces little change in the radiographic appearance of a periodontal site (Lang and Hill, 1977). In this context, it is instructive to consider the case history cited by Goodson et al (1984), in which an infrabony defect, undetectable by conventional radiographic analysis, and associated with an increase of 5 mm in the attachment level measurement, was demonstrated by direct surgical access. These phenomena occur most frequently in the molar and premolar regions because of the wide alveolar crest.

In a study of the pattern of periodontal osseous lesions on dried mandibles, Stoner (1972) found that small, craterlike defects often occurred in the center of the alveolar crest. These defects were located at a midpoint between the buccal and lingual cortical plates, which obscured their radiographic detection. Thus, it appears that medullary bone loss can be obscured by intact cortical plates and the bone loss disclosed by radiography is primarily related to a change in the vertical dimension of the cortical bone plates.

Extraoral panoramic radiographs may also be used for screening alveolar bone loss in individuals (Figs 385 and 386).

Pepelassi and Kipioti (unpublished data, 1994) compared radiographic (panoramic and

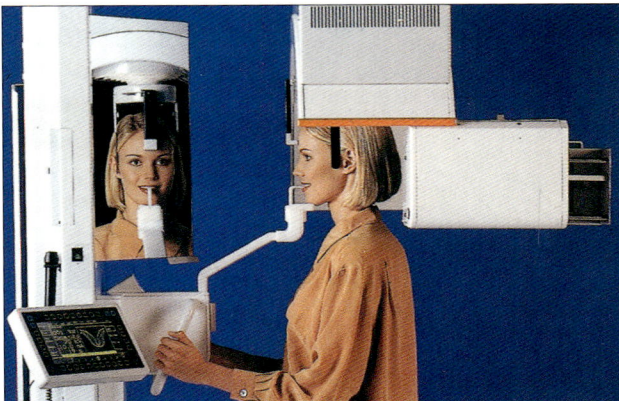

Fig 385 Sensorex (Sirona Dental, Germany) equipment for panoramic radiography.

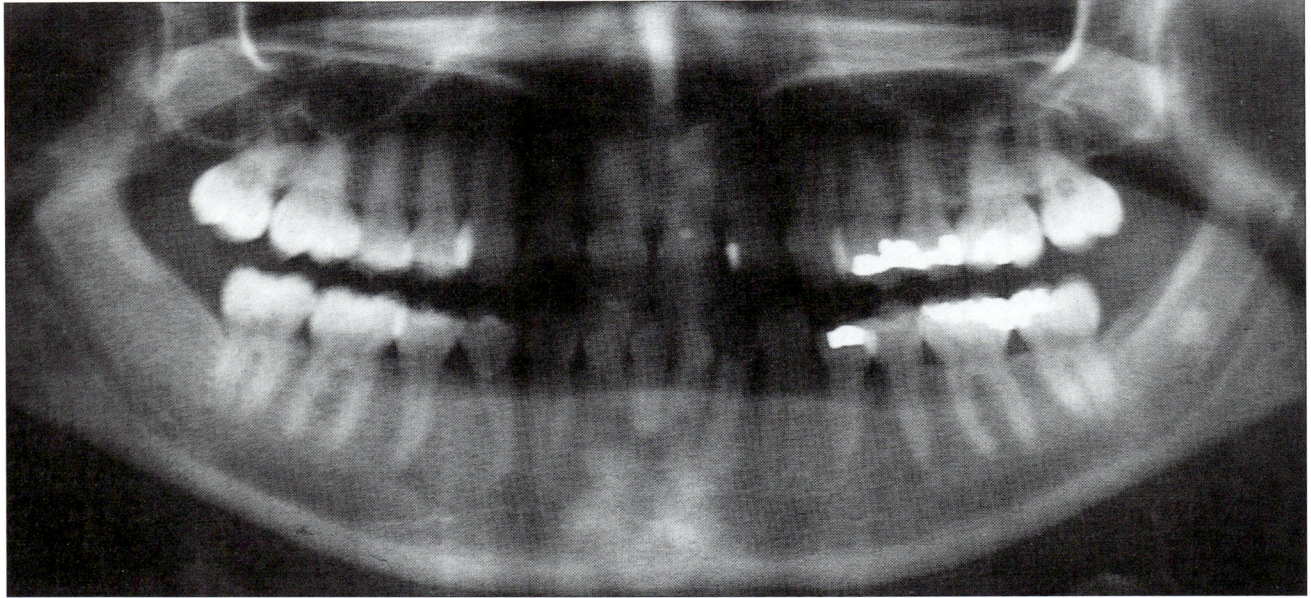

Fig 386 Extraoral panoramic radiograph, used to screen for alveolar bone loss.

periapical radiography) measurements of bone loss with direct measurements taken during surgery to correct endosseous defects. Factors such as tooth group, tooth surface, jaw location, number of osseous walls, and dimensions and volume of the defects were studied in relation to radiographic detection and accurate imaging of the defects. In all, 1,324 interproximal and/or buccal or lingual defects were studied in 100 patients.

Statistical evaluation of the data revealed the following:

- Only 233 of 1,324 defects were detected by both types of radiography.
- Periapical radiography was statistically significantly more effective for detecting defects, especially incipient defects. For the mandibular teeth, this difference between the two types of radiography was related to the group of teeth studied (anterior or premolars and molars), but was not influenced by the maxillary or mandibular location of the defect.
- The most critical factors for radiographic de-

tection of endosseous defects were their depth and buccolingual width, while variables such as the mesiodistal width, the volume of the defect, and the number of osseous walls had little or no influence.

- Compared to direct measurement of the defects during surgery, both periapical and panoramic radiographs resulted in errors of measurement, and the differences between the two were not statistically significant.
- On periapical radiographs, depth was underestimated in medium defects and overestimated in deep defects and in defects of large volume.
- In defects of medium mesiodistal width, this dimension was underestimated by periapical radiography.
- Three-wall defects of small buccolingual width were found to be statistically significantly deeper when assessed surgically than when they were assessed radiographically.

In a follow-up study on 5,072 approximal surfaces, Pepelassi et al (2000) again showed that periapical radiography was superior to panoramic radiography in detecting and accurately imaging periodontal osseous destruction. However, the ability of both methods to detect periodontal osseous defects was relatively low when compared with the gold standard of diagnosis by open flap surgery.

The potential and limitations of intraoral radiography to depict loss of supporting periodontal tissues have been reviewed extensively by Lang and Hill (1977) and Benn (1990). Table 25 recommends steps to take to improve clinical intraoral radiographs.

Digital subtraction radiography

A single radiograph does not indicate the rate or presence of active bone or attachment loss or whether past episodes of destruction and healing have occurred. This requires comparison of two or more carefully exposed radiographs with identical projections taken at different examinations.

In current clinical practice, bone loss is usually assessed by interpretation, that is, visual comparison of the radiographs. The radiograph contains so much information that it is difficult for the human eye to detect small changes in bone support against background noise comprising the teeth, cortical bone, and trabecular bone. It is difficult for clinicians to see changes that they do not expect or for their eyes to discern small changes in gray level (eg, small osseous changes superimposed on a root surface). Changes to interproximal bone are more readily apparent than are changes occurring buccally and lingually. The fact that it is difficult to see the

Table 25 Improving clinical intraoral radiographs for periodontal assessment*	
Action	**Reason**
Use vertical bite-wing views where possible.	Decrease patient exposure compared with complete-mouth series. Directs X-ray beam perpendicular to alveolar crest. Reduces examination time.
Use 90 kV(p).	Increased gray-level information in film improves ability to see changes in bone height. Decreases radiation dose to tissues.
Use superimposed millimeter grid.	Facilitates detection of bone loss over time.
Use root length ruler.	Facilitates detection of bone loss over time.
*From Jeffcoat et al (1995). Reprinted with permission.	

changes does not mean that the information is not recorded on the film.

Over the past 15 years, subtraction radiography has been applied with increasing frequency for detailed longitudinal evaluation of the outcome of periodontal therapy in experimental studies (Gröndahl and Gröndahl, 1983; Gröndahl et al, 1987; Gröndahl, 1997). The technique is especially useful for studies of regeneration and for evaluation of therapy in furcation involvement in mandibular molars (Brägger et al, 1988). For general clinical application, there are two major obstacles: the price and the influence of variations in projection geometry on the detectability of periodontal bone lesions (Gröndahl et al, 1987). To avoid a high rate of error, only very small differences between clinical radiographs, corresponding to an angulation error of less than 1 degree, can be tolerated; ie, the method requires special equipment that will produce identical periodical radiographs.

With computer processing of radiographic images, the clinical researcher can glean full information from the radiographic image. The first misconception about radiographs is that the bone loss must be advanced to be apparent on a radiograph. This may be true for visual interpretation: The film contains so much information that the clinician cannot generally detect bone loss until there is a change in mineral content of 30% to 50%. The fact that the clinician did not see the change, however, does not mean that it was not recorded in the gray levels of the radiographic film.

Computer programs are able to analyze the information in the source radiographs and present it in a form that can be more readily interpreted by the clinician or may provide a quantitative measure of the amount of bone loss or gain. Such methods are termed *image-processing techniques*. Computer image processing of high-quality images makes it possible to detect bone change of less than 5% with better than 90% sensitivity, specificity, and overall accuracy (Hausmann et al, 1985; Jeffcoat, 1992a, 1992b, 1993; Jeffcoat and Reddy, 1991, 1993). These changes may be de-

tected in interproximal spaces, over the buccal or lingual roots, or in furcations.

A study using probing and digital subtraction radiography to compare the progression of periodontitis has revealed a significant association between the presence of progressive PAL measured by an electronic probe and progressive alveolar bone loss (Jeffcoat and Reddy, 1991). Other studies have shown a significant correlation between probing attachment level gain and bone changes measured by digital subtraction radiography but not changes assessed on conventional radiographs (Wenzel and Sewerin, 1991).

Image-processing techniques have been developed to enhance the detection of small osseous changes over short periods of time. These include digital subtraction radiography and computer-assisted densitometric image analysis. Digital radiography is especially useful for detecting small changes in hard tissues between examinations. All unchanged structures are subtracted from a set of two radiographs, leaving only the area of change. The image-processing procedure subtracts unchanging teeth, cortical bone, and trabecular pattern, leaving only the bone gain or loss standing out against a neutral gray background on the subtraction image. By convention, bone gain is shown as a light area and bone loss as a dark area.

In computer-assisted densitometric image analysis, the images are not always displayed, but the numeric values after subtraction in areas of interest are analyzed to detect osseous changes. Additional software can localize the area of bone change, determine the size or mass of the area of change, and superimpose it on the original radiograph to facilitate interpretation by a clinician.

The first step in subtraction is digitization, which simplifies the information in the radiograph to a form that can be understood by a computer, which then analyzes and displays the information. The use of subtraction radiography requires that the radiographs be taken with similar contrast, density, and angulation. Meticulous attention to detail is critical when radiographs are exposed for use in digital radiographic techniques.

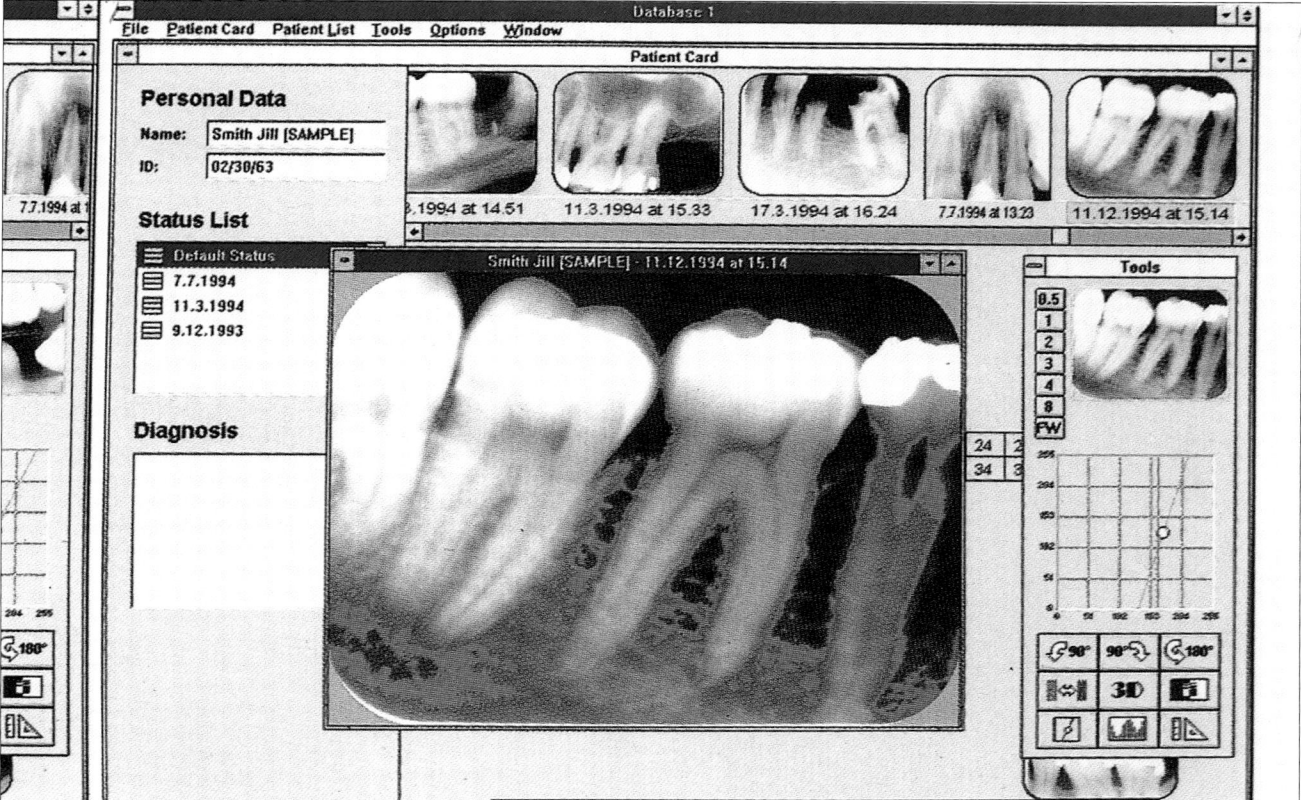

Fig 387 Digital intraoral radiography. By computer-aided digital subtraction radiography, bone loss or bone regeneration can be measured and visualized with color within 2 to 4 months.

Fortunately, the computer can aid in correction of errors. Computer algorithms have been developed to correct for variation in radiograph image density and contrast. The application of such algorithms is not limited to subtraction radiography. These programs may be readily applied in the clinical setting to pairs of conventional or direct digital radiography.

The subtraction images themselves may be assessed by interpretation or by measurement. Interpretation is a highly sensitive and specific method for detecting bone loss. As mentioned earlier, 5% loss of bone mineral may be detected with greater than 90% accuracy (Hausmann et al, 1982, 1985). Small osseous lesions may be detected with a sensitivity greater than 90% and a specificity greater than 96% (Jeffcoat et al, 1991; Jeffcoat and Reddy, 1993).

Color coding of the subtraction images improves the ability of clinicians inexperienced in reading subtraction images to detect bone loss or gain (Brägger and Pasquali, 1989; Reddy et al, 1991). This is exemplified by the Digora image plate system (Soredex Orion, Finland) for digital intraoral radiography (Fig 387), which reduces radiation exposure by as much as 90%, and by the Schick CDR system (Schick Technologies, Long Island City, NY) (Fig 388). Other systems for digital subtraction radiography are Sivision (Sirona Dental), Trophy Everest RVG system (Trophy radiology, France), DSR (Electro Medical Systems, Switzerland), Vista Ray (Dürr Dental, Germany), and the Sensa-Ray system (Regam Medical Systems, Sweden). In the color-coded images, bone gain may appear as shades of green and bone loss as shades of red.

347

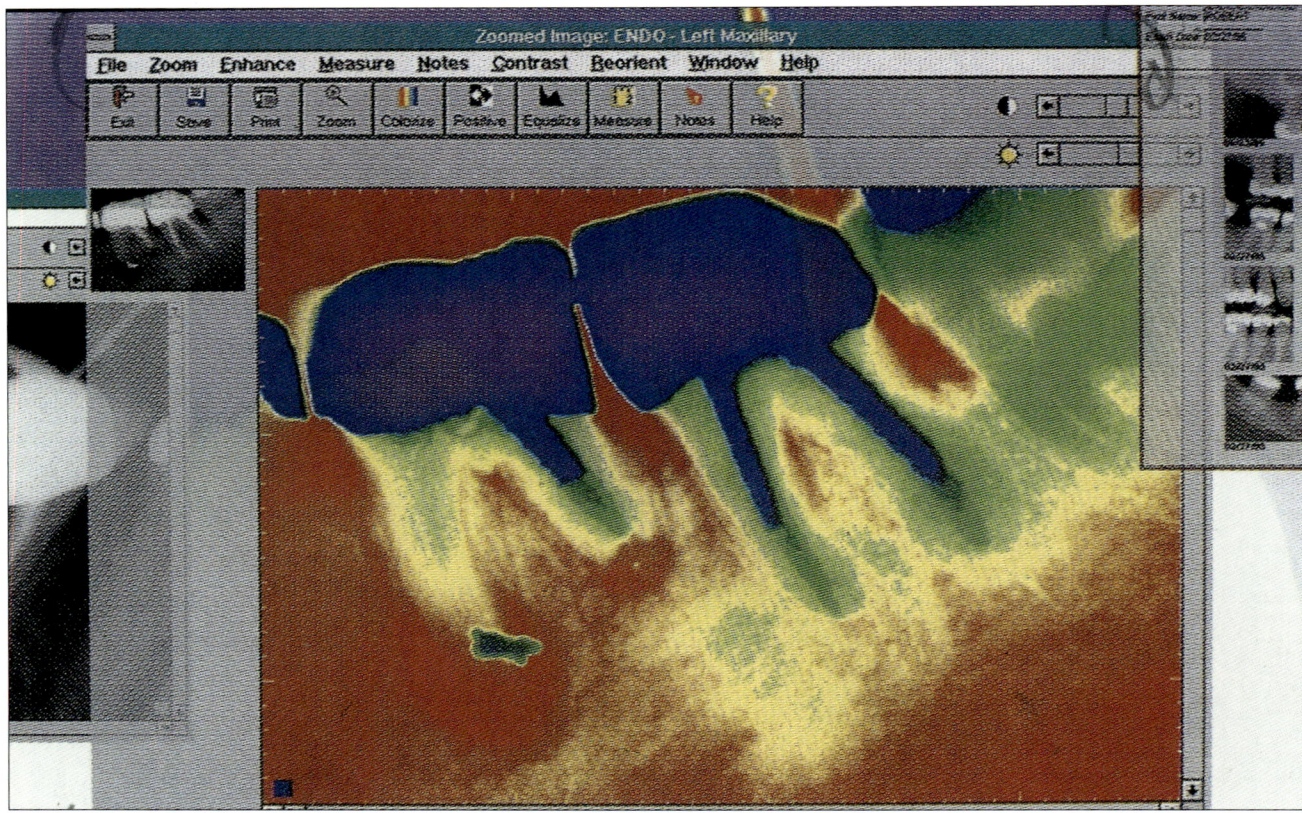

Fig 388 Color coding of subtraction radiographic images.

	Interpretation		Measurement	
			Progressive bone loss > 0.5 mm	Progressive bone loss < 0.5 mm
Method	Existing bone loss	Existing bone loss		
Periapicals: high-quality routine clinical film	X	X	X	
Bite-wings: high-quality routine clinical films	X	X	X	
Periapicals: standardized	X	X	X	X
Vertical bite-wings: standardized	X	X	X	X
Direct digital radiographs	X	X	X	X
Panoramic radiographs (screening only)				

Table 26 Summary of radiographic methods for detecting periodontitis*

*Modified from Jeffcoat et al (1995). Reprinted with permission.

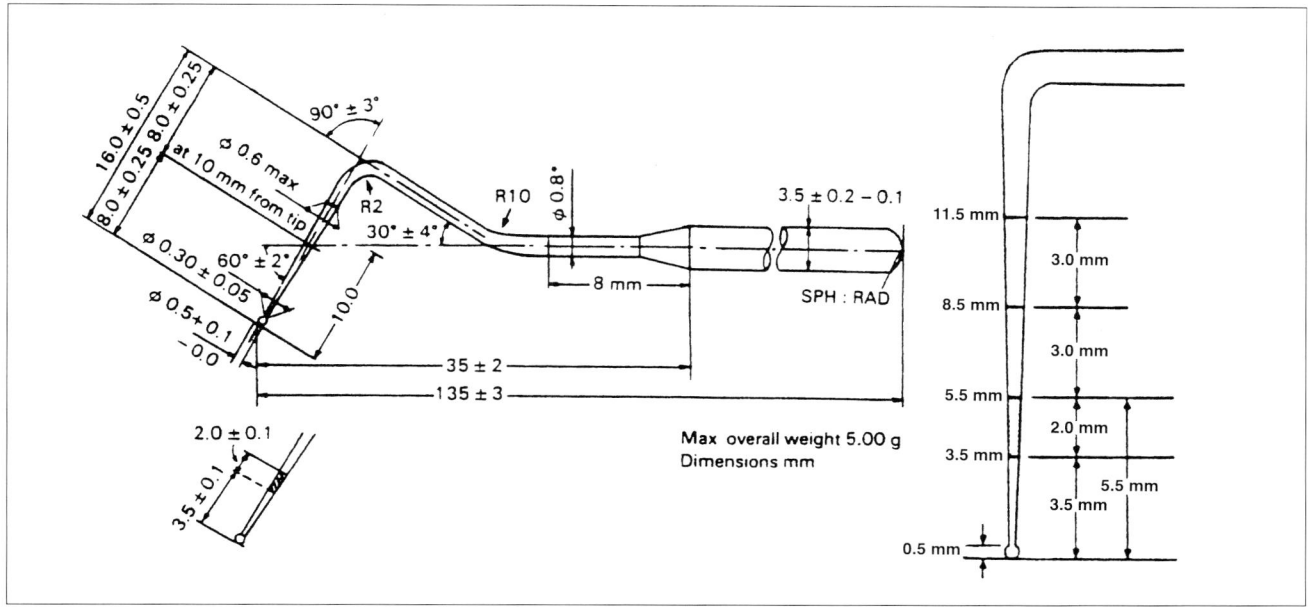

Fig 389 Probe designed for assessment of Community Periodontal Index of Treatment Needs.

In the ideal subtraction image, the teeth are nearly invisible, but the clinician has to identify tooth sites undergoing bone loss or gain to correlate the radiographic findings with clinical data and other tests for periodontal disease activity. Identification of the site is facilitated by superimposing the area of change disclosed by subtraction radiography on the original radiograph.

Interpretation of the subtraction image does not fully exploit the information it contains. The subtraction image itself can be used to make direct measurements, in millimeters, of bone change along the root surface. In addition, the mass of the region of bone change can be calculated by incorporating a reference wedge in the original radiographic image. Software permits the actual milligrams of bone loss or gain to be quantified.

Table 26 is an overview of available radiographic methods and their usefulness in diagnosis of alveolar bone loss associated with periodontitis. For reviews on radiography for diagnosis of periodontal diseases, see Jeffcoat et al (1995) and Hausmann (2000).

ASSESSMENT OF PERIODONTAL TREATMENT NEEDS

The Community Periodontal Index of Treatment Needs was developed jointly by the Fédération Dentaire Internationale and the World Health Organization in 1977 (Ainamo et al, 1982). The CPITN is now an established index for indicating levels of periodontal conditions for which specific interventions might be considered in populations. To date, national surveys based on the CPITN have been conducted in more than 100 countries.

To standardize measurement of the CPITN, a special probe has been designed (Fig 389) (Emslie, 1980). The approved basic probe is suitable for general use in epidemiology and for routine screening of patients in general practice. This new type of "tactile" probing or sensor instrument should be regarded as an extension of the examiner's fingers. A "sensing" force, which should not exceed 20 g, is used both to determine probing depth and to detect calculus. The direction of the probe during insertion should be, whenever pos-

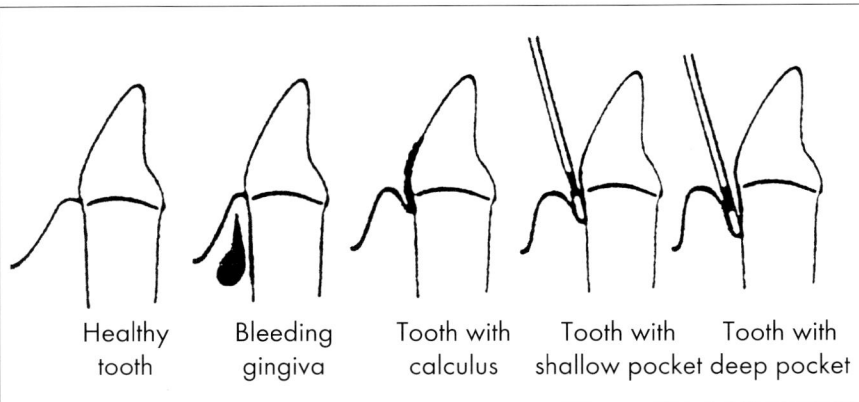

Fig 390 Clinical signs of periodontal disease recorded by the Community Periodontal Index of Treatment Needs.

Healthy tooth | Bleeding gingiva | Tooth with calculus | Tooth with shallow pocket | Tooth with deep pocket

sible, in the same plane as the long axis of the tooth. The ball-point tip should be kept in contact with the root surface. Discomfort and pain to the patient during probing indicates excessive force. Briefly, the CPITN method involves the use of the specially designed periodontal probe to score the dentition in sextants; all teeth or index teeth in each sextant may be scored. In most epidemiologic surveys, only the highest score for each sextant is recorded. However, for clinical application in the individual patient, every site (the mesial, buccal, distal, and lingual surfaces of every tooth) in the dentition should be recorded, to evaluate the "true" current treatment needs. Treatment needs based on the highest score at the sextant or even the tooth level are considerably overestimated.

The following are the CPITN scores (Fig 390):

- Code 0 = Healthy periodontal tissues
- Code 1 = Bleeding after gentle probing
- Code 2 = Supragingival or subgingival calculus or defective margin of restoration or crown
- Code 3 = Pathologic pocket of 4 to 5 mm
- Code 4 = Pathologic pocket of 6 mm or deeper
- Code x = Only one tooth or no teeth present in a sextant (third molars excluded unless they function in place of second molars)

The code numbers recorded indicate the following types of periodontal treatment needs:

- Code 0 = There is no need for periodontal treatment.
- Code 1 = Oral hygiene education is required.
- Codes 2 and 3 = Professional mechanical tooth cleaning (PMTC), scaling, and root planing are required in addition to oral hygiene education. Scaling and root planing includes elimination of subgingival plaque biofilms and plaque-retentive margins of restorations and crowns.
- Code 4 = Complex treatment is required in addition to PMTC scaling, root planing, and oral hygiene education.

DIAGNOSIS OF PERIODONTAL STATUS OF INDIVIDUAL TEETH

In the Gothenburg system, the periodontal status of every tooth is diagnosed. Proper diagnosis of periodontal disease should be based on examination and recording of the condition of the various periodontal structures (the gingiva, the periodontal membrane, the root cementum, and the alveolar bone). For detailed treatment planning, it is often an advantage to give each tooth in the dentition an individual diagnosis.

Four different diagnoses are used: gingivitis, periodontitis levis, periodontitis gravis, and periodontitis complicata.

Gingivitis

One or several gingival units around a particular tooth bleed on probing. Probing depth, attachment level measurements, and radiographic analysis fail to indicate loss of supporting tissues. Pseudopockets may be present.

Periodontitis levis

Probing depth, attachment level measurements, and radiographic analysis indicate even (horizontal) loss of supporting tissues not exceeding one third of the length of the root. Inflammation is indicated by bleeding on probing to the base of the pocket.

Periodontitis gravis

Probing depth, attachment level measurements, and radiographic analysis indicate even (horizontal) loss of supporting tissues exceeding one third of the length of the root. Bleeding on probing to the base of the pocket must be present.

Periodontitis complicata

This diagnosis is applied *(1)* when an angular bony defect (an infrabony pocket or interdental osseous crater) is present adjacent to a tooth, *(2)* when a tooth exhibits grade 3 mobility (see next section) and *(3)* for a multirooted tooth in which furcation involvements of grade II or III have been identified. Bleeding on probing to the base of the pocket must be present.

When an angular bony defect is present, the level of the root surface at which the base of the defect is located should also be defined. Hence, a tooth with this kind of osseous defect is often given a combined diagnosis: periodontitis levis et

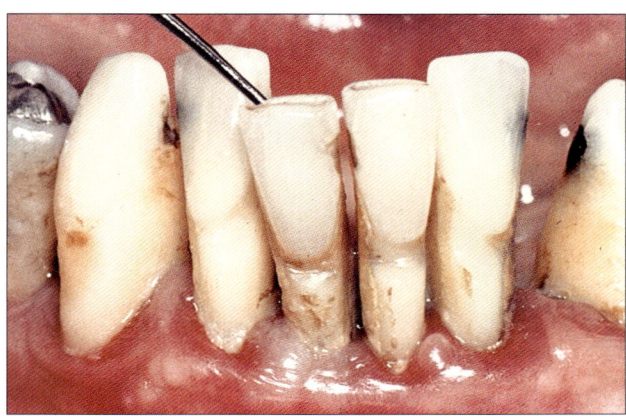

Fig 391 *Extremely mobile mandibular right central incisor.*

complicata when the apical termination of the angular bony defect is located at the levis level on the root surface and periodontitis gravis et complicata when it is located at the gravis level.

ASSESSMENT OF TOOTH MOBILITY

Pathologic migration of teeth is a common sequela to severe loss of periodontal support. When the functional forces on a tooth exceed the ability of the supporting tissues to resist them, the tooth becomes mobile and sometimes migrates (Fig 391). If not held in place by occlusal contacts or other forces (such as those exerted by the lips and tongue), teeth with extensive bone loss may move out of their original position. This is most common in the maxillary incisors. Although tooth migration, or drifting, is a feature of the late stages of periodontitis, for the patient it may be the very first sign of a problem, and it is not unusual for a patient to present with a chief complaint of, "My teeth have moved."

Increased tooth mobility can be caused by a variety of factors, such as orthodontic tooth movement, heavy functional loads (such as from prosthetic appliances), occlusal discrepancies, loss of

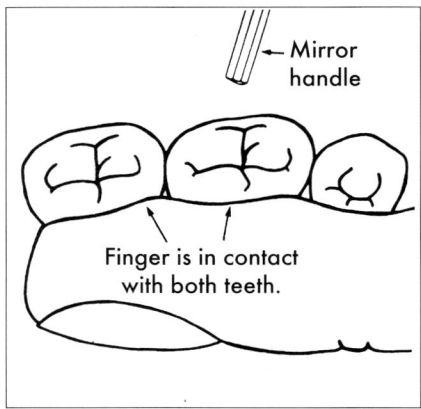 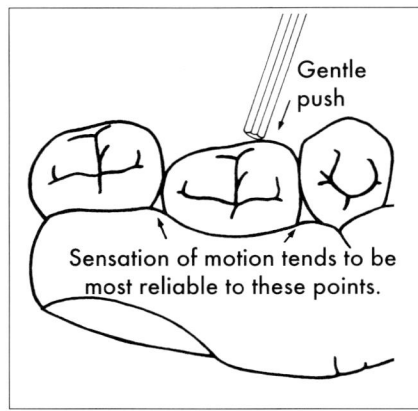

Figs 392 and 393 Steps in the clinical evaluation of tooth mobility.

alveolar bone secondary to endodontic problems, and periodontitis. Because periodontitis is not the only cause of tooth hypermobility, careful evaluation is necessary to determine the underlying cause. Although a logical first step is to determine the tooth's clinical attachment, other causes for the mobility should also be sought.

The clinical importance of increased tooth mobility is frequently overestimated. It has clearly been shown in animal experiments that, if plaque-induced inflammation is controlled, increased tooth mobility has no effect on the level of the connective tissue attachment (Ericsson and Lindhe, 1977; Lindhe and Ericsson, 1976). Several reports indicate that a similar conclusion is warranted for humans. Hypermobility of a tooth does not necessarily mean that it has a poor prognosis, and the mobility frequently persists after successful periodontal treatment (Lindhe and Nyman, 1975, 1984). Nevertheless, increasing tooth mobility over time should alert the clinician to a possible deterioration of periodontal support, and such teeth require careful evaluation for loss of clinical attachment.

In clinical practice, the extent of tooth mobility is most often subjectively graded on a scale of 1 to 3 using a system similar to the following (Lindhe et al, 1997):

- Grade 1: Slight mobility; movement of the tooth in a horizontal direction by approximately 0.2 to 1.0 mm.

- Grade 2: Moderate mobility; movement of the tooth in a horizontal direction by > 1.0 mm, but no evidence of vertical mobility.
- Grade 3: Marked mobility; movement of the tooth freely in both the horizontal and vertical directions.

Figures 392 and 393 illustrate the steps in clinical evaluation of tooth mobility. Although such procedures are adequate for routine clinical practice, a more objective method is required for research. A recent development is the Periotest system (Siemens, Germany) for objective assessment of tooth mobility; the tooth is rapidly percussed 16 times (four times per second) and then the rebound attenuation patterns emanating from the tooth are electronically recorded.

RECORDING OF CLINICAL EXAMINATIONS

Figure 394 shows a chart, modified from the Swedish Public Dental Health Service, for manual recording of clinical periodontal examination of patients. The following data are entered:

- Disclosed plaque, 24-hour free plaque reaccumulation (PFRI), and gingival bleeding on prob-

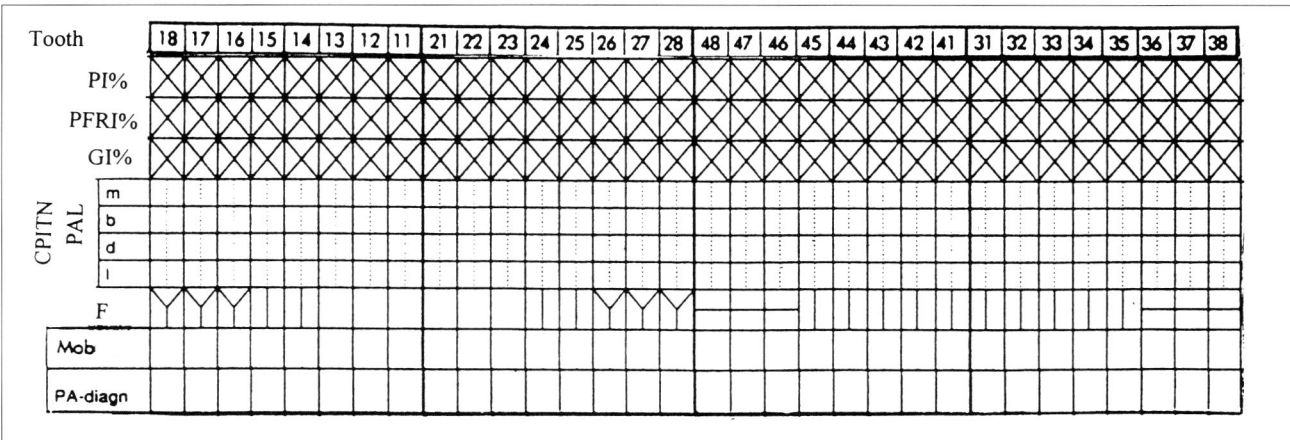

Fig 394 Chart, modified from the Swedish Public Dental Health Service, used for manual recording of clinical periodontal examinations. PI% = Disclosed plaque; PFRI% = Plaque Formation Rate Index; GI% = Gingival bleeding on probing; m = Mesial; b = Buccal; d = Distal; l = Lingual; F = Furcation involvement; Mob = Mobility; PA-diagn = Periodontal diagnosis.

T	18			17			16			15			14			13			12			11			21			22			23			24			25			26			27			28		
VAR	A	L	F	C	A	L	F	C	A	L	F	C	A	L	F	C	A	L	F	C	A	L	F	C	A	L	F	C	A	L	F	C	A	L	F	C	A	L	F	C	A	L	F	C	A	L	F	C	A	L	F	C	A	L	F	C	A	L	F	C	A	L	F	C
MES																																														
DIST																																														
BCC																																														
LING																																														
TOT																																														
CPITN																																														

T	48			47			46			45			44			43			42			41			31			32			33			34			35			36			37			38		
VAR	A	L	F	C	A	L	F	C	A	L	F	C	A	L	F	C	A	L	F	C	A	L	F	C	A	L	F	C	A	L	F	C	A	L	F	C	A	L	F	C	A	L	F	C	A	L	F	C	A	L	F	C	A	L	F	C	A	L	F	C	A	L	F	C
MES																																														
DIST																																														
BCC																																														
LING																																														
TOT																																														
CPITN																																														

AL MES = ☐☐	F SCORE 1 = ☐	CPITN SCORE 1 = ☐
AL BCC = ☐☐	F SCORE 2 = ☐	CPITN SCORE 2 = ☐
AL DIST = ☐☐	F SCORE 3 = ☐	CPITN SCORE 3 = ☐
AL LING = ☐☐		CPITN SCORE 4 = ☐
AL TOT = ☐☐		CPITN MEAN = ☐

Fig 395 Matrix for computer-aided analysis. T = Tooth number; VAR = Variable; AL = Probing attachment level; F = Furcation involvement; C = CPITN; MES = Mesial; DIST = Distal; BCC = Buccal; LING = Lingual; TOT = Total.

ing on the mesial, buccal, distal, and lingual surfaces or the mesiobuccal, buccal, distobuccal, mesiolingual, lingual, and distolingual surfaces

• Community Periodontal Index of Treatment Needs and probing attachment level on the mesial, buccal, distal, and lingual surfaces

- Furcation involvement on the mesial, buccal, and distal surfaces of maxillary molars, the mesial and distal surfaces of maxillary premolars, and the buccal and lingual surfaces of mandibular molars
- Mobility
- Tooth-related periodontal status: healthy, gingivitis, periodontitis levis, periodontitis gravis, or periodontitis complicata

Figure 395 shows a matrix for computer-aided analytic epidemiology of periodontal diseases as well as for examination of individual patients. Probing attachment level, furcation involvement, and the CPITN are recorded at the surface level (mesially, buccally, distally, and lingually).

> **Box 22** Prognostic risk factors for further periodontal attachment loss
>
> - Presence of subgingival biofilms and high levels of specific periopathogens subgingivally
> - Recent increase in probing depth and clinical attachment loss
> - Loss of compact bone from the alveolar crest
> - Bleeding on probing
> - Increase in periodontal pocket temperature
> - Increase in volume of gingival crevicular fluid
> - Presence of purulent exudate in smokers with genetic interleukin-1 polymorphism
> - Increase in levels of markers of periodontal disease activity: prostaglandin E_2, matrix metalloproteinases, and proinflammatory cytokines (particularly interleukin-1β) in the gingival crevicular fluid

DIAGNOSIS OF DISEASED PERIODONTAL POCKETS AND ACTIVE LESIONS

Together the features listed in Box 22 are not only very important signs of diseased periodontal pockets and active lesions, but also a guarantee for further rapid breakdown of the periodontal tissues; ie, they may be regarded as prognostic risk factors for further periodontal attachment loss.

Presence of subgingival biofilms and specific periopathogens

The periodontal diseases are indisputably infectious: The sole etiologic factor is the microbial challenge, and a prerequisite for development of the diseased pocket and an active lesion is the presence of subgingival periopathogens. Most of the subgingival microflora is attached to the root surface as plaque (biofilm), but the depths of the pocket also harbor many nonattaching, motile species, particularly various sizes and forms of spirochetes.

In the biofilms (see Fig 39 in chapter 1) the microorganisms live in well-organized symbiosis, supplied with nutrients via microchannels through the plaque matrix and inaccessible to phagocytozing leukocytes (PMNLs and macrophages), chemical plaque control agents, and antibiotics. The presence of subgingival plaque may be demonstrated by cautious insertion of the tip of a periodontal curette to the base of the pocket and debridement of the root surface in a coronal direction. To facilitate this procedure, the pocket may be distended with a plane instrument.

At the 1996 World Workshop in Periodontics, it was concluded that human periodontitis is caused mainly by *Actinobacillus actinomycetemcomitans, Porphyromonas gingivalis,* and *Bacteroides forsythus. P gingivalis* and *A actinomycetemcomitans* are regarded as exogenous, transmissible periopathogens, while *B forsythus* is considered to be endogenous and opportunistic (American Academy of Periodontology, 1996c). Recently, Machtei et al (1997) showed that, in deep periodontal pockets, high levels of *B forsythus* increase the risk for further loss of periodontal attachment sevenfold. Other species of

Fig 396 Root fracture and localized alveolar bone loss with bacteria in the fracture, inaccessible for mechanical cleaning and antibiotics.

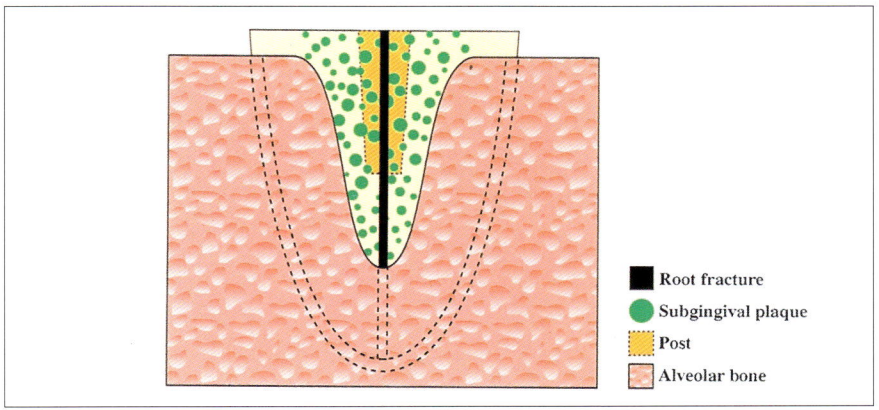

■ Root fracture
● Subgingival plaque
▮ Post
▢ Alveolar bone

opportunistic endogenous periopathogens are *Prevotella intermedia* and *Treponema denticola.* The presence and levels of subgingival periopathogens can be evaluated by subgingival sampling, with a sterile curette or paper point, and DNA probe analyses, conventional anaerobic culture techniques, or chairside tests. For details see chapter 1.

Recent increases in probing depth and clinical attachment loss

Although recent increases in probing depth and clinical attachment loss are evidence of disease activity in the recent past, but not necessarily of ongoing disease, they are highly indicative of diseased pockets, active lesions, and further loss of attachment. Recent loss of attachment is the outcome of interactions among etiologic factors and external and internal modifying factors. Most clinicians would agree that very few periodontal pockets deeper than 5 mm are healthy. For example, isolated deep pockets on the buccal or lingual surfaces of endodontically treated teeth restored with posts are usually associated with untreatable root fractures (Fig 396).

Like caries and other infectious diseases, the periodontal diseases may be characterized by pe-

riods of exacerbation and quiescence. This was demonstrated in a study by Goodson et al (1982): In untreated subjects with existing periodontal pockets, PAL was measured every month for 1 year. During this period, 83% of the sites did not change significantly, 6% exhibited significant further loss of attachment, and 11% exhibited less loss of attachment. Figure 397 exemplifies the patterns of attachment level and probing depth at three different sites from the study.

Other studies have confirmed that sites showing evidence of destructive periodontal activity may subsequently show no further activity or may be subject to one or more exacerbations. During the lifetime of an individual, there may be relatively short periods in which many sites undergo periodontal destruction, followed by extensive periods of remission (Socransky et al, 1984). Exceptions to this pattern of disease are the patients most susceptible to periodontitis: smokers and those with genetic interleukin-1 (IL-1) polymorphism and type 1 diabetes. Such patients may exhibit aggressive periodontitis more frequently than others and without efficient treatment and intensive supportive care they will more or less continuously lose periodontal attachment.

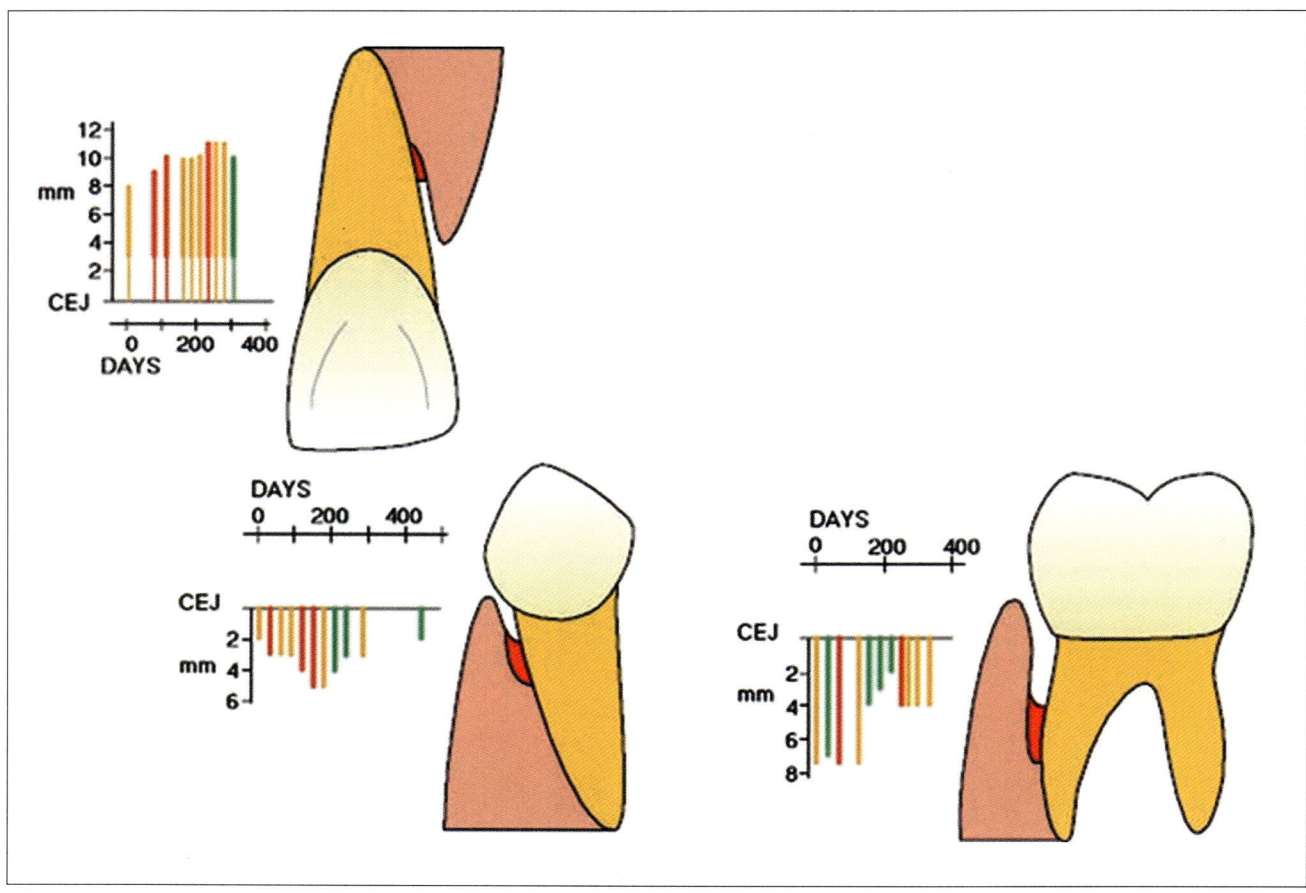

Fig 397 Progression and regression of attachment loss. The distance from the CEJ to the base of the pocket reveals the alterations in periodontal attachment during the period. (Modified from Goodson et al, 1982. Reprinted with permission.)

Loss of compact bone from the alveolar crest

Loss of compact bone from the alveolar crest or a diffuse lamina dura indicates active bone resorption. In the posterior interproximal areas, this can readily be screened on four vertical bite-wing radiographs (see Figs 377 to 383). It should also be possible to identify active periodontal lesions by monitoring bone loss over a period of 2 to 4 months, using computer-aided digital subtraction radiography (see Figs 387 and 388).

Presence of bleeding on probing

The absence of bleeding on probing is a reliable parameter of periodontal stability, provided that the assessment procedure is standardized (Lang et al, 1990). Bleeding on standardized probing indicates the presence of gingival inflammation. Whether bleeding on probing at repeated examinations over time will predict progression of a lesion is, however, questionable (Lang et al, 1986; 1990; Vanooteghem et al, 1987). Numerous studies have shown that a 30% probability for future attachment loss may be predicted for sites that repeatedly exhibit bleeding on probing (Badersten et al, 1985d, 1990; Claffey et al, 1990; Lang et al, 1986; Vanooteghem et al, 1987, 1990).

Bleeding on probing is sensitive to different forces applied to the probe. In a study of healthy young adults, Lang et al (1991) showed an almost linear relationship between probing force and the percentage of bleeding sites. At probing forces of greater than 0.25 N (25 g), bleeding is the result of tissue trauma, rather than a sign of inflammation. To assess the "true" percentage of sites bleeding because of inflammation, the probing force should be 0.25 N or less, clinically a light probing force. This has also been confirmed in patients who have experienced loss of attachment, ie, with successfully treated advanced periodontitis (Karayannis et al, 1991; Lang et al, 1991).

Because the absence of bleeding on probing at 0.25 N indicates periodontal stability, with a negative predictive value of 98% to 99% (Lang et al, 1990), this is the most reliable clinical variable for monitoring patients' progress in daily practice. Nonbleeding sites may be considered periodontally stable: Bleeding sites seem to be at increased risk for progression of periodontitis, especially when the same site consistently bleeds at repeated examinations (Claffey et al, 1990; Lang et al, 1986). Sites that bleed on probing at a constant force of 0.25 N should therefore be registered dichotomously: This not only allows calculation of mean bleeding on probing for the patient but also provides a topographic chart of the bleeding sites. Repeated scores during maintenance will indicate the surfaces at higher risk for loss of attachment.

Increase in periodontal pocket temperature

The five classic signs of tissue inflammation include rubor (redness), calor (increased temperature), tumor (swelling or edema), dolor (pain), and functio laesa (loss of function). Redness and increased temperature are related to vascular changes.

Regeneration of most human pathogenic microorganisms is retarded at increased temperature: Fever is one of the nonspecific host responses to local and general infections. Because body temperature has long been used to evaluate the occurrence and severity of infectious diseases, it seems logical to include measurement of the subgingival temperature in the evaluation of diseased periodontal pockets and active periodontal lesions. This was the rationale underlying the innovation of a digital "microthermometer," combined with a flat, thin periodontal probe, to identify diseased periodontal pockets (Axelsson, 1982). Commercial devices have been introduced in recent years (eg, PerioTemp System, ABIODENT, Danvers, MA).

The PerioTemp System has been described by Kung et al (1990). The device is about the size and shape of a periodontal probe and uses a small thermistor bead to determine temperature. The probe tip is housed in a casing with low thermal conductivity so that the probe itself does not alter the ambient temperature. The probe is sensitive to 0.1°C and assesses the temperature rapidly so that the entire mouth (6 sites per tooth, 168 sites for 28 teeth) can be evaluated quickly. The device is linked to a computer. In the initial report of the device, sites from patients with advanced chronic periodontitis and healthy subjects were examined. Advanced disease was associated with a mean increase of 0.65°C at a site, and an anterior (cooler) to posterior (warmer) temperature gradient was observed.

A series of reports has provided an in-depth analysis of the relationship of subgingival temperature to periodontal disease (Haffajee et al, 1992a, 1992b, 1992c). The use of the device depends on referencing the subgingival temperature to the core, or sublingual, temperature, which is generally higher than the mean subgingival temperature. In patients with varying degrees of existing periodontal disease, the mean subgingival temperature was correlated with clinical measures, including occurrence of plaque, redness, bleeding on probing, and probing depth. The temperature increased with the presence of plaque (0.5°C difference). Similarly, the temperature increased sequentially when sites were stratified as shallower than 4 mm (mean = 34.6°C), 4 to 6 mm (35.2°C), and deeper than 6 mm (35.8°C). This study allowed verification of the algorithm that is the basis for the color coding of the diode display: Normal temperature is indicated by emission of a green light, slightly elevated temperature by a yellow light, and marked elevation of temperature by a red light.

When the device was used to predict the risk of future PAL (Haffajee et al, 1992b), the most obvious difference was observed for shallow sites (less than 4 mm). It was found that 8.9% of such sites with bleeding on probing and markedly elevated temperature lost 2.0 mm of PAL, compared to only 1.4% of sites that did not bleed and were in the normal temperature range.

A study of the relationship of temperature to the subgingival microflora revealed that elevated subgingival temperature was associated with the presence of some putative pathogens (Haffajee et al, 1992c). Subjects with elevated temperatures had significantly higher percentages of *P intermedia* and *Peptostreptococcus micros,* and lower mean percentages of *Capnocytophaga* species. Sites with elevated temperatures harbored higher percentages of *P intermedia* I and II, *A actinomycetemcomitans* serotypes a and b, and *P gingivalis* more frequently than did sites with lower temperatures, while *Capnocytophaga* species were elevated more often at cooler sites. Other studies have confirmed these findings. In a study by Fedi and Killoy (1992), the temperature of pockets more than 5 mm deep with bleeding on probing was 1.0°C to 1.8°C higher than that of pockets less than 3 mm deep without bleeding. In another study (Meyerov et al, 1991), the pocket temperature increased consistently with probing depth.

The PerioTemp system has recently been used in two other studies with different aims. In the first study, subgingival temperature was evaluated in smokers (more than 20 cigarettes a day) and nonsmokers with periodontitis (Dinsdale et al, 1997). Mean sublingual and site temperatures were calculated for smokers and nonsmokers, and mean temperature differentials (ΔT) between the sublingual temperature and the site temperature

were calculated for each site. Smokers had a higher mean sublingual temperature than did nonsmokers. The mean subgingival site temperature was 0.4°C higher in smokers than it was in nonsmokers, a statistically significant difference ($P <$ .01). The mean temperatures for both healthy and diseased sites were higher in smokers than in nonsmokers ($P <$ .01). When the mean ΔT between healthy and diseased sites were compared across each group, significant differences were also found. For healthy sites, the smokers had a mean ΔT 0.2°C lower ($P <$ .01) than did the nonsmokers, representing warmer sites, which indicates less vascular flow in smokers. In diseased sites, however ΔT was 0.3°C higher ($P <$ .01) in smokers, which indicates more severely diseased pockets in smokers than in nonsmokers.

In the second study, subgingival temperature was evaluated in relation to the degree of periodontal health, gingival crevicular fluid, enzymes, cytokines, and subgingival plaque microorganisms (Wolff et al, 1997). The results showed a correlation between subgingival temperature and *(1)* clinical status (healthy sites, gingivitis, and diseased pockets), *(2)* the GCF volume, *(3)* enzyme levels, and *(4)* specific plaque microorganisms associated with periodontal diseases.

Niederman et al (1995) evaluated the correlation of three different subgingival measurements to healthy and diseased periodontal pockets compared to bleeding on probing. The data indicated that all three subgingival temperature assessment methods differentiated between clinically defined periodontal health and disease ($P <$ .02). All three measurements also correlated significantly ($P <$ .02), but modestly ($r > 0.49$) with bleeding on probing. Obviously subgingival temperature assessment is superior to bleeding on probing in the identification of diseased periodontal pockets.

In a study by Buchmann et al (unpublished data, 1994), another sensitive periodontal temperature probe (Thermcoax TKA 05/10) was used for measuring subgingival site temperature prior to periodontal therapy and up to 6 months afterward, for detection of sites of disease progression. Posttherapy sites were classified as unchanging or as having a further increase in probing depth or periodontal attachment loss, indicative of sites at risk for ongoing periodontal disease within the 6-month monitoring period (test group, n = 127, 70.6%). Baseline subgingival temperature and bleeding on probing measurements were recorded to differentiate stable and progressive periodontitis sites. Sites with reduced probing depths and PAL gain of greater than 2 mm served as disease-inactive controls (n = 53, 29.4%). Site temperatures were calculated as the difference between subgingival and baseline subgingival temperature measurements. The mean site temperature was significantly higher in active sites than in inactive sites ($P < .001$). The sensitivity for prediction of periodontal progression was 85%, and the positive and negative predictive values were 87% and 53%, respectively.

Using a different concept (Fig 398) for measuring subgingival temperature, Lindskog et al (1994) reported that the difference in temperature between the outer surface of the free gingiva and within the gingival crevice was about 0.5°C in healthy sites and more than 1.5°C in diseased pockets. Because the mean subgingival temperature at healthy posterior teeth is normally some degrees higher than it is at healthy anterior teeth, this seems to be a promising approach.

The findings from all these studies are in accordance with existing knowledge of temperature increase in inflamed tissues and might improve the diagnostic potential for disclosing sites at relative periodontal risk. To date, the temperature probe has not been widely applied by either general practitioners or periodontists. This may relate to the configuration of the probe and the additional time required to use the device in posterior sites. However, in the near future, it is likely that inexpensive, simple, efficient subgingival temperature probes will become standard diagnostic tools, and the clinician will record pocket temperature along with other clinical variables. In addition, simple devices for self-diagnosis will soon be available, enabling patients themselves to monitor risk sites and seek professional consultation in cases of "pocket fever."

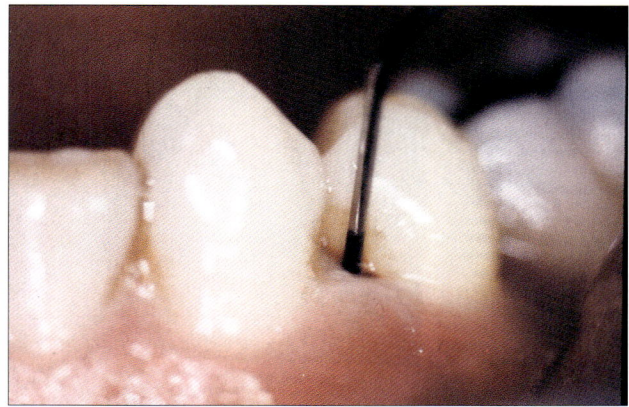

Fig 398 Measurement of subgingival temperature.

Increase in gingival crevicular fluid volume

Gingival crevicular fluid is a serumlike exudate that bathes the gingival sulcus or periodontal sulcus and follows an osmotic gradient within local tissues. Since 1960, numerous studies have indicated that the volume of gingival crevicular fluid that can be collected from inflamed gingiva has a statistically significant association ($P < .05$) with clinical assessments of gingivitis and histometric measures of gingival inflammation (Björn et al, 1965; Daneshmand and Wade, 1976; Egelberg, 1964; Hancock et al, 1979; Lindhe and Rylander, 1975; Rudin et al, 1970).

The strong statistical association between the volume of gingival crevicular fluid and the extent of gingival inflammation has led to the widespread use of measurements of gingival crevicular fluid as an objective assessment of gingival inflammation in clinical research studies. However, the conditions under which gingival crevicular fluid is collected greatly affect the amount of fluid obtained. It is therefore important to stabilize both conditions of collection and the method used to quantify the fluid obtained.

Gingival crevicular fluid is usually collected by inserting filter paper strips with standardized dimensions just within the gingival crevice for a fixed amount of time (Brill and Krasse, 1958). The

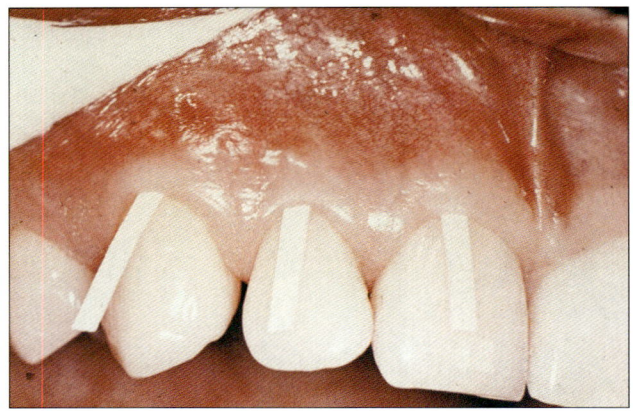

Fig 399 Insertion of paper strips to collect gingival crevicular fluid.

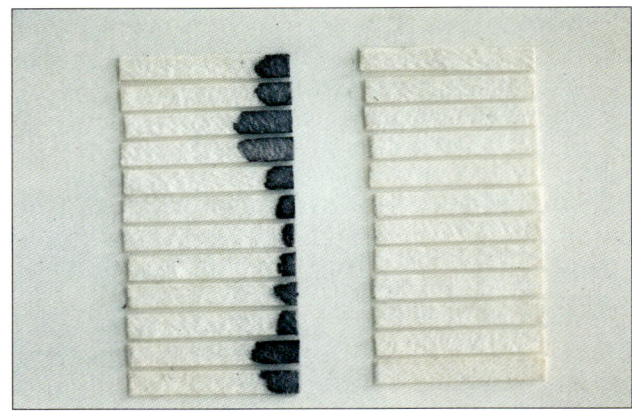

Fig 400 Amount of fluid collected, expressed as the distance, in millimeters, that the gingival crevicular fluid has traveled along the paper strip.

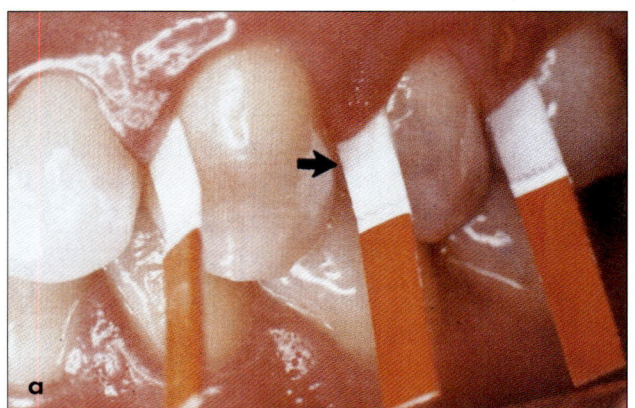

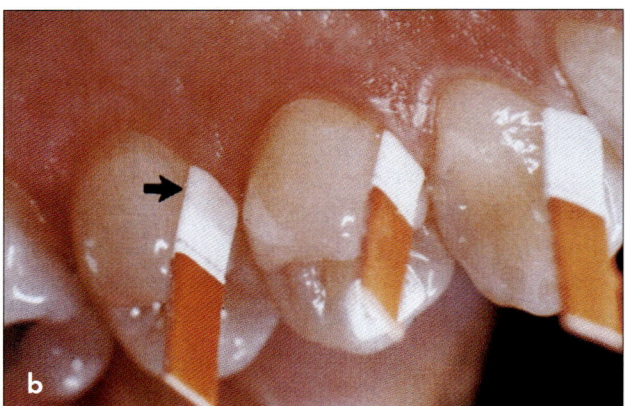

Figs 401a and 401b Technique for intracrevicular collection with precut filter paper strips. Buccal and palatal strips are usually placed at the same time, angled so that the leading edges meet at the midpoint of the mesial surface of the tooth. The strips are left in place for 30 seconds. *Arrows* = Gingival crevicular fluid accumulating on the strips.

fluid is absorbed by the filter paper through capillary action (Fig 399). In earlier studies, the strips were air dried and then stained with ninhydrin, which detects the presence of amino acids. With this method, the amount of fluid collected can be expressed as the distance (millimeters) that the gingival crevicular fluid has traveled along the filter paper strip (Fig 400).

The technique usually involves subgingival insertion, eg, from the buccal and lingual or palatal aspects of the mesial surface of the teeth. In the clinical setting, the buccal (Fig 401a) and the palatal (Fig 401b) strips would be inserted at the same time and angled so that the leading edges meet at the midpoint of the mesial surface of the tooth. The strips are left in place for 30 seconds. This procedure allows the two strips to be processed separately for analysis of the amount of GCF as well as different mediators. Experimentally, patients have ingested a fluorescent dye prior to collection of gingival crevicular fluid. The fluorescent dye would then be collected when the crevicular fluid was harvested.

At present, the volume of gingival crevicular fluid collected on a precut filter paper strip is determined by a Periotron 8000, an electronic device that measures the change in capacitance across the wetted strip. This change is converted to a digital readout, which can be correlated to the volume of gingival crevicular fluid. Some potential sources of error were associated with the use of the earlier model of the Periotron (the results can be affected by the room temperature and humidity, and placement of the filter paper strip within the jaws of the machine must be standardized).

However, the improved device (Periotron 8000, Pro Flow, Amityville, NY) is generally recognized as providing accurate and reproducible results. The new Periotron 8000 provides automatic calibration to true volume, an interface with a computer for storage, retrieval and display of data, and measures larger volumes of fluid (up to 3 µl). Although GCF flow is only approximately 20 µL/hour, the pocket volume is approximately 0.5 µL, with a wide range related to the probing depth. As a result, the total pocket volume is exchanged about 40 times an hour.

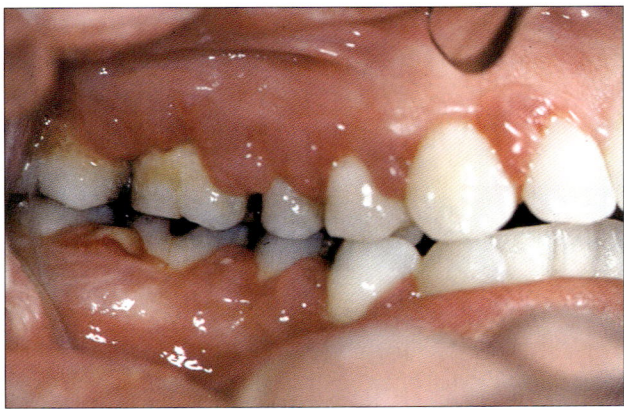

Fig 402 Spontaneous interdental suppuration in the mandibular posterior teeth.

amined the association between the presence of purulent exudate and progression of periodontitis. A strong association with the risk of disease progression was reported by Armitage et al (1994). In subjects with untreated periodontitis, disease progression was monitored after 6 months; the criterion for progression was additional bone loss, assessed by subtraction radiography. The sites with suppuration at baseline (25% of the total sites) were at a threefold higher risk of further bone loss during the following 6 months.

Presence of suppuration (purulent exudate)

Suppuration (purulent exudate or pus) is a common feature of periodontal inflammation, especially in cases of advanced, untreated periodontitis (Fig 402). An early term for periodontitis was *pyorrhea alveolaris,* literally a flow of pus from the alveolus. Suppuration can be readily detected with gentle application of digital pressure (in a coronal direction) to the gingival surface.

Conceptually, purulent exudate can be regarded as a PMNL-rich variant of gingival crevicular fluid. Clinically, suppuration is an important sign of ongoing infection. Few studies have ex-

Increase in levels of markers of periodontal disease activity

Since the work of Brill (1960), the gingival crevicular fluid has been studied for its potential to provide clinicians with diagnostic data on periodontal disease. Although available only in microliter quantities, it is easily accessible by painless, noninvasive techniques that can be repeated relatively frequently, allowing longitudinal, site-specific monitoring.

Analysis of GCF for disease markers has numerous advantages because, unlike serum and saliva, it is site specific, conveniently sampled, and contains components derived from both the host—in the form of plasma, connective tissue, and cellular components—and the microbial dental plaque. Gingival crevicular fluid has the potential to reflect the intricacies of the bacteria-host interaction and could provide not only information about the balance between the two but also specific details about the mechanisms of pathogenesis.

In a review article, Curtis (1991) clearly differentiated disease markers as *(1)* indicators of current disease, *(2)* predictors of future disease progression, and *(3)* predictors of future disease at currently healthy sites. In searching for markers that could predict susceptibility to periodontal diseases, or further periodontal breakdown in those with disease, a reasonable hypothesis is that disease progression reflects changes in susceptibility, at either the systemic or local level. Because the GCF reflects the influences of both host systemic responses and local modulation of those responses arising from interaction with a specific bacterial burden, it would appear to be an "ideal" biologic sample in which to seek such indicators or predictors. However, a distinction must be made between the presence of host-produced molecules associated with inflammation alone, such as reversible gingivitis, and those associated with destructive disease activity, ie, longitudinal attachment loss and bone resorption. Furthermore, consideration must be given to whether biochemical mediators are risk markers of disease activity or true risk factors.

The GCF is regarded as a serum transudate because most serum proteins are present in concentrations similar to those in serum itself (Cimasoni, 1983); it thus broadly reflects the systemic immunoglobulin and complement status of the host. However, GCF is modified by the local environment associated with the periodontal crevice or pocket.

As the GCF migrates from the host microcirculation, through inflamed tissues, and into the periodontal pocket, it acquires mediators involved in the destructive host response, and byproducts of local tissue metabolism as well as PMNLs, microorganisms, and their products from the periodontal pocket. Thus the composition of GCF is altered by the local tissue and bacteria, which may add or delete factors. For example, serum contains only subpicomolar levels of PGE_2, partly because of its rapid metabolism, but large amounts are synthesized by the local inflammatory cell infiltrate associated with a periodontal lesion (Offenbacher et al, 1984). In contrast, there is less complement protein C3 in GCF than in serum, because bacteria in the crevice activate the complement cascade, leading to depletion of C3 (Schenkein and Genco, 1977).

Because the "gold standard" for assessment of disease activity is progressive loss of connective tissue, analysis of the products of tissue breakdown in GCF would be expected to yield useful data. Evidence from many sources suggests that a strong host response is associated with tissue destruction (for review see Lamster, 1997). Specifically, pronounced cellular activity by the predominant inflammatory cells associated with periodontal disease (PMNLs and macrophages) is now considered to contribute to the active phase of disease, and increased levels of mediators derived from these cells are being examined as the basis of potential diagnostic tests for active periodontal disease. In this context, the following four mediators in GCF have been investigated extensively for their potential application in diagnosis of active periodontal disease and prediction of further loss of periodontal support: Prostaglandin E_2, β-glucuronidase (βG), neutrophil elastase (NE), and aspartate aminotransferase (AST).

Prostaglandin E_2

Prostaglandin E_2, a metabolite of arachidonic acid, is formed mainly when macrophages are stimulated by bacterial lipopolysaccarides but is also released by neutrophils (PMNLs) and fibroblasts (Fig 403). Prostaglandin E_2 has been shown to have many proinflammatory effects, including increased vasodilation, enhanced responsiveness of receptors to painful stimuli, release of collagenase by inflammatory cells, and activation of osteoclasts (for details see chapter 5).

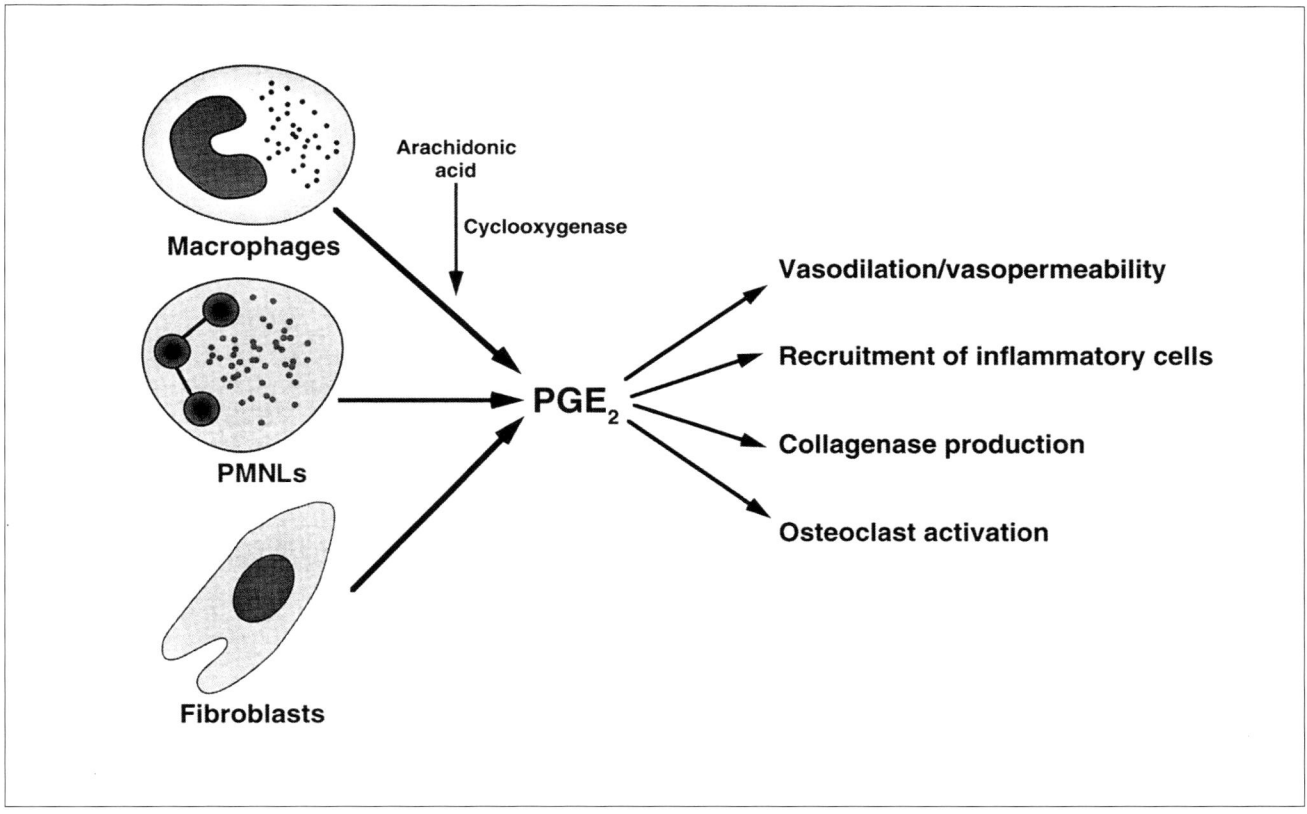

Fig 403 Effects of prostaglandin E$_2$ (PGE$_2$), which is released by macrophages, neutrophils (PMNLs), and fibroblasts. (From Lamster, 1997. Reprinted with permission.)

Crevicular fluid levels of PGE$_2$ are significantly elevated in persons affected by periodontitis, although considerable variation occurs both within and among diseased patients (Offenbacher et al, 1981). In an initial report, crevicular fluid samples from subjects with chronic and aggressive periodontitis were contrasted (Offenbacher et al, 1984). The latter, representing a risk group more likely to experience rapid disease progression, exhibited PGE$_2$ levels three times those of the cohort with chronic periodontitis.

Following these promising results, a prospective longitudinal trial was initiated to correlate disease progression and PGE$_2$ in crevicular fluid (Offenbacher et al, 1986). Patients with periodontitis and healthy patients were monitored with sequential manual probing and GCF sampling every 3 months for a period of 18 to 36 months. Con-

centrations of PGE$_2$ were quantified for individual sites and averaged per patient. Patients with disease activity at one or more sites exhibited significantly elevated mean concentrations of PGE$_2$ in GCF at the time of demonstrable attachment loss. Although GCF from sites of active disease contained a mean PGE$_2$ concentration of 305.6 µg/mL, a significantly lower mean concentration of 65.7 µg/mL was recorded in GCF from contralateral inactive sites. When PGE$_2$ results and disease progression were categorized, disease activity and stability were correctly identified with a sensitivity of 76% and a specificity of 96%. Similarly, positive and negative predictive values were calculated as 93% and 85%, respectively.

In a recent 5-year longitudinal maintenance study on selected smokers and nonsmokers with refractory periodontal disease, Söder (1998a)

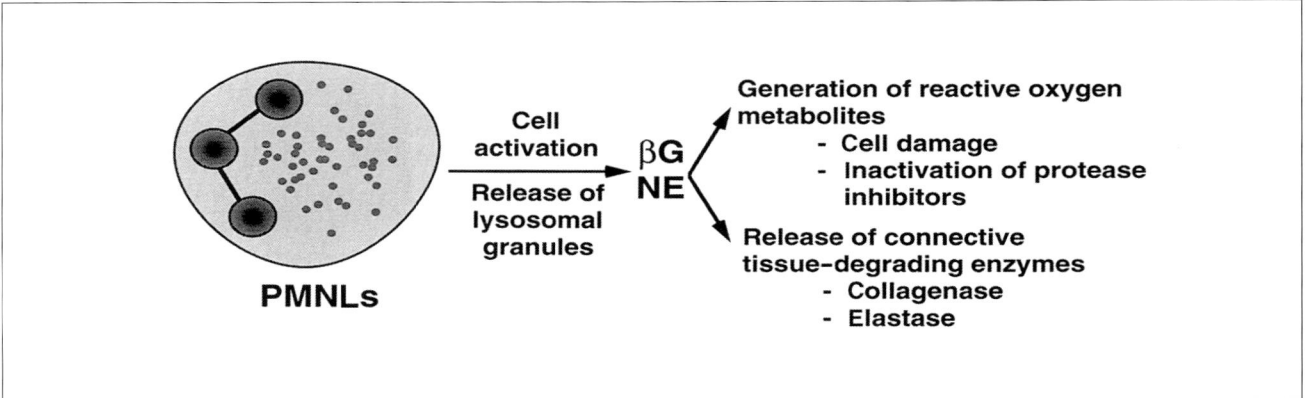

Fig 404 PMNL-derived lysosomal enzymes β-glucuronidase (βG) and neutrophil elastase (NE) in gingival crevicular fluid. An exuberent PMNL response is associated with release of reactive oxygen metabolites and tissue-degrading enzymes. (From Lamster, 1997. Reprinted with permission.)

showed that PGE_2 levels were significantly higher ($P < .001$) in sites with high levels of matrix metalloproteinase 8 derived from PMNLs, than they were in sites with low levels of matrix metalloproteinase 8, in both smokers and nonsmokers. A statistically significant correlation also was found between probing depth and levels of PGE_2 in nonsmokers ($P < .05$).

A rapid enzyme immunoassay similar to enzyme-linked immunosorbent assay (ELISA) has been described for quantifying PGE_2 in GCF (Nelson et al, 1992). Preliminary data indicate that this prototype reliably measures concentrations as low as 10 pg/mL.

β-Glucuronidase

The phagocytozing PMNLs (neutrophils) may release several types of enzymes from their lysosomes during phagocytosis as well as cellular necrosis. Two such enzymes, β-glucuronidase and neutrophil elastase (Fig 404), have frequently been used as GCF markers of active periodontal lesions.

β-Glucuronidase is a lysosomal enzyme involved in the degradation of the connective tissue ground substance. This acid glycohydrolase has been used as a marker for primary granule release

from PMNLs, and βG in GCF has been shown to be correlated with the number of PMNLs in the crevice.

The basis for evaluating βG as a diagnostic test for periodontal disease derives from a number of lines of evidence. First, the PMNLs are the predominant leukocytes in the gingival crevice (more than 90%) and are observed in the crevice during all stages of periodontal disease. Second, there is a historical association between abscess formation and suppuration, suppuration representing a large accumulation of PMNLs and bacteria that have lysed because of the failure of the PMNL influx to control the infection.

Host tissue can be damaged by the extracellular release of lysosomal contents (ie, collagenase, elastase) as well as the generation of reactive oxygen metabolites, which can both damage cells and inactivate protease inhibitors. Proper functioning of protease inhibitors is therefore critical for controlling the pathologic consequences of extracellular lysosomal enzyme release. Results of numerous cross-sectional studies suggest that the presence of βG in GCF may have diagnostic significance for periodontal disease.

Harper et al (1989) observed that total βG activity in GCF was significantly correlated with the occurrence of subgingival periodontal pathogens associated with more severe periodontal disease;

however, after they controlled for variation in disease severity, the correlations were not overwhelmingly strong. This finding suggested individual variation in the subgingival PMNL response to the subgingival microbial challenge.

The results of the first longitudinal trial monitoring the relationship of βG to clinical attachment level were published by Lamster et al (1988). Patients were monitored for clinical attachment level over a 6-month period. Samples of GCF were collected from the mesiobuccal crevice of all teeth except third molars. The total amounts of βG in GCF at baseline and 3 months later were related to clinical attachment level over the 6 months of the trial. Enzyme analysis was conducted at both the patient and the site levels. The results showed that analysis of enzyme activity in gingival crevicular fluid could identify patients with chronic periodontitis who were at risk for future disease progression. The authors concluded that persistently elevated levels of this enzyme, which in gingival crevicular fluid could serve as a marker for PMNL activity in the crevice, were associated with loss of probing attachment.

These findings were subsequently confirmed in a continuation and expansion of the first study, as the patients were followed for 12 months (Lamster et al, 1994b). The sensitivity and specificity of β-glucuronidase as a screening test for future PAL in patients with existing chronic periodontitis was better than 80%. In addition, a multicenter trial examining βG activity in gingival crevicular fluid as a measure of identifying patients at risk for future disease activity has been completed (Lamster et al, 1995a). This study focused on previously treated patients and indicated that persistently elevated levels of βG in gingival crevicular fluid were associated with an increase of 6 to 14 times in the risk for PAL during the monitoring period.

Neutrophil elastase

The assessment of neutrophil (PMNL) elastase in GCF provides another marker of intracrevicular PMNL activity (see Fig 404). Neutrophil elastase

(NE) is a serine endopeptidase found in primary granules and is a powerful proteolytic enzyme that can attack many substrates. The relationship of NE to the severity of periodontal disease has been studied during the past 10 years. NE activity is higher in GCF from patients with periodontitis than it is in GCF from patients with gingivitis; NE in GCF increases with the development of experimental gingivitis (Listgarten and Levin, 1981); and periodontal therapy tends to reduce NE activity in the fluid (Listgarten, 1992). For reviews see Lamster (1997).

A rapid spectrofluorometric assay for crevicular elastase has been developed and assessed in 30 untreated adults with periodontitis, who were followed longitudinally for 6 months (Palcanis et al, 1992). Crevicular fluid was collected on test strips impregnated with human polymorphonuclear leukocyte elastase substrate, and the presence of elastase, indicated by fluorescence, was graded on a scale of 0 to 4. Additionally, progression of periodontitis was assessed with sequential automated probing and computer-assisted digital radiography. Mean elastase scores were significantly higher at sites demonstrating progressive disease changes. Using a threshold value of 2 for elastase response, the test exhibited a sensitivity of 84% and a specificity of 66% in predicting periodontitis progression.

Armitage et al (1994) found that baseline NE is significantly higher at approximal sites exhibiting progressive bone loss during the experimental period. In a 5-year longitudinal maintenance study in patients with severe periodontitis, Jin et al (1995a, 1995b) showed that increased levels of NE are associated with disease progression and can be used to monitor response to the maintenance program (Jin et al, 1995b). NE also serves as a diagnostic marker for patients with refractory (nonresponding) periodontitis (Jin et al, 1995a). Recently, Söder (1998a) showed that, in sites with matching probing depths, NE activity is significantly higher ($P < .001$) in smokers than in nonsmokers.

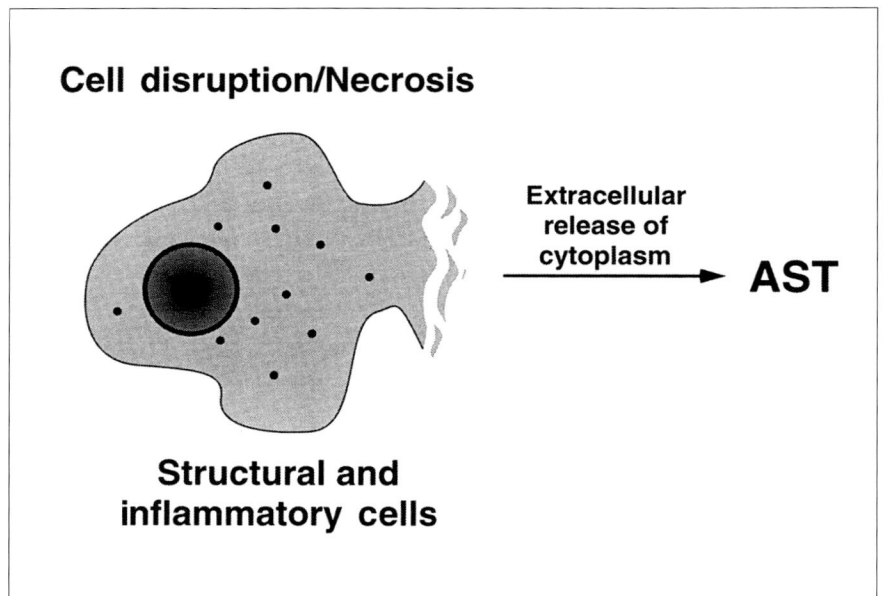

Cell disruption/Necrosis

Extracellular
release of
cytoplasm → **AST**

**Structural and
inflammatory cells**

Fig 405 Extracellular release of aspartate aminotransferase (AST), associated with cellular damage and necrosis. (From Lamster, 1997. Reprinted with permission.)

Aspartate aminotransferase

Because loss of tooth-supporting tissue is characteristic of periodontitis, markers of tissue destruction in gingival crevicular fluid have been examined for their potential application in diagnostic tests. Those investigated most extensively are cytoplasmic enzymes, such as lactate dehydrogenase and particularly aspartate aminotransferase (AST), which is present in many body tissues, with pronounced distribution in heart, liver, and skeletal muscle. The extracellular release of AST and other cytoplasmic enzymes is associated with cellular damage and cellular death (Fig 405).

Chambers et al (1984) evaluated changes in the level of AST in GCF during the development of experimental periodontitis in beagle dogs. A pronounced period of attachment loss was observed in the 3 weeks following ligation, and a peak in the AST concentration in GCF was noted 2 weeks following ligation. The concentration of AST in GCF was 10 to 100 times greater than the concentration in serum.

Recently, a series of studies in humans examined the relationship between AST activity in GCF and existing periodontal disease and between AST and periodontal disease progression. In a cross-sectional study, crevicular AST correlated with disease severity, as measured by probing depth, attachment level, bleeding on probing, Gingival Index, and Plaque Index (Imrey et al, 1991). Although crevicular levels of AST consistently decrease with repeated sampling, a 30-second sample appears to yield the most repeatable AST activity levels (Persson and Page, 1990).

Subsequent investigations have focused on monitoring crevicular AST levels in patients with periodontitis. In a 2-year study, Persson et al (1990) monitored 25 previously treated patients by reexamination every 3 months. Compared to stable sites, those sites losing 2 mm or more of clinical attachment exhibited significantly elevated levels of AST in GCF.

The sensitivity and specificity of the AST test in diagnosing active disease were similar for concentration thresholds of 800, 1,000, and 1,200 mIU, but clearly superior to 600 mIU. At the 800 mIU threshold, sensitivity and specificity were calculated as 93% and 68%, respectively, and the odds ratio as 15.4. In a similar longitudinal study of patients with periodontitis, only 2.6% of sites underwent attachment loss of 2 mm or more. The sites that met this rigid criterion for disease activity had higher concentrations of AST in crevicular fluid (Chambers et al, 1984).

Recently, a preprobing chairside test (Pocket Watch, Steri-Oss, Yorba Linda, CA) for AST in the GCF has been introduced (Fig 406). The GCF is sampled for 30 seconds. A reagent fluid is added to the GCF sample on the paper strip; within 10 minutes, a color change indicates the level of AST.

Other host-derived markers

Despite the evidence strongly suggesting the association of both β-glucuronidase and neutrophil elastase with active periodontal disease, as assessed by PAL, the association between other PMNL indicators and active disease is not as clear. Leukotriene B_4, which forms as a result of the action of lipoxygenase on arachidonic acid, is believed to be a product of PMNLs, and its identification in gingival crevicular fluid has been proposed as a marker of PMNL activity, particularly during the acute phases of gingival inflammation and periodontal disease. The levels of leukotriene B_4 in tissues affected by periodontitis are four times higher than the levels in healthy tissue, and the levels in gingival crevicular fluid from sites in patients with localized aggressive periodontitis are significantly elevated compared to healthy sites.

In addition, levels of the important enzyme collagenase have been examined in gingival crevicular fluid for its relationship to disease progression. In an experimental periodontitis model, Kryshtalskyj et al (1986) studied both collagenolytic activity and enzyme inhibitors in gingival crevicular fluid. Active disease was associated with elevated collagenolytic activity and reduced inhibitor activity, while the opposite applied to gingival crevicular fluid from healthy sites. Collagenase activity in gingival crevicular fluid from patients with various forms of periodontal disease has also been studied. Gingival crevicular fluid from patients with localized aggressive periodontitis has been shown to have a greater

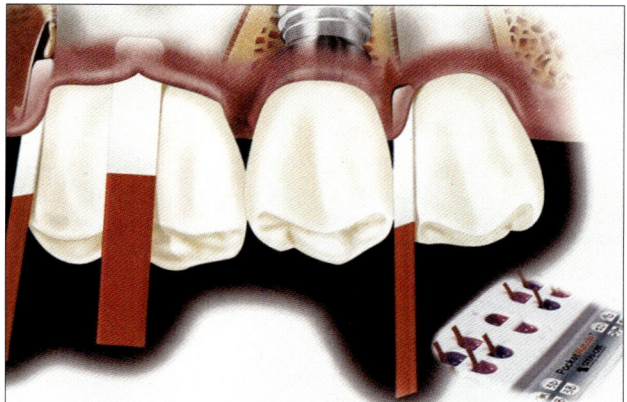

Fig 406 Preprobing chairside test for AST.

amount of both total collagenase and collagenase in the active form, as well as less inhibitor activity, than gingival crevicular fluid from age-matched healthy controls (Larivee et al, 1986). Again, the collagenase was seen to be mammalian (or host) in origin.

Similar methods were used to study collagenase activity in gingival crevicular fluid from patients with a healthy periodontium, gingivitis, chronic periodontitis, and localized aggressive periodontitis (Villela et al, 1987). The levels generally correlated with clinical measures of existing disease, and analysis confirmed the predominance of the mammalian form of the enzyme.

Many cellular types in the periodontium can produce collagenase, but a study of the specific origin of this enzyme in gingival crevicular fluid has suggested that PMNLs are the major source (Sorsa et al, 1988). A positive relationship between collagenase activity in gingival crevicular fluid and PAL has been reported (Lee et al, 1991).

A rapid chairside version of the collagenase test (Periocheck, Advanced Clinical Technologies, Westwood, MA) has been described and approved by some regulatory agencies as a tissue monitor (Bowers and Zarhadnik, 1989). The test protocol involves collection of crevicular fluid from pocket orifices for 15 seconds, utilizing filter paper strips. Individual strips are then incubated at 43°C on collagen gels. Enzyme activity, if present, releases a conjugated blue dye, which is absorbed into positive strips. Comparing color intensity and area to test standards, strip responses are scored on a scale of 0 to 2. Although healthy subjects exhibit a mean collagenase score of 0.17 cross sectionally, patients with periodontitis score significantly higher, with a mean of 0.93 (Bowers and Zarhadnik, 1989).

The local release of prostaglandins coincides with a number of other immunoinflammatory events, such as secretion of cytokines, collagenases, and other proteases that escalate periodontal destruction (Offenbacher et al, 1993; Page, 1991). Cytokines, a heterogenous group of host peptides including interleukin-1α (IL-1α), interleukin-1β (IL-1β), and interleukin-6 (IL-6), incite a series of immunoinflammatory events, including lymphocyte activation, macrophage chemotaxis, prostaglandin production, and osteoclastic bone resorption (for details see chapter 5). Although IL-1α and IL-1β can be isolated from human crevicular fluid, concentrations are higher in patients with periodontitis than in patients with gingivitis and in healthy patients (Masada et al, 1990). Interleukin in human GCF appears to increase significantly with severe, refractory disease (Reinhardt et al, 1993).

Diagnostic tests based on IL-1 might best be applied in untreated or recall populations with periodontitis. In a recent study, Gamonal et al (2000) showed that the amount of crevicular IL-1β, IL-8, and IL-10 was associated with periodontal status. However, Engebretson et al (1999) showed that the amount of IL-1 was 2.5 times higher in GCF and 3.5 times higher in gingival tissues before periodontal treatment in patients with genetic IL-1β polymorphism compared to patients without genetic polymorphism, which indicates that the levels of IL-1β are typical of a given patient. These data may explain why Figueredo et al (1999) found that the levels of IL-1β in GCF were increased in samples from periodontitis patients, regardless of the severity of disease at the sampled site, suggesting once again that the levels of IL-1β are typical of a given patient. In this context, it is of interest to note that a new Periodontal Suscep-tibility Test (PST) recently has been introduced for diagnosis of genetic polymorphism of IL-1 (for details see chapter 3).

Antibody titers

Specific antibody in gingival crevicular fluid is most often examined by enzyme-linked immunosorbent assay. Ebersole et al (1987) showed that, compared with the serum concentration, 9% of gingival crevicular fluid samples had an elevated antibody titer to a putative pathogen and 91% of patients had either the same or a lower titer. In adolescent and adult patients with aggressive periodontitis, the titer of antibody to *A actinomycetemcomitans* and *P gingivalis* was observed to be higher in gingival crevicular fluid than in serum.

A different approach to evaluating the relationship of the antibody response to active periodontal disease is to examine the levels of immunoglobulin G (IgG) subclasses in gingival crevicular fluid (Reinhardt et al, 1989). Sites undergoing PAL of at least 2 mm during the previous 3-month interval were sampled, and elevated levels of IgG4 compared with healthy or stable sites were detected. The switch to IgG4 may indicate the progression of the inflammatory infiltrate to one that is more chronic. Immunoglobulin G4 does not efficiently activate complement or bind to inflammatory cells and may indicate that the host is not able to mount a successful response to the microbial challenge (Reinhardt et al, 1989).

Recent evidence suggests that immunoglobulin A (IgA) in gingival crevicular fluid may have a role in periodontal homeostasis. A study in patients with chronic periodontitis revealed that reduced concentrations of IgA in gingival crevicular fluid are associated with an increased risk for PAL (Lamster et al, 1994). Supporting evidence for this was seen in a cross-sectional study of mediators of immunity and inflammation in gingival crevicular fluid from patients with a variety of forms of periodontitis (Ebersole et al, 1993). The study of IgA in gingival crevicular fluid may help to identify a protected patient.

Table 27 Host-derived mediators in gingival crevicular fluid that have been proposed as diagnostic tests for periodontal disease*

Mediator	Source	Relationship to disease activity in humans (references)
Prostaglandin E$_2$	Macrophages; PMNLs	Yes (Offenbacher et al, 1986, 1991; Söder, 1998a)
Collagenase	PMNLs	Yes (Lee et al, 1991)
		No (Birkedal-Hanson et al, 1993)
β-Glucuronidase	PMNLs	Yes (Lamster, 1991; Lamster et al, 1988, 1995a)
Neutrophil elastase	PMNLs	Yes (Jin et al, 1995a, 1995b; Palcanis et al, 1992; Söder, 1998a)
Aspartate aminotransferase	Cytoplasmic enzyme; many	Yes (Chambers et al, 1991; Persson et al, 1990)
Alkaline phosphatase	Many	Yes (Binder et al, 1987)
Immunoglobulin G4	Plasma cells	Yes (Reinhardt et al, 1989)
Immunoglobulin A	Plasma cells	Yes (Lamster et al, 1994)
Interleukin-1β	Macrophages	Yes (Gamonal et al, 2000; Figueredo et al, 1999)

*Modified from Lamster and Grbic (1995). Reprinted with permission.

Table 27 illustrates the various host-derived mediators in the gingival crevicular fluid that have been proposed as diagnostic tests for periodontal diseases. For reviews on the analysis of GCF, see Ebersole and Taubman (1994), Lamster and Grbic (1995), Lamster (1997), and Williams and Paquette (1997).

Conclusions

The adult population can broadly be described as comprising a great majority likely to experience gingivitis and a minority susceptible to periodontitis. There is also an intermediate group. After several years of poor gingival plaque control and irregular maintenance care, even individuals of limited susceptibility will develop periodontitis. This is the main reason why the prevalence of gingivitis may be relatively high and the prevalence of periodontitis extremely low in children and young adults (only about 0.1% in Scandinavia with high standard of oral hygiene and dental care) but much higher in the dentate elderly.

Diagnosis of clinically healthy and inflamed gingiva

Clinically healthy gingiva is characterized by a pale pink color, a stippled surface texture resembling orange peel, a thin gingival margin, free gingiva that is attached to the tooth surface, and elastic resilience. Clinical signs of inflamed gingiva (gingivitis) are redness, swelling (edema), loss of stippling, calor, bleeding on probing, secretion of gingival crevicular fluid, and a free gingival margin that is detached from the tooth surface. In the most advanced forms, spontaneous bleeding and ulceration may occur. The most common indices for diagnosis of gingivitis are the Gingival Index by Löe and Silness (1963; Löe, 1967), the Gingival Bleeding Index by Ainamo and Bay (1975), and the Papillary Bleeding Index by Saxer and Mühlemann (1975).

Diagnosis of periodontal attachment loss

Diagnosis of periodontitis must include not only clinical signs of inflammation and disease activity but also loss of periodontal support. Loss of periodontal support is mostly diagnosed by a combination of probing of attachment loss and radiographic evaluation of alveolar bone loss.

In single-rooted teeth, loss of periodontal attachment occurs only vertically along the root. In multirooted teeth, loss of attachment can also occur horizontally, indicating furcation involvement. Vertical loss of attachment is the distance between the cementoenamel junction and the base of the pocket and can be measured manually with a millimeter-graded probe. Several automated (computer-aided) and controlled-force probes are also available, some with resolutions of 0.1 to 0.5 mm. However, probing depth cannot be related to measurement of vertical PAL.

Horizontal PAL may be diagnosed with curved, slim, double-ended curettes or special furcation probes. Furcation involvement is classified as one of three different grades: I = horizontal loss of supporting tissues not exceeding one third of the width of the tooth; II = loss of support exceeding one third of the width of the tooth, but not encompassing the total width of the furcation area; III = through-and-through destruction of the supporting tissues in the furcation.

Radiographic diagnosis

For detailed analysis of the alveolar bone, the usual method is conventional intraoral complete-mouth radiography, supplemented with four vertical bite-wing radiographs, taken with a standardized technique, such as film holders attached to the long cone. The normal threshold for no loss of alveolar bone is 1.5 to 2.0 mm from the cementoenamel junction. However, considerable probing loss of periodontal attachment in the posterior interproximal regions may be undetected on radiographs because the spongiform bone has a much lower mineral content than does the compact bone.

The eye cannot observe differences in mineral loss less than 30% to 50% on radiographs. Therefore, the new computer-aided digital subtraction radiographic techniques offer much greater potential to diagnose even small differences (about 5%) of bone loss or bone gain, which may occur over brief intervals. The subtraction images may be color coded, enabling the clinician to identify where change has occurred.

Assessment of treatment needs

The Community Periodontal Index of Treatment Needs is a simplified index for estimation of existing periodontal treatment needs, based on clinical examination at the individual and sextant levels for epidemiologic surveys. However, at the surface level, it is also useful for clinical evaluation of treatment needs in patients.

Diagnosis of individual teeth

In the Gothenburg system, the periodontal status of every tooth is diagnosed, based on recording at examination of the status of the periodontal structures (the gingiva, the periodontal membrane, the root cementum, and the alveolar bone). To facilitate treatment planning, each tooth is given an individual diagnosis: gingivitis, periodontitis levis, periodontitis gravis, or periodontitis complicata.

Assessment of tooth mobility

Increased tooth mobility can be caused by a variety of factors, such as orthodontic tooth movement, heavy functional loads (such as from prosthetic appliances), occlusal discrepancies, and loss of alveolar bone secondary to endodontic problems or periodontitis. Because periodontitis is not the only cause of tooth hypermobility, a loose tooth should be carefully evaluated to determine the underlying cause: A logical first step is careful determination of the clinical attachment.

Recording of diagnoses

To facilitate detailed periodontal examination of the patient in clinical practice, a chart designed for manual or computer-aided recording of the most important diagnoses at the tooth and surface levels is of great importance.

Diagnosis of active lesions

Together, the following features are not only very important signs of diseased periodontal pockets and active periodontal lesions but also a guarantee of further rapid breakdown of the periodontal tissues; they may be regarded as prognostic risk factors for further periodontal attachment loss:

- The presence of subgingival biofilms and high levels of specific periopathogens subgingivally
- A recent increase in pocket depth and clinical attachment loss
- The loss of compact bone on the alveolar crest
- The presence of bleeding on probing
- An increase in periodontal pocket temperature
- An increase in volume of gingival crevicular fluid
- An increase of PGE_2, endogenous matrix metalloproteinases, proinflammatory cytokine levels, etc in the GCF

CHAPTER 7

EPIDEMIOLOGY
OF PERIODONTAL DISEASES

Epidemiology may be descriptive or analytic. Descriptive epidemiology deals with the occurrence, severity, and distribution of diseases and the mortality in any selected population. Analytic epidemiology seeks to discern, directly or indirectly, the causes of a disease, and to evaluate any public health consequences of intervention. Until about 20 years ago, it was generally accepted within the dental profession that:

- All individuals eventually become susceptible to severe periodontitis.
- Gingivitis progresses to periodontitis: There is continuous, linear loss of periodontal support and finally tooth loss.
- Susceptibility to periodontitis increases with age.

A more recent approach is to dichotomize the adult population, differentiating between those who are healthy or have gingivitis and those who are susceptible to periodontitis. The prevalence of gingivitis and mild or moderate forms of periodontitis is strongly correlated to the standard of gingival plaque control and dental care habits. However, periodontitis is the result of a complex interplay of bacterial challenge, host response, and other modifying factors, and, despite extreme variations in oral hygiene standards, the prevalence of severe periodontitis in adults is about 5%

to 15% in both industrialized and developing countries (Ånerud et al, 1983; Hugoson and Jordan, 1982; Löe et al, 1986; for review see Burt, 1996; Pilot, 1998). Among children and young adults, the prevalence of aggressive periodontitis (localized or generalized) is as low as 0.1% in the Scandinavian countries, about 1% in the United States, and as high as 5% in some developing countries (Källestål and Matsson, 1990; Källestål et al, 1990; Löe and Brown, 1991; Sjödin et al, 1993; for review see Armitage and Van Dyke, 1996).

A major dilemma in epidemiology of periodontal diseases is that, apart from the Community Periodontal Index of Treatment Needs (CPITN), there are still no international standards or recommendations. Retrospective comparison of data on periodontal status in different surveys and studies is very difficult. Gingivitis, probing depth, clinical attachment level, and radiographically assessed alveolar bone loss have all been used as criteria, quite inconsistently. The threshold values adopted for "deep" or "pathologic" periodontal pockets, or for the clinical attachment levels and alveolar bone scores required for the assumption that "true" loss of periodontal tissue support has occurred, have varied considerably from study to study. In addition, the number of "affected" tooth surfaces required for designating an individual subject as a "case," ie, as suffering from periodontal disease, has varied. These inconsistencies in the definitions inevitably affect the figures describing the distribution of the disease.

Any measure of prevalence of periodontitis is dependent on how the disease is defined, ie, the definition of a periodontitis case. For example, data from a US national survey show that, if the disease is defined as the identification of at least one site with probing attachment loss (PAL) of 2 mm or more, about 80% of all adults, and more than 90% of those aged 55 to 64 years, are affected (US Public Health Service, 1987). When the definition of a case is at least one site with PAL of 4 mm or more, the prevalence drops to below 10%. Even when allowance is made for the uncertainty regarding definitions of what constitutes a case, it is clear that mild to moderate periodontitis is so prevalent that the milder forms are almost universal. The severe manifestations of the disease, ie, those which lead to tooth loss, or at least threaten it, are less prevalent. These examples demonstrate that prevalence data are of little value if they do not specify the relevant definition of a case and the age group to which they apply.

Trends in prevalence and severity of periodontal diseases are not easy to ascertain, because the philosophic basis for their measurement has changed with the disease model. Even so, national survey data for the United States suggest that the prevalence of gingivitis has declined over the last 30 years or so and that, while there has been little change in the prevalence of periodontitis, the severity has decreased (Capilouto and Douglas, 1988). Similar improvements in periodontal health have been reported in Scandinavia (Axelsson et al, 2000; Hansen et al, 1990; Hugoson et al, 1992).

Apart from bleeding on probing and probing depth, the standard clinical variable measured to assess periodontal status is PAL. Probing attachment loss expresses accumulated disease at a site rather than current activity and is a diagnostic "gold standard" for periodontitis. However, lack of consensus on how best to apply PAL for case definition continues to hamper clinical and epidemiologic research. In descriptive as well as analytic epidemiologic studies, PAL should be the variable of choice for evaluation of loss of periodontal support by destructive periodontal diseases. Such studies should be conducted in randomized indicator age groups instead of selected groups of individuals with different age intervals. Thorough examination of periodontal status should include circumferential probing assessments around all teeth.

However, in various studies, PAL and CPITN have been measured on all teeth and surfaces, all teeth in two quadrants, the worst teeth in each sextant, and selected index teeth. Measurements have been made on six, four, two, and one sites per tooth, and simple clinical diagnostic methods as well as high-technology diagnostic equipment (eg, computerized probes, computer-aided digital subtraction radiography), analyses of markers in the gingival crevicular fluid, and genetic tests have been used. However, the debate over which method is the most appropriate is still ongoing.

As one illustration of this problem, it has been suggested that the 1985–1986 National Survey of Oral Health in US Employed Adults and Seniors (Miller et al, 1987a) may have underestimated the national prevalence of periodontitis because it measured only two sites per tooth (mesiobuccal and midbuccal) in one maxillary and one mandibular quadrant. Because the survey protocol did not include the most susceptible sites, furcations, and lingual areas, disease was probably underestimated. From the epidemiologic perspective, another source of underestimation in the national surveys is likely to be the necessary sampling restrictions: The subjects in the 18- to 64-year-old group included only employed people, mostly from small businesses, and the seniors were those who attended senior centers. This sample was probably biased toward individuals with better periodontal health.

The epidemiologic studies of periodontal diseases conducted in more than 100 national surveys were based on the highest CPITN score at the individual or sextant level. This is far from the "true" treatment need at all remaining tooth surfaces and provides no information about lost periodontal support.

Fig 407 Mean loss of probing attachment by age group in the county of Värmland, Sweden, in 1988 and 1998. (From Axelsson et al, 2000. Reprinted with permission.)

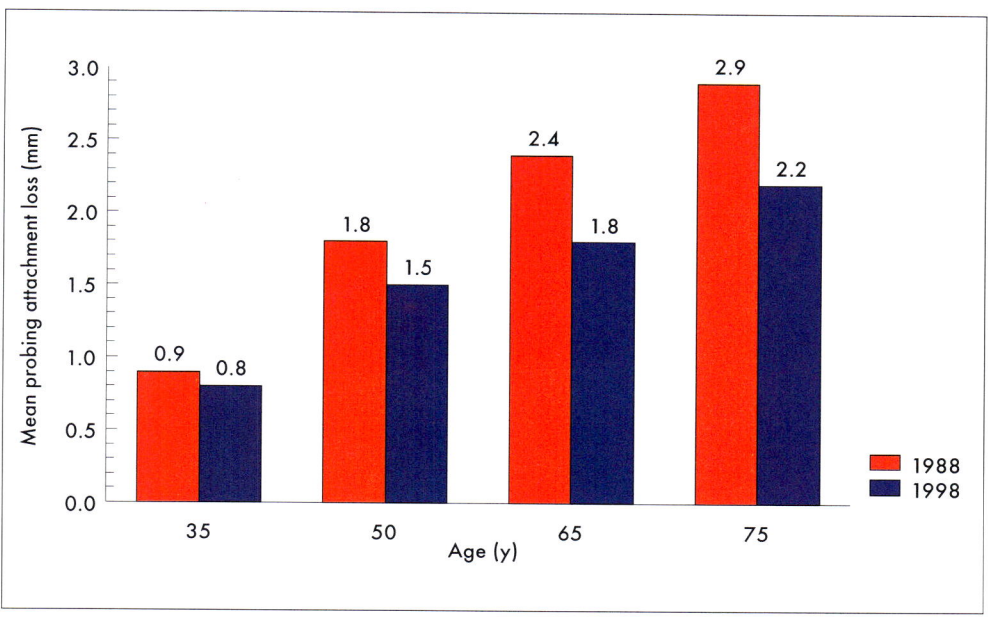

PREVALENCE OF PERIODONTAL DISEASES: PROBING ATTACHMENT LOSS

Probing attachment loss can be measured vertically as well as horizontally (furcation involvement). To date, there are very few epidemiologic studies based on vertical PAL (Axelsson et al, unpublished data, 1990; Axelsson et al, 1998, 2000; Baelum et al, 1986, 1988a, 1988b; Brown et al, 1990; Löe et al, 1978, 1986; Okamoto et al, 1988; Yoneyama et al, 1988; for review, see Burt, 1991, 1996; Papapanou 1994, 1996; Papapanou and Lindhe, 1997). Only three of these studies were carried out on randomized indicator age groups (35-, 50-, 65-, and 75-year-old Swedes) and included horizontal PAL (furcation involvement), as well as vertical PAL and CPITN, on all tooth surfaces (Axelsson et al, unpublished data, 1990; Axelsson et al, 1998, 2000). Particularly in Scandinavia, several studies on periodontal prevalence and incidence have assessed alveolar bone loss or bone scores diagnosed on radiographs (Björn et al, 1969b; Hugoson and Laurell, 2000; Hugoson et al, 1998b; Papapanou et al, 1988; Papapanou and Wennström, 1989; Salonen et al, 1991; for review

see Jeffcoat et al, 1995; Papapanou, 1994, 1996; Papapanou and Lindhe, 1997, and chapter 6).

In adults, tooth loss and loss of periodontal support vary markedly among different countries, selected subgroups of populations, ages, individuals, and teeth. In the classic study, "The Natural History of Periodontal Disease," Löe et al (1978, 1986) compared the prevalence of PAL in a randomly selected group of Norwegian students and academics and Sri Lankan tea workers who practiced no oral hygiene and lacked access to dental care. At 40 years of age, the mean loss of probing attachment was only 1.5 mm in the Norwegian subjects and 4.5 mm in the Sri Lankan subjects.

Probing attachment loss related to age

Periodontal prevalence is strictly age related because loss of periodontal attachment is cumulative, although not necessarily linear, throughout life. Figure 407 shows the mean loss of probing attachment in randomly selected 35, 50, 65, and 75 year olds from the county of Värmland, Sweden in 1988 and 1998. The true differences between the four age groups are probably much

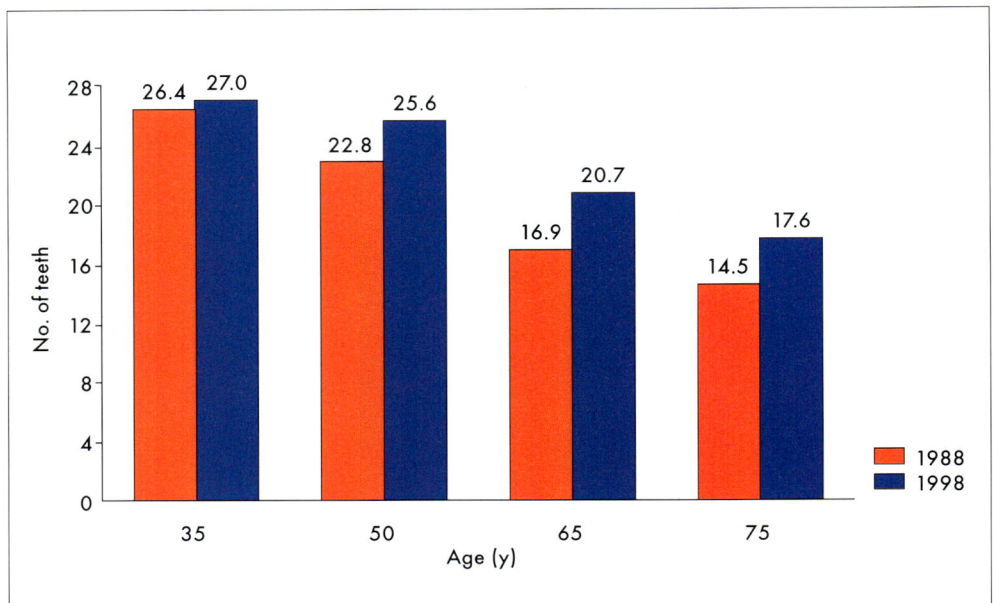

Fig 408 Mean number of teeth (excluding third molars) by age group in the county of Värmland in 1988 and 1998. (From Axelsson et al, 2000. Reprinted with permission.)

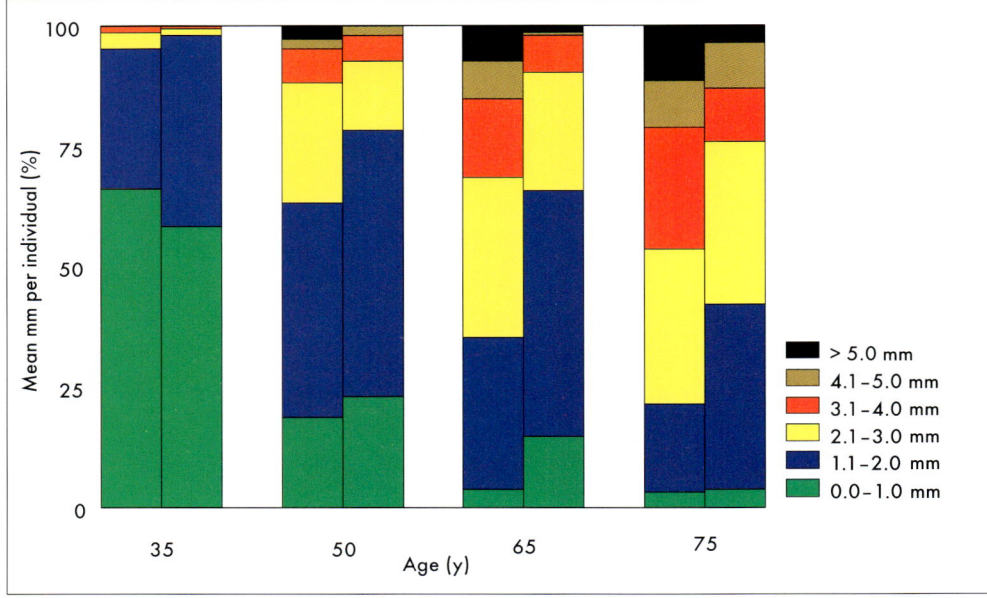

Fig 409 Frequency distribution (%) of different mean levels of probing attachment loss at mesial sites per individual by age group in 1988 and 1998. (From Axelsson et al, 2000. Reprinted with permission.)

greater, because, after exclusion of third molars, in the 75 year olds the teeth lost are more diseased compared with those lost by the 35 and 50 year olds. However, the overall number of remaining teeth increased significantly from 1988 to 1998, particularly in 65 and 75 year olds (Fig 408), while PAL was significantly reduced (see Fig 407) as an effect of the preventive program introduced to the entire adult population in 1985 (Axelsson et al, 2000). However, in patients up to the age of 50 years, the buccal surfaces exhibit more PAL than do the approximal surfaces in a well-maintained toothbrushing populatioon as an iatrogenic effect of frequent toothbrushing (see the section on pattern of attachment loss later in this chapter). In our analytic epidemiology, there was no

Fig 410 Frequency distribution (%) of probing attachment loss at mesial sites by age group in 1988 and 1998. (From Axelsson et al, 2000. Reprinted with permission.)

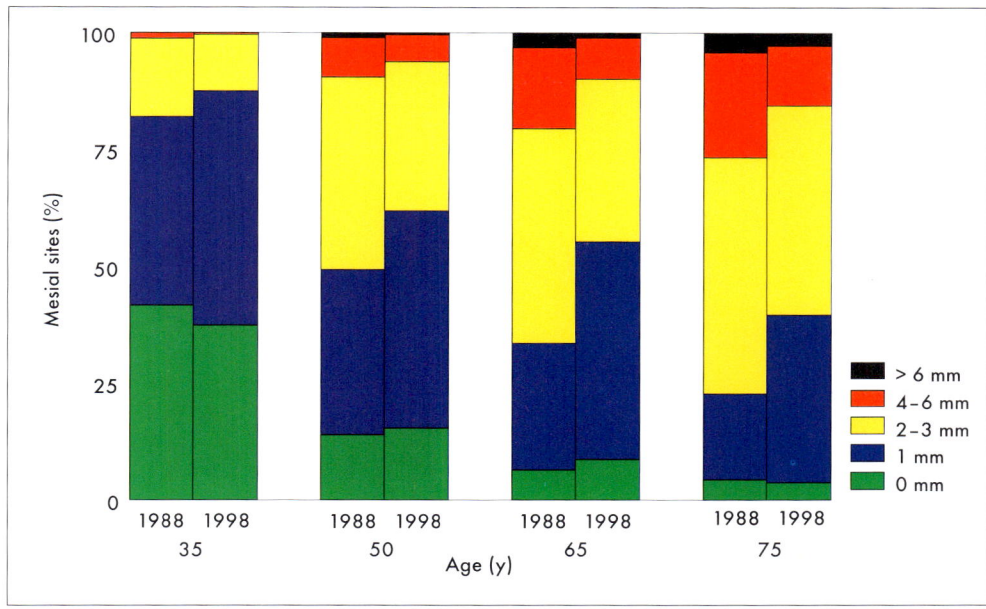

difference between mean values of PAL on mesial versus distal surfaces, but the reliability of measurement was higher on the mesial surfaces. As a consequence, the "true" prevalence of PAL on mesial sites is presented here. The amount of attachment loss varied considerably among individuals as well as tooth surfaces. For example, in the 50-year-old group, which was expanded (n = 450) for a longitudinal study, only 7% of the individuals exhibited a mean of 3 to 5 mm PAL in 1998 while about 80% had a mean PAL of only 0 to 2 mm (Fig 409). Figure 410 shows the frequency distribution of varying amounts of PAL for the total number of sites examined (more than 100,000) in the four different age groups in 1988 and 1998. In 1998, > 85% of the sites in 35 year olds had 0 or 1 mm of PAL, and no sites exhibit 4 mm or greater of PAL. In 65 and 75 year olds respectively, only 10% and 15% of the sites had 4 mm or more of PAL in 1998.

Figure 411 illustrates the age-specific severity of PAL based on epidemiologic data from various populations. Figure 412, from a study of adult dentate populations in the United States in 1985 (Miller et al, 1987b), shows the subjects grouped according to the most severe loss of attachment and age group.

In the 1985 to 1986 US national survey, the proportion of adults with at least one site of PAL measuring 2 mm or more exceeded 70%, even among adults aged 35 to 44 years; the proportion was more than 90% among those aged 55 to 64 (Fig 413). The presence of at least one site with PAL of 4 mm or more increased steadily from 13.8% of 25 to 34 year olds to 53.6% of 55 to 64 year olds. When the minimum threshold for PAL was set at 7 mm, there was again a steady increase with age, from 3.8% of 35 to 44 year olds to 9.3% of 55 to 64 year olds affected. Probing depth is also related to age, although less directly than PAL. The 1985 to 1986 US national survey found probing depths of 4 to 6 mm in 13.4% of all adults, and more frequently in older groups (Brown et al, 1990).

As discussed previously, the long-held assumption that periodontitis is a disease of aging has been challenged in recent years (Burt, 1994). The current view sees the greater periodontal destruction in the elderly as a reflection of lifetime accumulation of disease rather than as an age-specific condition. A relatively low prevalence of severe (as opposed to moderate) loss of periodontal support among the elderly was first shown in Sweden (Hugoson and Jordan, 1982) and has since been demonstrated elsewhere (see

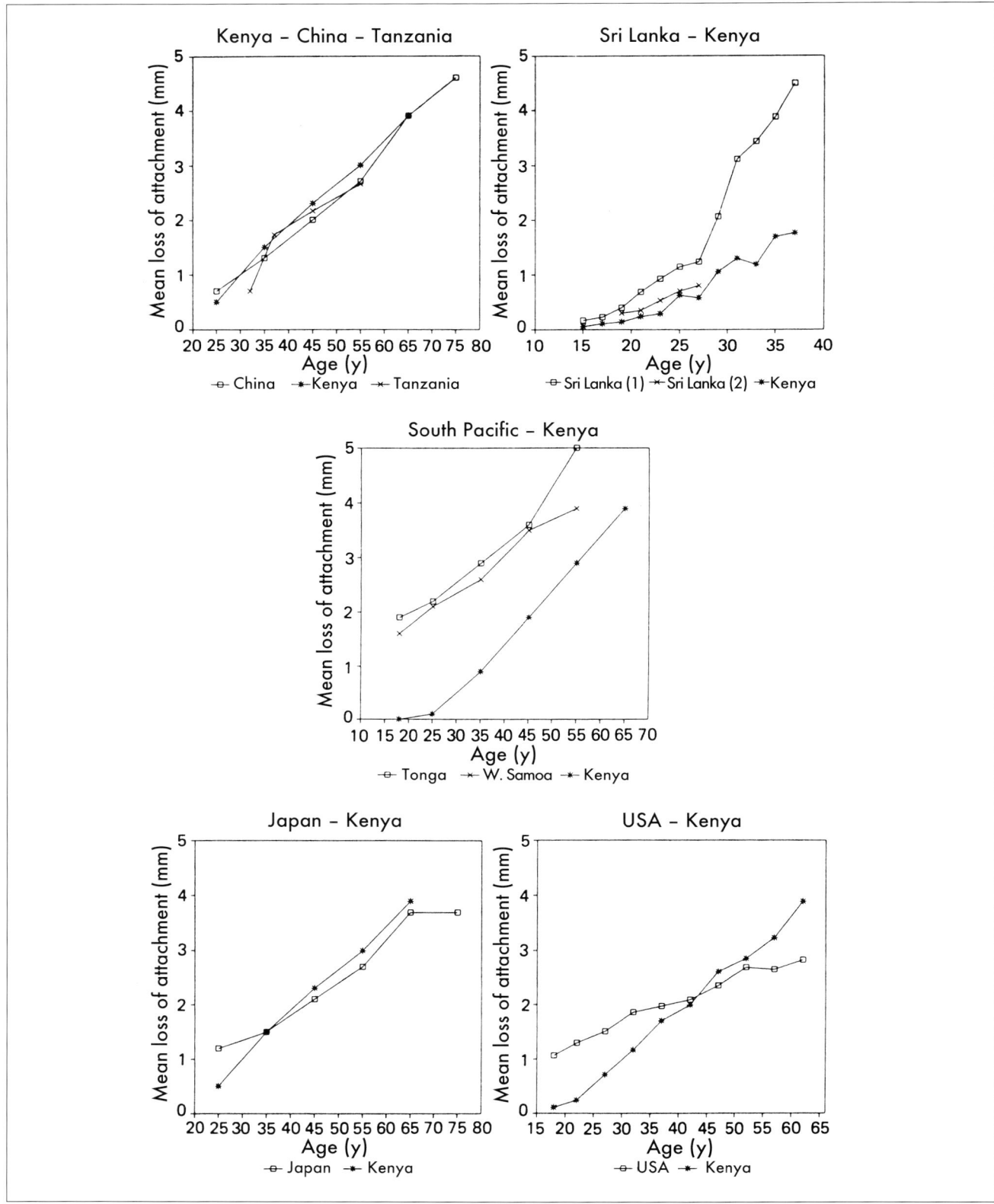

Fig 411 Age-specific severity of probing attachment loss in various populations. (From Baelum et al, 1991. Reprinted with permission.)

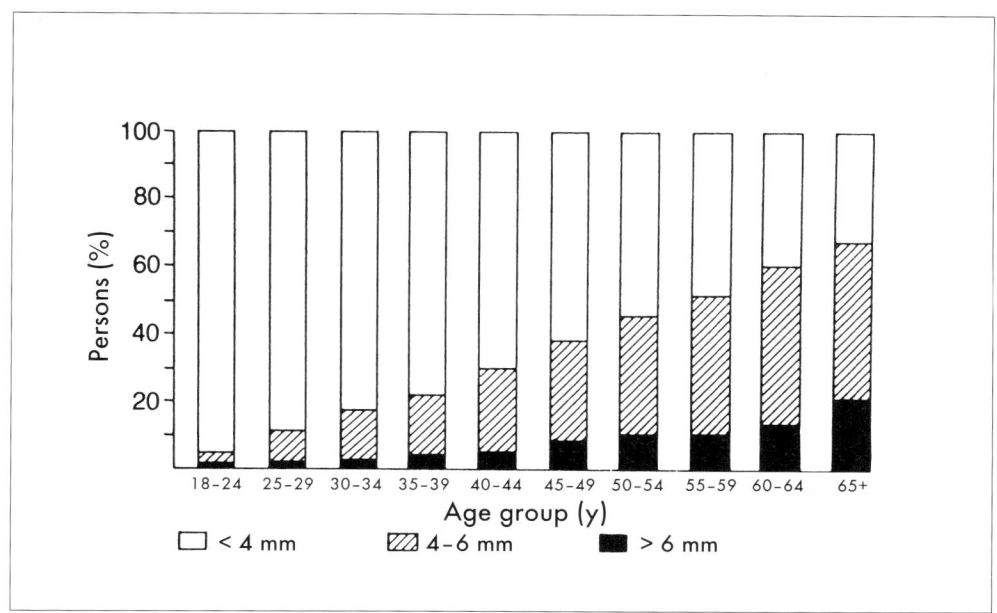

Fig 412 Percentage of individuals with severe loss of attachment by age group in adult dentate populations in the US in 1985. (From Miller et al, 1987b. Reprinted with permission.)

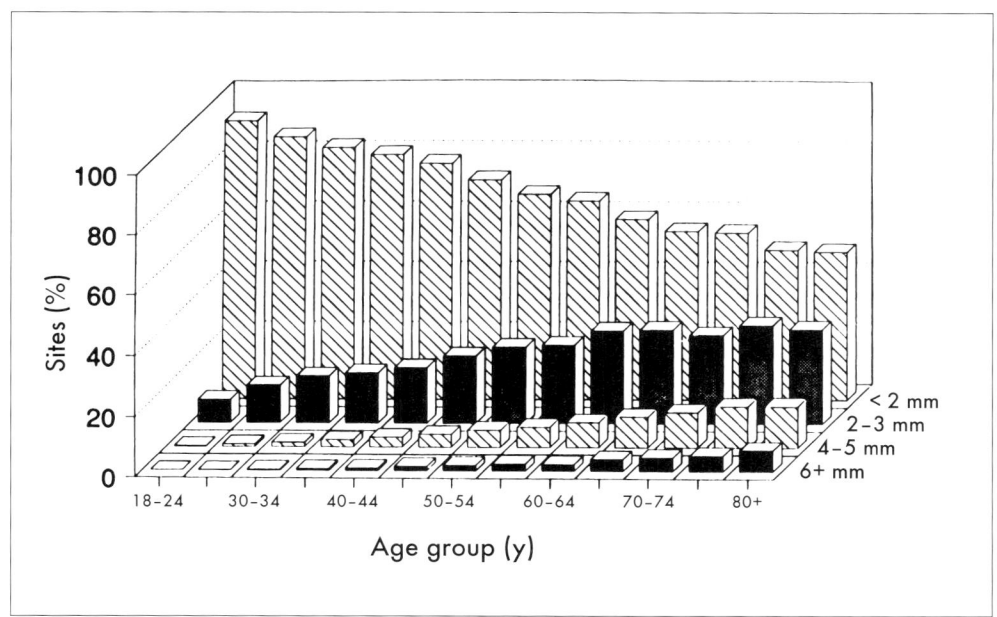

Fig 413 Percentage of sites with attachment loss, by severity, in 1986 to 1987 national survey of US adults. (From Miller et al, 1987b. Reprinted with permission.)

Figs 407 to 410). Surveys of older people in the United States, Canada, and Australia have found that PAL or probing depths of 6 mm or more was prevalent in some 15% to 30% of persons examined (Hunt et al, 1990; Locker and Leake, 1993a; Slade et al, 1993). In all these studies, PAL of 4 to 6 mm was common. Higher estimates of periodontal destruction came from a cross-sectional New England study of community-living elderly people (Douglass et al, 1993; Fox et al, 1994). The New England study was of persons aged 70 to 96 years, older than those examined in the 1985 to 1986 US national survey, and the results could reflect cohort effects (ie, results specific to the generation studied and that may not be found in subsequent generations). All these reports agree that PAL increases with age, but most did not find extensive loss of function in the affected teeth.

Periodontitis frequently begins in youth and early adulthood, rather than later in adulthood. Some degree of PAL in youth is well documented in population studies (Ånerud et al, 1983; Clerehugh and Lennon, 1986; Hoover et al, 1981; Källestål and Matsson, 1990; Källestål et al, 1990). However, as stated already, the prevalence of aggressive periodontitis in children and young adults is very low in European populations. Among 16 year olds in Finland and Switzerland, only 0.1% exhibit loss of alveolar bone adjacent to permanent first molars (Kronauer et al, 1986; Saxén, 1980). Similar data have also been reported for schoolchildren in England (Saxby, 1987). Retrospective studies by Sjödin et al (1989, 1993) and Cogen et al (1992), however, indicate that 75% to 90% of all subjects with aggressive periodontitis had previously experienced loss of alveolar bone around the primary teeth.

In a study of more than 11,000 young adults (aged 14 to 17 years) in the United States, 50 (0.53%) were found to have localized aggressive periodontitis (LAP) with attachment loss of greater than 3 mm on at least one first molar and one incisor or second molar, and an additional 14 (0.13%) had generalized aggressive periodontitis (GAP). When the data were weighted to represent the racial mixture of this age group in the United

States, about 87,000 cases of LAP and GAP were estimated among 13 million 14 to 17 year olds. More second molars and premolars than incisors were found to have PAL of greater than 3 mm. Incidental attachment loss of more than 3 mm on one or more teeth was found in 175 subjects, or 1.61% of the population examined.

Epidemiologic studies have largely overlooked GAP. There has been some agreement on the diagnostic criteria, eg, at least eight teeth must exhibit 3-mm PAL and 5-mm probing depths. Löe et al (1986) reported that 8% of Sri Lankan tea workers had GAP. Of 5,849 persons aged 18 to 34 in the National Institute of Dental Research Adult Survey, 212 (3.6%) had moderate GAP with PAL of more than 3 mm on eight teeth (Löe and Brown, 1991; Oliver et al, 1998). The rationale for using PAL of more than 3 mm as a threshold was that eight teeth with that amount of PAL in persons aged 18 to 34 years would be atypical of chronic periodontitis and more likely to represent GAP. This represents 1.8 million of 46.6 million people in the United States aged 18 to 34 years. Only 17 subjects had advanced GAP with PAL of more than 5 mm on eight teeth. The prevalence of moderate GAP increased from 1.3% in 18 to 24 year olds to 5.7% in those aged 30 to 34 years. A similar age-related increase in advanced GAP was found. Subgingival calculus was almost always present (Oliver et al, 1998). (For details on the new classification of GAP, see chapter 5.) In some developing countries, the prevalence of aggressive periodontitis in children and young adults may be higher because of inadequate oral hygiene, nutritional deficiencies, genetics, race, etc (Löe et al, 1986).

Hypothetically, the more susceptible members of the population are those in whom periodontitis begins in youth, in which case the relatively low prevalence of severe PAL among many dentate elderly could be partly a survival phenomenon; ie, those most susceptible to severe periodontitis have already lost several or all of their teeth. The most rapid disease progression is observed in the relatively small number of people in whom the disease starts young. Despite widespread assumptions, it is not yet clear whether this type of disease is associated with leukocyte defects: virtually no epidemiologic data are available. (For details on aggressive periodontitis, see chapters 3 and 5.)

It is uncommon for elderly people with reasonably intact dentitions to exhibit sudden bursts of periodontitis (Page, 1984). Tooth retention, good oral hygiene, and periodontal health (expressed as little gingival inflammation and few deep pockets) are closely associated, regardless of age (Abdellatif and Burt, 1987; Axelsson et al, 1991, 2000; Burt et al, 1985). The New England studies (Fox et al, 1994) raised the question of whether periodontal destruction becomes more severe among the very elderly, while the Piedmont studies (Locker et al, 1991) showed highly variable levels of periodontal destruction among the elderly. An issue to be addressed, especially with an increasingly dentate aging population, is the minimum standard of periodontal health compatible with an acceptable quality of life in the elderly.

Probing attachment loss related to determinants

In addition to age, factors such as gender, socioeconomic status (particularly educational level), dental care habits, and place of residence (urban or rural), the so-called determinants, are also related to the prevalence of clinical attachment loss. Clinical attachment loss of all levels of severity is generally more prevalent in males than in females. This has been a consistent finding in all national surveys in the United States since the first (1960 to 1962) as well as in several other studies (Axelsson et al, unpublished data, 1990; Axelsson et al, 2000). Oral hygiene standards are usually higher in women than in men: Men have more calculus and plaque deposits (Abdellatif and Burt, 1987). In a study of dentate persons aged 65 and older in Iowa, age was negatively related to the proportion of teeth classified as periodontally healthy in men, but positively related to that proportion in women (Levy et al, 1987).

The reasons underlying these gender differences have not been explored in detail but are thought to be related to poorer oral hygiene and dental attendance habits among men rather than any genetic factor. Hormonal changes may be reflected in such transient conditions as pregnancy- and puberty-associated gingivitis. In a study by Norderyd et al (1993), 50- to 64-year-old women who were receiving estrogen replacement therapy had less gingival bleeding than did controls, even after the researchers allowed for higher educational levels and lower plaque accumulation.

Historically, levels of periodontal disease have been related to lower socioeconomic status. Gingivitis and poor oral hygiene are clearly related to lower socioeconomic status, but the relationship between periodontitis and socioeconomic status is less direct. The 1985–1986 US national survey found that the prevalence of PAL at all levels of severity was not closely related to household income (Brown et al, 1996a; Oliver et al, 1991). Probing attachment loss of 4 mm or more and 7 mm or more in at least one site were both closely correlated with educational levels; the relationship was much weaker with PAL of 2 mm or more because this measure was so common.

The association between high socioeconomic status and gingival health is a function of better oral hygiene among the more educated and a greater frequency of dental attendance among the more dentally aware and those with dental insurance (who are more likely to be white-collar employees, ie, those with more education) (Axelsson et al, unpublished data, 1990; Paulander et al, 2002; for details see chapter 2). Although racial and ethnic differences in periodontal status have been demonstrated many times, it is still not clear whether these are true genetic differences or whether socioeconomic status, a complex and multifaceted variable that can include a variety of cultural factors, confounds these relationships.

In a randomized sample of almost six hundred 50 to 55 year olds in the county of Värmland, Sweden, the number of remaining teeth and loss of periodontal attachment on the mesial surfaces were evaluated in relation to residential area, sex, dental care habits, educational level, and smoking and snuffing habits (see Figs 103 and 104 in chapter 2) (Axelsson and Paulander, 1994). From this cross-sectional part of the study, irregular dental care, followed by smoking and low education, were the most important risk indicators for loss of periodontal attachment. Other factors, such as occupation, employment versus unemployment, systemic diseases, medication, salivary secretion rate, dietary and oral hygiene habits, attitudes and opinions related to oral health, plaque scores, lifestyle (regular or irregular exercise, etc), and body mass index, will also be evaluated. The 50 year olds of this randomized sample (n = 448) have been followed longitudinally for 10 years to evaluate these variables as possible risk factors and prognostic risk factors for dental caries, periodontal diseases, and other oral diseases. Irregular dental care, followed by smoking and high plaque values, was the most important risk factor for tooth loss (see Fig 123 in chapter 2) and PAL (Axelsson et al, 2000). Further evaluation by multivariate analysis is ongoing. The goal of this analysis is to describe the characteristics and ranking order of factors that explain why the subset representing 25% the healthiest subjects lost no further PAL, while there was considerable loss in the 25% of subjects with the most serious cases. For details on external modifying factors see chapter 2.

Extent and Severity Index

In clinical practice, PAL is usually measured at four (mesial, buccal, distal, and lingual) or six sites (mesiobuccal, midbuccal, distobuccal, mesiolingual, midlingual, and distolingual). In epidemiologic studies, however, the number of probing assessments per tooth has varied from two to six, while the examination may include all teeth (complete-mouth examination) or a subset of index teeth (partial-mouth examination).

Carlos et al (1986) proposed a bivariate Extent and Severity Index (ESI) for recording loss of peri-

odontal tissue support in individuals. The extent component describes the proportion of tooth sites that show signs of destructive periodontitis, and the severity component, expressed as a mean value, describes the amount of PAL at the diseased sites. Sites at which PAL is greater than 1 mm are denoted as diseased. Although arbitrary, this threshold value serves a dual purpose: It readily discloses the proportion of sites affected by disease at levels exceeding the error inherent in clinical measurement of PAL, and it prevents the inclusion of unaffected sites in assessment of the mean value for attachment loss in the individual subject. To limit the number of measurements required per subject, a partial examination, comprising the midbuccal and mesiobuccal aspects of the maxillary right and mandibular left quadrants, is recommended.

The bivariate nature of the index facilitates a description of PAL patterns: For example, an ESI of 85, 3.0 in 65 year olds suggests a generalized but rather mild form of destructive disease, in which 85% of the tooth sites are affected by an average PAL of 3 mm. In contrast, an ESI of 25, 6.0 describes a severe, localized form of disease.

This system is being used increasingly and has been applied in a number of recent cross-sectional studies of elderly subjects (Fox et al, 1994; Oliver et al, 1998). However, in randomized samples of subjects up to 50 years of age, PAL on the buccal sites is at least comparable to that on the approximal sites (Axelsson et al, unpublished data, 1990). In toothbrushing populations, most buccal PAL is an iatrogenic effect. It should also be noted that the ESI index does not include values for lingual sites.

Frequency distribution of periodontal diseases

Recent epidemiologic surveys in industrialized countries indicate that gingivitis affects most adolescents and 40% to 50% of adults. As stated earlier, surveys also show that aggressive periodontitis in children and young adults is rare (0.1% to 0.5%) (Källestål and Matsson, 1990; Källestål et al, 1990; Löe and Brown, 1991; Saxén, 1980; Sjödin et al, 1993; for review see Armitage and Van Dyke, 1996). Most adults are affected by moderate periodontitis; the severe, generalized form of aggressive periodontitis is clustered in only 5% to 15% of any population (Ånerud et al, 1983; Löe et al, 1986; for review see Pilot, 1998).

The methods of investigation and the clinical variables used in the various studies are neither uniform nor standardized, as discussed earlier. Clinical measurements may be recorded at one or several of sites per tooth, and clinical assessment may be based on either partial- or complete-mouth recordings. These differences are particularly important because partial-mouth recording has been shown to influence the outcome of prevalence and severity studies of the disease in a population (Beck and Löe, 1993; Papapanou, 1994). Discrepancies in findings from different studies should therefore be interpreted with caution.

Most surveys report the prevalence of probing depth and attachment loss. Although increased probing depth is certainly of importance in clinical practice, probing measurements alone do not disclose the full extent of destruction and may be a poor indicator of disease in certain cases or populations (Axelsson et al, unpublished data, 1990; Axelsson et al, 2000; Baelum et al, 1986, 1988a, 1988b; Yoneyama et al, 1988). These surveys showed that loss of attachment is accompanied by gingival recession and that destructive periodontal disease can occur with limited pocketing.

Loss of attachment is generally accepted as the gold standard for periodontal destruction. However, the level of attachment in normal and diseased states has not been clearly defined; consequently, levels of attachment loss ranging from more than 2 mm to more than 6 mm have been used. As a cutoff point in epidemiologic studies, an attachment loss of 4 mm has been proposed, because it represents a serious condition (Axelsson et al, 2000; Burt, 1991); it is only above this

level of attachment loss that the function of the tooth may be compromised and the risk of tooth loss increases.

As discussed earlier, another unresolved issue is the definition of a case (Beck and Löe, 1993; Burt, 1991). This is more complicated for periodontal disease than for other infectious processes. Clinical data are collected from numerous sites in the mouth of each subject, and each unit or site can readily be denoted as healthy or diseased. However, because multiple measurements are available for each subject, it is more difficult to define a case, ie, a diseased subject. This will largely depend on the criteria, the threshold levels chosen, and the proportion of affected sites selected.

Data from a US national survey (Miller et al, 1987a) have clearly shown that varying the threshold for attachment loss can have a dramatic effect on the distribution. At a low threshold (2 mm), a high prevalence of disease was observed in the study population, whereas at higher thresholds (4 or 6 mm) the distribution became skewed. With respect to defining cases there is no real consensus on the threshold for attachment loss or the number of affected sites within a mouth (see Fig 409, which illustrates the frequency distribution of mean PAL per individual).

A recent review by Baehni and Bourgeois (1998) revealed how the outcome of epidemiologic surveys is influenced by the variables and cutoff points selected (Table 28). However, for most countries, only limited epidemiologic data are available to date. Information on disaggregated measures is often fragmented and confined to regions, to selected groups of individuals, or to certain age categories. With few exceptions, national surveys using precise clinical measurements are simply nonexistent. In addition, the data available from the World Health Organization's Global Oral Health Data Bank are outdated for some countries.

Hugoson et al recently presented data on the distribution of periodontal disease in a Swedish adult population, based on randomized samples of 20, 30, 40, 50, 60, and 70 year olds in 1973, 1983, and 1993 (Hugoson et al, 1998a; Hugoson and

Laurell, 2000). Based on the clinical and radiographic findings, all dentate individuals were classified according to the following criteria (Hugoson and Jordan, 1982):

- Group 1: Healthy or almost healthy gingival units and normal alveolar bone height; fewer than 12 bleeding gingival units in the molar-premolar regions
- Group 2: Gingivitis; more than 12 bleeding gingival units in the molar-premolar regions; normal alveolar bone height
- Group 3: Alveolar bone loss around the majority of the teeth, not exceeding one third of the length of the roots

- Group 4: Alveolar bone loss around the majority of the teeth, ranging between one third and two thirds of the length of the roots
- Group 5: Alveolar bone loss around the majority of the teeth, exceeding two thirds of the length of the roots; presence of angular bony defects and/or furcation defects

During the last 20 years of the study, there was an increase in the number of individuals with no alveolar bone, loss, independent of age; ie, the number of healthy individuals or individuals with gingivitis (groups 1 and 2) increased from 49% in 1973 to 60% in 1993 (Fig 414). In addition, there was a decrease in the number of individuals with

Table 28 Periodontal profile in adult populations using disaggregated measures*

Country	Sample	Results
Canada (Locker and Leake, 1993a)	671 persons (50–65 y and older)	Attachment loss > 4 mm: 88% Attachment loss > 7 mm: 25%
Greece (Anagnou-Vareltzides et al, 1996)	563 persons (25–64 y)	Probing depths > 6 mm: 35–44 y: 48.0% rural; 33.3% urban 55–64 y: 43.9% rural; 25.0% urban Attachment loss > 6 mm: 35–44 y: 68.5% rural; 71.2% urban 55–64 y: 68.4% rural; 31.8% urban 14.4% (rural) and 9.5% (urban) of the subjects accounted for 75% of all sites with attachment loss > 6 mm.
Japan (Yoneyama et al, 1988)	319 persons (20–79 y)	Attachment loss > 2 mm (one site): 80%–98% of subjects Attachment loss > 5 mm (one site): 20–29 y: 5% of subjects 40–49 y: 35% 70–79 y: 68%
Sweden (Hugoson et al, 1992)	597 persons (20–70 y)	Healthy (23% of subjects): 20 y: 58% 40 y: 17% 60 y: 12% Severe disease (2% of subjects): 20 y: 0% 40 y: 1% 60 y: 6%

moderate alveolar bone loss (group 3). Groups 4 and 5, accounting for 13% to 14% of the population studied, showed generally no change from 1983 to 1993. These two groups had been considerably smaller in 1973.

This observation is in agreement with other published epidemiologic studies in Sweden (Axelsson et al, 2000; Papapanou et al, 1988, 1989; Wennström et al, 1993). Similar distributions of periodontal disease have been reported in other industrialized countries with well-organized dental care (Brown and Löe, 1993). In the 1985 to 1986 survey of employed 18- to 64-year-old adults in the United States, 12.8% of the individuals showed severe periodontal disease, expressed as a loss of attachment greater than 5 mm (Brown et al, 1990). In developing countries with minimal dental resources, the proportion of the population exhibiting severe periodontal disease is also minor (Baelum et al, 1986, 1988a, 1988b; Löe et al, 1986).

Pattern of attachment loss

In analytic epidemiology, it is important to identify not only individuals at risk, but also teeth and surfaces at risk. The pattern of tooth loss and attachment loss in different age groups should

Table 28 (cont'd)

Country	Sample	Results
Switzerland (Schürch et al, 1992)	556 persons (20–89 y)	Probing depths > 6 mm: 0%–4% of sites: 73.6% of subjects 30% of sites: 11.5% of subjects
Scotland (Jenkins and Kinane, 1989)	880 persons (16–73 y and older)	Advanced bone loss (> 50% bone height): 25–29 y: 4.3% of subjects 40–49 y: 33.3% 50–73 y: 54.1% Generalized advanced bone loss: 25–29 y: 0.0% of subjects 40–49 y: 3.9% 50–73 y: 5.4%
United States (Brown et al, 1996a)	7447 persons (13–65 y and older)	Probing depths > 4 mm: 29.2% of subjects (19.8%–37.2%) Probing depths > 6 mm: 3.9% of subjects 18–24 y: 0.7% 35–44 y: 3.8% 55–64 y: 7.9% Attachment loss > 3 mm: 39.7% of subjects (2.1%–81.5%) Attachment loss > 5 mm: 14.7% of subjects: 18–24 y: 0.3% 35–44 y: 12.3% 55–64 y: 35.1% Recession > 3 mm: 14.6% of subjects (0.4%–45.5%)
United States (Dolan et al, 1997)	761 persons (50–65 y and older)	Attachment loss > 4 mm (one site): 92% of subjects Attachment loss > 7 mm (one site): 35% of subjects

*From Baehni and Bourgeois (1998). Reprinted with permission.

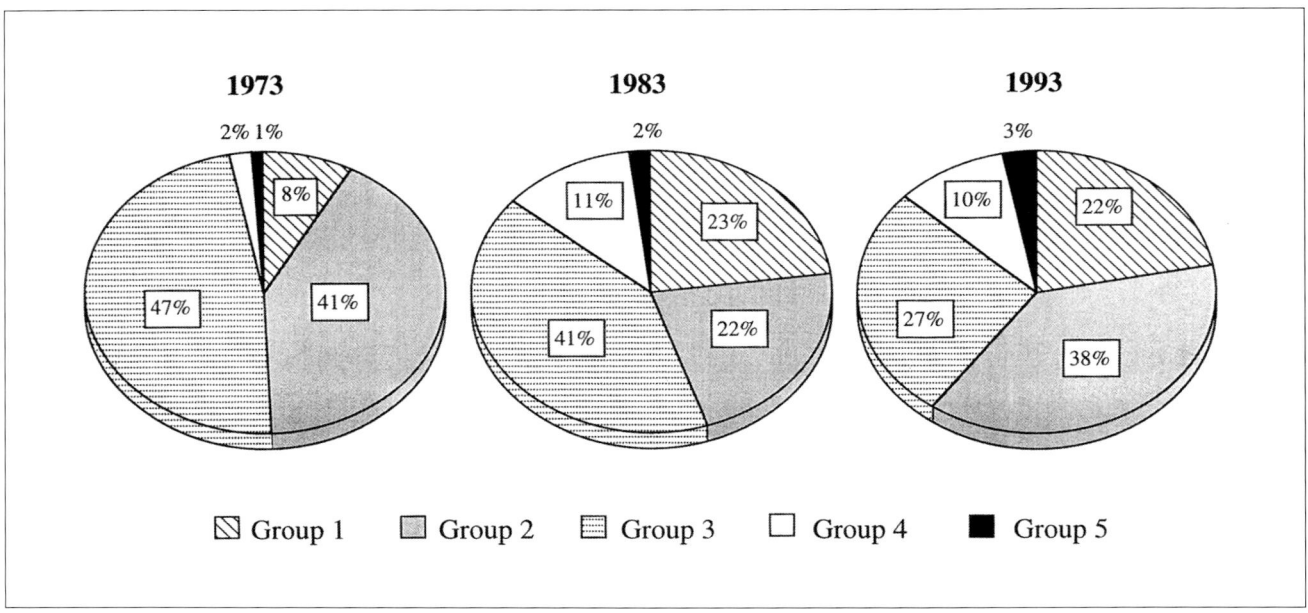

Fig 414 Distribution of Swedish adults, according to the severity of their periodontal disease in 1973, 1983, and 1993. Group 1 = Healthy gingiva; Group 2 = Gingivitis; Group 3 = Bone loss of less than one third; Group 4 = Bone loss of one third to two thirds; Group 5 = Bone loss of more than two thirds. (From Hugoson et al, 1998a. Reprinted with permission.)

therefore be analyzed cross sectionally as well as longitudinally. Analytic epidemiologic studies revealed the pattern of remaining teeth in a randomized sample of 35 year olds (Fig 415). There were very few missing teeth, except for some premolars extracted for orthodontic reasons (Axelsson et al, unpublished data, 1990). On the other hand, only 5% to 10% of the first molars remained in 75 year olds, and the highest percentage of teeth remaining were mandibular anterior teeth and maxillary canines (Fig 416). In 50 year olds, 30% to 40% of molars have already been lost. The molars, followed by the maxillary premolars, are undoubtedly at greatest risk for tooth loss (Axelsson et al, unpublished data, 1990). However, as discussed earlier, in adult populations up to the age of 50 years most tooth loss is directly or indirectly caused by caries in industrialized countries. However, in a 10-year longitudinal study of a randomized sample of more than three hundred 50 year olds, the number of lost teeth and associated causes were: periodontal disease—109, dental

caries—39, iatrogenic reasons (root fracture in nonvital teeth with posts)—68, unknown reasons—16 (Axelsson et al, 2000).

Most buccal PAL in subjects up to the age of 50 years is attributable to toothbrush abrasion, whereas almost all approximal PAL is unquestionably caused by the gingival microflora. From a preventive aspect, it is therefore of interest to compare the pattern of approximal PAL with the pattern of tooth loss in randomly selected age groups (Figs 415 to 418). In 35 year olds, PAL on the distal surfaces of the maxillary first molars was already about twice that on the mesial surfaces (see Fig 417) (Axelsson et al, unpublished data, 1990). This is of consequence for the risk of furcation involvement on the "inaccessible" distal surfaces and could have been prevented if these surfaces had been the target of gingival plaque control from early adulthood. In 75 year olds, PAL was still greater on the distal surfaces of the remaining maxillary first molars, despite 90% of loss of these teeth (see Figs 416 and 418). Clini-

Fig 415 Frequency distribution of remaining teeth (third molars excluded) in 35 year olds (Fédération Dentaire Internationale [FDI] tooth-numbering system).

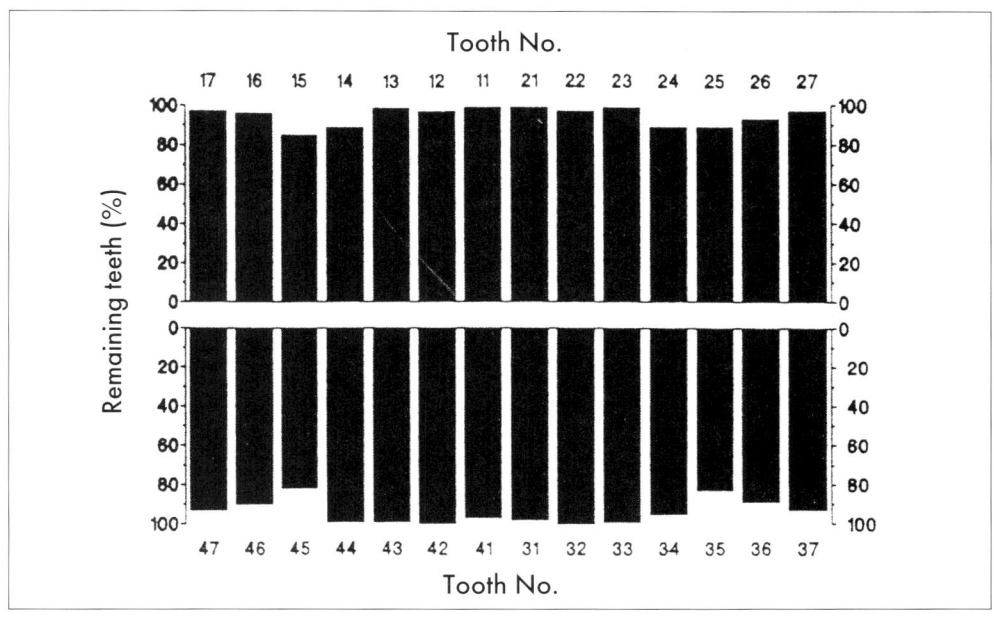

Fig 416 Frequency distribution of remaining teeth (third molars excluded) in 75 years olds (FDI tooth-numbering system).

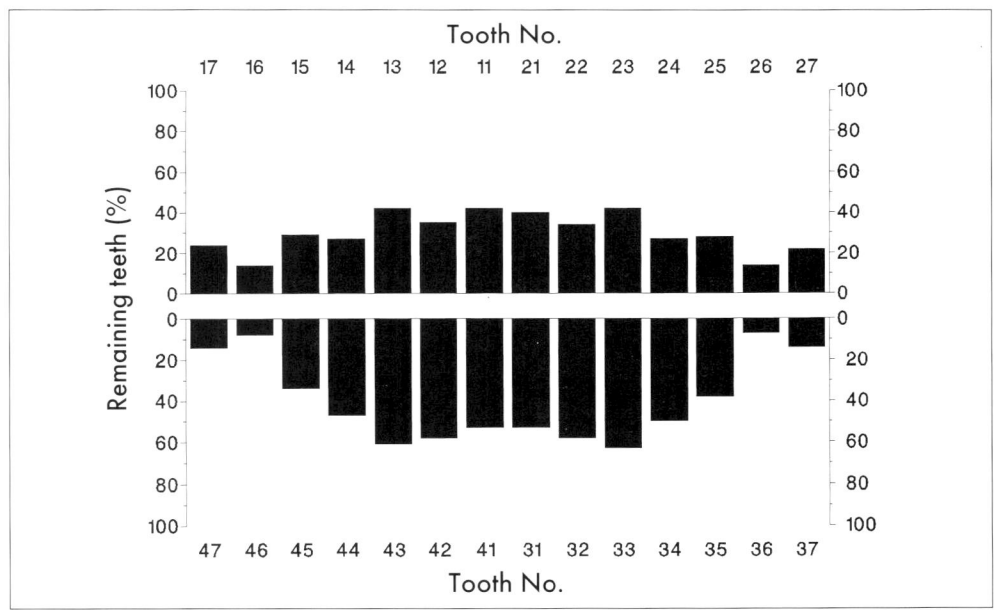

cal attachment loss on the mandibular central and lateral incisors in 35 year olds may be partly explained by local factors such as plaque retention associated with heavy supragingival calculus formation, abnormal frenum, smoking, thin alveolar bone, and crowded and rotated teeth.

The patterns of PAL on the buccal and lingual surfaces in 35 year olds are shown in Figs 419 and 420. The greater PAL on the buccal surfaces is attributable to toothbrush abrasion and is in accordance with the results of early studies on the pattern of abrasive defects (Sangnes, 1975).

387

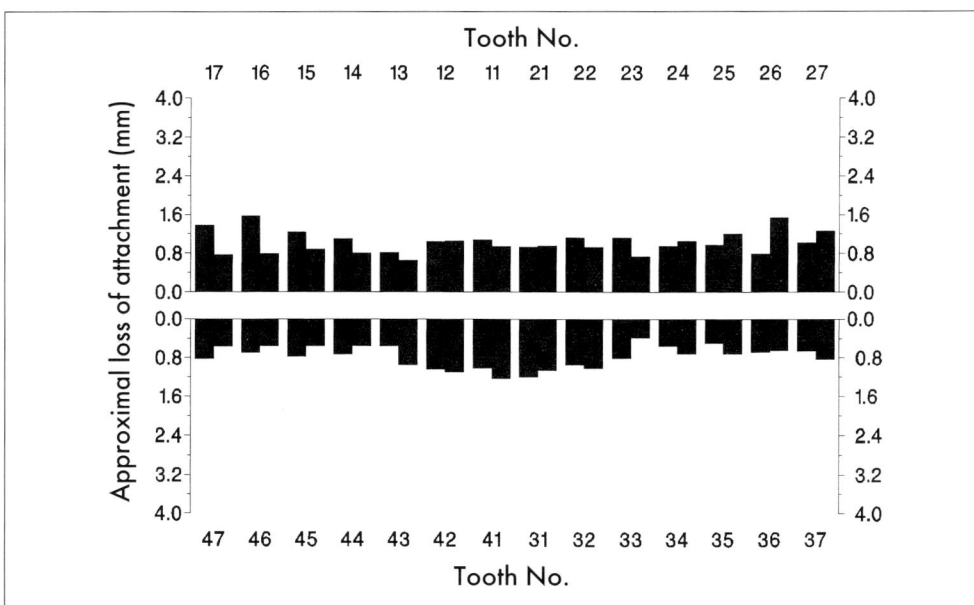

Fig 417 Prevalence and pattern of approximal loss of attachment in 35 year olds (FDI tooth-numbering system).

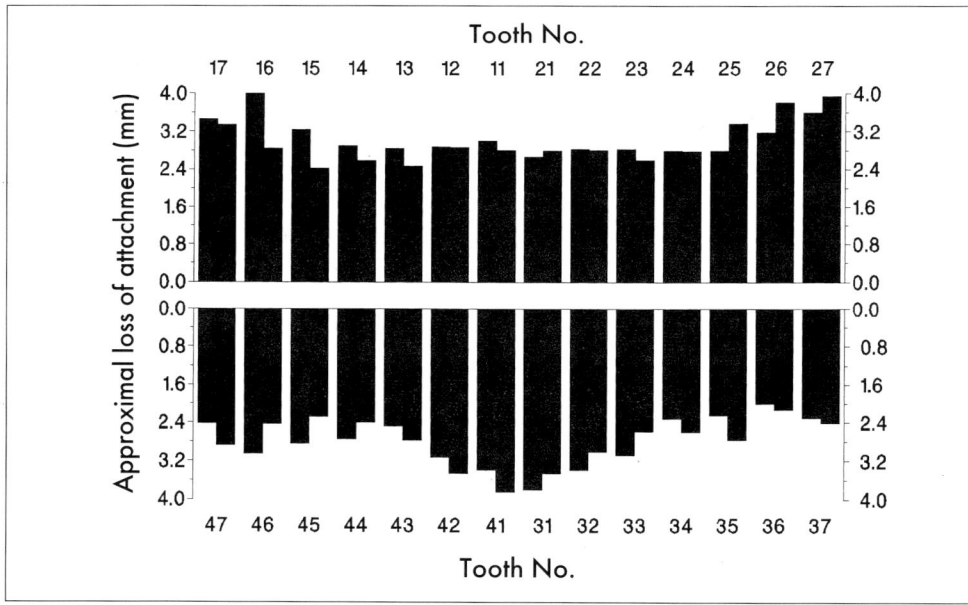

Fig 418 Prevalence and pattern of approximal loss of attachment in 75 year olds (FDI tooth-numbering system).

Treatment of teeth with furcation involvement is much more complicated than is treatment of diseased pockets in single-rooted teeth. Therefore, diagnosis and analytic epidemiology on the pattern of furcation involvement are important. Figures 421 and 422 show the frequency distrib-ution of noninvolved and furcation-involved surfaces in randomly selected 50 and 75 year olds. In 50 year olds, grades II and III furcation involvement are most frequent on the distal surfaces of the maxillary first molars while grade I is most common on the buccal surfaces of the

Fig 419 Prevalence and pattern of buccal loss of attachment in 35 year olds (FDI tooth-numbering system).

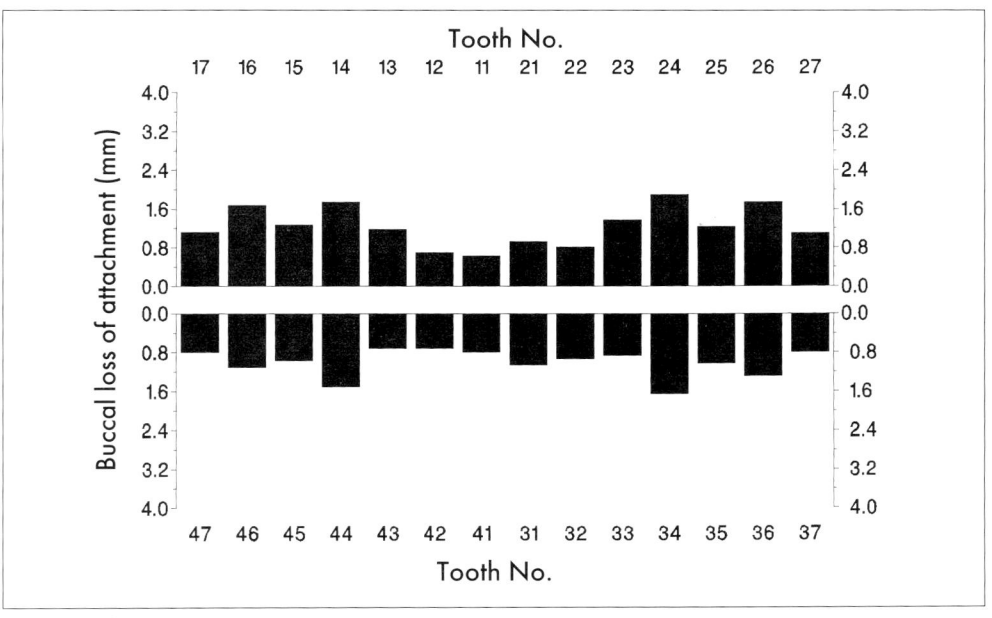

Fig 420 Prevalence and pattern of lingual loss of attachment in 35 year olds (FDI tooth-numbering system).

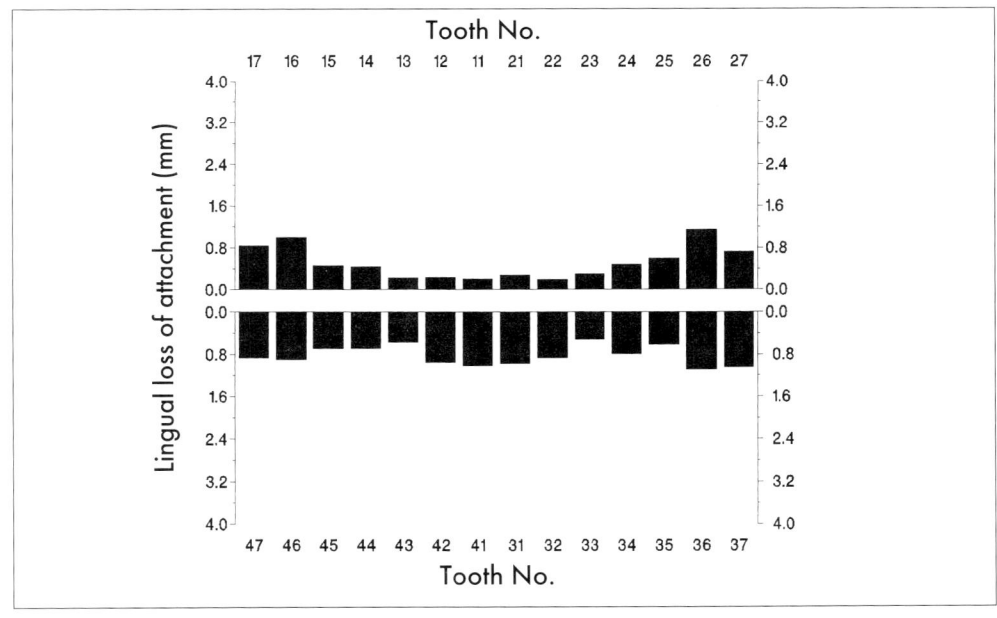

mandibular first molars (Axelsson et al, unpublished data, 1990).

In the previously mentioned study, "Natural History of Periodontal Disease," Löe et al (1978) compared the prevalence of PAL in a randomly selected group of Norwegian students and aca-demics with that of Sri Lankan tea workers (Fig 423 and 424). The maxillary molars of the Sri Lankan group were the key-risk teeth. Most of the maxillary molars exhibited grade III (through-and-through) furcation involvement. In addition, an average of seven teeth had been

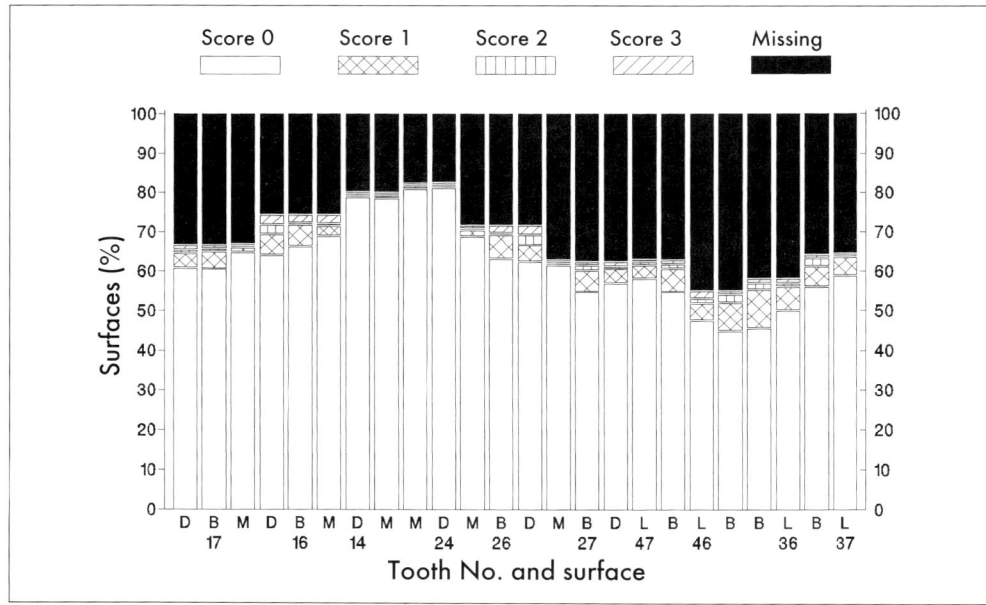

Fig 421 The pattern and frequency distribution of furcation involvement in 50 year olds (FDI tooth-numbering system). Score 0 represents uninvolved surfaces; scores 1 to 3 represent varying grades of furcation involvement (see chapter 6). D = Distal; B = Buccal; M = Mesial; L = Lingual.

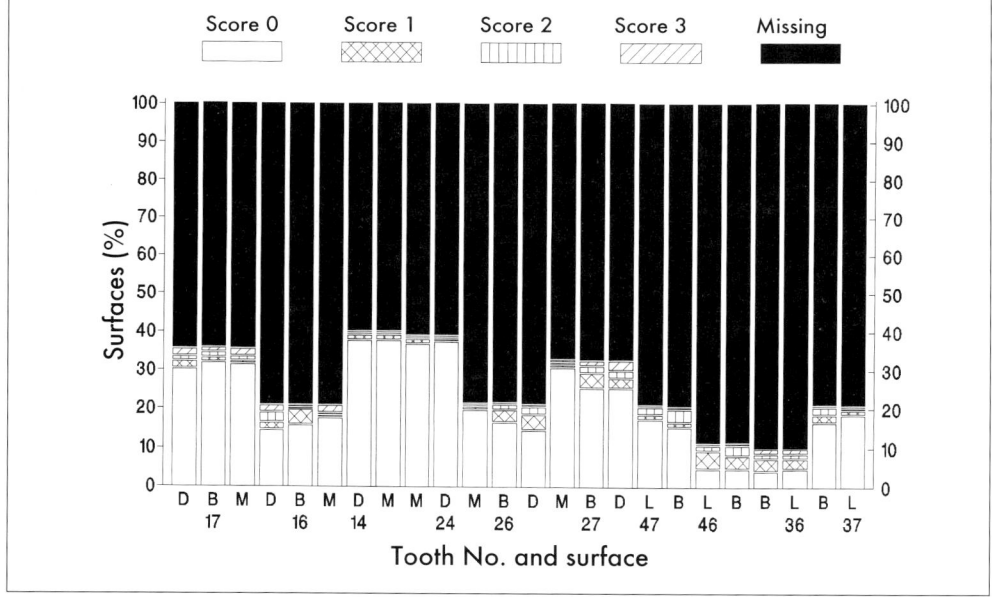

Fig 422 The pattern and frequency distribution of furcation involvement in 75 year olds (FDI tooth-numbering system). Score 0 represents uninvolved surfaces; scores 1 to 3 represent varying grades of furcation involvement (see chapter 6). D = Distal; B = Buccal; M = Mesial; L = Lingual.

lost per subject; 8% of the group had lost 20 teeth each.

An epidemiologic study in a Japanese population by Okamoto et al (1988) examined the mean probing attachment levels at different teeth and distal, buccal, and mesial surfaces for six different age groups (Fig 425). There was increasing loss of attachment with increasing age and a tendency in most age groups for more loss in the molar and incisor tooth regions.

In the healthy dentition, the location of the alveolar bone margin is normally 1.5 to 2.0 mm from

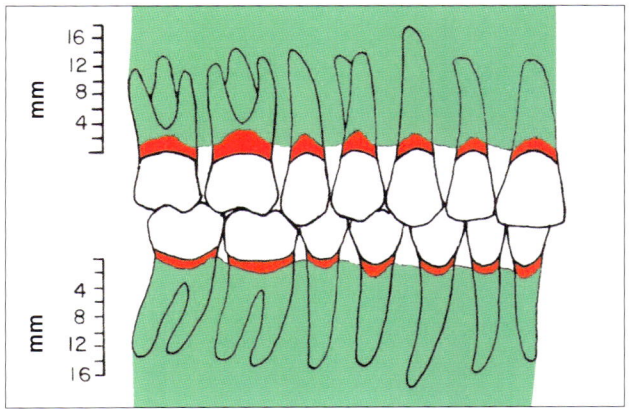

Fig 423 Average pattern of attachment loss in Norwegian students and academics. At 40 years of age, the mean loss of attachment is 1.5 mm. (Modified from Löe et al, 1978. Reprinted with permission.)

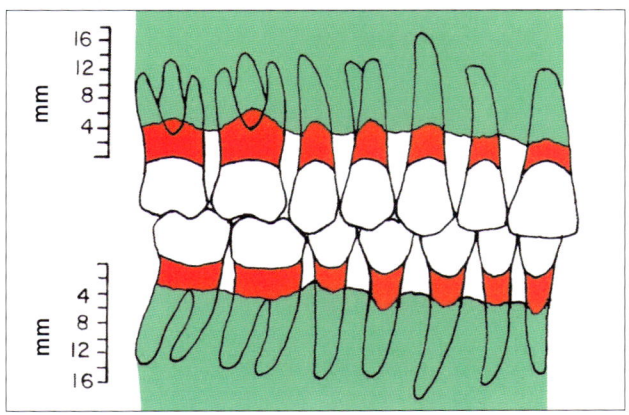

Fig 424 Average pattern of attachment loss in Sri Lankan tea workers. At 40 years of age, the mean loss of attachment is 4.5 mm. (Modified from Löe et al, 1978. Reprinted with permission.)

Fig 425 Mean probing attachment levels at different teeth and distal, buccal, and mesial (DBM) surfaces in six age groups: 20 to 29 years old; 30 to 39 years old; 40 to 49 years old; 50 to 59 years old; 60 to 69 years old; and 70 to 79 years old (FDI tooth-numbering system). CEJ = Cementoenamel junction. (From Okamoto et al, 1988. Reprinted with permission.)

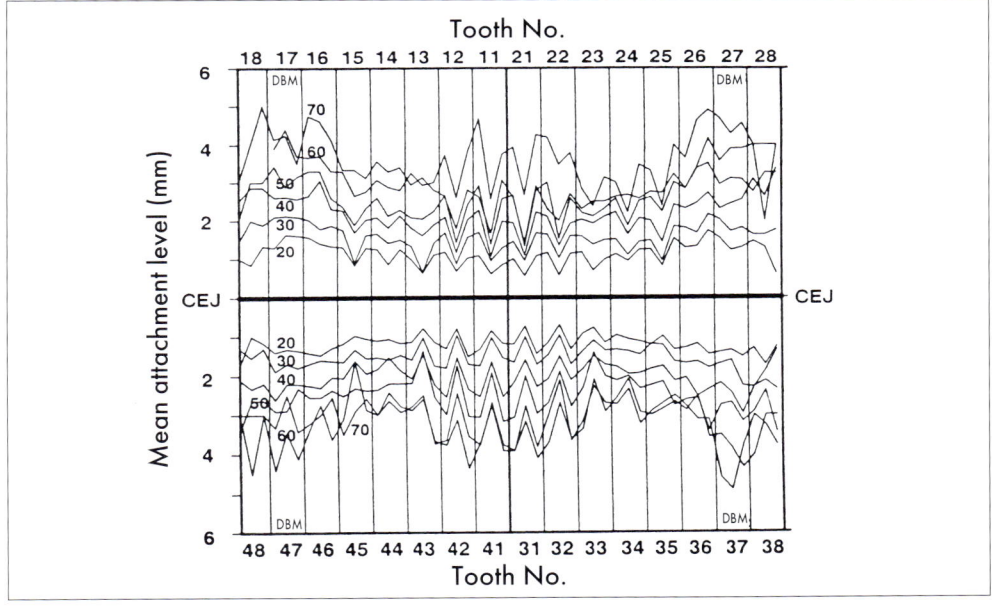

the cementoenamel junction: Where there is loss of periodontal support, measurements of probing attachment level on the approximal surfaces should therefore be 1.5 to 2.0 mm less than the alveolar bone level. However, infrabony pockets may sometimes be undetected on radiographs; at such sites, PAL may exceed alveolar bone loss. Papapanou and Wennström (1989) compared the pattern of alveolar bone loss and PAL on the approximal surfaces (Figs 426 and 427).

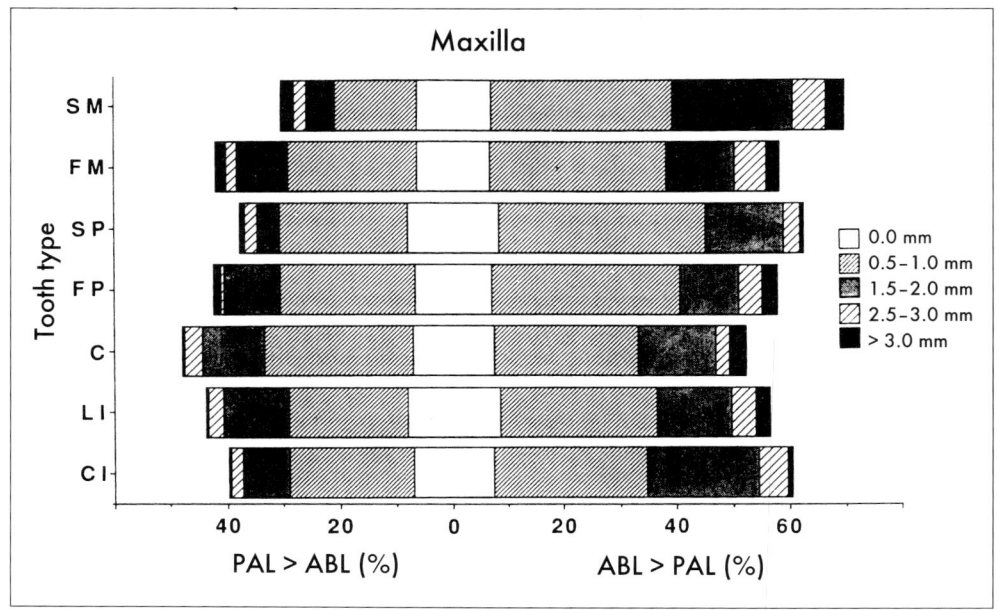

Fig 426 Maxillary pattern of the differences (mm) between PAL and alveolar bone loss (ABL), by tooth type. SM = Second molar; FM = First molar; SP = Second premolar; FP = First premolar; C = Canine; LI = Lateral incisor; CI = Central incisor. (From Papapanou and Wennström, 1989. Reprinted with permission.)

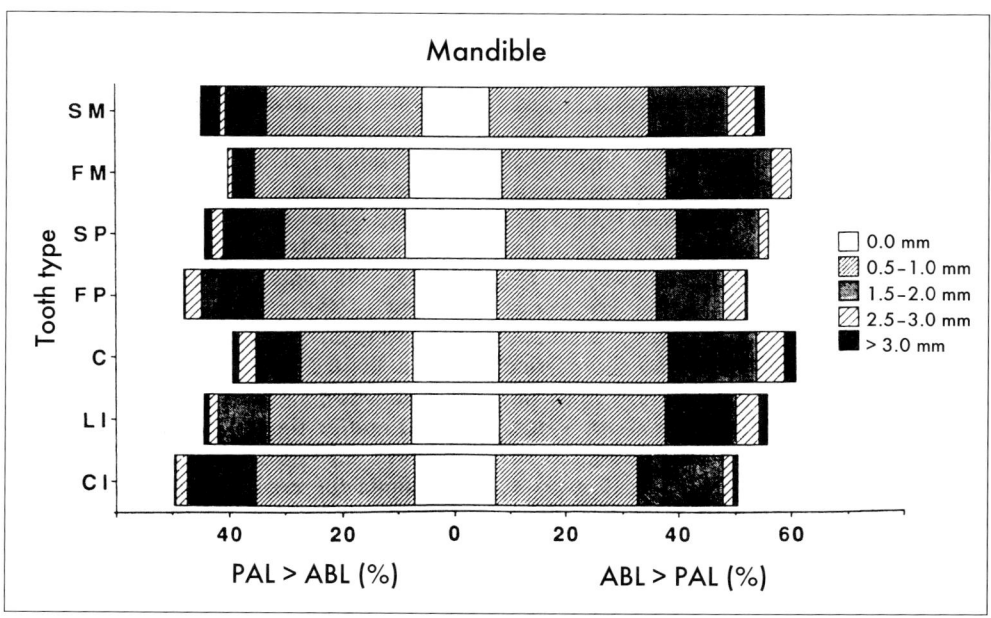

Fig 427 Mandibular pattern of the differences (mm) between PAL and ABL, by tooth type. SM = Second molar; FM = First molar; SP = Second premolar; FP = First premolar; C = Canine; LI = Lateral incisor; CI = Central incisor. (From Papapanou and Wennström, 1989. Reprinted with permission.)

INCIDENCE OF PERIODONTAL DISEASES: ANNUAL LOSS OF PERIODONTAL SUPPORT

The incidence of periodontal diseases is conventionally expressed as annual loss of periodontal support, calculated from data on clinical probing of attachment loss or radiographic evaluation of alveolar bone loss. However, although epidemiologic data reveal that the prevalence of periodontal diseases is strongly age related (Axelsson et al, unpublished data, 1990; Axelsson et al, 2000; for review, see Burt, 1991, 1996; Papapanou, 1994, 1996; Papapanou and Lindhe, 1997), the rate of loss of periodontal support is not linear at the individual or site level.

As in caries and other infectious diseases, in periodontal disease the incidence may be influenced by periods of exacerbation and quiescence. Goodson et al (1982) measured PAL monthly, for a year, in untreated subjects with existing periodontal pockets: They reported that 83% of the sites did not change significantly, 6% exhibited significant further loss of attachment, and 11% exhibited less loss of attachment (see Fig 397 in chapter 6). These results suggest that the disease is dynamic and characterized by exacerbation, remission, and periods of inactivity. Over a subject's life span, there may be relatively short periods during which many sites undergo periodontal destruction followed by long intervals of remission (Socransky et al, 1984).

The incidence of periodontal disease differs significantly among different populations and individuals. In their classic study, Löe et al (1978, 1986) described the initiation and the rate of progression of periodontal disease and subsequent tooth loss in a population of tea workers in Sri Lanka who had never received any dental treatment or prevention. From 1970 to 1977, the mean annual probing loss of attachment on the mesial surfaces was about 0.25 mm in 17- to 37-year-old Sri Lankan men and less than 0.10 mm in age-matched Norwegian academics who received regular dental care (Löe et al, 1986). From 1970 to

1985, 8% of the Sri Lankan men lost, on average, 9 to 13 mm periodontal attachment (the rapidly progressive group) and 12 to 20 teeth because of periodontal disease. Eighty-one percent of the subjects, with a mean loss of attachment of 4 to 7 mm, were regarded as a moderately progressive group (Löe et al, 1986).

In a study of adolescents with aggressive periodontitis, Brown et al (1996b) documented the pattern of progression of the disease and changes in its extent and severity over 6 years. In a national survey of the oral health of US children in 1986 to 1987, periodontal attachment loss was recorded from clinical examinations of 14,013 adolescents. Those with aggressive periodontitis were identified and categorized as having LAP, GAP, or incidental attachment loss.

The subjects, aged 13 to 20 years at baseline, were recalled 6 years later for clinical examination and were reclassified according to their current periodontal status (Figs 428 and 429). The severity and extent of the diseases had continued to increase; sites already diseased at baseline showed lesion progression to deeper involvement of the periodontium, and sites that had been unaffected at baseline showed loss of attachment at follow-up, thus changing the disease characteristics and the basis for the clinical classification. Of the individuals classified with LAP at baseline, 62% still had LAP 6 years later, but 35% had developed GAP. Of those initially classified with GAP, 82% retained this classification at follow-up. In the group with incidental attachment loss, 28% had developed LAP or GAP, and 30% were reclassified as having no attachment loss. In all three groups, the teeth most often affected were the molars and incisors (Fig 430).

These findings highlight the limitations of current morphologic criteria for the classification of aggressive periodontitis, and further suggest that the difference between LAP and GAP lies in the number and type of teeth involved: Progression of the two conditions is similar, and some cases of LAP develop into GAP. For details see chapter 5.

In another 10-year longitudinal study, Baelum et al (1997a) evaluated the progression of de-

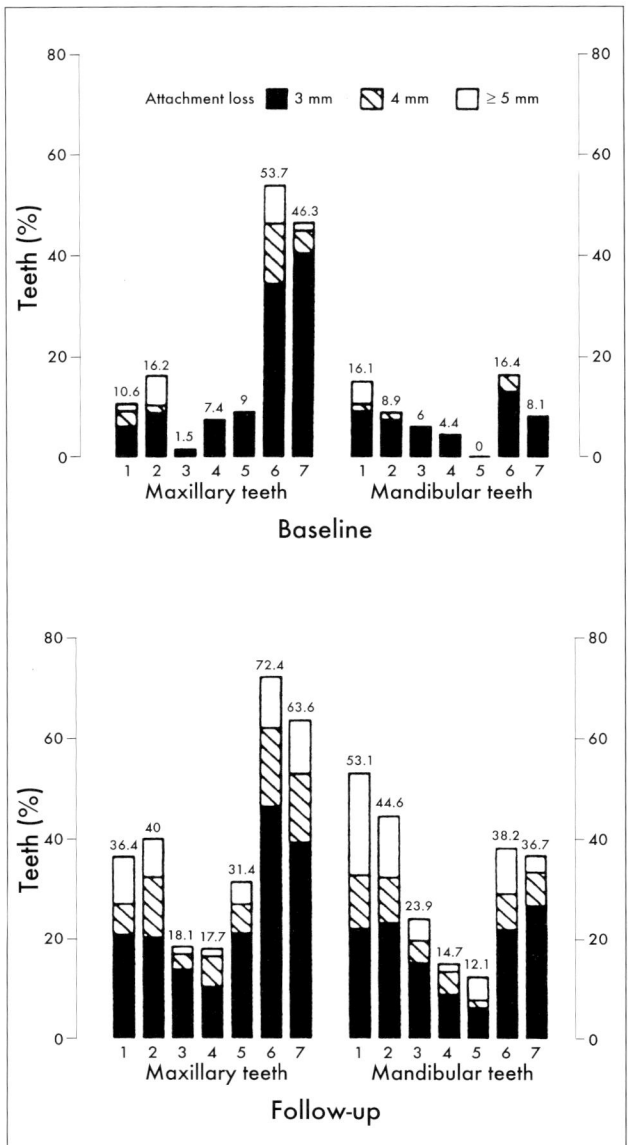

Fig 428 Frequency distribution of attachment loss, by tooth type, at baseline and 6-year follow-up in subjects with localized aggressive periodontitis. 1 = Central incisors; 2 = Lateral incisors; 3 = Canines; 4 = First premolars; 5 = Second premolars; 6 = First molars; 7 = Second molars. (From Brown et al, 1996b. Reprinted with permission.)

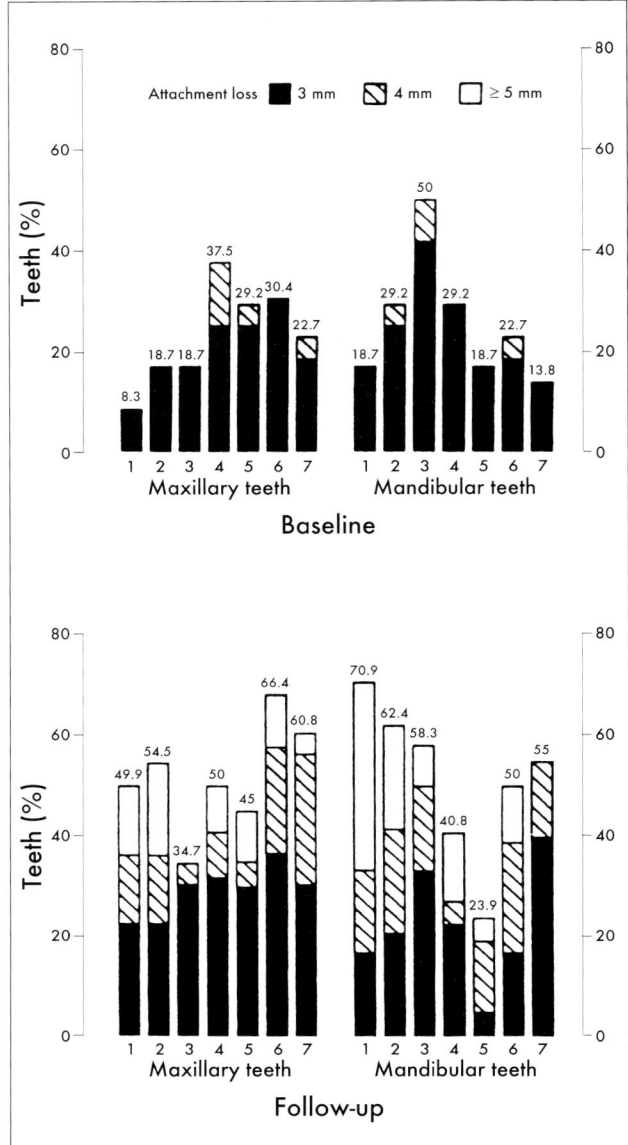

Fig 429 Frequency distribution of attachment loss, by tooth type, at baseline and 6-year follow-up in subjects with generalized aggressive periodontitis. 1 = Central incisors; 2 = Lateral incisors; 3 = Canines; 4 = First premolars; 5 = Second premolars; 6 = First molars; 7 = Second molars. (From Brown et al, 1996b. Reprinted with permission.)

structive periodontal disease among 20- to 80-year-old Chinese with limited access to dental health facilities and traditionally minimal oral hygiene habits. The aim was to determine whether the rates of disease progression differed marked-

ly from those in toothbrushing populations with adequate resources for dental care. At baseline, the participants were examined for tooth mobility, plaque, calculus, gingival conditions, attachment levels, and probing depths at four sites of

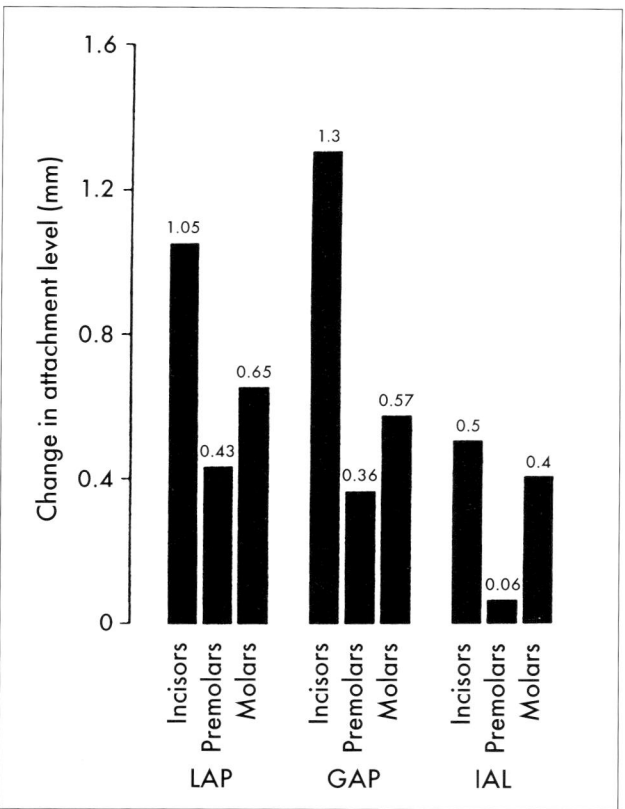

Fig 430 Mean changes in attachment level in incisors, premolars, and molars, over 6 years, in subjects with localized aggressive periodontitis (LAP), generalized aggressive periodontitis (GAP), or incidental attachment loss (IAL). (From Brown et al, 1996b. Reprinted with permission.)

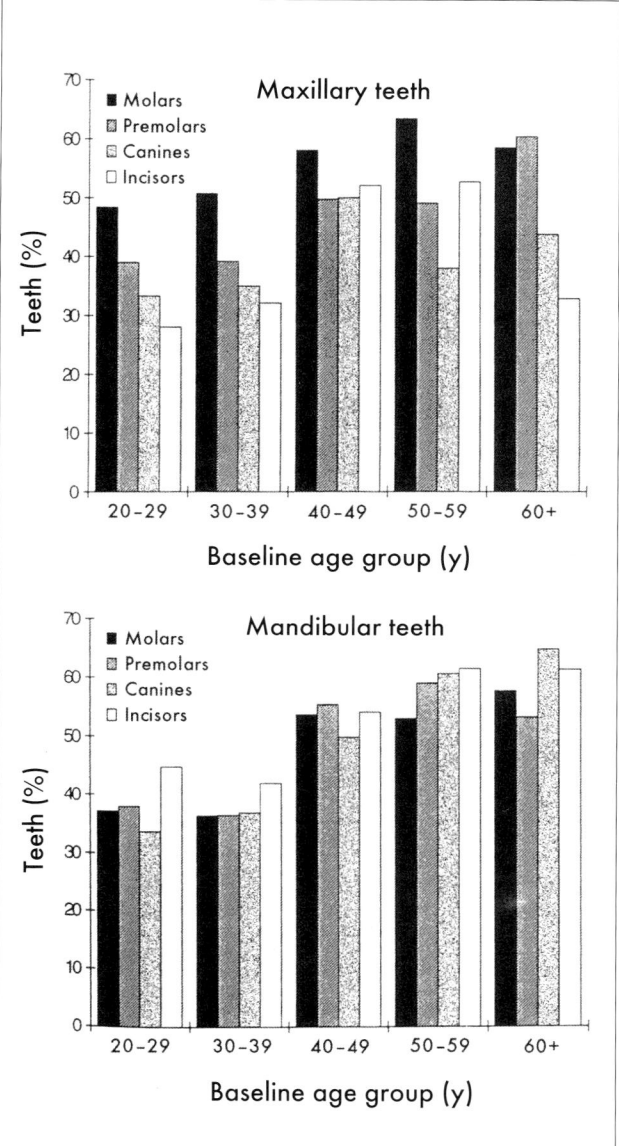

Fig 431 Frequency distribution of maxillary and mandibular teeth with attachment loss of 3 mm or more over 10 years. (From Baelum et al, 1997b. Reprinted with permission.)

each tooth present. At the 10-year follow-up, probing depth and attachment level recordings were repeated, excluding the third molars.

A total of 398 persons remained dentate at follow-up. Virtually all subjects had experienced 2 mm or more of attachment loss, frequently at a large proportion of sites. Attachment loss of 3 mm or more was also widespread, but the distribution of individuals on this basis was positively skewed in all age groups. Positive skew was even more pronounced for attachment loss of 4 mm or more. Some types of teeth, such as mandibular incisors and maxillary molars, had higher progression

rates than, for example, maxillary incisors (Fig 431). The mean individual rates of attachment loss did not differ significantly between age groups and were remarkably similar to those in toothbrushing populations with ready access to dental care (Baelum et al, 1997b).

In the longest study to date, Ismail et al (1990) evaluated attachment loss over 28 years in a group of US adults. Attachment loss of 3 mm or more was recorded in 15% of sites and in 88% of the subjects. In another 10-year longitudinal study in Swedish adults, Papapanou et al (1989), using radiographic evidence, recorded 2 mm or more of crestal bone loss at 15% of sites. A similar 6-year Norwegian study of radiographic bone loss reported stability at 90% of the sites; bone loss was reported at 3% of sites during the first 3 years, 6% of sites during the second 3-year period, and 10% of sites overall. High rates of periodontal disease progression were found in 5% of subjects, while about 70% demonstrated very few or no sites with bone loss. In addition, significantly different rates of bone loss were disclosed relative to tooth type and initial bone loss (Albandar, 1990a). Haffajee et al (1983a, 1983b) also studied progression of moderate periodontitis over 6 years. At any given site, progression was slow, and rapid progression was limited to a small number of individuals.

Recently Hugoson and Laurell (2000) presented data from a 17-year longitudinal study of a randomized sample (n = 429) of dentate Swedish subjects aged 15 to 60 years at baseline. Starting at the age of 20 years, there was a general pattern of bone height reduction over time corresponding to an annual loss of approximately 0.1 mm. At the age of 30 years, about 80% of the population had one or more sites with bone loss equal to 10% or more of root length. Seventeen percent had 6 or more such sites, indicating destructive periodontal disease. These individuals and sites could not be identified in advance based only on previous periodontal disease prevalence. Very few individuals (about 5%) exhibited an individual bone loss of 2 mm or more.

In another recent Swedish longitudinal study, Axelsson et al (2000) evaluated over a 10-year period the incidence of periodontal disease in a randomized sample (n = 314) of 50 year olds in the county of Värmland (ie, subjects were 60 years of age at the end of the study). Because of a well-organized dental care program for all children and adults, which also included preventive pro-

grams based on the individual needs, the mean alveolar bone loss was only 0.4 mm per individual over the 10-year period. That means the mean annual alveolar bone loss was only 0.04 mm. The percentage of subjects with 0, 1, 2, 3, 4, 5, 6, or 7 or more mesial sites exhibiting 2 mm or more PAL during the 10-year period was 24%, 24%, 17%, 11%, 9%, 5%, 3%, and 7% respectively (Fig 432).

In a 3-year North Carolina study of almost 500 adults aged 65 to 80 years, ie, a sample with extensive attachment loss at baseline, no further loss was recorded in 50% of subjects. Attachment loss of 3 mm or more occurred in one or more teeth in only 12% of subjects at the 18-month and 3-year examinations (Beck et al, 1994). Attachment loss was attributed to recession at 42% of the sites and increased probing depth at 58% of the sites.

However, in longitudinal studies based on excellent gingival plaque control it has been shown that, irrespective of the patient's age, further loss of clinical attachment can be prevented for years. In a 15-year longitudinal study (Axelsson et al, 1991), adults in three different age groups visited a dental hygienist for oral hygiene education and professional mechanical tooth-cleaning, at needs-related intervals, one to three times a year. Initially, the test groups were compared with age-matched control groups who were receiving only "traditional dental care" annually. After the first 6 years, the test groups had achieved an average gain in probing attachment per individual of 0.2 mm, and there was a corresponding loss of about 1.0 mm in the control groups. For ethical reasons, the control groups were therefore also offered a similar preventive program. To analyze cost effectiveness, the three test groups are being maintained in a needs-related preventive program. The 30-year reexamination is scheduled for 2002.

At the 15-year reexamination, the oldest group was aged 66 to 85 years. Figure 433 shows the average effect on probing attachment level, from 1972 to 1987. The average probing gain of attachment on the approximal surfaces (0.4 to 0.5 mm) suggests that many approximal infrabony pockets present at baseline underwent "repair."

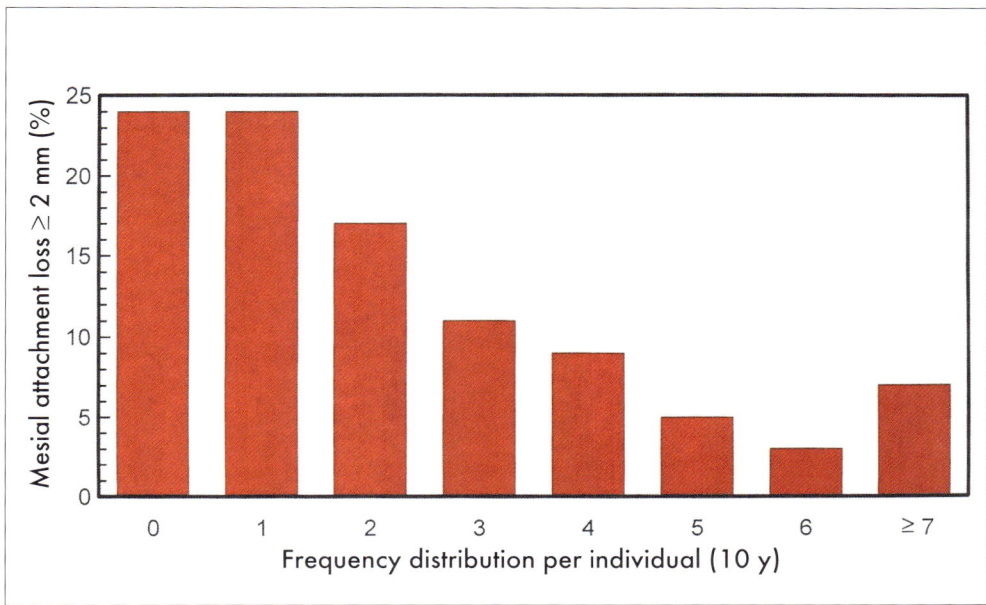

Fig 432 Frequency distribution of individuals who lost ≥ 2 mm periodontal attachment from 1988 to 1998 at 0 to 7 or more mesial sites. (From Axelsson et al, 2000. Reprinted with permission.)

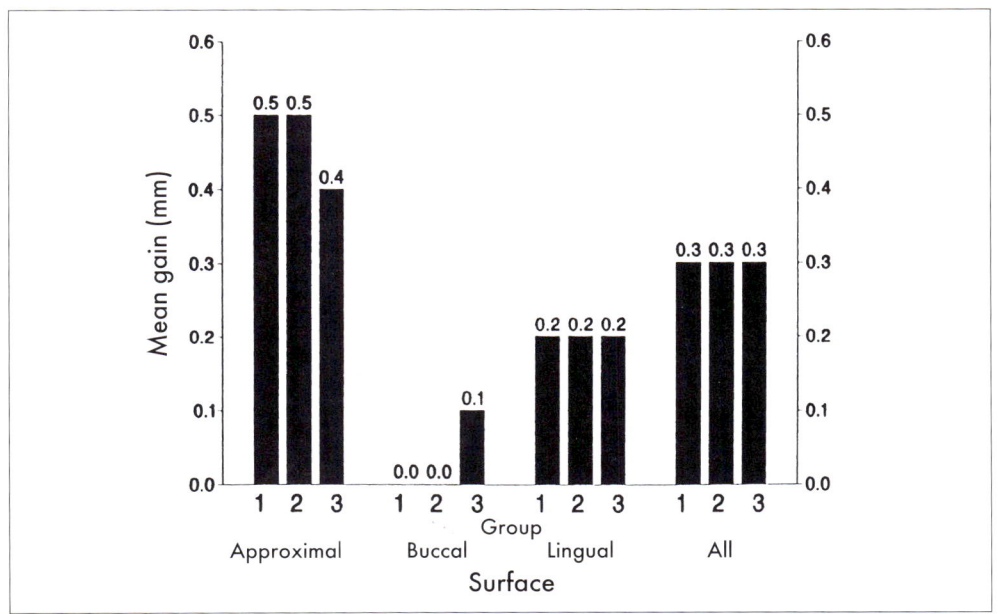

Fig 433 Gain in attachment level over 15 years (1972 to 1987), by age group. Group 1 was 20 to 35 years at baseline, group 2 was 36 to 50 years at baseline, and group 3 was 51 to 70 years at baseline. (From Axelsson et al, 1991. Reprinted with permission.)

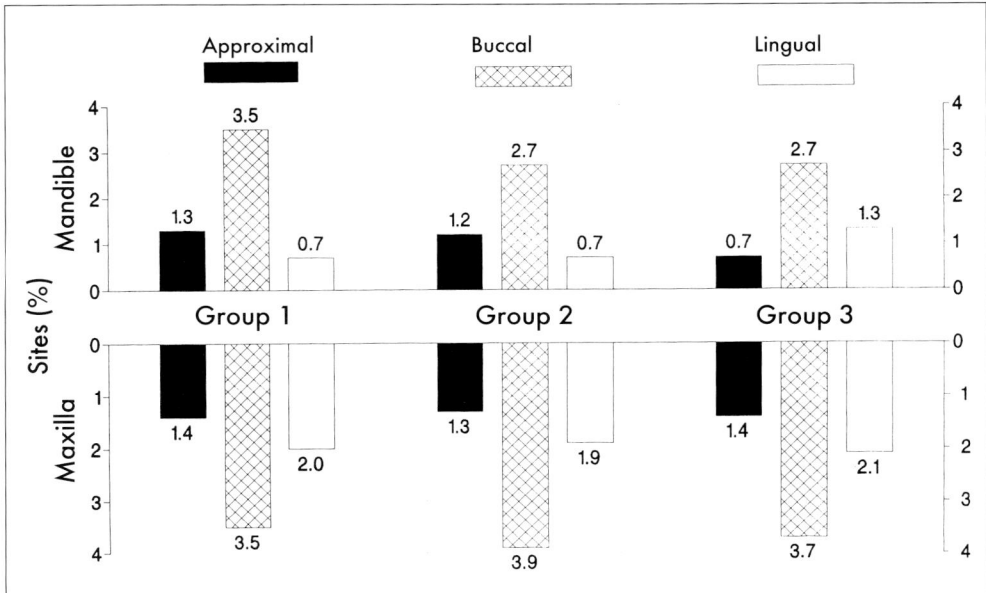

Fig 434 Frequency of sites with attachment loss of greater than 1 mm over 15 years, by age group. Group 1 was 20 to 35 years at baseline, group 2 was 36 to 50 years at baseline, and group 3 was 51 to 70 years at baseline. (From Axelsson et al, 1991. Reprinted with permission.)

Figure 434 shows the frequency of the very few sites with more than 1.0 mm of attachment loss over the 15 years (Axelsson et al, 1991). For the 15-year-period, the average number of teeth lost per subject was only 0.2; during the same period, randomized samples of the adult Swedish population recorded a loss of 3.0 teeth per individual.

Periodontal Treatment Needs

According to recommendations of the World Health Organization, the Community Periodontal Index of Treatment Needs (see chapter 6) is used at the individual and sextant levels for estimating periodontal treatment needs in population surveys (Ainamo et al, 1982; Cutress et al, 1987). To date, more than 200 surveys have been undertaken in more than 100 different countries.

Miyazaki et al (1991a) presented an overview of 103 CPITN surveys on adolescents (15 to 19 years old) from more than 60 countries (Fig 435). The most frequent finding was the presence of calculus, with or without bleeding (score 2), which was much more prevalent in subjects from nonindustrialized countries than in those from industrialized countries. Probing depths of 4 to 5 mm (score 3) were present in about two thirds of the populations examined. However, probing depths of greater than 5 mm (score 4) were infrequent.

Data from almost 100 CPITN surveys in 35 to 44 year olds conducted in more than 50 countries showed that, at both the individual and sextant levels, calculus and shallow pocketing (scores 2 and 3) were the most frequently observed findings (Miyazaki et al, 1991b). With few exceptions, both the percentage of subjects and the mean number of sextants per subject with score 4 were low (Figs 436 and 437).

The CPITN data are updated regularly, and new studies are added to the database on publication. However, for some countries, no new entries have been made in recent years, and the information available is based on surveys conducted more than 10 years ago. The value of the CPITN as an epidemiologic tool has been questioned (Baelum et al, 1995; Schürch et al, 1990). Although the profession now has a better under-

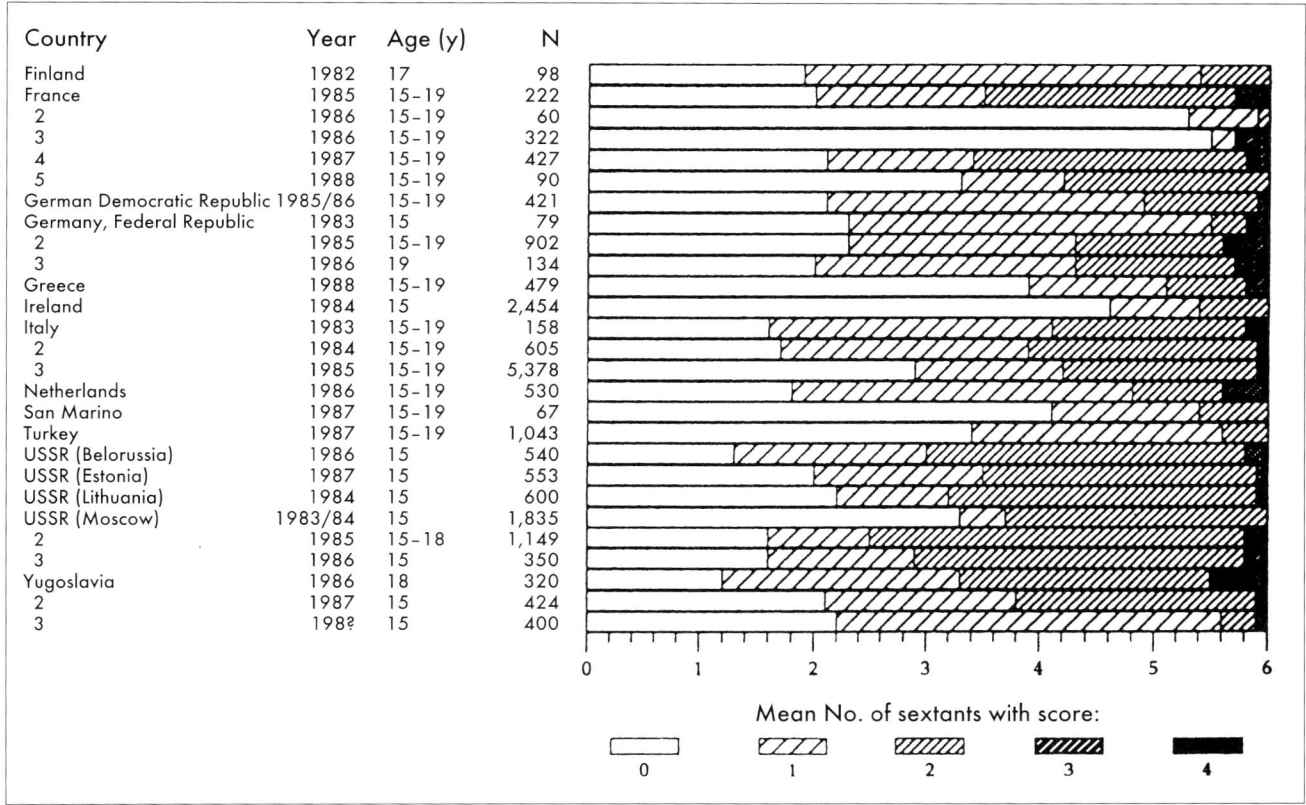

Fig 435 Mean number of sextants with CPITN scores 0 to 4 (see chapter 6) in 15- to 19-year-old Europeans. (From Miyazaki et al, 1991a. Reprinted with permission.)

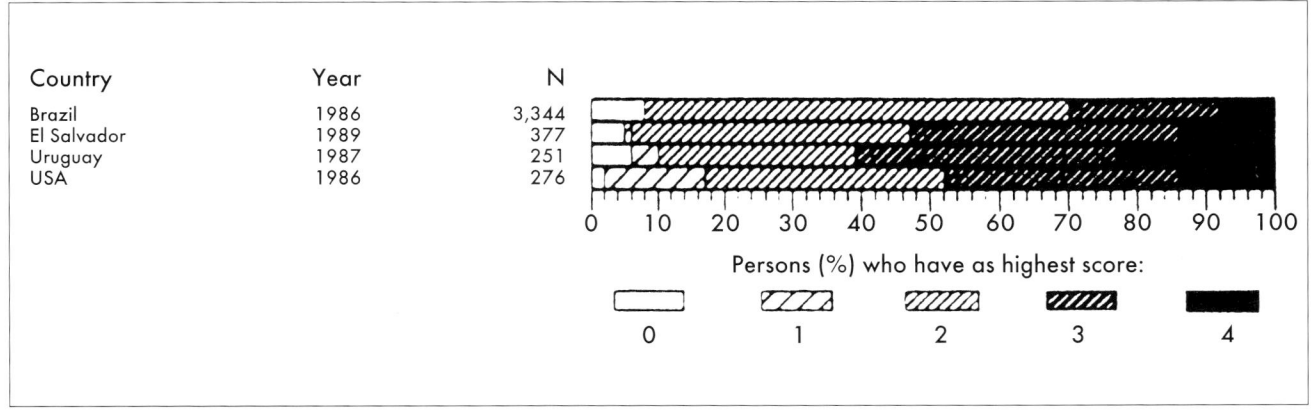

Fig 436 Percentages of North and South American 35 to 44 year olds exhibiting a particular CPITN score (0 to 4) as their highest score. (From Miyazaki et al, 1991b. Reprinted with permission.)

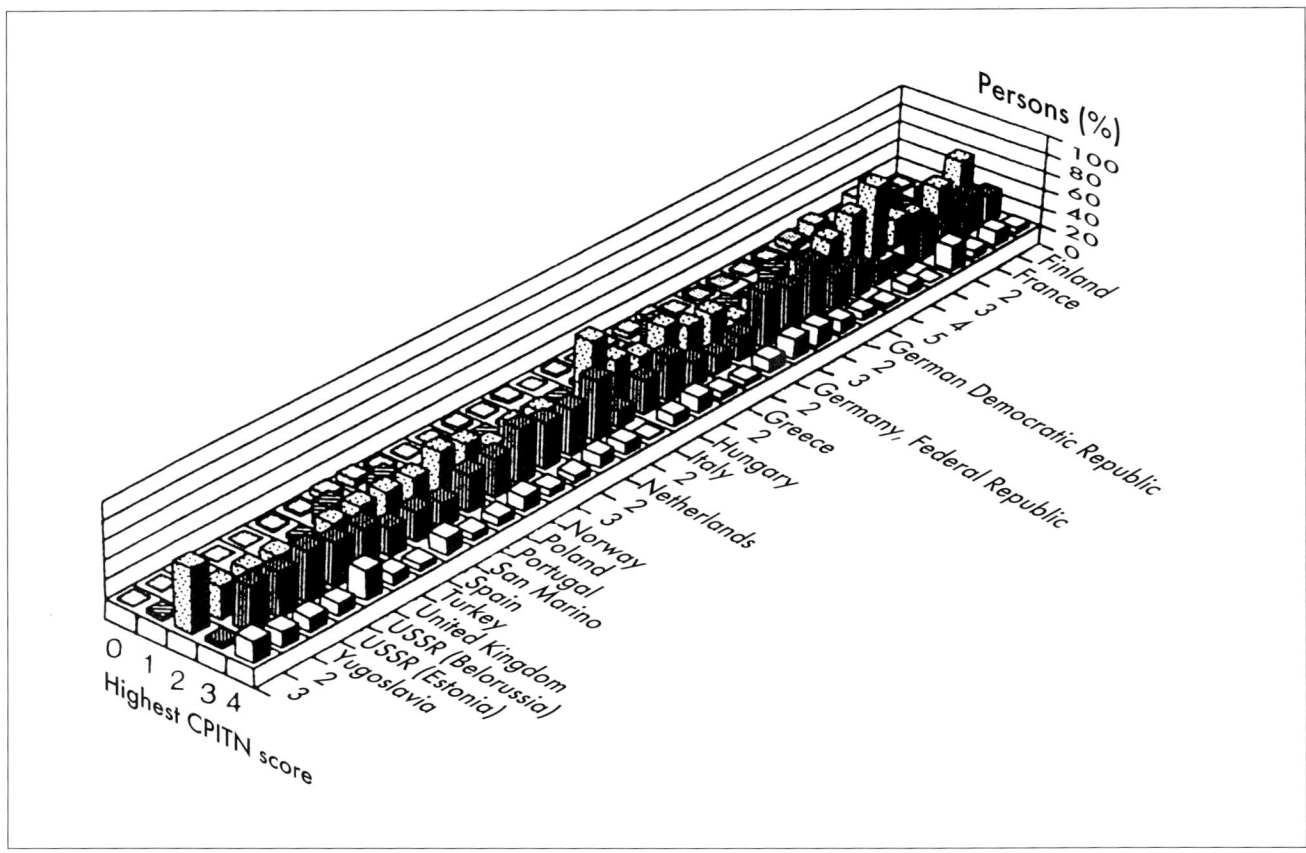

Fig 437 Percentages of European 35 to 44 year olds exhibiting a particular CPITN score (0 to 4) as their highest score. (From Miyazaki et al, 1991b. Reprinted with permission.)

standing of the global nature of the problem, the view of the periodontal status of populations in some regions or countries is fragmented.

Tables 29 and 30 summarize findings from CPITN surveys, showing scores 0 and 4 in Organization for Economic Corporation and Development (OECD) countries and former Eastern European countries (with economies in transition), respectively (Miyazaki et al, 1991a, 1991b; Pilot et al, 1987; Pilot and Miyazaki 1991, 1994; World Health Organization, 1997). Deep pockets (≥ 6 mm) were rare in the youngest group and more frequent in the older groups. Among 15 to 19 year olds, deep pockets were recorded in only 4 of 34 studies and in only a small percentage of the population. Among 35 to 44 year olds, the prevalence of deep pockets was lower in the

OECD countries (2% to 28%) than in Eastern Europe (2% to 40%).

It is important to recognize that use of the highest CPITN score at the individual, sextant, and even tooth level, according to the hierarchical principle, grossly overestimates periodontal treatment need. In both analytic cross-sectional epidemiologic studies (Axelsson et al, unpublished data, 1990; Axelsson et al, 2000) and longitudinal studies (Axelsson et al, 1991, 2000) CPITN scores were evaluated and compared at the individual, sextant, tooth, and surface levels. Sextants, teeth, and sites were stratified as CPITN scores 1, 2, 3, 4, or missing, similar to the decayed, missing, or filled teeth (DMFT) and decayed, missing, or filled surface (DMFS) indices in caries epidemiology. Edentulous sex-

Table 29 Periodontal profile in OECD countries; highest scores for periodontal conditions measured by CPITN: healthy (score 0) and probing depths ≥ 6 mm (score 4)

Country	Age 15–19 y				Age 35–44 y				Age 65–74 y			
			Score (%)				Score (%)				Score (%)	
	Year	n	0	4	Year	n	0	4	Year	n	0	4
Australia	1985	461	2	0	1988	176	0	28				
Canada	1989	187	17	0								
Finland					1982–1988	318	2	6	1982–1988	306	2	27
France	1992	956	45	0	1993	1,000	12	2	1995	600	16	3
Germany	1987–1989	2,505	7	3	1991	567	5	3	1991	397	4	6
Greece	1988	479	30	0	1985	741	8	14				
Hungary					1991	824	4	2				
Ireland	1984	2,454	43	0	1989	419	6	2				
Italy	1985	5,386	26	0	1985	21,352	3	12				
Japan					1991–1999	660	3	9	1991–1999	422	1	19
Korea	1995	600	6	0	1995	600	17	5	1995	600	3	19
Netherlands	1986	530	6	1	1986	473	4	7	1986	416	1	15
New Zealand	1982	267	58	0	1989	606	11	4	1989	186	10	7
Norway					1983	768	0	8				
Poland	1989	705	21	0	1990	685	9	6	1990	776	10	4
Portugal	1993	541	25	0	1984	616	3	8				
Spain	1987	1,037	26	0	1993	533	3	11	1993	479	2	17
Turkey					1987	494	3	6				
United Kingdom					1988	603	4	13				
United States	1986	358	17	5	1991	439	1	16	1989	422	5	32

Source: WHO Global Oral Health Bank.
There are no available data in the WHO Global Oral Health Data Bank for CPITN conditions in the following countries: Austria, Belgium, Czech Republic, Denmark, Iceland, Luxembourg, Mexico, Sweden, and Switzerland.
From Baehni and Bourgeois (1998). Reprinted with permission.

Table 30 Periodontal profile in Eastern Europe; highest scores of periodontal conditions measured by CPITN: healthy score (0) and probing depths ≥ 6 mm (score 4)

Country	Age 15–19 y		Score (%)		Age 35–44 y		Score (%)		Age 65–74 y		Score (%)	
	Year	n	0	4	Year	n	0	4	Year	n	0	4
Armenia	1987	262	11	0								
Belarus	1986	540	2	0	1986	327	0	31				
Croatia	1992	376										
Estonia	1987	553	2	0	1987	434	0	13	1987	274	0	69
Israel	1984	241	40	0								
Kyrgystan	1987	548	1	0	1987	449	0	31	1987	4,139	0	91
Latvia					1993	1,082	1	7	1993	1,082	0	11
Lithuania	1984	600	6	0								
Malta					1986	286	0	2				
Russian Federation	1986	350	12	0								
Slovenia	1986	400	8	1	1987	406	4	19				
Tajikistan	1987	430	0	0	1987	357	0	30				
Turkmenistan	1987	509	2	0	1987	377	0	40				
Yugoslavia	1987	424	2	0	1987	439	1	16				

Source: WHO Global Oral Health Data Bank

From Baehni and Bourgeois (1998). Reprinted with permission.

Fig 438 Frequency distribution, at the sextant level, of CPITN scores 0 to 4 and missing teeth, by age group in 1988 and 1998. (From Axelsson et al, 2000. Reprinted with permission.)

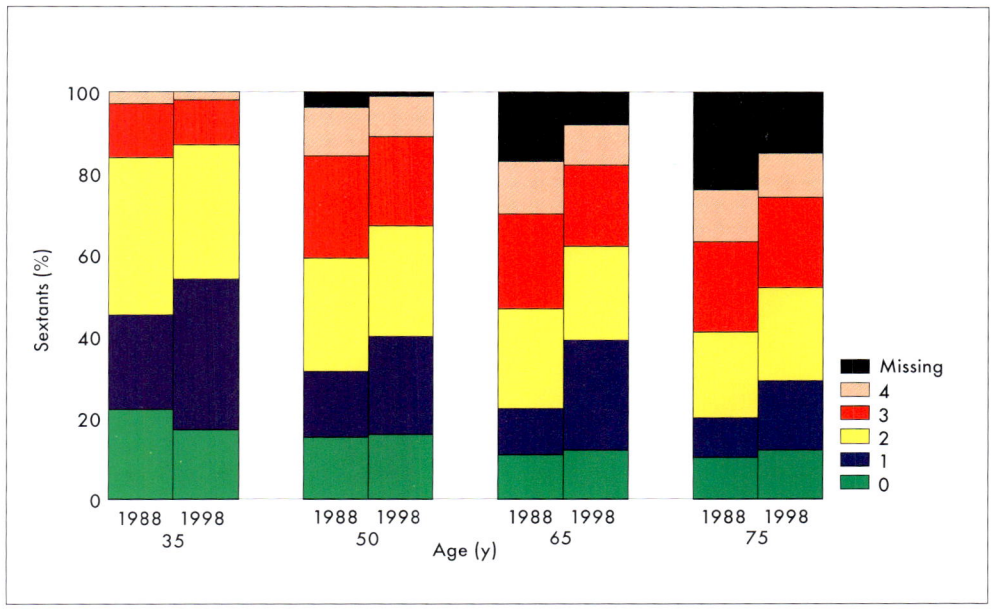

Fig 439 Frequency distribution, at the site level, of CPITN scores 0 to 4 and missing teeth, by age group in 1988 and 1998. (From Axelsson et al, 2000. Reprinted with permission.)

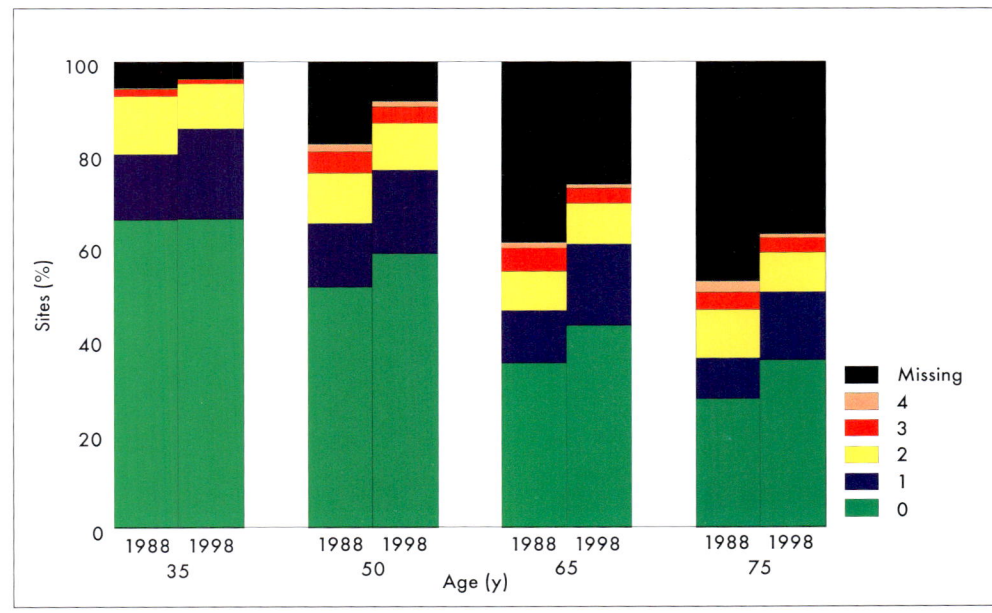

tants and lost teeth and sites will have had no periodontal treatment needs for several years. By using the CPITN at the site level and excluding missing sites, "true" periodontal treatment needs can be evaluated in individuals as well as in groups and populations.

Figure 438 shows the frequency distribution of CPITN scores 0 to 4 and missing teeth, at the sextant level, in a randomized sample of adults in the county of Värmland, Sweden in 1988 and 1998. For comparison, Fig 439 shows the frequency distribution of CPITN scores in more than 110,000

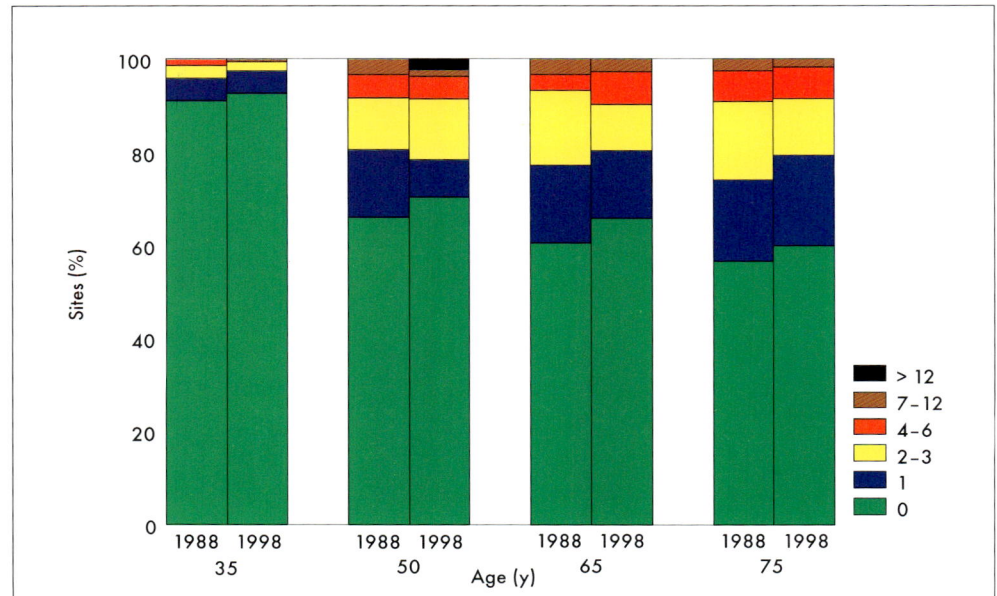

Fig 440 Frequency distribution (%) of individuals with 0, 1, 2 to 3, 4 to 6, 7 to 12, and >12 sites with CPITN score 4, by age group in 1988 and 1998. (From Axelsson et al, 2000. Reprinted with permission.)

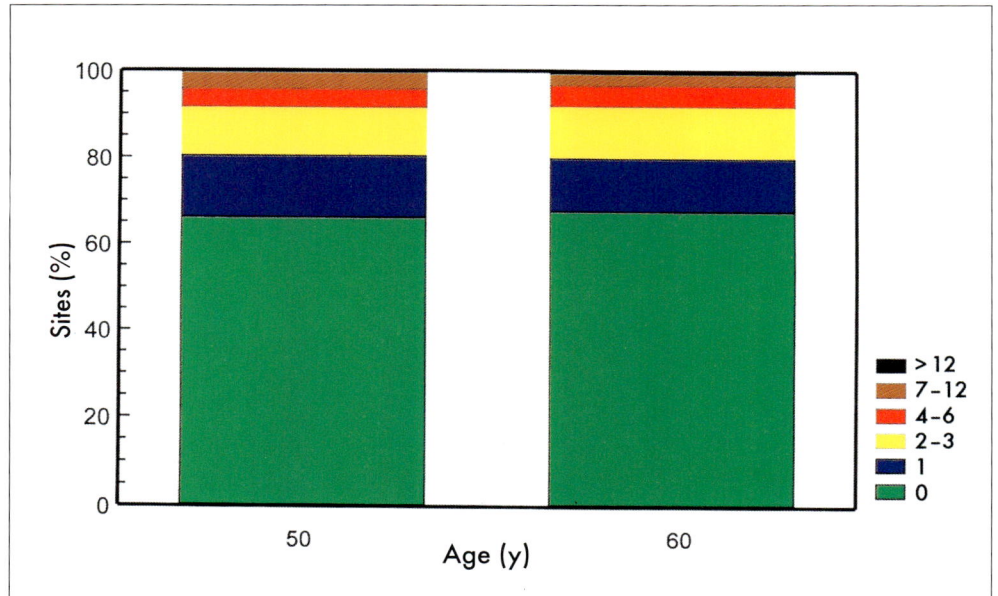

Fig 441 Frequency distribution (%) of individuals with 0, 1, 2 to 3, 4 to 6, 7 to 12, and >12 sites with CPITN score 4 in 1988 (50 year olds) and 1998 (60 year olds). (From Axelsson et al, 2000. Reprinted with permission.)

sites, representing true periodontal treatment needs (Axelsson et al, 2000). Obviously the existing periodontal treamtent based on CPITN was reduced from 1988 to 1998 at sextant as well as site levels. However, at the sextant level, treatment needs are overestimated, even when edentulous sextants are excluded. An unexpected finding was that only 2% to 3% of all sites in 75 year olds had a CPITN score of 4, and about 60% of the remaining sites were healthy. Figure 440 shows the frequency distribution of individuals in the four age groups who exhibited 0, 1, 2 to 3, 4 to 6, 7 to 12,

Fig 442 Frequency distribution of missing teeth and mesial surfaces with CPITN scores 0 to 4 in 50 year olds (FDI tooth-numbering system). (From Axelsson, 1998. Reprinted with permission.)

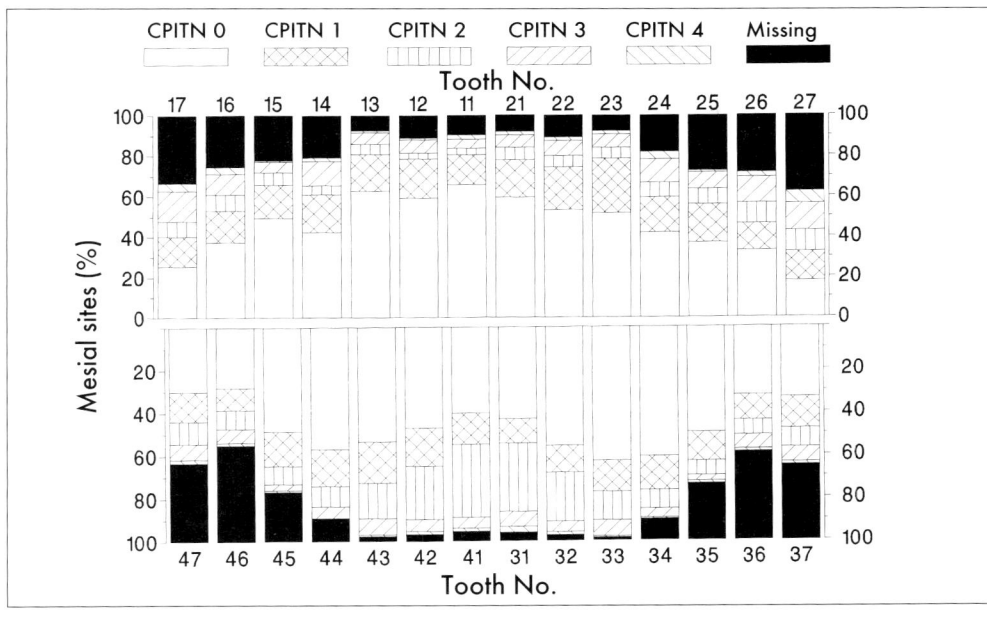

Fig 443 Frequency distribution of missing teeth and lingual surfaces with CPITN scores 0 to 4 in 50 year olds (FDI tooth-numbering system). (From Axelsson, 1998. Reprinted with permission.)

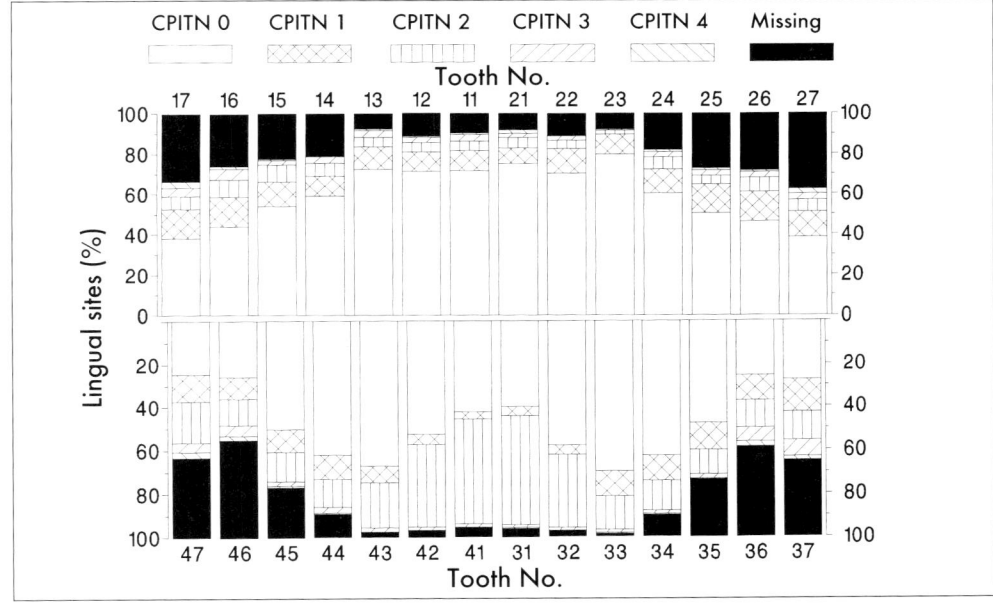

or more than 12 sites with a CPITN score of 4 in 1988 and 1998. In 1998, about 95%, 70%, 65%, and 60% of the 35, 50, 65, and 75 year olds, respectively, had no single site deeper than 5 mm (CPITN score of 4), reaffirming the high quality of the Swedish dental care system for both younger adults and the elderly. The randomized sample of 50 year olds in 1988 were followed longitudinally and reexamined in 1998 at the age of 60 years. Fig 441 shows that the percentage of individuals without any sites with a CPITN score of 4 had increased during the 10-year period, while the num-

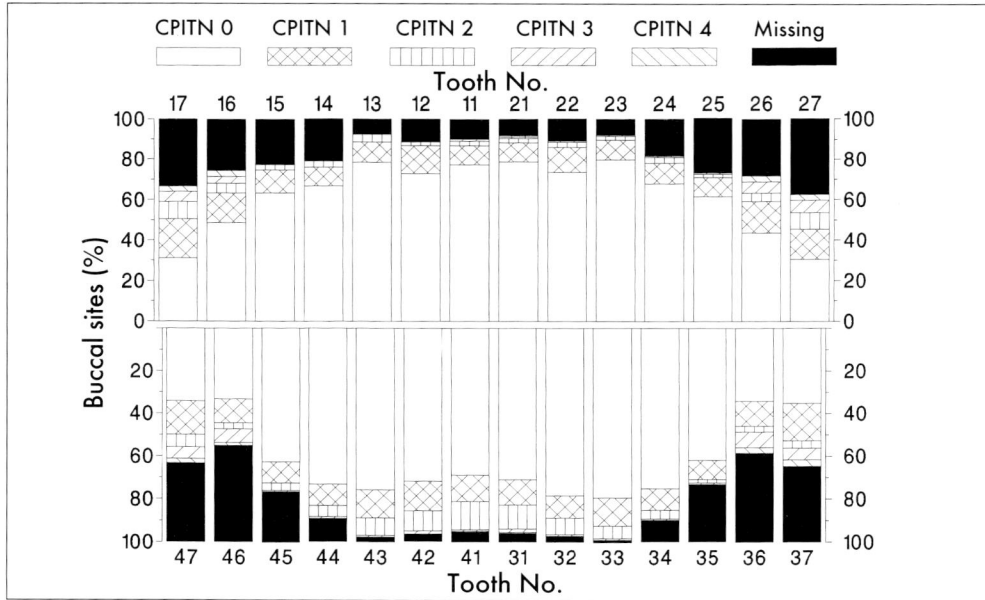

Fig 444 Frequency distribution of missing teeth and buccal surfaces with CPITN scores 0 to 4 in 50 year olds (FDI tooth-numbering system). (From Axelsson, 1998. Reprinted with permission.)

ber of individuals with 7 to 12 sites with a CPITN score of 4 was reduced by about 50%.

To plan an efficient preventive strategy, it is essential to have data on the pattern of disease in the dentition at the surface level. Figures 442 to 444 show the pattern of CPITN scores and missing teeth on different tooth surfaces in the randomized sample of 50 year olds in 1988. Score 4 is almost negligible, and score 3 is limited mainly to the mesial and distal surfaces of the maxillary molars, ie, the key-risk surfaces. The mesial and lingual surfaces of the mandibular incisors have the highest percentages of score 2, indicating supragingival calculus that requires removal (Axelsson et al, unpublished data, 1990; Axelsson, 1998).

CONCLUSIONS

Descriptive epidemiology deals with the occurrence, severity, and distribution of diseases and mortality in any selected population. Analytic epidemiology seeks to discern, directly or indi-rectly, the causes of a disease and to evaluate any public health consequences of intervention. Until about 20 years ago, it was generally accepted within the dental profession that:

- All individuals eventually become susceptible to severe periodontitis.
- Gingivitis progresses to periodontitis: There is continuous, linear loss of periodontal support and finally tooth loss.
- Susceptibility to periodontitis increases with age.

A more recent approach is to dichotomize the adult population, differentiating between those who are healthy or have gingivitis and those who are susceptible to periodontitis. The prevalence of gingivitis and mild or moderate forms of periodontitis is strongly correlated with the standard of gingival plaque control and dental care habits. Periodontitis, however, is the result of a complex interplay of bacterial challenge, host response, and other modifying factors. Despite extreme variations in oral hygiene standards, the prevalence of severe periodontitis in adults is about 5% to 15% in both industrialized and developing countries.

A major dilemma in epidemiology of periodontal diseases is that, apart from the Community Periodontal Index of Treatment Needs, there are still no international standards or recommendations. Retrospective comparison of data on periodontal status in different surveys and studies is very difficult. Gingivitis, probing depth, clinical attachment level, and radiographically assessed alveolar bone loss have all been used as criteria, quite inconsistently. The threshold values adopted for classification of "deep" or "pathologic" periodontal pockets, or for probing attachment loss and alveolar bone scores that indicate "true" loss of periodontal tissue support, have varied considerably from study to study. In addition, the number of "affected" tooth surfaces required for designating an individual subject as a case, ie, as suffering from periodontal disease, has varied. These inconsistencies in the definitions inevitably affect the figures describing the distribution of the disease. Data from different epidemiologic studies can therefore be compared and extrapolated only with great caution.

Although tooth loss in individuals younger than 50 years in industrialized countries is mainly the result of dental caries, either directly or indirectly (root fractures in nonvital teeth with posts), among the elderly an estimated 40% to 60% of tooth loss is attributable to periodontal disease. However, in some developing countries with low or very low caries prevalence (India, China, and some African countries), periodontal diseases are the main reason for tooth loss in adults: the molars predominate, followed by the maxillary premolars.

Prevalence

The prevalence of periodontal diseases should measure the accumulated loss of periodontal support in different age groups at the individual, tooth, and surface levels. Progress is not linear, and the prevalence expresses the cumulative sum of all episodes of exacerbation, remission, and re-gression. The prevalence of periodontal diseases is therefore strictly age related.

In epidemiologic studies, loss of periodontal support (prevalence) is usually based on vertical PAL. However, most of the Scandinavian studies are based on radiographic measurements of alveolar bone loss. Most epidemiologic studies are conducted on samples that are selected or randomized and stratified into age intervals. Loss of periodontal support is usually assessed on the basis of recordings of vertical PAL on the mesiobuccal and midbuccal sites of part of the dentition (partial-mouth examination). Up to the age of 50 years, most buccal PAL is attributable to toothbrush abrasion. By contrast, approximal PAL is mainly caused by periodontal disease. Horizontal clinical attachment loss (furcation involvement) may occur in multirooted teeth. The most reliable data for studies of prevalence are those based on complete-mouth measurements of vertical and horizontal PAL at all available sites, on randomized samples of indicator age groups. To date, very few such studies have been conducted. Periodontitis is not a disease of adulthood but begins during childhood among those most susceptible (at high risk) to periodontal diseases. Aggressive periodontitis starts at a very early age: In most industrialized countries, prevalence is very low (about 0.1%), but prevalence is higher in some developing countries where malnutrition and poor oral hygiene are common.

Analytic epidemiologic studies have shown that poorly educated rural men who receive irregular dental care lose about twice as much periodontal support as do well-educated, urban women who receive regular dental care.

In the Extent and Severity Index (ESI), the extent component describes the proportion of tooth sites that show signs of destructive periodontitis, and the severity component, expressed as a mean value, describes the amount of clinical attachment loss at the diseased sites.

Analytic epidemiologic studies on the pattern of loss of periodontal attachment among adults at the surface level reveal that the most loss occurs at the distal surfaces of the maxillary first molars and the approximal and lingual surfaces of the mandibular incisors. This may be explained by local factors, such as the presence of dental plaque that is inaccessible to toothbrushing on the distal surfaces of the maxillary first molars and the presence of plaque-retaining supragingival calculus on the mandibular incisors. Attachment loss on the buccal surfaces is mainly attributable to toothbrush abrasion in patients 50 years of age or younger.

Incidence

At both the individual and site levels, the progression (incidence) of periodontitis is irregular, involving exacerbations and so-called burnouts. However, at the group and population levels, the incidence is usually expressed in annual loss of periodontal support. Only a few epidemiologic studies on the incidence of periodontal diseases have been conducted. In the classic study on the natural history of periodontal diseases in Sri Lankan tea workers without access to dental care, the annual loss of periodontal support was 0.25 mm; annual loss of periodontal support was only 0.1 mm in age-matched Norwegian academics who received regular dental care. However, in a recent 10-year longitudinal Swedish study of a randomized sample of 50 year olds (more than 90% of whom received regular dental care), the annual loss of periodontal support was only 0.04 mm. The incidence would be considerably higher among groups selected as specifically susceptible to periodontal disease than it would be in randomized samples. In the US national survey, se-

lected subgroups of individuals with LAP and GAP lost 0.45 mm and 1.1 mm, respectively, per individual over a 6-year period. On the other hand, a 15-year longitudinal study showed that further progression of periodontitis could be prevented, irrespective of the patient's age (the oldest group was 65 to 85 years), in unselected subjects maintained in a needs-related preventive program.

Studies on the pattern of incidence have revealed that progression rates are higher for maxillary molars and mandibular incisors than, for example, maxillary incisors and mandibular premolars. This explains why the greatest loss of periodontal support occurs in the maxillary molars and the mandibular incisors.

Treatment Needs

Periodontal treatment needs have been estimated in more than 150 national surveys based on the Community Periodontal Index of Treatment Needs, applied at the individual and sextant levels. However, the highest CPITN score—not only at the individual and sextant levels but also at the tooth level—considerably overestimates the "true" treatment need at the surface level. Moreover, missing sites (ie, teeth extracted several years previously) should be excluded. The gold standard for evaluation of true treatment needs should be based on data at the surface level (for reviews on the epidemiology of periodontal diseases, see Armitage and Van Dyke, 1996; Baehni and Bourgeois, 1998; Baelum et al, 1991; Burt, 1991, 1996; Brown and Löe, 1993; Papapanou, 1994, 1996; Papapanou and Lindhe, 1997; Pilot, 1998).

REFERENCES

Abbate SL, Brunzell JD (1990). Pathophysiology of hyperlipidemia in diabetes mellitus. J Cardiovasc Pharmacol 16(suppl 9):1–7.

Abdellatif HM, Burt DA (1987). An epidemiological investigation into the relative importance of age and oral hygiene status as determinants of periodontitis. J Dent Res 66:13–18.

Abiko Y, Shimizu N, Yamaguchi M, Suzuki H, Takiguchi H (1998). Effect of aging on functional changes of periodontal tissue cells. Ann Periodontol 3:350–369.

Adriaens PA, Loesche WJ, de Boever JA (1986). Bacteriological study of the microbial flora invading the radicular dentin of periodontally diseased caries-free human teeth. In: Lehner T, Cimasoni G (eds). Borderland Between Caries and Periodontal Disease III. Geneva: Editions Médecine et hygiène: 383.

Adriaens PA, de Boever JA, Loesche WJ (1988a). Bacterial invasion in root cementum and radicular dentine of periodontally diseased teeth in humans: A reservoir of periodontopathic bacteria. J Periodontol 59:222–230.

Adriaens PA, Edwards CA, de Boever JA, Loesche WJ (1988b). Ultrastructural observations on bacterial invasion in cementum and radicular dentine of periodontally diseased human teeth. J Periodontol 55:493–503.

Agarwal S, Huang JP, Piesco N, Suzuki JB, Riccelli AE, Johns LP (1996). Altered neutrophil function in localized juvenile periodontitis: Intrinsic or induced? J Periodontol 67:337–344.

Ah MKB, Johnson GK, Kaldahl WB, Patil KD, Kalkwarf KL (1994). The effect of smoking on the response to periodontal therapy. J Clin Periodontol 21:91–97.

Ainamo J (1970). Concomitant periodontal disease and dental caries in young adult males. Suom Hammaslaak Toim 66:303–366.

Ainamo J, Bay I (1975). Problems and proposals for recording gingivitis and plaque. Int Dental J 25:229–235.

Ainamo J, Barmes D, Beagrie G, Cutress T, Martin J, Sardo-Infirri J (1982). Development of the WHO community periodontal index of treatment needs (CPITN). Int Dent J 32:281–291.

Albandar JM, Rise J, Abbas D (1987). Radiographic quantification of alveolar bone level changes. Predictors of longitudinal bone loss. Acta Odontol Scand 45:55–59.

Albandar JM (1990a). A 6-year study on the pattern of periodontal disease progression. J Clin Periodontol 17:467–471.

Albandar JM (1990b). Some predictors of radiographic alveolar bone height reduction over 6 years. J Periodontal Res 25:186–192.

Albandar JM, Axelsson P, Buischi Y, Mayer M (1994). Long-term effect of two preventive programs on the incidence of plaque and gingivitis in adolescents. J Periodontol 65:605–610.

Albandar JM, Buischi Y, Axelsson P (1995). Caries lesions and dental restorations as predisposing factors in the progression of periodontal diseases in adolescents—A 3-year longitudinal study. J Periodontol 66:249–254.

Albandar JM, Brown L, Brunelle J, Löe H (1996). Gingival state and dental calculus in early-onset periodontitis. J Periodontol 67:953–959.

Albandar JM, Brown L, Genco R, Löe H (1997). Clinical classification of early-onset periodontitis in adolescents and young adults. J Periodontol 68:545–555.

References

Albandar JM, Kingman A, Brown L, Löe H (1998). Gingival inflammation and subgingival calculus as determinants of disease progression in early-onset periodontitis. J Clin Periodontol 25:231–237.

Albandar JM, Kingman A (1999). Gingival recession, gingival bleeding, and dental calculus in adults 30 years of age and older in the US, 1988-1994. J Periodontol 70:30–43.

Albandar JM, Brunelle JA, Kingman A (1999). Destructive periodontal disease in adults 30 years of age and older in the United States, 1988-1994. J Periodontol 70:13–29.

Albandar JM, Streckfus CF, Adesanya MR, Winn DM (2000). Cigar, pipe and cigarette smoking as risk factors for periodontal disease and tooth loss. J Periodontol 71:1874–1881.

Albandar JM (2002). Periodontal diseases in North America. Periodontol 2000 (in press).

Aldridge JP, Lester V, Watts TLP, Collins A, Viberti G, Wilson RF (1995). Single-blind studies of the effects of improved periodontal health on metabolic control in type 1 diabetes mellitus. J Clin Periodontol 22:271–275.

Ali RW, Martin L, Haffajee A, Socransky S (1997). Detection of identical ribotypes of *Porphyromonas gingivalis* in patients residing in the United States, Sudan, Romania and Norway. Oral Microbiol Immunol 12:106–111.

Alpar B, Leyhausen G, Sapotnick A, Gunay H, Geurtsen W (1998). Nicotine-induced alterations in human primary periodontal ligament and gingiva fibroblast cultures. Clin Oral Investig 2:40–46.

American Academy of Periodontology (1989). Proceedings of the World Workshop in Clinical Periodontics. Chicago: American Academy of Periodontology: 1/23–1/24.

American Academy of Periodontology (1996a). Epidemiology of periodontal diseases. J Periodontol 67:935–945.

American Academy of Periodontology (1996b). Tobacco use and the periodontal patient. J Periodontol 67:51–56.

American Academy of Periodontology (1996c). Consensus report. Periodontal diseases: Pathogenesis and microbial factors. Ann Periodontol 1:926–932.

American Academy of Periodontology (1996d). Diabetes and periodontal disease. J Periodontol 67:166–176.

American Diabetes Association (1997). Report of the Expert Committee on the Diagnosis and Classification of Diabetes Mellitus. Diabetes Care 20:1183–1197.

Anagnou-Vareltzides A, Diamanti-Kipioti A, Afentoulidis N, et al (1996). A clinical survey of periodontal conditions in Greece. J Clin Periodontol 23:758–763.

Andersson D, Springer T (1987). Leukocyte adhesion deficiency: an inherited defect in the Mac-1, LFA-1, and p150,95 glycoproteins. Annu Rev Med 38:175–194.

Ånerud KE, Robertson P, Löe H, Anerud A, Boysen H, Patters RM (1983). Periodontal disease in three young adult populations. J Periodontal Res 18:655–668.

Araujo MG, Berglundh T, Albrektsson T, Lindhe J (1999). Bone formation in furcation defects. J Clin Periodontol 26:643–652.

Armitage GC, Jeffcoat M, Chadwick D (1994). Longitudinal evaluation of elastase as a marker for the progression of periodontitis. J Periodontol 65:120–128.

Armitage GC (1995). Clinical evaluation of periodontal diseases. Periodontol 2000 7:39–53.

Armitage GC (1996). Periodontal diseases: Diagnosis. Ann Periodontol 1:37–215.

Armitage GC, Van Dyke TE (1996). Periodontal diseases of children and adolescents. J Periodontol 67:57–62.

Armitage GC (1999). Development of a classification system for periodontal diseases and conditions. Ann Periodontol 4:1–6.

Armitage GC, Wu Y, Wang HY, Sorrell J, di Giovine FS, Duff GW (2000). Low prevalence of a periodontitis-associated interleukin-1 composite genotype in individuals of Chinese heritage. J Periodontol 71:164–171.

Armitage GC (2001). Adverse pregnancy outcomes and periodontitis: Discussion, conclusions, and recommendations. Ann Periodontol 6:189–192.

Arno A, Waerhaug J, Lövdal A, Schei O (1958). Incidence of gingivitis as related to sex, occupation, tobacco consumption, toothbrushing and age. Oral Surg Oral Med Oral Pathol 11:587–595.

Arno A, Schei O, Lovdal A, Waerhaug J (1959). Alveolar bone loss as a function of tobacco consumption. Acta Odontol Scand 17:3–10.

Ashimoto A, Chen C, Bakker I, Slots J (1996). Polymerase chain reaction detection of 8 putative periodontal pathogens in subgingival plaque of gingivitis and advanced periodontitis lesions. Oral Microbiol Immunol 11:266–273.

Asikainen S, Alaluusua S, Saxén L (1991a). Recovery of *A. actinomycetemcomitans* from teeth, tongue, and saliva. J Periodontol 62:203–206.

Asikainen S, Lai C-H, Alaluusua S, Slots J (1991b). Distribution of *Actinobacillus actinomycetemcomitans* serotypes in periodontal health and disease. Oral Microbiol Immunol 6:115–118.

Asikainen S, Chen C, Slots J (1995). *Actinobacillus actinomycetemcomitans* genotypes in relation to serotypes and periodontal status. Oral Microbiol Immunol 10:65–68.

Atkinson MA, Maclaren NK (1990). What causes diabetes? Sci Am 263:62–63, 66–71.

Attström R, van der Velden U (1994). Consensus report of session I. In: Lang N, Karring T (eds). Proceedings of the 1st European Workshop on Periodontics, 1993. London: Quintessence: 120–126.

Axelsson P, Lindhe J (1974). The effect of a preventive programme on dental plaque, gingivitis and caries in schoolchildren. Results after one and two years. J Clin Periodontol 1:126–138.

Axelsson P, Lindhe J (1977). The effect of a plaque control programme on gingivitis and dental caries in schoolchildren. J Dent Res 56 (special issue): C142–C148.

Axelsson P, Lindhe J (1978). Effect of controlled oral hygiene procedures on caries and periodontal disease in adults. J Clin Periodontol 5:133–151.

Axelsson P, Lindhe J (1981a). Effect of controlled oral hygiene procedures on caries and periodontal disease in adults—Results after six years. J Clin Periodontol 8:239–248.

Axelsson P, Lindhe J (1981b). The significance of maintenance care in the treatment of periodontal disease. J Clin Periodontol 8:281–294.

Axelsson P (1982). Periodontal probe. US Patent 4,364,730.

Axelsson P (1987). Placknybildningsindex PFRI—Indikator för karies- och parodontitprevention, munhygien-frekvens och ytrelaterad munhygien. Tandlakartidningen 79:387–391.

Axelsson P, Kristoffersson K, Karlsson R, Bratthall D (1987). A 30-month longitudinal study of the effects of some oral hygiene measures on *Streptococcus mutans* and approximal dental caries. J Dent Res 66:761–765.

Axelsson P (1991). A fourpoint scale for selection of caries risk patients, based on salivary *S. mutans* levels and plaque formation rate index. In: Johnson NW (ed). Risk Markers for Oral Diseases Caries, vol 1. Cambridge, NY: Cambridge UP: 158–170.

Axelsson P, Lindhe J, Nyström B (1991). On the prevention of caries and periodontal disease. Results of a 15-year-longitudinal study in adults. J Clin Periodontol 13:182–189.

Axelsson P (1993). New ideas and advancing technology in prevention and nonsurgical treatment of periodontal disease. Int Dent J 43:223–238.

Axelsson P (1994). Mechanical plaque control. In: Lang N, Karring T (eds). Proceedings of the 1st European Workshop on Periodontics, 1993. London: Quintessence: 219–243.

Axelsson P, Paulander J (1994). The oral health status in 50-55-year-olds in the county of Värmland. Värmland, Sweden: County Council of Värmland.

Axelsson P, Buischi YAP, Barbosa MFZ, Karlsson R, Pradi MCB (1994). The effect of a new oral hygiene training program on approximal caries in 12-15-year-old Brazilian children: Results after three years. Adv Dent Res 8:278–284.

Axelsson P (1998). Needs-related plaque control measures based on risk prediction. In: Lang NP, Attström R, Löe H (eds). Proceedings of the European Workshop on Mechanical Plaque Control. Berlin: Quintessence: 190–247.

Axelsson P, Paulander J, Lindhe J (1998). Relationship between smoking and dental status in 35-, 50-, 65-, and 75-year-old individuals. J Clin Periodontol 25:297–305.

Axelsson P, Paulander J, Svärdström G, Kaijser H (2000). Effects of population based preventive programs on oral health conditions. J Parodontol Implantol Orale 19:255–269.

Axelsson P, Paulander J, Nordström L, Jonsson AS, Appel B (2001). The Role of Genetic Interleukin-1 Polymorphism on Tooth Loss and Periodontal Support Loss in 50- to 60-year-old Smokers and Nonsmokers [abstract]. Gothenburg, Sweden: Scientific Congress, Dept of Periodontology, Univ of Gothenburg.

Axtelius B, Söderfeldt B, Edwardsson S, Attström R (1997). Therapy-resistant periodontitis (II). Compliance and general and dental health experiences. J Clin Periodontol 24:646–653.

Axtelius B, Söderfeldt B, Nilsson A, Edwardsson S, Attström R (1998). Therapy-resistant periodontitis. Psychosocial characteristics. J Clin Periodontol 25:482–491.

Baab DA, Öberg PÅ (1987). The effect of cigarette smoking on gingival blood flow in humans. J Clin Periodontol 14:418–424.

Badersten A, Nilvéus R, Egelberg J (1981). Effect of nonsurgical periodontal therapy. I. Moderately advanced periodontitis. J Clin Periodontol 8:57–72.

Badersten A, Nilvéus R, Egelberg J (1984a). Effect of nonsurgical periodontal therapy. II. Severely advanced periodontitis. J Clin Periodonol 11:63–76.

References

Badersten A, Nilvéus R, Egelberg J (1984b). Effect of nonsurgical periodontal therapy. III. Single versus repeated instrumentation. J Clin Periodontol 11:114–124.

Badersten A, Nilvéus R, Egelberg J (1985a). Effect of nonsurgical periodontal therapy. IV. Operator variability. J Clin Periodontol 12:190–200.

Badersten A, Nilveus R, Egelberg J (1985b). Effect of nonsurgical periodontal therapy. V. Patterns of probing attachment loss in non-responding sites. J Clin Periodontol 12:270–282.

Badersten A, Nilvéus R, Egelberg J (1985c). Effect of nonsurgical periodontal therapy VI. Localization of sites with probing attachment loss. J Clin Periodontol 12:351–359.

Badersten A, Nilvéus R, Egelberg J (1985d). Effect of nonsurgical periodontal therapy. VII. Bleeding, suppuration and probing depth in sites with probing attachment loss. J Clin Periodontol 12:432–440.

Badersten A, Nilvéus R, Egelberg J (1987a). Effect of nonsurgical periodontal therapy.VIII. Probing attachment changes related to clinical characteristics. J Clin Peridontol 14:425–432.

Badersten A, Nilvéus R, Egelberg J (1987b). 4-year observations of basic periodontal therapy. J Clin Periodontol 14:438–444.

Badersten A, Nilvéus R, Egelberg J (1990). Scores of plaque, bleeding, suppuration and probing depth to predict probing attachment loss. 5 year of observation following nonsurgical periodontal therapy. J Clin Periodontol 17:102–107.

Baehni P, Bourgeois D (1998). Epidemiology of dental health and disease. In: Lang NP, Attström R, Löe H (eds). European Workshop on Mechanical Plaque Control. Berlin: Quintessence: 19–34.

Baelum V, Fejerskov O, Karring T (1986). Oral hygiene, gingivitis and periodontal breakdown in adults Tanzanians. J Periodontal Res 21:221–232.

Baelum V, Fejerskov O, Manji F (1988a). Periodontal diseases in adult Kenyans. J Clin Periodontol 15:445–452.

Baelum V, Luan W, Fejerskov O, Xia C (1988b). Tooth mortality and periodontal conditions in 60-80-year-old Chinese. Scand J Dent Res 96:99–107.

Baelum V, Manji F, Fejerskov O (1991). The distribution of periodontal destruction in populations in non-industrialized countries: Evidence for the existence of high risk groups and individuals. In: Johnson NW (ed). Risk Markers for Oral Diseases. Vol 3: Periodontal diseases. Cambridge, NY: Cambridge UP: 27–74.

Baelum V, Manji F, Wanzala P, Fejerskov O (1995). Relationship between CPITN and periodontal attachment loss findings in an adult population. J Clin Periodontol 22:146–152.

Baelum V, Luan W, Chen X, Fejerskov O (1997a). Predictors of destructive periodontal disease incidence and progression in adult and elderly Chinese. Community Dent Oral Epidemiol 25:265–272.

Baelum V, Luen WM, Chen X, Fejerskov O (1997b). A 10-year study of the progression of destructive periodontal disease in adult and elderly Chinese. J Periodontol 68:1033–1042.

Bagdade JD, Stewart M, Walters E (1978). Impaired granulocyte adherence. A reversible defect in host defense in patients with poorly controlled diabetes. Diabetes 27:677–681.

Bakdash B (1994). People at risk for periodontitis—Oral hygiene and compliance. J Periodontol 65:539–544.

Baker E, Grook G, Schwabacher E (1961). Personality correlates of periodontal disease. J Dent Res 40:396–403.

Ballieux RE (1991). Impact of mental stress on the immune response. J Clin Periodontol 18:427–430.

Barco CT (1991). Prevention of infective endocarditis: A review of the medical and dental literature. J Periodontol 62:510–523.

Barnes GP, Parker W, Lyon T, Fultz R (1986). Indices used to evaluate signs, symptoms and etiologic factors associated with diseases of the periodontium. J Periodontol 57:643–651.

Bartlett JG, O'Keefe P, Tally FP, Louie TJ, Gorbach SL (1986). Bacteriology of hospital-acquired pneumonia. Arch Intern Med 146:868–871.

Bayliss R, Clarke C, Oakley CM, Somerville W, Whitfield A, Young SE (1983). The microbiology and pathogenesis of infective endocarditis. Br Heart J 50:513–519.

Beck JD, Koch GG, Rozier RG, Tudor GE (1990). Prevalence and risk indicators for periodontal attachment loss in a population of older community-dwelling blacks and whites. J Periodontol 61:521–528.

Beck JD, Löe H (1993). Epidemiological principles in studying periodontal diseases. Periodontol 2000 2:34–45.

Beck JD (1994a). People at risk for periodontitis—Risk assessment and multifactorial models. J Periodontol 65:464–467.

Beck JD (1994b). Methods of assessing risk for periodontitis and developing multifactorial models. J Periodontol 65:468–478.

Beck JD, Koch G, Offenbacher S (1994). Attachment loss trends over 3 years in community-dwelling older adults. J Periodontol 65:737–743.

Beck JD (1995). Issues in assessment of diagnostic tests and risk for periodontal diseases. Periodontol 2000 7:100–108.

Beck JD, Koch G, Offenbacher S (1995). Incidence of attachment loss over 3 years in older adults–New and progressiong lesions. Community Dent Oral Epidemiol 23:291–296.

Beck J, Garcia R, Heiss G, et al (1996). Periodontal disease and cardiovascular disease. J Periodontol 67(suppl):1123–1137.

Beck J (1998). Risk revisited. Community Dent Oral Epidemiol 26:220–225.

Beck J, Offenbacher S, Williams R, Gibbs P, Garcia R (1998). Periodontitis: A risk factor for coronary heart disease? Ann Periodontol 3:127–141.

Beck JD, Offenbacher S (2001). The association between periodontal diseases and cardiovascular diseases: A state-of-the-science review. Ann Periodontol 6:9–15.

Belting CM, Hiniker JJ, Dummett CO (1964). Influence of diabetes mellitus on the severity of periodontal disease. J Periodontol 35:476–480.

Benn DK (1990). A review of the reliability of radiographic measurements in estimating alveolar bone change. J Clin Periodontol 17:14–21.

Bennet KR, Read P (1982). Salivary immunoglobulin A levels in normal subjects, tobaccor smokers and patients with minor aphthous ulceration. Oral Surg Oral Med Oral Pathol 53:461–465.

Bergström J, Floderus-Myrhed B (1983). Co-twin control study of the relationship between smoking and some periodontal disease factors. Community Dent Oral Epidemiol 11:113–116.

Bergström J, Eliasson S (1987). Cigarette smoking and alveolar bone height in subjects with a high standard of oral hygiene. J Clin Periodontol 14:466–469.

Bergström J (1989). Cigarette smoking as risk factor in chronic periodontal disease. Commununity Dent Oral Epidemiol 17:245–247.

Bergström J (1990). Oral hygiene compliance and gingivitis expression in cigarette smokers. Scand J Dent Res 98:497–503.

Bergström J, Eliasson S, Preber H (1991). Cigarette smoking and periodontal bone loss. J Periodontol 62:242–246.

Bergström J, Preber H (1994). People at risk for periodontitis–Tobacco as a risk factor. J Periodontol 65:545–550.

Bergström J (1999). Tobacco smoking and supragingival dental calculus. J Clin Periodontol 26:541–547.

Bergström J, Eliasson S, Dock J (2000). Exposure to tobacco smoking and periodontal health. J Clin Periodontol 27:61–68.

Bernzweig E, Payne JB, Reinhardt RA, Dyer JK, Patil KD (1998). Nicotine and smokeless tobacco effects on gingival and peripheral blood mononuclear cells. J Clin Periodontol 25:246–252.

Bevenius J, Linder L, Hultenby K (1994). Site-related streptococcal attachment to buccocervical tooth surfaces. A correlative micromorphologic and microbiologic study. Acta Odontol Scand 52:294–302.

Binder TA, Goodson JM, Socransky SS (1987). Gingival fluid levels of acid and alkaline phosphatase. J Periodontal Res 22:14–19.

Birkedal-Hansen H (1993). Role of cytokines and infammatory mediators in tissue destruction. J Periodontal Res 28:500–510.

Bissada N, Manouchehr-Pour M, Haddow M, Spagnuolo P (1982). Neutrophil functional activity in juvenile and adult onset diabetic patients with mild and severe periodontitis. J Periodontal Res 17:500–502.

Björn A-L, Koch G, Lindhe J (1965). Evaluation of gingival fluid measurements. Odontol Revy 16:300–307.

Björn A-L, Björn H, Grkovic B (1969a). Marginal fit of restorations and its relation to periodontal bone level. Part I: Metal fillings. Odontol Revy 20:311–322.

Björn H, Halling A, Thybetg H (1969b). Radiographic assessment of marginal bone loss. Odont Revy 20:165–179.

Björn A-L, Björn H, Grkovic B (1970). Marginal fit of restorations and its relation to periodontal bone level. Part II: Crowns. Odontol Revy 21:337–346.

Blann AD, McCollum CN (1987). Adverse influence of cigarette smoking on endothelium. Thromb Haemost 70:47–53.

Blasi F, Denti F, Erba M, et al (1996). Detection of Chlymadia pneumoniae but not Helicobacter pylori atheroslerotic plaques of aortic aneurysms. J Clin Microbiol 34:2766–2769.

Blieden TM (1999). Tooth-related issues. Ann Periodontol 4:91–96.

Blix I, Hars R, Preus H, Helgeland K (1992). Entrance of *Actinobacillus actinomycetemcomitans* into Hep-2 cells in vitro. J Periodontol 63:723–728.

Blom L, Dahlquist G (1985). Epidemiological aspects of the natural history of childhood diabetes. Acta Paediatr Scand Suppl 320:20–25.

Bloom A, Ireland J (1980). A colour atlas of diabetes. Holland: Wolfe Medical Publications.

Blume R, Wolff S (1972). Chediak-Higashi syndrome: Study in 4 patients and a review of the literature. Medicine (Baltimore) 51:247–80.

413

References

Bolin A, Lavstedt S, Henrikson C (1986a). Proximal alveolar bone loss in a longitudinal radiographic investigation. III. Some predictors with possible influence on the progress in an unselected material. Acta Odontol Scand 44:257–262.

Bolin A, Lavstedt S, Frithiof L, Henriksson CO (1986b). Proximal alveolar bone loss in a longitudinal radiographic investigation. IV. Smoking and other factors influencing the progress in a material of individuals with at least 20 remaining teeth. Acta Odontol Scand 44:263–268.

Bolin A, Eklund G, Frithiof L, Lavstedt S (1993). The effect of changed smoking habits on marginal alveolar bone loss. A longitudinal study. Swed Dent J 17:211–216.

Bosman CW, Powell RN (1977). The reversal of localized experimental gingivitis. A comparison between mechanical toothbrushing procedures and a 0.2% chlorhexidine mouth rinse. J Clin Periodontol 4:161–172.

Boström L, Linder LE, Bergström J (1998). Influence of smoking on the outcome of periodontal surgery—A 5-year follow-up. J Clin Periodontol 25:194–201.

Bowers JE, Zarhadnik RT (1989). An evaluation of a chairside protease test for use in periodontal diagnosis. J Clin Dent 1:106–109.

Bradshaw DJ, Marsh PD, Watson G, Cummins D (1993). The effects of Triclosan and zinc citrate, alone and in combination, on a community of oral bacteria grown in vitro. J Dent Res 73:25–30.

Bragd L, Dahlén G, Wikström M, Slots J (1987). The capability of *Actinobacillus actinomycetemcomitans, Bacteroides gingivalis* and *Bacteroides intermedius* to indicate progressive periodontitis: A retrospective study. J Clin Periodontol 14:95–99.

Brägger U, Pasquali L, Rylander H, Carners D, Kornman K (1988). Computer assisted densitometric image analysis in periodontal radiography. A methodological study. J Clin Periodontol 15:29–39.

Brägger U, Pasquali L (1989). Color conversion of alveolar bone density changes in digital subtraction images. J Clin Periodontol 16:209–214.

Bredius RGM, de Vries CEE, Troelstra A, et al (1993). Phagocytosis of *Staphylococcus aureus* and *Haemophilus influenzae* type Bna opsonized with polyclonal human IgG1 and IgG2 antibodies. Functional hFc-gamma-R11a polymorphism to IgG2. J Immunol 151:1463–1472.

Brill N, Krasse B (1958). The passage of tissue fluid into the clinically healthy gingival pocket. Acta Odontol Scand 16:233–245.

Brill N (1960). Gingival conditions related to flow of tissue fluid into gingival pockets. Acta Odontol Scand 18:421–446.

Brown L, Meskin LH (1988). Sociodemographic differences in tooth loss patterns in US employed adults and seniors, 1985–86. Gerodontics 4:345–362.

Brown L, Oliver RC, Löe H (1990). Evaluating periodontal status of US employed adults. J Am Dent Assoc 121:226–232.

Brown LJ, Löe H (1993). Prevalence, extent, severity and progression of periodontal disease. Periodontol 2000 2:57–71.

Brown L, Garcia R (1994). People at risk for peridontitis—Utilization of dental services. J Periodontol 65:551–563.

Brown L, Brunelle J, Kingman A (1996a). Periodontal status in the US 1988–1991. Prevalence, extent and demographic variations. J Dent Res 75:672–683.

Brown L, Albandar J, Brunelle J, Löe H (1996b). Early-onset periodontitis: progression of attachment loss during 6 years. J Periodontol 67:960–967.

Brownlee M (1994). Glycation and diabetic complications. Diabetes 43:836–841.

Brunsvold M, Lane J (1990). The prevalence of overhanging dental restorations and their relationship to periodontal disease. J Clin Periodontol 17:67–72.

Buischi YAP, Axelsson P, Oliveira LB, Mayer MPA, Gjermo P (1994). The effect of two preventive programs on oral health knowledge and habits among Brazilian schoolchildren. Community Dent Oral Epidemiol 22:41–46.

Burt BA, Ismail AI, Eklund SA (1985). Periodontal disease, tooth loss and oral hygiene among older Americans. Community Dent Oral Epidemiol 13:93–96.

Burt BA (1991). The distribution of periodontal destruction in the populations of industrialized countries. In: Johnson NW (ed). Risk Markers for Oral Diseases. Vol 3: Periodontal diseases. Cambridge, NY: Cambridge UP: 9.

Burt BA (1994). Periodontitis and ageing: Reviewing recent evidence. J Am Dent Assoc 125:273–279.

Burt BA (1996). Epidemiology of periodontal diseases. Position paper. J Periodontol 67:935–945.

Caffesse RG, Sweeney PL, Smith BA (1986). Scaling and root planing with and without periodontal flap surgery. J Clin Periodontol 13:205–210.

Cairo M, Vandeven C, Toy C, Tischler D, Sender L (1988). Fluorescent cytometric analysis of polymorphonuclear leukocytes in Chediak-Higashi syndrome: Diminshed C3Bi expression (OKM1) with normal granular cell density. Pediatr Res 24:673–676.

Capilouto ML, Douglas CW (1988). Trends in the prevalence and severity of periodontal diseases in the US: A public health problem? J Public Health Dent 48:245–251.

Carlos J, Wolfe M, Kingman A (1986). The extent and severity index: A simple method for use in epidemiologic studies of periodontal disease. J Clin Periodontol 13:500–505.

Carlos J, Wolfe M, Zambon J, Kingman A (1988). Periodontal disease in adolescents: Some clinical and microbiologic correlates of attachment loss. J Dent Res 67:1510–1514.

Carlsson J, Egelberg J (1965). Effect of diet on early plaque formation in man. Odontol Revy 16:112–125.

Chambers D, Crawford J, Mukherjee S, Cohen R (1984). Aspartate aminotransferase increases in crevicular fluid during experimental periodontitis in beagle dogs. J Periodontol 55:526–530.

Chambers D, Imbrey PB, Cohen RC, Crawford JM, Alves MEAF, McSwiggin TA (1991). A longitudinal study of apartate aminotransferase in human gingival crevicular fluid. J Periodontal Res 26:65–74.

Charon J, Mergenhagen S, Gallin J (1985). Gingivitis and oral ulceration in patients with neutrophil destruction. J Oral Pathol 14:150–155.

Chen J, Burch J, Beck F, Horton J (1987). Periodontal attachment loss associated with proximal tooth restorations. J Prosthet Dent 57:416–420.

Chen C, Dunford P, Reynolds H, Zambon J (1989). *Eikenella corrodens* in human oral cavity. J Periodontol 60:611–616.

Chen H, Johnson B, Sims T, et al (1991). Humoral immune responses to *Porphyromonas gingivalis* before and following therapy in rapidly progressive periodontitis patients. J Periodontol 62:781–791.

Chen X, Wolff L, Aeppli D, et al (2001). Cigarette smoking, salivary/gingival crevicular fluid cotinine and periodontal status. A 10-year longitudinal study. J Clin Periodontol 28:331–339.

Christen AG (1970). The clinical effects of tobacco on oral tissue. J Am Dent Assoc 81:1378–1382.

Christen AG, Armstrong WR, McDaniel RK (1979). Intraoral leukoplakia, abrasion, periodontal breakdown, and tooth loss in a snuff dipper. J Am Dent Assoc 98:584–586.

Christersson LA, Slots J, Rosling B, Genco R (1985a). Microbiological and clinical effects of surgical treatment of localized juvenile periodontitis. J Clin Periodontol 12:465–476.

Christersson LA, Slots J, Zambon J, Genco R (1985b). Transmission and colonization of *Actinobacillus actinomycetemcomitans* in localized juvenile periodontitis patients. J Periodontol 56:127–131.

Christersson LA, Zambon J (1993). Suppression of subgingival *Actinobacillus actinomycetemcomitans* in localized juvenile periodontitis by systemic tetracycline. J Clin Periodontol 20:395–401.

Christgau M, Pallitzsch K, Schmalz G, Kreiner U, Frenzel S (1998). Healing response to non-surgical periodontal therapy in patients with diabetes mellitus: Clinical, microbiological and immunologic results. J Clin Periodontol 25:112–124.

Chuba P, Pelz K, Krekeler G, DeIsele T, Gobel U (1988). Synthetic oligodeoxynucleotide probes for the rapid detection of bacteria associated with human periodontitis. J Gen Microbiol 134:1931–1938.

Chung H-J, Chung C-P, Son S-H, Nisengard R (1989). *Actinobacillus actinomycetemcomitans* serotypes and leukotoxicity in Korean localized juvenile periodontitis. J Periodontol 60:506–511.

Ciancio SG, Yaffe S, Catz C (1972). Gingival hyperplasia and diphenylhydantoin. J Periodontol 43:411–414.

Cimasoni G (1983). Crevicular fluid updated. Monogr Oral Sci 12:103–123.

Claffey N, Nylund K, Kiger R, Garrett S, Egelberg J (1990). Diagnostic predicability of scores of plaque, bleeding, suppuration and probing depth for probing attachment loss. 3.5 years of observation following initial periodontal therapy. J Clin Periodontol 17:108–114.

Clark R, Page R, Wilde G (1977). Defective neutrophil chemotaxis in juvenile periodontitis. Infect Immun 18:94–700.

Clerehugh V, Lennon M (1986). A 2-year longitudinal study of early periodontitis in 14- to 16-year-old schoolchildren. Community Dent Health 3:135–141.

Clinton SK, Fleet JC, Loppnow H, et al (1991). Interleukin 1 gene expression in rabbit vascular tissue in vivo. Am J Pathol 138:1005–1014.

Cogen R, Stevens AW, Cohen-Cole SA, Kirk K, Freeman A (1983). Leukocyte function in the etiology of acute necrotizing ulcerative gingivitis. J Periodontol 54:402–407.

Cogen R, Wright J, Tate A (1992). Destructive periodontal disease in healthy children. J Periodontol 63:761–765.

Coldiron NB, Yukna RA, Weir J, Caudill RF (1990). A quantitative study of cementum removal with hand curettes. J Periodontol 6:293–299.

Collins JG, Windley H, Arnold R, Offenbacher S (1994). Effects of a *Porphyromonas gingivalis* infection on inflammatory mediator response and pregnancy outcome in hamsters. Infect Immun 62:4356–4361.

Colombo A, Haffajee A, Dewhirst F, et al (1998). Clinical and microbiological features of refractory periodontitis subjects. J Clin Periodontol 35:169–180.

References

Combs A, Lopatin D, Shelburne C (1999). Induction and expression of the Hsp90 homologue in *Porphyromonas gingivalis* [abstract 3211]. J Dent Res 78(special issue):507.

Corey LA, Nance WE, Hofstede P, Schenkein H (1993). Periodontal disease in a Virginia twin population. J Periodontol 64:1205–1208.

Costerton JW, Lewandowski Z, DeBeer D, Caldwell D, Korber D, James G (1994). Biofilms, the customized microniche. J Bacteriol 176:2137–2142.

Costerton JW, Lewandowski Z, Caldwell D, Korber D, Lappin-Scott H (1995). Microbial biofilms. Ann Rev Microbiol 49:711–745.

Croucher R, Marcenes WS, Torres MCMB, Hughes WS, Sheiham A (1997). The relationship between life-events and periodontitis. A case-control study. J Clin Periodontol 24:39–43.

Cuff MJ, McQuade MJ, Scheidt MJ, Sutherland DE, van Dyke TE (1989). The presence of nicotine on root surfaces of periodontally diseased teeth in smokers. J Periodontol 60:564–569.

Cumming BR, Löe H (1973). Consistency of plaque distribution in individuals without special home care instruction. J Periodontal Res 8:94–100.

Cummins D (1991). Zinc citrate/triclosan: A new antiplaque system for the control of plaque and the prevention of gingivitis: Short term clinical and mode of action studies. J Clin Periodontol 18:455–461.

Cunea E, Axelsson P (1997). Plackbildungsrateindex bei 3- bis 19-jährigen. Phillip J 7–8:237–239.

Cunningham MD, Seachord C, Ratcliffe K, Bainbridge B, Aruffo A, Darveau RP (1996). *Helicobacter pylori* and *Porphyromonas gingivalis* lipopolysaccharides are poorly transferred to recombinant soluble CD14. Infect Immun 64:3601–3608.

Curtis M (1991). Markers of periodontal disease susceptibility and activity derived from gingival crevicular fluid: Specific vs non-specific analyses. In: Johnson NW (ed). Risk Markers for Oral Diseases. Vol 3: Periodontal diseases. Cambridge, NY: Cambridge UP: 254.

Curtis MA, Slaney JM, Carman RJ, Johnson NW (1991). Identification of major surface protein antigens of *Porphyromonas gingivalis* using IgG antibody reactiity of periodontal case-control serum. Oral Microbiol Immunol 6:321–326.

Cutler C, Ekle P, Arnold R, van Dyke T (1991). Defective neutrophil function in an insulindependent diabetes mellitus patients. A case report. J Periodontol 62:394–401.

Cutler C, Shinedling A, Nunn M, et al (1999). Association between periodontitis and hyperlipidemia: Cause or effect? J Periodontol 70:1429–1434.

Cutress TW, Ainamo J, Sardo-Infirri J (1987). The Community Periodontal Index of Treatment Needs (CPITN) procedure for population groups and individuals. Int Dent J 37:222–233.

Dahlén G (1994). Microbial test methods for evaluation of periodontal activity. In: Hjørting-Hanssen E (ed). Odontology. Copenhagen: Munksgaard: 51–62.

Dahlén G, Wikström M (1995). Occurrence of enteric rods, staphylococci and Candida in subgingival samples. Oral Microbiol Immunol 10:42–46.

Dahlén G, Wikström M, Renvert S (1996). Treatment of periodontal disease based on microbiological diagnosis. A 5-year follow-up on individual patterns. J Periodontol 67:79–887.

Danesh J, Collins R, Peto R (1997). Chronic infections and coronary heart disease: Is there a link? Lancet 350:430–436.

Daneshmand H, Wade A (1976). Correlation between gingival fluid measurements and macroscopic and microscopic characteristics of gingival tissue. J Periodontal Res 11:35–46.

Daniell H (1976). Osteoporosis of the slender smoker. Arch Intern Med 136:298–337.

Danielsen B, Manji F, Nagelkerke N, Fejerskov O, Baelum V (1990). Effect of cigarette smoking on the transition dynamics in experimental gingivitis. J Clin Periodontol 17:59–164.

Darveau RP, Cunningham M, Bailey T, et al (1995). Ability of bacteria associated with chronic inflammatory disease to stimulate E-selectin expression and promote neutrophil adhesion. Infect Immun 63:1311–1317.

Darveau RP, Tanner A, Page R (1997). The microbial challenge in periodontitis. Periodontol 2000 14:12–32.

da Silva AM, Newman HN, Oakley DA (1995). Psychosocial factors in inflammatory periodontal diseases. A review. J Clin Periodontol 22:516–526.

Dawes C, Jenkins GN, Tonge CH (1963). The nomenclature of the integuments of the enamel surface of teeth. Br Dent J 16:65–68.

Delima AJ, Oates T, Assuma R, et al (2001). Soluble antagonists to interleukin-1 (IL-1) and tumor necrosis factor (TNF) inhibits loss of tissue attachment in experimental periodontitis. J Clin Periodontol 28:233–240.

Demolon IA, Persson GR, Moncla BJ, Johnson RH, Ammons WF (1993). Clinical and bacterial investigation of the guided tissue regeneration procedure. J Periodontol 64:609–616.

De Nardin E (2001). The role of inflammatory and immunological mediators in periodontitis and cardiovascular disease. Ann Periodontol 6:30–40.

Dennison DK, Gottsegen R, Rose LF (1996). Diabetes and periodontal diseases. J Periodontol 67:166–176.

Dennison DK, Van Dyke T (1997). The acute inflammatory response and the role of phagocytic cells in periodontal health and disease. Periodontol 2000 14:54–78.

DeStefano F, Anda R, Kahn H, Williamson D, Russell C (1993). Dental disease and risk of coronary heart disease and mortality. Br Med J 306:688–691.

Diabetes Control and Complications Trial Research Group (1993). The effect of intensive treatment of diabetes on the developmen and progression of long-term complications in insulin-dependent diabetes mellitus. N Engl J Med 329:977–986.

Dinsdale CRJ, Rawlinson A, Walsh TF (1997). Subgingival temperature in smokers and non-smokers with periodontal disease. J Clin Periodontol 24:761–766.

Di Rienzo JM (1991). Probe-specific DNA fingerprinting applied to the epidemiology of periodontal bacteria and disease activity of periodontitis. In: Hamada S, Holt S, McGhee J (eds). Periodontal Disease Pathogens and Host Immune Responses. Tokyo: Quintessence: 379–393.

Di Rienzo JM, Slots J, Sixou M, Sol M, Harmon R, McKay T (1994). Specific genetic variants of Actinobacillus actinomycetemcomitans correlate with disease and health in a regional population of families with localized juvenile periodontitis. Infect Immun 62:3058–3065.

Dolan TA, Gilbert GH, Ringelberg ML, et al (1997). Behavioral risk indicators of attachment loss in adult Floridians. J Clin Periodontol 24:223–232.

Donahue RP, Wu T (2001). Insuline resistance and periodontal disease: An epidemiologic overview of research needs and future directions. Ann Periodontol 6:119–124.

Donoghue H (1990). Can the colonisation resistance of the oral microflora be enhanced? Microb Ecol Health Dis 3:1–4.

Dougherty M, Slots J (1993). Periodontal diseases in young individuals. J Calif Dent Assoc 21:55–69.

Douglass CW, Jette A, Fox C, et al (1993). Oral health status of the elderly. N Engl J Gerontol 48:39–46.

Drangsholt MT (1998). A new causal model of dental diseases associated with endocarditis. Ann Periodontol 3:184–196.

Duncan A, Carman R, Harper F, Griffiths G, Curtis M (1992). Porphyromonas gingivalis: Presence of a species-specific antigen which is discriminatory in chronic inflammatory adult periodontal disease. Microb Ecol Health Dis 5:15–20.

Duncan M, Nakao S, Skobe Z, Xie H (1993). Interactions of P. gingivalis with epithelial cells. Infect Immun 61:2260–2265.

Dzink J, Socransky S, Ebersole J, Frey D (1983). ELISA and conventional techniques for identification of black-pigmented Bacteroides isolated from periodontal pockets. J Periodontal Res 18:369–374.

Dzink J, Tanner A, Haffajee A, Socransky S (1985). Gram-negative species associated with active destructive periodontal lesions. J Clin Periodontol 12:648–659.

Dzink J, Socransky S, Haffajee A (1988). The predominant cultivable microbiota of active and inactive lesions of destructiove periodontal diseases. J Clin Periodontol 15:316–323.

Ebersole J, Frey DE, Taubman MA, Haffajee AD, Socransky SS (1987). Dynamics of systemic antibody responses in periodontal disease. J Periodontal Res 22:184–186.

Ebersole J, Holt S (1991). Immunological procedures for diagnosis and risk assessment in periodontal diseases. In: Johnson NW (ed). Risk Markers for Oral Diseases. Vol 3: Periodontal diseases. Cambridge, NY: Cambridge UP: 203.

Ebersole J, Singer RE, Steffensen R, Filloon T, Kornman KS (1993). Inflammatory mediators and immunoglobulins in GCF from healthy, gingivitis and periodontitis sites. J Periodontal Res 28:543–546.

Ebersole J, Taubman M (1994). The protective nature of host responses in periodontal diseases. Periodontol 2000 5:112–141.

Egelberg J (1964). Gingival exudate measurements for evaluation of inflammatory changes of the gingivae. Odontol Revy 15:381–398.

Eggert F, Drewell L, Bigelow J, Speck J, Goldner M (1991). The pH of gingival crevices and periodontal pockets in children, teenagers and adults. Arch Oral Biol 36:233–238.

Ehnevid H, Jansson L, Lindskog S, Blomlöf L (1993a). Periodontal healing in teeth with periapical lesions. J Clin Periodontol 20:254–258.

Ehnevid H, Jansson L, Lindskog S, Blomlöf L (1993b). Periodontal healing in relation to radiographic attachment and endodontic infection. J Periodontol 64:1199–1204.

Ehnevid H (1995). Local Factors Modifying Marginal Periodontal Healing [thesis]. Stockholm, Sweden: Karolinska Institute.

Ehnevid H, Jansson L, Lindskog S, Weintraub A, Blomlöf L (1995). Endodontic pathogens: Propagation of infection through patent dentinal tubules in traumatized monkey teeth. Endod Dent Traumatol 11:229–234.

References

Ehnevid H, Jansson L, Lindskog S, Blomlöf L (1997). Periodontal healing in horizontal and vertical defects following surgical or non-surgical therapy. Swed Dent J 21:137–147.

Eichel B, Sharik H (1969). Tobacco smoke toxicity: Loss of human oral leukocyte function and fluid cell metabolism. Science 166:1424–1426.

Eid M (1986). Relationship between overhanging amalgam restorations and periodontal disease. Odontostomatol Trop 9:220–225.

Eklund S, Burt B (1994). Risk factors for total tooth loss in the US: Longitudinal analysis of national data. J Public Health Dent 54:5–14.

Emingil G, Buduneli E, Aliyev A, Akili A, Atilla G (2000). Association between periodontal disease and acute myocardial infarction. J Periodontol 71:1882–1886.

Emrich L, Shlossman M, Genco R (1991). Periodontal disease in non-insulin dependent diabetes mellitus. J Periodontol 62:123–130.

Emslie RD (1980). The 621 periodontal probe. Int Dent J 30:287–288.

Engebretson SP, Lamster IB, Herrera-Abreu M, et al (1999). The influence of interleukin gene polymorphism on expression of interleukin-1β and tumor necrosis factor-α in periodontal tissue and gingival crevicular fluid. J Periodontol 70:567–573.

Enwonwu C (1972). Epidemiological and biochemical studies of necrotizing ulcerative gingivitis and noma (cancrum oris) in Nigerian children. Arch Oral Biol 17:1357–1371.

Enwonwu C (1985). Infectious oral necrosis (cancrum oris) in Nigerian children: A review. Community Dent Oral Epidemiol 13:190–194.

Enwonwu C (1994). Cellular and molecular effects of malnutrition and their relevance to periodontal diseases. J Clin Periodontol 21:643–657.

Ericsson I, Lindhe J (1977). Lack of effect of trauma from occlusion on the recurrence of experimental periodontitis. J Clin Periodontol 4:115–127.

Ernster VL, Grady DG, Greene JC, et al (1990). Smokeless tobacco use and health effects among baseball players. JAMA 264:218–224.

Esposito C, Gerlach H, Brett J, Stern D, Vlassara H (1992). Endothelial receptor-mediated binding of glucose-modified albumin is associated with increased monolayer permeability and modulation of cell surface coagulant properties. J Exp Med 170:1387–1407.

Fang MA, Frost PJ, Iida-Klein A, Hahn TJ (1991). Effects of nicotine on cellular function in UMR 106-01 osteoblast-like cells. Bone 12:283–286.

Fedi PF Jr, Killoy WJ (1992). Temperature differences at periodontal sites in health and disease. J Periodontol 63:24–27.

Feldman RS, Bravacos JS, Rose CL (1983). Association between smoking different tobacco products and periodontal disease indexes. J Periodontol 54:481–487.

Figueredo C, Ribeiro M, Fischer R, Gustafsson A (1999). Increased interleukin-1β concentration in gingival crevicular fluid as a characteristic of periodontitis. J Periodontol 70:1457–1463.

Fischman SL (1986). Current status of indices of plaque. J Clin Periodontol 13:371–374.

Fleisher HC, Mellonig JT, Brayer WK, Gray JL, Barnett JD (1989). Scaling and root planing efficacy in multirooted teeth. J Periodontol 60:402–409.

Fleming TF (1999). Periodontitis. Ann Periodontol 4:32–37.

Folsom AR, Rosamond WD, Sharar E, et al (1999). Prospective study of markers of hemostatic function with risk of ischemic stroke. The Atherosclerosis Risk in Community (ARIC) Study Investigators. Circulation 100:736–742.

Fox CH, Jette AM, McGuire S, Feldman H, Douglass C (1994). Periodontal disease among New England elders. J Periodontol 65:676–684.

Frank RM, Voegel J (1978). Bacterial bone resorption in advanced cases of human periodontitis. J Periodontal Res 13:251–261.

Frank RM (1980). Bacterial penetration in the apical pocket wall of advanced human periodontitis. J Periodontal Res 15:563–573.

Freeman R, Goss S (1993). Stress measures as predictors of periodontal disease—A preliminary communication. Community Dent Oral Epidemiol 21:176–177.

French CK, Savitt E, Simon S, et al (1986). DNA probe detection of periodontal pathogens. Oral Microbiol Immunol 1:58–62.

Furuichi Y, Lindhe J, Ramberg P, Volpe AR (1992). Patterns of de novo plaque formation in the human dentition. J Clin Periodontol 19:423–433.

Furuichi Y (1998). Some Antiplaque and Antiinflammatory Agents in the Prevention and Treatment of Periodontal Disease [thesis]. Göteborg, Sweden: Göteborg Univ.

Galan JE (1996). Molecular genetic bases of Salmonella entry into host cells. Mol Microbiol 20:263–271.

Gamonal J, Acevedo A, Bascones A, Jorge O, Silva A (2000). Levels of interleukin-1β, -8, and -10 and RANTES in gingival crevicular fluid and cell populations in adult periodontitis patients and the effect of periodontal treatment. J Periodontol 71:1535–1545.

Garcia R, Nunn ME, Vokonas PS (2001). Epidemiologic associations between periodontal disease and chronic obstructive pulmonary disease. Ann Periodontol 6:71–77.

Garnick J, Silverstein L (2000). Periodontal probing: Probe tip diameter. J Periodontol 71:96–103.

Gemmell E, Marshall R, Seymour G (1997). Cytokines and prostaglandins in immune homeostasis and tissue destruction in periodontal disease. Periodontol 2000 14:112–143.

Genco RJ, Slots J (1984). Host responses in periodontal diseases. J Dent Res 63:441–451.

Genco RJ (1992). Host responses in periodontal diseases: Current concepts. J Periodontol 53:338–355.

Genco RJ, Löe H (1993). The role of systemic conditions and disorders in periodontal disease. Periodontol 2000 2:98–116.

Genco RJ (1996). Current view of risk factors for periodontal diseases. J Periodontol 67:1041–1049.

Genco RJ, Chadda S, Grossi S, et al (1997). Periodontal disease is a predictor of cardiovascular disease in a Native American population [abstract 3158]. J Dent Res 76(special issue):408.

Genco RJ, Wu T, Grossi S, et al (1999a). Periodontal microflora related to risk for myocardial infarction: A case control study [abstract 2811]. J Dent Res 78(special issue):457.

Genco RJ, Ho AW, Grossi SG, Dunford RG, Tedesco LA (1999b). Relationship of stress, distress and inadequate coping behaviors to periodontal disease. J Periodontol 70:711–723.

Geraci JE, Wilson JR (1982). Symposium on infective endocarditis III. Endocarditis due to Gram-negative bacteria. Report of 56 cases. Mayo Clin Proc 57:145–148.

Gibbons RJ, Van Houte J (1980). Bacterial adherence and the formation of dental plaques. In: Beachey E (ed). Bacterial Adherence, vol 6, Receptors and Recognition Series B. London: Chapman and Hall:60–104.

Gibbs RS, Romero R, Hillier SL, Eschenbach DA, Sweet RL (1992). A review of premature birth and subclinical infection. Am J Obstet Gynecol 166:1515–1528.

Gillespie J, De Nardin E, Radel S, Kuracina J, Smutko J, Zambon J (1992). Production of an extracellular toxin by the oral pathogen Campylobacter rectus. Microb Pathog 12:69–77.

Gilmore N, Scheiham A (1971). Overhanging dental restorations and periodontal disease. J Periodontol 42:8–12.

Glantz P (1969). On wettability and adhesiveness. A study of enamel, dentine, some restorative materials and dental plaque. Odontol Revy 20(suppl):17.

Glavind L, Lund B, Löe H (1968). The relationship between periodontal disease, diabetes duration, insulin dosage and retinal changes. J Periodontol 39:341–347.

Glick M, Garfunkel AA (1992). Common oral findings in two different diseases—Leukemia and AIDS. Part 1. Compendium 13:432, 434, 436.

Glick M, Muzyka BC, Lurie D, Salkin LM (1994). Oral manifestations associated with HIV-related disease as markers for immune suppression and AIDS. Oral Surg Oral Med Oral Pathol Oral Radiol Endod 94:344–349.

Gmür R, Strub J, Guggenheim B (1989). Prevalence of *Bacteroides forsythus* and *Bacteroides gingivalis* in subgingival plaque of prosthodontically treated patients on short recall. J Periodontal Res 24:113–120.

Goldstein S (1984). Cellular and molecular biological studies on diabetes mellitus. Pathol Biol 32:99–106.

Golub LM, Schneir M, Ramamurthy N (1978). Enhanced collagenase activity in diabetic rat gingiva: in vitro and in vivo evidence. J Dent Res 57:520–525.

Golub LM, Nicoll GA, Iacono VJ, Ramamurthy NS (1982). In vivo crevicular leukocytes response to a chemotactic challenge: Inhibition by experimental diabetes. Infect Immun 37:1013–1020.

Gonzalez Y, De Nardin A, Grossi S, et al (1996). Serum cotinine levels, smoking and periodontal attachment loss. J Dent Res 75:796–802.

Goodson JM, Tanner ACR, Haffajee AD, Sornberger GC, Socransky SS (1982). Patterns of progression and regression of advanced destructive periodontal disease. J Clin Periodontol 9:472–481.

Goodson JM, Haffajee AD, Socransky SS (1984). The relationship between attachment level loss and alveolar bone loss. J Clin Periodontol 11:348–359.

Goultschin J, Sgan-Cohen HD, Donchin M, Brayer L, Soskolne WA (1990). Association of smoking with periodontal treatment needs. J Periodontol 61:364–367.

Grbic JT, Lamster IB (1992). Risk indicators for future clinical attachment loss in adult periodontitis. Tooth and site variables. J Periodontol 63:262–269.

Greene J, Vermillion J (1960). Oral hygiene index: A method for classifying oral hygiene status. J Am Dent Assoc 61:172–179.

Greene J, Vermillion J (1964). The simplified oral hygiene index. J Am Dent Assoc 68:7–13.

Gröndahl HG, Gröndahl K (1983). Subtraction radiography for the diagnosis of periodontal bone lesions. Oral Surg Oral Med Oral Pathol 55:208–213.

Gröndahl K, Gröndahl HG, Wennström J, Heijl L (1987). Examiner agreement in estimating changes in periodontal bone from conventional and subtraction radiographs. J Clin Periodontol 14:74–79.

Gröndahl HG (1997). Radiographic examination. In: Lindhe J, Karring T, Lang N (eds). Clinical Periodontology and Implant Dentistry. Copenhagen: Munksgaard.

Grossi S, Zambon JJ, Ho AW, et al (1994). Assessment of risk for periodontal disease. I. Risk indicators of attachment loss. J Periodontol 65:260–267.

Grossi S, Genco R, Machtei E, et al (1995). Assessment of risk for periodontol disease. II. Risk indicators for alveolar bone loss. J Periodontol 66:23–29.

Grossi S, Skrepcinski F, De Caro T, Zambon J, Cummins D, Genco R (1996). Response to periodontal therapy in diabetics and smokers. J Periodontol 67:1094–1102.

Grossi S, Skrepcinski F, DeCaro T, et al (1997). Treatment of periodontal disease in diabetics reduces glycated hemoglobin. J Periodontol 68:713–719.

Grossi S, Genco R (1998). Periodontal disease and diabetes mellitus: A two-way relationship. Ann Periodontol 3:51–61.

Grossi S (2001). Treatment of periodontal disease and control of diabetes: An assessment of the evidence and need for future research. Ann Periodontol 6:138–145.

Gruica B, Buser D, Lang NP (2002). Impact of the Il-1 genotype and smoking on dental implant prognosis. J Dent Res (in press).

Gunaratnam M, Smith GLF, Socransky SS, Smith CM, Haffajee AD (1992). Enumeration of subgingival species on primary isolation plates using colony lifts. Oral Microbiol Immunol 7:14–18.

Gunsolly J, Quinn S, Tew J, Gooss C, Brooks C, Schenkein H (1998). The effect of smoking on individuals with minimal periodontal destruction. J Periodontol 69:165–170.

Gupta S, Leatham EW, Carrington D, et al (1997). Elevated Chlamydia pneumoniae antibodies, cardiovascular events, and azithromycin in male survivors of myocardial infarction. Circulation 96:404–407.

Haber J, Kent R (1992). Cigarette smoking in a periodontal practice. J Periodontol 63:100–106.

Haber J, Wattles J, Crowby M, Mandell R, Kaunudi J, Kent R (1993a). Evidence for cigarette smoking as a major risk factor for periodontitis. J Periodontol 64:16–23.

Haber J, Brinnell C, Crowley M, Mandell R, Joshipura K, Kent R (1993b). Antibodies to periodontal pathogens in cigarette smokers [abstract]. J Dent Res 71:297.

Haber J (1994). Smoking is a major risk factor for periodontitis. Curr Opin Periodontol: 12–18.

Haffajee AD, Socransky S, Goodson J (1983a). Clinical parameters as predictors of destructive periodontal disease activity. J Clin Periodontol 10:257–265.

Haffajee AD, Socransky SS, Goodson J (1983b). Comparison of different data analyses for detecting changes in attachment level. J Clin Periodontol 10:298–310.

Haffajee AD, Socransky S, Ebersole J, Smith D (1984). Clinical, microbiological and immunological features associated with the treatment of active periodontosis lesions. J Clin Periodontol 11:600–618.

Haffajee AD, Dzink J, Socransky S (1988a). Effect of modified Widman flap surgery and systemic tetracyclines on subgingival microbiota of periodontal lesions. J Clin Periodontol 15:255–262.

Haffajee AD, Socransky SS, Dzink JL, Taubman MA (1988b). Clinical, microbiological and immunological features of subjects with refractory periodontal diseases. J Clin Periodontol 15:240–246.

Haffajee AD, Socransky SS, Lindhe J, Kent RL, Okamoto H, Yoneyama T (1991a). Clinical risk indicators for periodontal attachment loss. J Clin Periodontol 18:117–125.

Haffajee AD, Socransky SS, Smith C, Dibart S (1991b). Relation of baseline microbial parameters to future periodontal attachment loss. J Clin Periodontol 18:744–750.

Haffajee AD, Socransky S, Smith C, Dibart S (1991c). Microbial risk indicators for periodontal attachment loss. J Periodontal Res 26:293–296.

Haffajee AD, Socransky SS, Goodson JM (1992a). Subgingival temperature (I). Relation to baseline clinical parameters. J Clin Periodontol 19:401–408.

Haffajee AD, Socransky SS, Goodson JM (1992b). Subgingival temperature (II). Relation to future periodontal attachment loss. J Clin Periodontol 19:409–416.

Haffajee AD, Socransky SS, Goodson JM (1992c). Subgingival temperature (III). Relation to microbial count. J Clin Periodontol 19:417–422.

Haffajee AD, Socransky S (1994). Microbial etiological agents of destructive periodontal diseases. Periodontol 2000 5:78–111.

Haffajee AD, Cugini M, Socransky S (1997). The effect of SRP on the clinical and microbiological parameters of periodontal diseases. J Clin Periodontol 24:324–334.

Haffajee AD, Cugini M, Tanner A, et al (1998). Subgingival microbiota in healthy well-maintained elder and periodontitis subjects. J Clin Periodontol 25:346–353.

Haffajee AD, Socransky SS (2001). Relationship of cigarette smoking to attachment level profiles. J Clin Periodontol 28:283–295.

Håkansson R (1991). Dental Care Habits and Dental Status in 1974–1985 Among Adults in Sweden. Comparative Cross-Sectional and Longitundinal Investigations [thesis]. Lund, Sweden: Lund University.

Hakkaranein K, Ainamo J (1980). Influence of overhanging posterior tooth restorations on alveolar bone height in adults. J Clin Periodontol 7:114–120.

Hall W (1969). Dilantin hyperplasia: A preventable lesion. J Periodontal Res 4(suppl 4):36–37.

Hallmon WW (1999). Occlusal trauma: Effect and impact on the periodontium. Ann Periodontol 4:102–108.

Hammarström L (1997). Enamel matrix, cementum development and regeneration. J Clin Periodontol 24:658–668.

Hancock E, Cray R, O'Leary T (1979). The relationship between gingival crevicular fluid and gingival inflammation. A clinical and histological study. J Periodontol 50:13–19.

Hanes P, Schuster G, Lubas S (1991). Binding, uptake and release of nicotine by human gingival fibroblasts. J Periodontol 62:147–152.

Hanioka T, Tanaka M, Ojima M, Takaya K, Matsumeri Y, Shizukuishi S (2000). Oxygen suffiency in the gingiva of smokers and non-smokers with periodontal disease. J Periodontol 71:1846–1851.

Hansen BF, Bjertness E, Gjermo P (1990). Changes in periodontal disease indicators in 35-year-old Oslo citizens from 1973 to 1984. J Clin Periodontol 17:249–254.

Hansen BF, Bjertness E, Gronnesby J (1993). A socio-ecologic model for periodontal diseases. J Clin Periodontol 20:584–590.

Hansen BF, Bjertness E, Grønnesby JK, Eriksen HM (1995). Changes in periodontal treatment needs. A follow-up study of Oslo citizens from the ages of 35 to 50 years. J Periodontal Res 30:410–417.

Haraszthy V, Zambon J, Trevisan M, Zeid M, Genco R (2000). Identification of periodontal pathogens in atheromatous plaques. J Periodontol 71:1554–1560.

Harper DS, Lamster I, Celenti R (1989). Relationship of subgingival plaque flora to lysosomal and cytoplasmic enzyme activity in gingival crevicular fluid. J Clin Periodontol 16:164–169.

Hart TC, Shapira L, Van Dyke TE (1994). People at risk for periodontitis—Neutrophil defects as risk factors. J Periodontol 65:521–529.

Hart TC, Kornman K (1997). Genetic factors in the pathogenesis of periodontitis. Periodontol 2000 14:202–215.

Hausmann E, Ortman L, McHenry K, Fallon J (1982). Relationship between alveolar bone measured by ^{125}I absorptiometry with analysis of standardized radiographs. I. Magiscan. J Periodontol 53:307–310.

Hausmann E, Christersson L, Dunford R, Wikesjö U, Phyo J, Genco R (1985). Usefulness of subtraction radiography in the evaluation of periodontal therapy. J Periodontol 56:4–7.

Hausmann E (2000). Radiographic and digital imaging in periodontal practice. J Periodontol 71:497–503.

Heins PJ, Fuller WW, Fries SE (1989). Periodontal probe use in general practice in Florida. J Am Dent Assoc 119:147–150.

Helöe L, Holst D, Rise J (1988). Development of dental status and treatment behavious among Norwegian adults 1973–1985. Community Dent Oral Epidemiol 16:52–57.

Hemmerle J, Frank RM (1991). Bacterial invasion of periodontal tissues after experimental immuno-suppressions in rats. J Biol Buccale 19:271–282.

Herulf G (1950). Om det marginale alveolarbenet hos ungdom i studiealderen—en röntgenstudie. Sver Tandlakarforb Tidn 43:42–82.

Herulf G (1951). On the marginal alveolar ridge in students. A roentgenografic study [abstract]. Acta Genet Stat Med 2.

Herulf G (1968). On the marginal alveolar ridge in adults. Sven Tandlak Tidskr 61:675–703.

Herzberg MC, MacFarlane GD, Gong K, et al (1992). The platelet interactivity phenotype of Streptococcus sanguis influences the course of experimental endocarditis. Infect Immun 60:4809–4818.

Herzberg MC, MacFarlane GD, Liu PX, et al (1994). The platelet as an inflammatory cell in periodontal disease: Interactions with Porphyromonas gingivalis. In: Genco RJ, Mergenhagen S, McGhee J, et al (eds). Molecular Basis for Pathogenesis and Molecular Targeting in Periodontal Disease. Washington DC: American Society for Microbiology: 247–255.

Herzberg MC, Meyer M (1998). Dental plaque, platelets and cardiovascular diseases. Ann Periodontol 3:151–160.

Herzberg MC (2001). Coagulation and thrombosis in cardiovascular disease: Plausible contributions of infectious agents. Ann Periodontol 6:16–19.

Hill HR, Sauls H, Dettloff JL, Quie PG (1974). Impaired leukotactic responsiveness in patients with juvenile diabetes mellitus. Clin Immunol Immunopathol 2:395–403.

Hillier SL, Martius J, Krohn MJ, Kiviat N, Holmes KK, Eschenbach DA (1988). A case control study of chorioamnionic infection and chorioamnionitis in prematurity. N Engl J Med 319:972–978.

Hillman J, Socransky S (1982). Bacterial interference in the oral ecology of *Actinobacillus actinomycetemcomitans* and its relationship to human periodontosis. Arch Oral Biol 27:75–77.

Hillman J, Socransky S (1989). The theory and application of bacterial interference to oral diseases. In: Myers HM (ed). New Biotechnology in Oral Research. Basel: Karger: 1–17.

Hirsch R, Clarke N, Shrikandi W (1989). Pulpal pathosis and severe alveolar lesions: A clinical study. Endod Dent Traumatol 5:48–54.

Hobbs HC, Rowe DJ, Johnson PW (1999). Periodontal ligament cells from insulin-dependent diabetics exhibit altered alkaline phosphatase activity in response to growth factors. J Periodontol 70:736–742.

Hollenbach KA, Barrett-Connor E, Edelstein SI, Holbrook T (1993). Cigarette smoking and bone mineral density in older men and women. Am J Public Health 83:1265–1270.

Holm G (1994). Smoking as an additional risk for tooth loss. J Periodontol 65:996–1001.

Holmstrup P, Westergaard J (1997). Necrotizing periodontal disease. In: Karring T, Lang N (eds). Clinical Periodontology and Implant Dentistry. Copenhagen: Munksgaard.

Holmstrup P (1999). Non-plaque-induced gingival lesions. Ann Periodontol 4:20–29.

Holt SC, Ebersole J, Felton J, Brunswold M, Kornman K (1988). Implantation of *Bacteroides gingivalis* in non-human primates initiates progression of periodontitis. Science 239:55–57.

Hoover JN, Ellegaard B, Attström R (1981). Radiographic and clinical examination of periodontal status of first molars in 15-16-year-old Danish schoolchildren. Scand J Dent Res 89:260–263.

Hoppichler F, Lechleitner M, Traweger C, et al (1996). Changes of serum antibodies to heat-shock protein 65 in coronary heart disease and acute myocardial infarction. Atherosclerosis 126:333–338.

Horning GM, Hatch CL, Cohen ME (1992). Risk indicators for periodontitis in a military treatment population. J Periodontol 63:297–302.

Horning GM, Cohen ME (1995). Necrotizing ulcerative gingivitis, periodontitis and stomatitis: Clinical staging and predisposing factors. J Periodontol 66:990–998.

Hugoson A, Jordan T (1982). Frequency distribution of individuals aged 20-70 years according to severity of periodontal disease. Community Dent Oral Epidemiol 10:187–192.

Hugoson A, Koch G, Bergendal T, et al (1986a). Oral health of individuals aged 3-80 years in Jönköping, Sweden, in 1973 and 1983 (I). A review of findings on dental care habits and knowledge of oral health. Swed Dent J 10:103–117.

Hugoson A, Koch G, Bergendal T, et al (1986b). Oral health of individuals aged 3-80 years in Jönköping, Sweden, in 1973 and 1983 (II). A review of clinical and radiographic findings. Swed Dent J 10:175–194.

Hugoson A, Thorstensson H, Falk J, Kuylenstierna J (1989). Periodontal conditions in insulin dependent diabetics. J Clin Periodontol 16:215–223.

Hugoson A, Laurell L, Lundgren D (1992). Frequency distribution of individuals aged 20-70 years according to severity of periodontal disease experience in 1973 and 1983. J Clin Periodontol 19:227–232.

Hugoson A, Norderyd O, Slotte C, Thorstensson H (1998a). Distribution of periodontal disease in a Swedish adult population 1973, 1983 and 1993. J Clin Periodontol 25:542–548.

Hugoson A, Norderyd O, Slotte C, Thorstensson H (1998b). Oral hygiene and gingivitis in a Swedish adult population 1973, 1983 and 1993. J Clin Periodontol 25:807–812.

Hugoson A, Laurell L (2000). A prospective longitudinal study on periodontal bone height changes in a Swedish population. J Clin Periodontol 27:665–674.

Hujoel PP, Drangsholt M, Spiekerman C, DeRouen TA (2000). Periodontal disease and coronary heart disease risk. JAMA 284:1406–1410.

Hunt RJ, Levy SM, Beck JD (1990). The prevalence of periodontal attachment loss in an Iowa population aged 70 and older. J Public Health Dent 50:251–256.

Iacopino AM, Cutler CW (2000). Pathophysiological relationships between periodontitis and systemic disease: Recent concepts involving serum lipids. J Periodontol 71:1375–1384.

Iacopino AM (2001). Periodontitis and diabetes interrelationships: Role of inflammation. Ann Periodontol 6:125–137.

Imrey P, Crawford J, Cohen R, Alves M, McSwiggen T, Chambers D (1991). A cross-sectional analysis of aspartate aminotransferase in human gingival crevicular fluid. J Periodontal Res 26:75–84.

International Agency for Research on Cancer (1986). Chemistry and analysis of tobacco smoke. In: IARC Working Group on the Evaluation of the Carcinogenic Risk of Chemicals to Humans. Tobacco Smoking, vol 38, IARC Monographs on the Evaluation of the Carcinogenic Risk of Chemicals to Humans. Lyon, France: IARC: 86–89.

Irving JT, Socransky S, Tanner A (1978). Histological changes in experimental periodontal disease in rats monoinfected with Gram-negative organisms. J Periodontal Res 13:326–332.

Ishikawa I, Nakashima K, Koseki T, et al (1997). Induction of the immune response to periodontopathic bacteria and its role in the pathogenesis of periodontitis. Periodontol 2000 14:9–111.

Isidor F, Karring T, Nyman S, Lindhe J (1985). New attachment-reattachment following reconstructive periodontal surgery. J Clin Periodontol 12:728–735.

Isidor F, Karring T (1986). Long-term effect of surgical and nonsurgical periodontal treatment. A 5-year clinical study. J Periodontal Res 21:462–472.

Ismail AI, Burt BA, Eklund SA (1983). Epidemiologic patterns of smoking and periodontal disease in the United States. J Am Dent Assoc 106:617–623.

Ismail AI, Morrison EC, Burt BA, Caffesse RG, Kavanagh MT (1990). Natural history of periodontal disease in adults: Findings from the Tecumseh Periodontal Disease Study, 1959-87. J Dent Res 69:430–435.

Iughetti L, Marino R, Bertolani MF, Bernasconi S (1999). Oral health in children and adolescents with IDDM—A review. J Pediatr Endocrinol Metab 12:603–610.

Jacobson L, Blomlöf J, Lindskog S (1994). Root surface texture after different scaling modalities. Scand J Dent Res 102:156–160.

James JA, Sayers NM, Drucker DB, Hull PS (1999). Effects of tobacco products on the attachment and growth of periodontal ligament fibroblasts. J Periodontol 70:578–525.

Jansson L, Ehnevid H, Lindskog S, Blomlöf (1993). Relationship between periapical and periodontal status. A clinical retrospective study. J Clin Periodontol 20:117–123.

Jansson L, Ehnevid H, Lindskog S, Blomlöf L (1994). Proximal restorations and periodontal status. J Clin Periodontol 21:577–582.

Jansson L (1995). Influence of endodontic infection on marginal periodontal status [thesis]. Stockholm, Sweden: Karolinska Inst.

Jeffcoat MK, Howell TH (1980). Alveolar bone destruction due to overhanging amalgam in periodontal disease. J Periodontol 51:599–602.

Jeffcoat M, Reddy M (1991). A comparison of probing and radiographic methods for detection of periodontal disease progression. Curr Opin Dent 1:45–51.

Jeffcoat M, Page R, Reddy M (1991). Use of digital radiography to demonstrate the potential of naproxen as an adjunct in the treatment of rapidly progressive periodontitis. J Periodontal Res 26:415–421.

Jeffcoat M (1992a). Radiographic methods for the detection of progressive alveolar bone loss. J Periodontol 63:367–372.

Jeffcoat M (1992b). Imaging techniques for the periodontium. In: Wilson T, Kornman K, Newman M (eds). Advances in Periodontics. Chicago: Quintessence: 47–57.

Jeffcoat M (1993). Bone loss in the oral cavity. J Bone Miner Res 8(suppl 2):467–474.

Jeffcoat M, Reddy M (1993). Digital subtraction radiography for longitudinal assessment of peri-implant bone change; method and validation. Adv Dent Res 7:196–201.

Jeffcoat MK, Chung Wang I, Reddy M (1995). Radiographic diagnosis in periodontics. Periodontol 2000 7:54–68.

Jeffcoat MK, Geurs NC, Reddy MS, Goldenberg RL, Hauth JC (2001). Current evidence regarding periodontal disease as a risk factor in preterm birth. Ann Periodontol 6:183–188.

Jenkins GN, Krebsbach P (1985). Experimental study of the migration of charcoal particles in the human mouth. Arch Oral Biol 30:697–699.

Jenkins WM, Kinane DF (1989). The "high risk" group in periodontitis. Br Dent J 167:168–171.

Jin LJ, Söder P, Åsman B, Söder B, Bergström K (1995a). Granulocyte elastase in gingival crevicular fluid: Improved monitoring of the site-specific response to treatment in patients with destructive periodontitis. J Clin Periodontol 22:240–246.

Jin LJ, Söder P, Åsman B, Söder B, Puriene A, Bergström K (1995b). Variations in crevicular fluid elastase levels in periodontitis patients on long-term maintenance. Eur J Oral Sci 103:84–89.

Johnson NW (1989). Detection of high-risk groups and individuals for periodontal diseases. Int Dent J 39:33–47.

Johnson NW (ed) (1991a). Risk Markers for Oral Diseases. Vol 3: Periodontal diseases. Cambridge, NY: Cambridge UP.

Johnson NW (1991b). Introduction: Current concepts of the nature and the natural history of the periodontal diseases and the need for disease markers. In: Johnson NW (ed). Risk Markers for Oral Diseases. Vol 3: Periodontal diseases. Cambridge, NY: Cambridge UP: 1–5.

Johnson V, Johnson BD, Sims T, Whitney C, Moncla B, Engel L (1993). Effects of treatment on antibody titer to *Porphyromonas gingivalis* in gingival crevicular fluid of patients with rapidly progressive periodontitis. J Periodontol 64:559–565.

Johnson NW (1994). Risk factors and diagnostic tests for destructive periodontitis. In: Lang N, Karring T (eds). Proceedings of the 1st European Workshop on Periodontics, 1993. London: Quintessence: 90.

Johnson NW, Curtis M (1994). Preventive therapy for periodontal diseases. Adv Dent Res 8:337–348.

Johnson GK, Slach NA (2001). Impact of tobacco use on periodontal status. J Dent Educ 65:313–321.

Jones CL, Saxton C, Ritchie J (1990). Microbiological and clinical effects of a dentifrice containing zinc citrate and triclosan in the human experimental gingivitis model. J Clin Periodontol 17:570–574.

Joshi N, O'Bryan T, Appelbaum PC (1991). Pleuropulmonary infections caused by *Eikenella corrodens*. Rev Infect Dis 13:1207–1212.

Joshipura KJ, Rimm EB, Douglass CW, Trichpoulos D, Ascherio A, Willet WC (1996). Poor oral health and coronary heart disease. J Dent Res 75:1631–1636.

Joshipura KJ, Douglass C, Willett W (1998). Possible explanations for the tooth loss and cardiovascular disease relationship. Ann Periodontol 3:175–183.

Jotikastihira NE, Lie T, Leknes KN (1992). Comparative in vitro studies of sonic, ultrasonic and reciprocating scaling instruments. J Clin Periodontol 19:560–569.

Kaldahl WB, Kalkwarf KL, Patil KD, Molvar MP (1990). Relationship of gingival bleeding, gingival suppuration and supragingival plaque to attachment loss. J Periodontol 61:347–351.

Kaldahl W, Johnson G, Patil K, Kalkwarf K (1996). Levels of cigarette consumption and response to periodontal therapy. J Periodontol 67:675–681.

Källestål C, Matsson L (1990). Periodontal conditions in a group of Swedish adolescents. II. Analysis of data. J Clin Periodontol 17:609–612.

Källestål C, Matsson L, Holm A-K (1990). Periodontal conditions in a group of Swedish adolescents (I). A descriptive epidemiologic study. J Clin Periodontol 17:601–608.

Kalra J, Chandhary A, Prasad K (1991). Increased production of oxygen free radicals in cigarette smokers. Int J Exp Pathol 72:1–7.

Karayannis A, Lang N, Joss A, Nyman S (1991). Bleeding on probing as it relates to probing pressures and gingival health in patients with a reduced but healthy periodontium. A clinical study. J Clin Periodontol 19:471–475.

Katz P, Wirthlin M, Szpunar S, et al (1991). Epidemiology and prevention of periodontal diseases in individuals with diabetes. Diabetes Care 14:375–385.

Kaye D (1994). Infective endocarditis. In: Isselbacher KJ, Braunwald E, Wilson JD, Martin JB, Fauci AS, Kasper DL (eds). Harrison´s Principles of Internal Medicine, ed 13. New York: McGraw-Hill: 520–526.

Keagle JG, Garnick JJ, Searle JR, King Ge, Morse PK (1989). Gingival resistance to probing forces. I. Determination of optimal diameter. J Periodontol 60:167–171.

Kenney EB, Kraal J, Saxe S, Jones J (1977). The effect of cigarette smoke on human oral polymorphonuclear leukocytes. J Periodontal Res 12:227–234.

Kerdvongbundit V, Wikesjö UM (2000). Effect of smoking on periodontal health in molar teeth. J Periodontol 71:433–437.

Keszthelyi G, Szabo I (1984). Influence of class II amalgam fillings on attachment loss. J Clin Periodontol 11:81–86.

Keyes PH, Rams T (1983). A rationale for management of periodontal diseases: rapid identification of microbial "theraputic targets" with phase-contrast microscopy. J Am Dent Assoc 106:803–812.

Kieser JB (1994). Non-surgical periodontal therapy. In: Lang NP, Karring T (eds). Proceedings of the 1st European Workshop on Periodontics, 1993. London: Quintessence: 131–158.

Kinane D, Lindhe J (1997). Pathogenesis of periodontitis. In: Lindhe J, Karring T, Lang N (eds). Clinical Periodontology and Implant Dentistry, ed 3. Copenhagen: Munksgaard: 189–225.

Kinane D (1998a). The role of interdental cleaning in effective plaque control (need for interdental cleaning in primary and secondary prevention). In: Lang NP, Attström R, Löe H (eds). Proceedings of the European Workshop on Mechanical Plaque Control. Berlin: Quintessence: 156–168.

Kinane D (1998b). Periodontal diseases' contributions to cardiovascular disease: an overview of potential mechanisms. Ann Periodontol 3:142–150.

Kinane D (1999). Periodontits modified by systemic factors. Ann Periodontol 4:54–63.

Kinane DF (2000). Genetic influences in the pathogenesis of destructive periodontal diseases and diagnostic implications. J Parodontol Implantol Orale 19:117–139.

Kirstein M, Aston C, Hintz R, Vlassara H (1992). Receptor-specific induction of insulin-like growth factor 1 in human monocytes by advanced glycosylation end product-modified proteins. J Clin Invest 90:439–446.

Kjersem H, Hilsted J, Madsbad S, Wandall JH, Johansen KS, Borregaard N (1988). Polymorphonuclear leucocyte dysfunction during short-term matabolic changes from normo- to hyperglycemia in type 1 (insulin dependent) diabetic patients. Infection 16:215–221.

Koch R (1884). Erste Konferenz zur Erörterung der Cholerafrage. Berl Klin Wochenschrift 30:20–49.

Köhler B, Andréen I, Jonsson B (1984). The effect of caries preventive measures in mothers on dental caries and the oral presence of the bacteria *Streptococcus mutans* and lactobacilli in their children. Arch Oral Biol 29:879–883.

Kois JC (1996). The restorative-periodontal interface: Biological parameters. Periodontol 2000 11:29–38.

Kolltveit KM, Eriksen HM (2001). Is the observed association between periodontitis and atherosclerosis causal? Eur J Oral Sci 109:2–7.

Komiya A, Kato T, Nakagawa T, et al (2000). A rapid DNA probe method for detection of *Porphyromonas gingivalis* and *Actinobacillus actinomycetemcomitans.* J Periodontol 71:760–767.

Kornman KS, Robertson PB (1985). Clinical and microbiological evaluation of therapy for juvenile periodontitis. J Periodontol 56:443–446.

Kornman KS, Löe H (1993). The role of local factors in the etiology of periodontal diseases. Periodontol 2000 2:83–97.

Kornman KS, Crane A, Wang H-Y, et al (1997a). The interleukin-1 genotype as a severity factor in adult periodontal disease. J Clin Periodontol 24:72–77.

Kornman KS, Page R, Tonetti M (1997b). The host response to the microbial challenge in periodontitis: assembling the players. Periodontol 2000 14:33–53.

Kornman KS, di Giovine F (1998). Genetic variations in cytokine expression: A risk factor for severity of adult periodontitis. Ann Periodontol 3:327–338.

Kornman KS, Pankow J, Offenbacher S, Beck J, di Giovine F, Duff GW (1999). Interleukin-1 genotypes and the association between periodontitis and cardiovascular disease. J Periodontal Res 34:353–357.

Kornman KS, Duff GW (2001). Candidate genes as potential links between periodontal and cardiovascular diseases. Ann Periodontol 6:48–57.

Kozai K, Wand D, Sandham J, Phillips H (1991). Changes in strains of mutans streptococci induced by treatment with chlorhexidine varnish. J Dent Res 70:1252–1257.

Kraal JH, Chancellor M, Bridges R, et al (1977). Variations in the gingival polymorphonuclear leukocyte migration rate induced by tobacco smoke. J Periodontal Res 12:242–249.

Krall EA, Dawson-Hughes B, Garvey A, Garcia R (1997). Smoking, smoking cessation and tooth loss. J Dent Res 76:1653–1659.

Krall EA, Garvey AJ, Garcia RI (1999). Alveolar bone loss and tooth loss in male cigar and pipe smokers. J Am Dent Assoc 130:57–64.

Krane S (1983). Hereditable diseases of connective tissue. In: Wagner B, Fleischmajer R, Kaufman N. Connective Tissue Diseases. Baltimore: Williams & Wilkins.

Kronauer E, Borsa G, Lang N (1986). Prevalence of incipient juvenile periodontitis at age 16 years in Switzerland. J Clin Periodontol 13:103–108.

Kryshtalskyj E, Sodek J, Ferrier JM (1986). Correlation of collagenoltic enzymes an inhibitors in gingival crevicular fluid with clinical and microscopic changes in experimental periodontitis in the dog. Arch Oral Biol 31:21–31.

Kung RT, Ochs B, Goodson JM (1990). Temperature as a periodontal diagnostic. J Clin Periodontol 17:557–563.

Kuramitsu HK, Qi M, Kang I, Chen W (2001). Role for periodontal bacteria in cardiovascular diseases. Ann Periodontol 6:41–47.

Kurer JR, Watts T, Weinman J, Gower D (1995). Psychological mood of regular dental attenders in relation to otal hygiene behaviour and gingival health. J Clin Periodontol 22:52–55.

Kuusela S, Honkala E, Kannas L, Tynjala J, Wold B (1997). Oral hygiene habits of 11-year-olds in 22 European countries and Canada in 1993-94. J Dent Res 76:1602–1609.

Kweider M, Lowe G, Murray G, Kinane D, McGowen D (1993). Dental disease, fibrinogen and white cell count: Links with myocardial infarction? Scott Med J 38:73–74.

LaCassin F, Hoen B, Leport C, et al (1995). Procedures associated with infective endocarditis in adults. A case control study. Eur Heart J 16:1968–1974.

Ladner J, Lin P, Beck F, Mitchell J, Horton J (1992). An SEM study of root surfaces following planing by hand and two distinct types of ultrasonic instruments [abstract]. J Dent Res 71(special issue):224.

Lai C-H, Listgarten M, Shirakawa M, Slots J (1987). *Bacteroides forsythus* in adult gingivitis and periodontitis. Oral Microbiol Immunol 2:152–157.

Lai C-H, Oshima K, Slots J, Listgarten M (1992). Wolinella recta in adult gingivitis and periodontitis. J Periodontal Res 27:8–14.

Lalla E, Lamster IB, Schmidt AM (1998). Enhanced interaction of advanced glycation end products with their cellular receptor RAGE: Implications for the pathogenesis of accelerated periodontal disease in diabetes. Ann Periodontol 3:13–19.

Lalla E, Lamster IB, Feit M, et al (2000). Blockade of RAGE suppresses periodontitis-associated bone loss in diabetic mice. J Clin Invest 105:1117–1124.

Lamont R, Chan A, Belton C, Izutsu K, Vasel D, Weinberg A (1995). *Porphyromonas gingivalis* invasion of gingival epithelial cells. Infect Immun 63:3878–3885.

Lamster IB, Oshrain R, Harper D, Celenti R, Hovliaras C, Gordon J (1988). Enzyme activity in crevicular fluid for detection and prediction of clinical attachment loss in patients with chronic adult periodontitis: 6 month results. J Periodontol 59:516–523.

Lamster IB (1991). Host-derived enzyme activities in gingival crevicular fluid as markers of periodontal disease susceptibility and activity: Historical perspective, biological significance and clinical implications. In: Johnson NW (ed). Risk Markers for Oral Diseases. Vol 3. Periodontal diseases. Cambridge, NY: Cambridge Press: 277.

Lamster IB, Smith QT, Celenti RS, Singer RE, Grbic JT (1994a). Development of a risk profile for periodontal disease: Microbial and host response factors. J Periodontol 65(5, suppl):511–520.

Lamster IB, Holmes LG, William Gross KB, et al (1994b). The relationship of β-glucuronidase activity in crevicular fluid to clinical parameters of periodontal disease. Findings from a multicenter study. J Clin Periodontol 21:118–127.

Lamster IB, Grbic JT (1995). Diagnosis of periodontal disease based on analysis of the host response. Periodontol 2000 7:83–99.

Lamster IB, Holmes L, William Gross K (1995a). The relationship of beta-glucuronidase activity in crevicular fluid to probing attachment loss in patients with adult periodontitis. Findings from a multicenter study. J Clin Periodontol 22:36–44.

Lamster IB, Grbic J, Fine J, et al (1995b). A critical review of periodontal disease as a manifestation of HIV infection. In: Greenspan J, Greenspan D (eds). Oral manifestation of HIV Infection [Proceedings of the 2nd international workshop on the oral manifestation of HIV infection, Jan 31-Feb 3 1993, San Fransisco, CA]. Chicago: Quintessence: 247–256.

Lamster IB (1997). Evaluation of components of gingival crevicular fluid as diagnostic tests. Ann Periodontol 2:123–137.

Lamster IB, Grbic JT, Bucklan RS, Mitchell-Lewis D, Reynolds HS, Zambon JJ (1997). Epidemiology and diagnosis of HIV-associated periodontal diseases. Oral Dis 3 (suppl 1):S141–S148.

Lamster IB, Grbic JT, Mitchell-Lewis DA, Begg MD, Mitchell A (1998). New concepts regarding the pathogenesis of periodontal disease in HIV infection. Ann Periodontol 3:62–75.

Lamster IB, Lalla E (2001). Periodontal disease and diabetes mellitus: Discussion, conclusions, and recommendations. Ann Periodontol 6:146–149.

Lang NP, Cumming BR, Löe H (1973). Toothbrushing frequency as it relates to plaque development and gingival health. J Periodontol 7:396–405.

Lang NP, Hill RG (1977). Radiographs in periodontics. J Clin Periodontol 4:16–28.

Lang NP, Cumming B, Löe H (1977). Oral hygiene and gingival health in Danish dental students and faculty. Community Dent Oral Epidemiol 5:237–242.

Lang NP, Joss A, Orsanic T, Gusberti FA, Siegrist BE (1986). Bleeding on probing. A predictor for the progression of periodontal disease? J Clin Periodontol 13:590–596.

Lang NP, Nyman S, Adler R, Joss A (1990). Absence of bleeding on probing—A predictor for periodontal health. J Clin Periodontol 17:714–721.

Lang NP (1991). Clinical markers of active periodontal disease. In: Johnson NW (ed). Risk Markers for Oral Diseases. Vol 3: Periodontal disease. Cambridge, NY: Cambridge UP: 179–202.

Lang NP, Nyman S, Senn C, Joss A (1991). Bleeding on probing as it relates to probing pressure and gingival health. J Clin Periodontol 18:257–261.

Lang NP, Karring T (1994). Proceedings of the 1st European Workshop on Periodontics, 1993. London: Quintessence.

Lang NP, Mombelli A, Attström R (1997). Dental plaque and calculus. In: Lindhe J, Karring T, Lang N, (eds). Clinical Periodontology and Implant Dentistry. Copenhagen: Munksgaard: 102–137.

Lang NP (1998). Commonly used indices to assess oral hygiene and gingival and periodontal health and diseases. In: Lang NP, Attström R, Löe H (eds). Proceedings of the European Workshop on Mechanical Plaque Control. Berlin: Quintessence: 50–71.

Lannan S, Mc Lean A, Drost E, et al (1992). Changes in neutrophil morphology and morphometry following exposure to cigarette smoke. Int J Exp Pathol 73:183–191.

Larivee J, Sodek J, Ferrier JM (1986). Collagenase and collagenase inhibitor activities in crevicular fluid of patients receiving treatment for localized juvenile periodontitis. J Periodontal Res 21:702–715.

Lavstedt S, Bolin A, Henriksson C, Carstensen J (1986). Proximal alveolar bone loss in a longitudinal radiographic investigation. I. Methods of measurement and partial recording. Acta Odontol Scand 44:149–157.

Lee W, Aitken S, Kulkarni G, et al (1991). Collagenase activity in recurrent periodontitis: relationship to disease progression and doxycylline therapy. J Periodontal Res 26:479–485.

Leeper SH, Kalkwarf KL, Strom EA (1985). Oral status of "controlled" adolescent type 1 diabetics. J Oral Med 40:127–133.

Leknes KN, Lie T, Wikesjö UME, Bogle GC, Selvig KA (1994). Influence of tooth instrumentation roughness on subgingival colonization. J Periodontol 65:303–308.

Leknes KN (1997). The influence of anatomic and iatrogenic root surface characteristics on bacterial colonization and periodontal destruction: A review. J Periodontol 68:507–516.

Leonhardt Å, Bergenlundh T, Ericsson I, Dahlén G (1992). Putative periodontal pathogens on titanium implants and teeth in experimental gingivitis and periodontitis in beagle dogs. Clin Oral Implants Res 3:112–119.

Leonhardt Å, Olsson J, Dahlén G (1995). Bacterial colonization on titanium, hydroxyapatite and amalgam surfaces in vivo. J Dent Res 74:1607–1612.

Leonhardt Å, Renvert S, Dahlén G (1999). Microbial findings at failing implants. Clin Oral Implants Res 10:339–345.

Levy SM, Heckert D, Beck J, Kohaut F (1987). Multivariate correlates of periodontally healthy teeth in an elderly population. Gerodontics 3:85–88.

Libby P, Egan D, Skarlatos S (1997). Role of infectious agents in atherosclerosis and restenosis: an assessment of the evidence and need for future research. Circulation 96:4095–4103.

Lie T, Meyer K (1977). Calculus removal and loss of tooth substance in response to different periodontal instruments. A scanning electron microscope study. J Clin Periodontol 4:250–262.

Lie T (1978). Ultrastructural study of early dental plaque formation. J Periodontal Res 13:391–409.

Lie T, Leknes KN (1985). Evaluation of the effect on root surfaces of air rubine scalers and ultrasonic instrumentation. J Periodontol 56:522–531.

Lien Y-H, Stern R, Fu J, Siegel R (1984). Inhibition of collagen fibril formation in vitro and subsequent cross-linking by glucose. Science 225:1489–1491.

Lindén GJ, Mullally B (1994). Cigarette smoking and periodontal destruction in young adults. J Periodontol 65:718–723.

Lindhe J, Nyman S (1975). The effect of plaque control and surgical pocket elimination on the establishment and maintenance of periodontal health. A longitudinal study of periodontal therapy in cases of advanced disease. J Clin Periodontol 2:67–79.

Lindhe J, Rylander H (1975). Experimental gingivitis in young dogs. Scand J Dent Res 83:314–326.

Lindhe J, Hamp SE, Löe H (1975). Plaque-induced periodontal disease in beagle dogs. J Periodontal Res 10:243–255.

Lindhe J, Ericsson I (1976). The influence of trauma from occlusion on reduced but healthy periodontal tissues in dogs. J Clin Periodontol 3:110–122.

Lindhe J, Haffajee AD, Socransky SS (1983). Progression of periodontal disease in adult subjects in the absence of periodontal therapy. J Clin Periodontol 10:433–442.

Lindhe J, Nyman S (1984). Long-term maintenance of patients treated for advanced periodontal disease. J Clin Periodontol 11:504–514.

Lindhe J, Okamoto H, Yoneyama T, Haffajee A, Socransky SS (1989a). Longitudinal changes in periodontal disease in untreated subjects. J Clin Periodontol 16:662–670.

Lindhe J, Okamoto H, Yoneyama T, Haffajee A, Socransky SS (1989b). Periodontal loser sites in untreated adult subjects. J Clin Periodontol 16:671–678.

Lindhe J, Karring T, Lang NP (1997). Clinical Periodontology and Implants in Dentistry. Copenhagen: Munksgaard.

Lindquist B, Emilson C, Wennerholm K (1989). Relationship between mutans streptococci in saliva and their colonization of tooth surfaces. Oral Microbiol Immunol 4:71–76.

Lindskog S, Blomlöf L (1983). Cementum hypoplasia in teeth affected by juvenile periodontitis. J Clin Periodontol 13:748–751.

Lindskog S, Blomlöf L (1992). Mineralized tissue-formation in periodontal wound healing. J Clin Periodontol 19:741–748.

Lindskog S, Blomlöf L, Håkanson H (1994). Differential periodontal temperature measurements in the assessment of periodontal disease activity: An experimental and clinical study. Scand J Dent Res 102:10–16.

Ling TY, Sims TJ, Chen H, et al (1993). Titer and subclass distribution of serum IgG antibody reactive with Actinobacillus actinomycetemcomitans in localized juvenile periodontitis. J Clin Immunol 13:100–111.

Lippke J, Peros W, Keville M, Savitt E, French C (1991). DNA probe detection of Eikenella corrodens, Wolinella recta and Fusobacterium nucleatum in subgingival plaque. Oral Microbiol Immunol 6:81–87.

Lissau I, Holst D, Friis-Hasche E (1990). Dental health behaviors and periodontal disease indicators in Danish youths. A 10-year epidemiological follow-up. J Clin Periodontol 17:42–47.

Listgarten MA, Socransky S (1964). Ultrastructural characteristics of a spirochete in the lesion of acute necrotizing ulcerative gingivostomatitis (Vincent´s infection). Arch Oral Biol 9:95–96.

Listgarten MA (1965). Electron microscopic observations of the bacterial flora of acute necrotizing gingivitis. J Periodontol 36:325–339.

Listgarten MA, Mayo H, Tremblay R (1975). Development of dental plaque on epoxy resin crowns in man. A light and electron microscopic study. J Periodontol 46:10–26.

Listgarten MA (1976). Structure of the microbial flora associated with periodontal health and disease in man. A light and electron microscopic study. J Periodontol 47:1–18.

Listgarten MA, Helldén L (1978). Relative distribution of bacteria at clinically healthy and periodontally diseased sites in humans. J Clin Periodontol 5:115–132.

Listgarten MA, Lindhe J, Helldén L (1978). Effects of tetracycline and/or scaling on human periodontal disease. Clinical, microbiological and histological observations. J Clin Periodontol 5:246–271.

Listgarten MA, Levin S (1981). Positive correlation between the proportions of subgingival spirochetes and motiel bacteria and susceptibility of human subjects to periodontal deterioration. J Clin Periodontol 8:122–138.

Listgarten M (1992). Microbiological testing in the diagnosis of periodontal disease. J Periodontol 63:332–337.

Listgarten MA, Lai CH, Young V (1993). Microbial composition and pattern of antibiotic resistance in subgingival microbial samples from patients with refractory periodontitis. J Periodontol 64:155–161.

Listgarten MA (1994). The structure of dental plaque. Periodontol 2000 5:52–65.

Locker D, Leake J, Hamilton M, Hicks T, Lee J, Main P (1991). The oral health status of older adults in four Ontario communities. J Can Dent Assoc 57:727–732.

Locker D, Leake JL (1993a). Periodontal attachment loss in independently living older adults in Ontario, Canada. J Public Health Dent 53:6–11.

Locker D, Leake JL (1993b). Risk indicators and risk markers for periodontal disease experience in older adults living independently in Ontario, Canada. J Dent Res 72:9–17.

Locker D, Ford J, Leake JL (1996). Incidence of and risk factors for tooth loss in a population of older Canadians. J Dent Res 75:783–789.

Löe H, Silness J (1963). Periodontal disease in pregnancy. I. Prevalence and severity. Acta Odontol Scand 21:533–551.

Löe H, Theilade E, Jensen SB (1965). Experimental gingivitis in man. J Periodontol 36:177–187.

Löe H (1967). The Gingival Index, the Plaque Index and the Retention Index System. J Periodontol 38:610–616.

Löe H, Ånerud Å, Boysen H, Smith M (1978). The natural history of periodontal disease in man. The rate of periodontal destruction before 40 years of age. J Periodontol 49:607–620.

Löe H, Anerud Å, Boysen H (1986). Natural history of periodontal disease in man: rapid, moderate and no loss of attachment in Sri Lankan laborers 14–46 years of age. J Clin Periodontol 13:431–440.

Löe H, Brown L (1991). Early-onset periodontitis in the USA. J Periodontol 62:608–616.

Löe H (1994). People at risk for periodontitis—Approach the year 2000. J Periodontol 65:464–467.

Loesche WJ (1976). Chemotherapy of dental plaque infections. Oral Sci Rev 9:65–107.

Loesche WJ, Syed SA (1978). Bacteriology of human experimental gingivitis: Effect of plaque and gingivitis score. Infect Immun 21:830–839.

Loesche WJ, Syed S, Laughon B, Stoll J (1982). The bacteriology of acute necrotizing ulcerative gingivitis. J Periodontol 53:223–230.

Loesche WJ, Gusberti F, Mettraux GR, Higgins T, Syed S (1983). Relationship between oxygen tension and subgingival bacterial flora in untreated human periodontal pockets. Infect Immun 42:659–667.

Loesche WJ, Syed S, Schmidt E, Morrison E (1985). Bacterial profiles of subgingival plaques in periodontitis. J Periodontol 56:447–456.

Loesche WJ, Lopatin DE, Giordano J, Alcoforado G, Hujoel P (1992). Comparison of the benzozyl-DL-arginine naphthylamide (BANA) test, DNA probes, and immunological reagents for ability to detect anaerobic periodontal infections due to *Porphyromonas gingivalis, Treponema denticola,* and *Bacteroides forsythus.* J Clin Microbiol 30:427–433.

Loesche WJ (1994). Periodontal disease as a risk factor for heart disease. Compend Contin Educ Dent 15:976–991.

Loesche WJ (1997). Association of the oral flora with important medical diseases. Curr Opin Periodontol 4:21–28.

Loesche WJ, Shork A, Terpenning MS, Chen YM, Domiguez L, Grossman N (1998a). Assessing the relationship between dental disease and coronary heart disease in elderly US veterans. J Am Dent Assoc 129:301–311.

Loesche WJ, Shork A, Terpenning MS, et al (1998b). The relationship between dental disease and cerebral vascular accident in elderly United States veterans. Ann Periodontol 3:161–174.

Loesche WJ (2000). Periodontal disease: Link to cardiovascular disease. Compendium 21:463–482.

Loos B, Claffey N, Egelberg J (1988). Clinical and microbiological effects of root debridement in periodontal furcation pockets. J Clin Periodontol 15:453–463.

Loos B, Nyland K, Claffey N, Egelberg J (1989). Clinical effects of root dibridement in molar and nonmolar teeth: a 2-year follow-up. J Clin Periodontol 16:498–504.

Loos B, Mayrand D, Genco R, Dickinson D (1990). Genetic heterogenety of *Porphyromonas (Bacteroides) gingivalis* by genomic DNA fingerprinting. J Dent Res 69:1488–1493.

Loos B, van Winkelhoff A, Dunford R, et al (1992). A statistical approach to the ecology of *Porphyromonas gingivalis.* J Dent Res 71:353–358.

Lopatin D, Blackburn E (1992). Avidity and titer of immunoglobulin G subclasses to *Porphyromonas gingivalis* in adult periodontitis patients. Oral Microbiol Immunol 7:332–337.

Lorenz KA, Weiss PJ (1994). Capnocytophagal pneumonia in a healthy man (letter). West J Med 160:79–80.

Lövdal A, Arno A, Schei O, Waerhaug J (1961). Combined effect of subgingival scaling and controlled oral hygiene on the incidence of gingivitis. Acta Odontol Scand 19:537–555.

Lowe GD (1998). Etiopathogenesis of cardiovascular disease: Hemostasis, thrombosis, and vascular medicine. Ann Periodontol 3:121–126.

Lowe GD (2001). The relationship between infection, inflammation, and cardiovascular disease: An overview. Ann Periodontol 6:1–8.

Lynch M, Jandinski J, Fenesey K, Murray P (1991). Crevicular fluid interleukin-1β levels in HIV-associated periodontal disease [abstract]. J Dent Res 70:1208.

MacFarlane GD, Herzberg MC, Wolff LF, Hardie NA (1992). Refractory periodontitis associated with abnormal polymorphonuclear leucocyte phagocytosis and cigarette smoking. J Periodontol 63:908–913.

Machtei EE, Dunford R, Hausmann E, et al (1997). Longitudinal study of prognostic factors in established periodontitis patients. J Clin Periodontol 24:102–109.

Madianos PN, Papapanou P, Nannmark U, Dahlén G, Sandros J (1996). *Porphyromonas gingivalis* FDC381 multiplies and persists within human oral epithelial cells in vitro. Infect Immun 64:660–664.

Madianos PN (1997). Interactions of *Porphyromonas gingivalis* with oral epithelial cells [thesis]. Göteborg, Sweden: Göteborg University.

Madianos PN, Papapanou P, Sandros J (1997). *Pophyromonas gingivalis* infection of oral epithelium inhibits neutrophil transepithelial migration. Infect Immun 65:3983–3990.

Madianos PN, Lieff S, Murtha AP, et al (2001). Maternal periodontitis and prematurity. Part II: Maternal infection and fetal exposure. Ann Periodontol 6:175–182.

Magnusson I, Lindhe J, Yoneyama T, Liljenberg B (1984). Recolonization of a subgingival microbiota following scaling in deep pockets. J Clin Periodontol 11:193–207.

Mahanonda R, Seymour G, Powell L, Good M, Halliday J (1991). Effect of initial treatment of chronic inflammatory periodontal disease on the frequency of peripheral blood T-lymphocytes specific to periodontopathic bacteria. Oral Microbiol Immunol 6:221–227.

Mandel ID (1991). Markers of periodontal disease susceptibility and activity derived from saliva. In: Johnson NW (ed). Risk Markers for Oral Diseases. Vol 3: Periodontal diseases. Cambridge, NY: Cambridge UP: 228–253.

Mandell RL, Socransky SS (1981). A selective medium for *Actinobacillus actinomycetemcomitans* and the incidence of the organism in juvenile periodontitis. J Periodontol 52:593–598.

Mandell RL (1984). A longitudinal microbiological investigation of *Actinobacillus actinomycetemcomitans* and *Eikenella corrodens* in juvenile periodontitis. Infect Immun 45:778–780.

Mandell RL, Tripodi L, Savitt E, Goodson J, Socransky SS (1986). The effect of treatment on *Actinobacillus actinomycetemcomitans* in localized juvenile periodontitis. J Periodontol 57:94–99.

Mandell RL, Ebersole J, Socransky SS (1987). Clinical immunologic and microbiologic features of active disease sites in juvenile periodontitis. J Clin Periodontol 14:534–540.

Mandell RL, Di Rienzo J, Kent R, Joshipura K, Haber J (1992). Microbiology of healthy and diseased periodontal sites in poorly controlled insulin-dependent diabetics. J Periodontol 63:274–279.

Marazita ML, Burmaster JA, Gunsolley JC, Koertge TE, Lake K, Schenkein HA (1994). Evidence for autosomal dominant inheritance and race-specific heterogenity in early-onset periodontitis. J Periodontol 65: 623–630.

Marazita ML, Lu H, Cooper M, et al (1996). Genetic segregation analyses of serum IgG2 levels. Am J Hum Genet 58:1042–1049.

Marcenes WS, Sheiham A (1992). The relationship between work stress and oral health status. Soc Sci Med 35:1511–1520.

References

Marcum JS (1967). The effect of crown margin depth upon gingival tissues. J Prosthet Dent 17:479.

Marcus AJ, Hajjar DP (1993). Vascular transcellular signaling. J Lipid Res 34:2017–2031.

Markkanen H, Paunio K, Tiekso J (1985). Regional differences and some background factors in relation to periodontal health in the Finnish population aged 30 years and over. Proc Finn Dent Soc 81:192–198.

Mariotti A (1999). Dental plaque-induced gingival diseases. Ann Periodontol 4:7–17.

Marsh PD (1989). Host defenses and microbial homeostasis: Role of microbial interactions. J Dent Res 68:1567–1575.

Marsh PD (1991). Sugar, fluoride, pH and microbia homeostasis in dental plaque. Proc Finn Dent Soc 87:515–525.

Marsh PD (1992). Microbiological aspects of the chemical control of plaque and gingivitis. J Dent Res 71:1431–1438.

Marsh PD (1994). Microbial ecology of dental plaque and its significance in health and disease. Adv Dent Res 8:263–271.

Martinez-Canut P, Lorca A, Magán R (1995). Smoking and periodontal disease severity. J Clin Periodontol 22:743–749.

Masada MP, Persson R, Kenny JS, Lee SW, Page RC, Allison AC (1990). Measurement of interleukin-1α and -1β in gingival crevicular fluid: Implications for the pathogenesis of periodontal disease. J Periodontal Res 25:156–163.

Mashimo PA, Yamamoto Y, Slots J, Park BH, Genco RJ (1983). The periodontal microflora of juvenile diabetics. Culture, immunofluorescence and serum antibody studies. J Periodontol 54:420–430.

Massler M, Ludwick W (1952). Relation of dental caries experience and gingivitis to cigarette smoking in males 17 to 21 years old. J Dent Res 31:319–322.

Matia JI, Bissada, NF, Maybury JE, Richetti P (1986). Efficiency of scaling of the molar furcation area with and without surgical access. Int J Periodontics Restorative Dent 6:25–35.

Mattila K, Nieminen M, Valtonen V, et al (1989). Association between dental health and acute myocardial infarction. Br Med J 298:779–782.

Mattila K (1993). Dental infections as a risk factor for acute myocardial infarction. Eur Heart J 14:51–53.

Mattila K, Valle M, Nieminen M, Valtonen V, Hietaniemi K (1993). Dental infections and coronary atherosclerosis. Arteriosclerosis 103:205–211.

McDermid AS, McKee AS, Marsh PD (1990). Interactions and pH optimal for growth of three black-pigmented *Bacteroides* species 8 [abstract]. J Dent Res 69:999.

McDonald HM, O'Loughlin JA, Jolley P, Vigneswaren R, McDonald PJ (1991). Vaginal infection and preterm labor. Br J Obstet Gynaecol 98:427–435.

McDonald HM, O'Loughlin JA, Jolley P, Vigneswaren R, McDonald PJ (1992). Prenatal microbiological risk factors associated wth preterm birth. Br J Obstet Gynaecol 99:190–196.

McFall WT (1982). Tooth loss in 100 treated patients with perodontal disease. J Periodontol 53:539–549.

McFall WT, Bader J, Rozier R, Ramsey D (1988). Presence of periodontal data in patient records of general practitioners. J Periodontol 59:445–449.

McGlynn FD, Gale E, Glaros A, LeResche L, Massoth DL, Weiffenbach JM (1990). Biobehavioral research in dentistry: some directions for the 1990s. Ann Behav Med 12:133–140.

McGuire JR, McQuade MJ, Rossmann JA, et al (1989). Cotininen in saliva and gingival crevicular fluid of smokers with periodontal disease. J Periodontol 60:176–181.

McGuire JR, Nunn ME (1999). Prognosis versus actual outcome. IV. The effectiveness of clinical parameters and IL-1 genotype in accurately predicting prognoses and tooth survival. J Periodontol 70:49–50.

McKaig RG, Patton LL, Thomas JC, Strauss RP, Slade GD, Beck JD (2000). Factors associated with periodontitis in an HIV-infected southeast USA study. Oral Dis 6:158–165.

McMullen J, Van Dyke T. Horoszewicz H, Genco R (1981). Neutrophil chemotaxis in individuals with advanced periodontal disease and a genetic predisposition to diabetes mellitus. J Periodontol 52:167–173.

Mealy B (2000). Diabetes and periodontal diseases. J Periodontol 71:664–678.

Ménard C, Mouton C (1995). Clonal diversity of the taxon *Porphyromonas gingivalis* assessed by random amplified polymorphic DNA fingerprinting. Infec Immun 63:2522–2531.

Mendez MV, Scott T, Lamorte W, Vokonas P, Menzoian JO, Garcia R (1998). Chronic inflammatory diseases are associated with peripheral vascualr disease. Am J Surg 176:153–157.

Meng HX (1999). Periodontal abscesses. Ann Periodontol 4:79–82.

Mengel R, Buns C, Steizel M, Flores-de-Jacoby L (1994). An in vitro study of oscillating instruments for root planing . J Clin Periodontol 21:513–518.

Mettraux GR, Gusberti F, Graf H (1984). Oxygen tension (pO_2) in untreated human periodontal pockets. J Periodontol 55:516–521.

Meyer K, Lie T (1977). Root surface roughness in response to periodontal instrumentation studied by combined use of microroughness measurements and scanning electron microscopy. J Clin Peridontol 4:77–91.

Meyerov R, Lemmer J, Cleaton-Jones P, Volchansky A (1991). Temperature measurements in periodontal pockets. J Periodontol 62:95–99.

Michalowicz BS, Aeppli D, Virag JG, et al (1991a). Periodontal findings in adult twins. J Periodontol 62:293–299.

Michalowicz BS, Aeppli D, Kuba RK, et al (1991b). A twin study of gentic variation in proportional radiographic alveolar bone height. J Dent Res 70:1431–1435.

Michalowicz BS (1993). Genetic and inheritance considerations in periodontal disease. Curr Opin Periodontol 1:11–17.

Michalowicz BS (1994). People at risk for periodontitis—Genetic and heritable risk factors. J Periodontal Res 65:479–488.

Michalowicz BS, Ronderos M, Camara-Silva R, Contreras A, Slots J (2000). Human herpes viruses and Porphyromonas gingivalis are associated with juvenile periodontitis. J Periodontol 71:981–988.

Miller A, Brunelle J, Carlos J, et al (1987a). Oral health of US adults. National findings 1985-86 [NIH Publication No 87-2878]. Bethesda, MD: National Institute of Dental Research.

Miller A, Brunelle J, Carlos J, Brown L, Löe H (1987b). National Institute of Dental Research. Oral Health in United States Adults. National Findings. The National Survey of Oral Health in US Employed Adults and Seniors 1985-1986 [NIH Publication 87-2868]. Washington, DC: US Department of Health and Human Services.

Miyazaki H, Pilot T, Leclercq MH, Barmes D (1991a). Profiles of periodontal conditions in adolescents measured by CPITN. Int Dent J 41:67–73.

Miyazaki H, Pilot T, Leclercq MH, Barmes D (1991b) Profiles of periodontal conditions in adults, measured by CPITN. Int Dent J 41:74–80.

Modeer T, Lavstedt S, Ahlund C (1980). Relation between tobacco consumption and oral health in Swedish schoolchildren. Acta Odontol Scand 38:223–227.

Molenaar D, Palumbo P, Wilson W, Ritts Jr R (1976). Leukocyte chemotaxis in diabetic patients and their non-diabetic first-degree relatives. Diabetes 35:880–883.

Mombelli A, Nicopoulou-Karayianni K, Lang NP (1990). Local differences in the newly formed crevicular microbiota. Schweiz Monatsschr Zahnmed 100:154–158.

Mombelli A (1996). Microbiological monitoring. J Clin Periodontol 23:251–257.

Mombelli A (1998). The role of dental plaque in the initiation and progression of periodontal diseases. In: Lang NP, Attström R, Löe H (eds). Proceedings of the European Workshop on the Mechanical Plaque Control. Berlin: Quintessence: 85–97.

Mombelli A, Schmid B, Rutar A, Lang NP (2000). Persistence patterns of Porphyromonas gingivalis, Prevotella intermedia/nigrescens, and Actinobacillus actinomycetemcomitans after mechanical therapy of periodontal disease. J Periodontol 71:14–21.

Moncla B, Motley S, Braham P, Ewing L, Adams T, Vermeulen M (1991). Use of synthetic oligonucleotide DNA probes for identification and direct detection of Bacteroides forsythus in plaque samples. J Clin Microbiol 29:2158–2162.

Mongardini C, van Steenberghe D, Dekeyser C, Quirynen M (1999). One stage full- versus partial-mouth disinfection in the treatment of chronic adult or generalized early-onset periodontitis. I. Long-term clinical observations. J Periodontol 70:632–645.

Mooney J, Adonogianaki E, Kinane D (1993). Relative avidity of serum antibodies to putative periodontopathogens in periodontal disease. J Periodontal Res 28:444–450.

Moore W, Holdeman L, Smibert R, Hash D, Burmeister J, Ranney R (1982). Bacteriology of severe periodontitis in young adult humans. Infect Immun 38:1137–1148.

Moore W, Holdeman L, Cato E, Smibert R, Burmeister J, Ranney R (1983). Bacteriology of moderate (chronic) periodontitis in mature adult humans. Infect Immun 42:510–515.

Moore W, Holdeman L, Cato E, et al (1985). Comparative bacteriology of juvenile periodontitis. Infect Immun 48:507–519.

Moore J, Wilson M, Kieser JB (1986). The distribution of bacterial lipopolysacccharide (endotoxin) in relation to periodontally involved root surfaces. J Clin Periodontol 13:748–751.

Moore W (1987). Microbiology of periodontal disease. J Periodontal Res 22:335–341.

Moore L, Johnson J, Moore W (1987a). Selenomonas noxia sp nov, Selenomonas flueggei sp nov, Selenomonas dianae sp nov and Selenomonas artemidis sp nov from the human gingival crevice. Int J Syst Bacteriol 36:271–280.

Moore L, Moore W, Cato E, et al (1987b). Bacteriology of human gingivitis. J Dent Res 66:989–995.

Moore W, Moore L, Ranney R, Smibert R, Burmeister J, Schenkein H (1991). The microflora of periodontal sites showing active destructive progression. J Clin Periodontol 18:729–739.

References

Moore L, Moore W, Riley C, Brooks C, Burmeister J, Smibert R (1993). Periodontal microflora of HIV positive subjects with gingivitis or adult periodontitis. J Periodontol 64:48–56.

Moore W, Moore L (1994). The bacteria of periodontal diseases. Periodontol 2000 5:66–77.

Moore PA, Weyant RJ, Mongelluzzo MB, et al (1999). Type 1 diabetes mellitus and oral health: Assessment of periodontal disease. J Periodontol 70:409–417.

Morris J, Sewll D (1994). Necrotizing pneumonia caused by mixed infection with *Actinobacillus actinomycetemcomitans* and *Actinomyces israelii*: Case report and review. Clin Infect Dis 18:450–452.

Morrison HI, Ellison LF, Taylor GW (1999). Periodontal disease and risk of fatal coronary heart and cerebrovascular diseases. J Cardiovasc Risk 6:7–11.

Moss ME, Beck JD, Kaplan BH, et al (1996). Exploratory case-control analysis of psychosocial factors and adult periodontitis. J Periodontol 67(suppl 1):1060–1069.

Mowat AG, Baum J (1971). Chemotaxis of polymorphonuclear leukocytes from patients with diabetes mellitus. N Engl J Med 284:621–627.

Mueller-Heubach E, Rubenstein DN, Schwarz SS (1990). Histological chorioamnionitis and preterm delivery in different patient populations. Obstet Gynecol 75:622–626.

Mullally BH, Lindén GJ (1996). Molar furcation involvement associated with cigarette smoking in periodontal referrals. J Clin Periodontol 23:658–661.

Mullally B, Breen B, Linden G (1999). Smoking and patterns of bone loss in early-onset periodontitis. J Periodontol 70:394–401.

Murayama Y, Kurihara H, Nagai A, Dompkowski D, Van Dyke T (1994). Acute necrotizing ulcerative gingivitis: Risk factors involving host defense mechanisms. Periodontol 2000 6:116–124.

Murray PA, Winkler J, Sadowski L, et al (1988). Microbiology of HIV-associated gingivitis and periodontitis. In: Robertson P, Greenspan J (eds). Perspectives on Oral Manifestations of AIDS. Littleton: PSG: 105–118.

Murray JJ (1989). The Prevention of Dental Diseases, ed 2. London: Oxford UP.

Murray PA, Winkler J, Peros W, French C, Lippke J (1991). DNA probe detection of periodontal pathogens in HIV-associated periodontal lesions. Oral Microbiol Immunol 6:34–40.

Murray PA (1994). Periodontal diseases in patients infected by human immunodeficiency virus. Periodontol 2000 6:50–67.

Nakib NM, Bissada NF, Simmelink JW, Goldstine SN (1982). Endotoxin penetration into rott cementum of periodontally healthy and diseased human teeth. J Periodontol 53:368–378.

Navarro R, Corell P (1976). Plaque control in gingival hyperplasia secondary to dilantin therapy: Report of a case. J Oral Med 31:27–28.

Nazzarro V, Blanchet-Bardon C, Mimoz C, Revuz J, Puissant A (1988). Papillon-Lefevre syndrome. Ultrastructural study and successful treatment with acitretin. Arch Dermatol 124:533–539.

Nelson S, Hynd B, Pickrum H (1992). Automated enzyme immunoassay to measure prostaglandin E_2 in gingival crevicular fluid. J Periodontal Res 27:143–148.

Newman MG, Socransky S, Savitt E, Propas D, Crawford A (1976). Studies of the microbiology of periodontosis. J Periodontol 47:373–379.

Newman MG, Socransky S (1977). Predominant cultivable microbiota in periodontosis. J Periodontal Res 12:120–128.

Newman MG, Kornman K, Holtzman S (1994). Association of clinical risk factors with treatment outcomes. J Periodontol 5:489–497.

Niederman R, Naleway C, Lu B-Y, Buyle-Bodin Y, Robinson P (1995). Subgingival temperature as a gingival inflammatory indicator. J Clin Periodontol 22:804–809.

Nieminen A, Asikainen S, Torkko H, Kari K, Uitto V-J, Saxén L (1996). Value of some laboratory and clinical measurements in the treatment lan for advanced periodontitis. J Clin Periodontol 23:572–581.

Nikias M, Fink R, Sollecito W (1977). Oral health status in relation to socioeconomic and ethnic characteristics of urban adults in the USA. Community Dent Oral Epidemiol 5:200–206.

Nishimura F, Takahashi K, Kurihara M, Takashiba S, Murayama Y (1998). Periodontal disease as a complication of diabetes mellitus. Ann Periodontol 3:20–29.

Noble RC, Penny B (1975). Comparison of leukocyte count and function in smoking and nonsmoking young men. Infect Immun 12:550–555.

Noiri Y, Ebisu S (2000). Identification of periodontal disease–associated bacteria in the "plaque-free zone." J Periodontol 71:1319–1326.

Nolte WA (1973). Oral ecology. In: Nolte WA (ed). Oral Microbiology, ed 2. St Louis: Mosby: 21.

Norderyd O, Grossi S, Machtei E (1993). Periodontal status of women taking postmenopausal estrogen supplementation. J Periodontol 64:957–962.

Norderyd O, Hugoson A (1998). Risk for severe periodontal disease in a Swedish adult population. A cross-sectional study. J Clin Periodontol 28:1022–1028.

Norderyd O, Hugoson A, Grusovin G (1999). Risk for severe periodontal disease in a Swedish adult population. A longitudinal study. J Clin Periodontol 26:608–615.

Nordland P, Garrett S, Vanooteghem R, Hutchens LH, Egelberg J (1987). The effect of plaque control and root debridement in molar teeth. J Clin Periodontol 14:231–236.

Novaes AB Jr, Pereira A, de Moraes N, Novaes AB (1991). Manifestations of insulin-dependent diabetes mellitus in the periodontium of young Brazilian patients. J Periodontol 62:116–122.

Novak MJ (1999). Necrotizing ulcerative periodontitis. Ann Periodontol 4:74–77.

Nowzari H, Slots J (1994). Microorganisms in polytetrafluoroethylene barrier membranes for guided tissue regeneration. J Clin Periodontol 21:203–210.

Nowzari H, Matian F, Slots J (1995). Periodontal pathogens on polytetrafluoroethylene membrane for guided tissue regeneration inhibit healing. J Clin Periodontol 22:469–474.

Nyman S, Rosling B, Lindhe J (1975). Effect of professional tooth-cleaning on healing after periodontal surgery. J Clin Periodontol 2:80–86.

Nyman S, Lindhe J, Rosling B (1977). Periodontal surgery in plaque-infected dentitions. J Clin Periodontol 4:240–249.

Nyman S, Gottlow J, Karring T, Lindhe J (1982a). The regenerative potential of the periodontal ligament. An experimental study in the monkey. J Clin Periodontol 9:257–265.

Nyman S, Lindhe J, Karring T, Rylander H (1982b). New attachment following surgical treatment of periodontal disease. J Clin Periodontol 9:290–296.

Nyman S, Gottlow J, Lindhe J, et al (1987). New attachment formation by guided tissue regeneration. J Periodontal Res 22:252–254.

Nyvad B, Kilian M (1987). Microbiology of the early colonization of human enamel and root surfaces in vivo. Scand J Dent Res 95:369–380.

Offenbacher S, Farr D, Goodson J (1981). Measurement of prostaglandin E in crevicular fluid. J Clin Periodontol 8:359–367.

Offenbacher S, Odle B, Gray R, Van Dyke T (1984). Crevicular fluid prostaglandin E levels as ameasure of the periodontal disease status of adult and juvenile periodontitis patients. J Periodontal Res 19:1–13.

Offenbacher S, Odle B, Van Dyke T (1986). The use of crevicular fluid prostaglandin E$_2$ levels as a predictor of periodontal attachment loss. J Periodontal Res 21:101–112.

Offenbacher S, Soskolne W, Collins J (1991). Prostaglandins and other eicosanoids in gingival crevicular fluid as markers of periodontal disease activity. In: Johnson NW (ed). Risk Markers for Oral Diseases. Vol 3: Periodontal diseases. Cambridge, NY: Cambridge UP: 313.

Offenbacher S, Heasman PA, Collins JG (1993). Modulation of host PGE$_2$ secretion as a determinant of periodontal disease expression. J Periodontol 64:432–444.

Offenbacher S, Collins JG, Yalda B, Haradon G (1994). Role of prostaglandins in high risk periodontitis patients. In: Genco RJ, Hamada S, Lehner T, Mghee J, Mergenhagen S (eds). Molecular pathogenesis of periodontal diseases. Washington, DC: ASM Press: 203–214.

Offenbacher S (1996). Periodontal diseases: Pathogenesis. Ann Periodontol 1:821–878.

Offenbacher S, Katz V, Fertik G, et al (1996). Periodontal infection as a risk factor for preterm low birth weight. J Periodontol 67(10, suppl):1103–1113.

Offenbacher S, Jared HL, O´Reilly PG, et al (1998). Potential pathogenic mechanisms of periodontitis-associated pregnancy complications. Ann Periodontol 3:233–250.

Offenbacher S, Madianos PN, Champagne CME, et al (1999). Periodontitis-atherosclerosis syndrome: An expanded model of pathogenesis. J Periodontal Res 34:346–352.

Offenbacher S, Lieff S, Boggess KA, et al (2001). Maternal periodontitis and prematurity. Part I: Obstetric outcome of prematurity and grwoth restriction. Ann Periodontol 6:164–174.

Ogawa T, McGhee M, Moldoveanu Z, et al (1989). Bacteroides-specific IgG and IgA subclass antibody-secreting cells isolated from chronically inflamed gingival tissues. Clin Exp Immunol 76:103–110.

Okamoto H, Yoneyama T, Lindhe J, Haffajee AD, Socransky SS (1988). Methods of evaluating periodontal disease data in epidemiological research. J Clin Periodontol 15:430–439.

O'Leary TJ, Drake RB, Naylor JE (1972). The plaque control record. J Periodontol 43:38–39.

Oliver R, Brown L, Löe H (1991). Variations in the prevalence and extent of periodontitis. J Am Dent Assoc 122:43–48.

Oliver RC, Tervonen T (1993). Periodontitis and tooth loss in diabetics: A comparison with employed adults. J Am Dent Assoc 124:71–76.

Oliver RC, Tervonen T (1994a). People at risk for periodontitis—Diabetes and periodontal disease. J Periodontol 65:530–538.

Oliver RC, Tervonen (1994b). Diabetes—A risk factor for periodontitis in adults? J Periodontol 65:539–548.

Oliver RC, Brown LJ, Löe H (1998). Periodontal diseases in the US population. J Periodontol 69:269–278.

Osborne JM, Chacko GW, Barndt JT, Anderson CL (1994). Ethnic variation in frequency of an allelic polymorphism of human Fc-gamma-R11A determined with allele specific oligonucleotide probes. J Immunol Methods 173:207–217.

Österberg T, Mellström D (1986). Tobacco smoking: A major risk factor for loss of teeth in three 70-year-old cohorts. Community Dent Oral Epidemiol 14:367–370.

Pabst M, Pabst K, Collier J, et al (1995). Inhibition of neutrophil and monocyte defensive functions by nicotine. J Periodontol 66:1047–1055.

Pack ARC, Coxhead LJ, McDonald BW (1990). The prevalence of overhanging margins in posterior amalgam restorations and periodontal consequences. J Clin Periodontol 17:145–154.

Page RC, Schroeder H (1976). Pathogenesis of inflammatory periodontal disease. A summary of current work. Lab Invest 33:235–249.

Page RC, Schroeder HE (1982). Periodontitis in man and other animals. Basel: Karger.

Page RC, Bowen T, Altman L, et al (1983). Prepubertal periodontitis. I. Definition of a clinical disease entity. J Periodontol 54:257–271.

Page RC (1984). Periodontal diseases in the elderly: A critical evaluation of current information. Gerodontology 3:63–70.

Page RC, Beatty P, Waldrop TC (1987). Molecular basis for the functional abnormality in neutrophils from patients with generalized prepubertal periodontitis. J Periodontal Res 22:182–183.

Page RC (1989). Review of the guidelines for acceptance of chemotherapeutic products for the control of supragingival dental plaque and gingivitis. J Dent Res 68:1640–1644.

Page RC (1991). The role of inflammatory mediators in the pathogenesis of periodontal disease. J Periodontal Res 26:230–242.

Page RC, Sjöström K, Ou J, Chen H (1993). Clinical and immunological aspects of periodontitis. Autoimmun Dis 13:487–508.

Page RC, Beck J (1997). Risk assessment for periodontal diseases. Int Dent J 47:61–87.

Page RC, Kornman K (1997). The pathogenesis of human periodontitis: An introduction. Periodontol 2000 14:9–11.

Page RC, Offenbacher S, Schroeder H, Seymour G, Kornman K (1997). Advances in the pathogenesis of periodontitis: Summary of developments, clinical implications and future directions. Periodontol 2000 14:216–217.

Page RC (1998). The pathobiology of periodontal diseases may affect systemic diseases: Inversion of a paradigm. Ann Periodontol 3:108–120.

Page RC (1999). Milestones in periodontal research and the remaining critical issues. J Periodontal Res 34:331–339.

Page RC (2001). Periodontitis and respiratory diseases: Discussion, conclusions, and recommendations. Ann Periodontol 6:87–90.

Palcanis KG, Larjava IK, Wells BR, et al (1992). Elastase as an indicator of periodontal disease progression. J Periodontol 63:237–242.

Palmer RM (1988). Tobacco smoking and oral health: Review. Br Dent J 164:258–260.

Papapanou PN, Wennström J, Gröndahl K (1988). Periodontal status in relation to age and tooth type. J Clin Periodontol 15:469–478.

Papapanou PN, Wennström J (1989). Radiographic and clinical assessments of destructive periodontal disease. J Clin Periodontol 16:609–612.

Papapanou PN, Wennström J, Gröndahl K (1989). A 10-year retrospective study of periodontal disease progression. J Clin Periodontol 16:403–411.

Papapanou PN, Wennström JL (1991). The angular bony defect as indicator of further alveolar bone loss. J Clin Periodontol 18:317–322.

Papapanou PN (1994). Epidemiology and natural history of periodontal disease. In: Lang N, Karring T (eds). Proceedings of the 1st European Workshop on Periodontics, 1993. London: Quintessence: 23–41.

Papapanou PN (1996). Periodontal diseases: Epidemiology. Ann Periodontol 1:1–36.

Papapanou PN, Lindhe J (1997). Epidemiology of periodontal diseases. In: Lindhe J, Karring T, Lang N (eds). Clinical Periodontology and Implant Dentistry, ed 3. Copenhagen: Munksgaard: 69–101.

Papapanou PN, Baelum V, Wen-Min L, et al (1997a). Subgingival microbiota in adult Chinese: Prevalence and relation to periodontal disease progression. J Periodontol 68:651–666.

Papapanou PN, Madianos PN, Dahlén G, Sandros J (1997b). "Checkerboard" versus culture: A comparison between two methods for identification of subgingival microbiota. Eur J Oral Sci 105:389–396.

Parkhill JM, Hennig BJW, Chapple ILC, Heasman PA, Taylor JJ (2000). Association of interleukin-1 gene polymorphisms with early-onset periodontitis. J Clin Periodontol 27:682–689.

Parr RW, Green E (eds) (1974). Examination and Diagnosis of Periodontal Disease / Produced by Section on Instructional System Design, Division of Periodontology, School of Dentistry, University of California at San Francisco [DHEW Publication No. (HRA) 74-36]. Bethesda, MD: US Dept of Health, Education, and Welfare, Public Health Service, Health Resources Administration, Bureau of Health Resources Development, Division of Dentistry.

Patton LL, McKaig R, Strauss R, Rogers D, Eron JJ (2000). Changing prevalence of oral manifestations of human immuno-deficiency virus in the era of protease inhibitor therapy. Oral Surg Oral Med Oral Pathol Oral Radiol Endod 89:299–304.

Paulander J, Axelsson P, Lindhe J (2002). Relationship between level of education and oral health status in 35-, 50-, 65- and 75-year-olds. J Clin Periodontol (in press).

Paunio K, Impivaara O, Tiesko J, Mäki J (1993). Missing teeth and ischaemic heart disease in men aged 45-64 years. Eur Heart J 14(Suppl K):54–56.

Pavicic M, Van Winkelhoff A, Douqué N, Steures R, De Graaff J (1994). Microbiological and clinical effects of metronidazole and amoxicillin in *Actinobacillus actinomycetemcomitans*-associated periodontitis. A 2-year evaluation. J Clin Periodontol 21:107–112.

Payne JB, Johnson GK, Reinhardt RA, Maze CR, Dyer JK, Patil KD (1994). Smokeless tobacco effects on monocyte secretion of PGE2 and IL-1beta. J Periodontol 65:937–941.

Payne JB, Johnson GK, Reinhardt R, et al (1996). Nicotine effects of PGE2 and IL-1 beta release by LPS-treated human monocytes. J Periodontal Res 31:99–104.

Pearce WH, Sweis I, Yao J, McCarthy W, Koch AE (1992). Interleukin-1beta and tumor necrosis factor-alpha release in normal and diseased human infrarenal aortas. J Vasc Surg 16:784–789.

Pepelassi EA, Tsiklakis K, Diamanti-Kipioti A (2000). Radiographic detection and assessment of the periodontal endosseous defects. J Clin Periodontol 27:224–230.

Persson GR, Page R (1990). Effect of sampling time and repetition on gingival crevicular fluid and aspartate aminotransferase activity. J Periodontal Res 25:236–242.

Persson GR, DeRouen T, Page R (1990). Relationship between gingival crevicular fluid levels of aspartate aminotransferase and active tissue destruction in treated chronic periodontitis patients. J Periodontal Res 25:81–87.

Persson GR, Engel D, Whitney C, et al (1994). Immunization against *Porphyromonas gingivalis* inhibits progression of experimental periodontitis in nonhuman primates. Infect Immun 62:1026–1031.

Petit MD, van Steenbergen T, Scholte LM, van der Velden U, de Graff J (1993). Epidemiology and transmission of *Porphyromonas gingivalis* and *Actinobacillus actinomycetemcomitans* among children and their family members. J Clin Periodontol 20:641–650.

Peto R, Lopez A, Boreham J, Thun M, Heath C Jr (1992). Mortality from tobacco in developed countries: Indirect estimations from national vital statistics. Lancet 339:1268–1278.

Pilot T, Barmes D, Leclercq M, McCombie B, Sardo Infirri J (1987). Periodontal conditions in adolescents, 15-19 years of age: an overview of CPITN data in the WHO Global Oral Data Bank. Community Dent Oral Epidemiol 15:336–338.

Pilot T, Miyazaki H (1991). Peridontal conditions in Europe. J Clin Periodontol 18:353–357.

Pilot T, Miyazaki H (1994). Global results: 15 years of CPITN epidemiology. Int Dent J 44:553–560.

Pilot T (1998). The periodontal disease problem. A comparison between industrialized and developing countries. Int Dent J 48(suppl 1):221–232.

Pindborg J (1947). Tobacco and gingivitis. I. Statistical examination of the significance of tobacco in the development of ulceromembranous gingivitis and in the formation of calculus. J Dent Res 26:261–264.

Pindborg J (1949). Tobacco and gingivitis. II. Correlation between consumption of tobacco, ulceromembranous gingivitis and calculus. J Dent Res 28:460–463.

Pindborg JJ, Holmstrupp P (1987). Necrotizing gingivitis related to HIV infection. Afr Dent J 1:5–8.

Plasschaert A, Folmer T, Van der Heuvel J, Jansen J, Van Opijnen L, Wouters S (1978). An epidemiologic survey of periodontal disease in Dutch adults. Community Dent Oral Epidemiol 6:65–70.

Plaut H (1894). Studien zur bacteriellen Diagnostik der Diphterie und der Anginen. Deutsche Med Wochenschr 20:920–923.

Pociot F, Briant L, Jongeneel CV, et al (1993). Association of tumor necrosis factor (TNF) and class II major histocompatibility complex alleles with the secretion of TNF-alpha and TNF-beta by human mononuclear cells: A possible link to insulin-dependent diabetes mellitus. Eur J Immunol 23:224–231.

Pontoriero R, Nyman S, Lindhe J (1988). The angular bony defect in the maintenance of the periodontal patient. J Clin Periodontol 15:200–204.

Poore T, Johnson G, Reinhardt R, Organ C (1995). The effects of smokeless tobacco on clinical parameters of inflammation and gingival crevicular fluid prostaglandin E_2, interleukin-1alpha and interleukin-1beta. J Periodontol 66:177–183.

Poulsen K, Theilade E, Lally E, Demuth D, Kilian M (1994). Population structure of *Actinobacillus actinomycetemcomitans*. A framework for studies of disease-associated properties. Microbiology 140: 2049–2060.

Prato GPP (1999). Mucogingival deformities. Ann Periodontol 4:98–100.

Preber H, Bergström J (1985). Occurrence of gingival bleeding in smoker and nonsmoker patients. Acta Odontol Scand 43:315–320.

Preber H, Bergström J (1986a). Cigarette smoking in patients referred for periodontal treatment. Scand J Dent Res 94:102–108.

Preber H, Bergström J (1986b). Effect of non-surgical treatment on gingival bleeding in smokers and non-smokers. Acta Odontol Scand 44:85–89.

Preber H, Bergström J (1986c). The effect of non-surgical treatment on periodontal pockets in smokers and non-smokers. J Clin Periodontol 13:319–323.

Preber H, Bergström J (1990). Effect of cigarette smoking on periodontal healing following surgical therapy. J Clin Periodontol 17:324–328.

Preber H, Bergström J, Linder L (1992). Occurence of periopathogens in smoker and non-smoker patients. J Clin Periodontol 19:667–671.

Preber H, Linder L, Bergström J (1995). Periodontal healing and periopathogenic microflora in smokers and non-smokers. J Clin Periodontol 22:946–952.

Preus HR, Morland B (1987). In vitro studies of monocyte function in two siblings with Papillon-Lefevre syndrome. Scand J Dent Res 95:59–64.

Preus HR (1988). Treatment of rapidly destructive periodontitis in Papillon-Lefevre syndrome. Laboratory and clinical observations. J Clin Periodontol 15:639–643.

Preus HR (1989). *Actinobacillus actinomycetemcomitans* in rapidly destructive periodontitis of Papillon-Lefevre syndrome [thesis]. Oslo, Norway: Univ of Oslo.

Progulske-Fox A, Kozarov E, Dorn B, Dunne Jr W, Burks J, Wu Y (1999). *Porphyromonas gingivalis* virulence factors and invasion of cells of the cardiovascular system. J Periodontal Res 34:393–399.

Quigley G, Hein J (1962). Comparative cleansing efficiency of manual and power brushing. J Am Dent Assoc 65:26–29.

Quinn S, Zhang J, Gunsolley J, Schenkein H, Tew J (1998). The influence of smoking and race on adult periodontitis and serum IgG2 levels. J Periodontol 69:171–177.

Quirynen M, Marechal M, Busscher HJ, Weerkamp AH, Darius PL, van Steenberghe D (1990). The influence of surface free energy and surface roughness on early plaque formation. An in vivo study in man. J Clin Periodontol 17:138–144.

Quirynen M, Dekeyser C, Van Steenberghe D (1991). The influence of gingival inflammation, tooth type, and timing on the rate of plaque formation. J Periodontol 62:219–222.

Quirynen M, Bollen C (1995). The influence of surface roughness and surface-free energy on supra- and subgingival plaque formation in man. A review of the literature. J Clin Periodontol 22:1–14.

Quirynen M, Bollen C, Vandekerckhove B, Dekeyser C, Papapanou W, Eyssen H (1995). Full- versus partial-mouth disinfection in the treatment of periodontal infections. Short-term clinical and microbiological observations. J Dent Res 74:1459–1467.

Ramberg P, Lindhe J, Dahlén G, Volpe AR (1994). The influence of gingival inflammation on de novo plaque formation. J Clin Periodontal 21:51–56.

Ramberg P, Axelsson P, Lindhe J (1995). Plaque formation at healthy and inflamed gingival sites in young individuals. J Clin Periodontol 22:85–88.

Ramfjord SP (1959). Indices for prevalence and incidence of periodontal disease. J Periodontol 30:51–59.

Ramfjord SP (1967). The periodontal disease index (PDI). J Periodontol 83:602–610.

Ramfjord SP, Emslie R, Greene J, Held A, Waerhaug J (1968). Epidemiological studies of periodontal diseases. Am J Public Health 58:1713–1722.

Ramfjord SP, Knowles JW, Nissle RR, et al (1973). Longitudinal study of periodontal therapy. J Periodontol 44:66–77.

Rams TE, Keyes P (1983). A rationale for the management of periodontal diseases: Effects of tetracycline on subgingival bacteria. J Am Dent Assoc 107:37–41.

Rams TE, Babalola OO, Slots J (1990). Subgingival occurrence of enteric rods, yeasts and staphylococci after systemic doxycycline therapy. Oral Microbiol Immunol 5:166–168.

Rams TE, Feik D, Slots J (1992). Ciprofloxacin/metronidazole treatment of recurrent adult periodontitis. J Dent Res 71:319.

Rams TE, Feik D, Slots J (1993). Campylobacter rectus in human periodontitis. Oral Microbiol Immunol 8:230–235.

Ranney R (1991). Diagnosis of periodontol disease. Adv Dent Res 5:21–36.

Ranney R (1993). Classification of periodontal diseases. Periodontol 2000 2:13–25.

Rateitschak KH, Wolf H, Hassel T (1989). Color atlas of dental medicine, ed 2. New York: Thieme Verlag.

Raulin L, MacPherson J, McQuade M, Hanson B (1988). The effect of nicotine on the attachment of human fibroblasts to glass and human root surfaces in vitro. J Periodontol 59:318–325.

Read T, Harris HW, Grunfeld C, et al (1993). The protective effect of serum lipoproteins against bacterial lipopolysaccharide. Eur Heart J 14(suppl K):125–129.

Reddy M, Bruch J, Jeffcoat M, Williams R (1991). Contrast enhancement as an aid to interpretation in digital subtraction radiography. Oral Surg Oral Med Oral Pathol 71:763–769.

Reddy M (1997). The use of periodontal probes and radiographs in clinical trials of diagnostic tests. Ann Periodontol 2:113–122.

Reddy M, Palcanis K, Geurs N (1997). A comparison of manual and controlled-force attachment-level measurements. J Clin Periodontol 24:920–926.

Rees TD, Otomo-Corgel J (1992). The diabetic patient. In: Wilson TG, Kornman KS, Newman MG (eds). Advances in Periodontics. Chicago: Quintessence: 278–295.

Rees TD (1994). The diabetic dental patient. Dent Clin North Am 38:447–463.

Reichard P (1990). Intensified Conventional Treatment in Insulin Dependent Diabetes Mellitus (IDDM)—Long Term Feasibility, Effects and Side Effects [thesis]. Stockholm, Sweden: Karolinska Institute.

Reife RA, Shapiro RA, Bamber BA, Berry KK, Mick GE, Darveau RP (1995). *Porphyromonas gingivalis* lipopolysaccharide is poorly recognized by molecular components of innate host defencse in a mouse model of early inflammation. Infect Immun 63:4686–4694.

Reinhardt RA, McDonald TL, Bolton RW, DuBois LM, Kaldahl WB (1989). IgG subclasses in gingival fluid from active versus stable periodontal sites. J Periodontol 60:44–50.

Reinhardt RA, Maze CA, Seagren-Alley CD, Dubois LM (1991). HLA-D types associated with type 1 diabetes and periodontitis [abstract]. J Dent Res 70:1190.

Reinhardt RA, Masada MP, Kaldahl WB, et al (1993). Gingival fluid IL-1 and IL-6 levels in refractory periodontitis. J Clin Periodontol 20:225–231.

Renvert S, Dahlén G, Wikström M (1998). The clinical and microbiological effects of non-surgical periodontal therapy in smokers and non-smokers. J Clin Periodontol 25:153–157.

Reynolds JJ, Meikle M (1997). Mechanisms of connective tissue matrix destruction in periodontitis. Periodontol 2000 14:144–157.

Ricci G, Rasperini G, Silvestri M, Cocconcelli PS (1996). In vitro permeability evaluation and colonization of membranes for periodontal regeneration by *Porphyromonas gingivalis.* J Periodontol 67:490–496.

Ridker PM, Cushman M, Stampfer MJ, Russell PT, Hennekens CH (1997). Inflammation, aspirin and the risk of cardiovascular disease in apparently healthy men. N Engl J Med 336:973–979.

Ritz L, Hefti AF, Rateitschak KH (1991). An in vitro investigation on the loss of substance in scaling with various instruments. J Clin Periodontol 18:643–647.

Riviere G, Wagoner M, Baker-Zander S, et al (1991a). Identification of spirochetes related to Treponema pallidum in necrotizing ulcerative gingivitis and chronic periodontitis. New Engl J Med 325: 539–543.

Riviere G, Weisz K, Simonson L, Lukehart S (1991b). Pathogen-related spirochetes identified within gingival tissue from patients with acute necrotizing ulcerative gingivitis. Infect Immun 59:2653–2657.

Riviere G, Weisz K, Adams D, Thomas D (1991c). Pathogen-related oral spirochetes from dental plaque are invasive. Infect Immun 59:3377–3380.

Riviere G, Elliot K, Adams D, et al (1992). Relative proportions of pathogens-related oral spirochetes (PROS) and Treponema denticola in supragingival and subgingival plaque from patients with periodontitis. J Periodontol 63:131–136.

Robertson PB, Walsh M, Greene J, Ernster V, Grady D, Hauck W (1990). Periodontal effects associated with the use of smokeless tobacco. J Periodontol 61:438–443.

Robertson PB, Ernster V, Walsh M, Greene J, Grady D, Hanck W (1992). Periodontal effects associated with the use of smokeless tobacco: Results after 1 year. In: Smokeless tobacco or health. An international perspective [DHHS Publication 92-3461]. Washington, DC: US Department of Health and Human Services: 78–86.

Robinson PJ, Vitek RM (1979). The relationship between gingival inflammation and resistance to probe penetration. J Periodontal Res 14:239–243.

Rodenburg JP, Van Winkelhoff A, Winkel E, Goene R, Abbas F, De Graaff J (1990). Occurrence of *Bacteroides gingivalis, Bacteroides intermedius* and *Actinobacillus actinomycetemcomitans* in severe periodontitis in relation to age and treatment history. J Clin Periodontol 17:392–399.

Rodriguez-Ferrer H, Strahan J, Newman H (1980). Effect on gingival health of removing overhanging margins of interproximal subgingival amalgam restorations. J Clin Periodontol 7:457–462.

Romero R, Baumann P, Gomez R, et al (1993). The relationship between spontaneous rupture of membranes, labor and microbial invasion of the amniotic cavity and amniotic fluid concentration of prostaglandins and thromboxane B2 in term pregnancy. Am J Obstet Gynecol 168:1654–1664.

Rosenberg ES, Torosian JP, Slots J (1991). Microbial differences in 2 clinically distinct types of failures of osseointegrated implants Clin Oral Implants Res 2:135–144.

Rosling B, Nyman S, Lindhe J (1976a). The effect of systematic plaque control on bone regeneration in infrabony pockets. J Clin Periodontol 3:38–53.

Rosling B, Nyman S, Lindhe J, Jern B (1976b). The healing potential of the periodontal tissues following different techniques of periodontal surgery in plaque-free dentitions. A 2-year clinical study. J Clin Periodontol 3:233–250.

Rosling B, Wannfors B, Volpe AR, Furuichi Y, Ramberg P, Lindhe J (1997a). The use of a triclosan/copolymer dentifrice may retard the progression of periodontitis. J Clin Periodontol 24:873–880.

Rosling B, Dahlén G, Volpe A, Furuichi Y, Ramberg P, Lindhe J (1997b). Effect of triclosan on the subgingival microbiota of periodontitis susceptible subjects. J Clin Periodontol 24:881–887.

Roulard-Bosma W, Van Dijk J (1986). Periodontal diseases in Down's syndrome: A review. J Clin Periodontol 13:64–73.

Rowland RW (1999). Necrotizing ulcerative gingivitis. Ann Periodontol 4:65–73.

Rudin HJ, Overdiek H, Rateitschak K (1970). Correlation between sulcus fluid rate and clinical and histological inflammation of the amrginal gingiva. Helv Odontol Acta 14:21–26.

Russell AL, Consolazio CF, White CL (1961). Periodontal disease and nutrition in Eskimo scouts of the Alaska national guard. J Dent Res 40:604–613.

Saarela M, Stucki A-M, von Troil-Lindén B, Alaluusua S, Jousimies-Somer H, Asikainen S (1993). Intra- and interindividual comparison of Porphyromonas gingivalis genotypes. FEMS Immunol Med Microbiol 6:99–102.

Saglie FR, Carranza F Jr, Newman M, Cheng L, Lewin K (1982a). Identification of tissue-invading bacteria in human periodontal disease. J Periodontal Res 17:452–455.

Saglie FR, Newman M, Carranza F, Pattison G (1982b). Bacterial invasion of gingiva in advanced periodontitis in humans. J Periodontol 53:217–222.

Saglie FR, Newman MG, Carranza Jr FA (1982c). A scanning electron microscope study of leukocytes and their interaction with bacteria in human periodontitis. J Periodontol 53:752–761.

Saglie FR, Carranza Jr FA, Newman MG (1985). The presence of bacteria within the oral epithelium in periodontal disease. I. A scanning and transmission electron microscopic study. J Periodontol 56:618–624.

Saglie FR, Johansen JR, Feo MF (1986a). Tooth surfaces after scaling and root planing: Stereo microscopic and scanning electron microscopic studies. Compend Contin Educ Dent 7:494–506.

Saglie FR, Smith C, Newman M, Carranza F Jr, Pertuiset J (1986b). The presence of bacteria in the oral epithelium in periodontal disease. II. Immunohistochemical identification of bacteria. J Periodontol 57:492–500.

Saglie FR, Pertuise JH, Rezende MT, Sabet MS, Raoufi D, Carranza FA Jr (1987). Bacterial invasion in experimental gingivitis in man. J Periodontol 58:837–846.

Saglie FR, Pertuiset J, Rezende M, Nestor M, Mafrany A, Cheng J (1988a). In situ correlative immuno identification of mononuclear infiltrates and invasive bacteria in diseased gingiva. J Periodontol 59:688–696.

Saglie FR, Marfany A, Camargo P (1988b). Intra-gingival occurrence of Actinobacillus actinomycetemcomitans and Bacteroides gingivalis in active destructive periodontal lesions. J Periodontol 59:259–265.

Saglie FR (1991). Bacterial invasion and its role in the pathogenesis of periodontal disease. In: Hamada S, Holt S, McGhee J (eds). Periodontal Disease: Pathogens and Host Immune Responses. Tokyo: Quintessence: 27–40.

Saikku P, Leinonen M, Mattila K, et al (1988). Serological evidence of an association of a novel Chlamydia, TWAR, with chronic coronary heart disease and acute myocardial infarction. Lancet 2:983–986.

Sakki TK, Knuuttila M, Vimpari S, Hartikainen M (1995). Association of lifestyle with periodontal health. Community Dent Oral Epidemiol 23:155–158.

Sakki TK, Knuuttila M, Anttila S (1998). Lifestyle, gender and occupational status as determinants of dental health behavior. J Clin Periodontol 25:566–570.

Salonen L, Frithiof L, Wouters F, Helldén L (1991). Marginal alveolar bone height in an adult Swedish population. A radiographic cross-sectional epidemiologic study. J Clin Periodontol 18:223–232.

Salvi GE, Lawrence HP, Offenbacher S, Beck J (1997a). Influence of risk factors on the pathogenesis of periodontitis. Periodontol 2000 14:173–201.

Salvi GE, Yalda B, Collins JG, et al (1997b). Inflammatory mediator response as a potential risk marker for periodontal diseases in insulin-dependent diabetes mellitus patients. J Periodontol 68:127–135.

Salvi GE, Beck J, Offenbacher S (1998). PGE$_2$, IL-1beta, and TNF-alpha responses in diabetics as modifiers of periodontal disease expression. Ann Periodontol 3:40–50.

Sandros J, Papapanou PN, Nannmark U, Dahlén G (1994). Porphyromonas gingivalis invades human pocket epithelium in vitro. J Periodontal Res 29:62–69.

Sandros J, Madianos P, Papapanous P (1996). Cellular events concurrent with Porphyromonas gingivalis invasion of oral epithelium in vitro. Eur J Oral Sci 104:363–371.

Sangnes G (1975). Effectiveness and adverse effects of toothbrushing procedures [thesis]. Oslo, Norway: Univ of Oslo.

Sastrowijoto SH, Hillemans P, van Steenbergen T, Abraham-Inpijn L, de Graaff J (1989). Periodontal condition and microbiology of healthy and diseased periodontal pockets in Type I diabetes mellitus patients. J Clin Periodontol 16:316–322.

Saunders LAM, Feldman RG, Voorhorst-Ogink MM, et al (1995). Human immunoglobulin G (IgG) Rc receptor IIA (CD32) polymorohism and IgG2-mediated bacterial phagocytosis by neutrophils. Infect Immun 63:73–81.

Savitt ED, Socransky S (1984). Distribution of certain subgingival microbial species in selected periodontal conditions. J Periodontal Res 19:111–123.

Savitt ED, Strzempko M, Vaccaro K, Peros W, French C (1988). Comparison of cultural methods and DNA probe analyses for the detection of *Actinobacillus actinomycetemcomitans, Bacteoides gingivalis* and *Bacteroides intermedius* in subgingival plaque samples. J Periodontol 59:431–438.

Saxby M (1987). Juvenile periodontitis: An epidemiological study in the west Midlands of the UK. J Clin Periodontol 14:594–598.

Saxe SR, Greene JC, Bohannan HM, Vermillon JR (1967). Oral debris, calculus and periodontal disease in the beagle dog. Periodontics 5:217–225.

Saxén L (1980). Prevalence of juvenile periodontitis in Finland. J Clin Periodontol 7:177–186.

Saxén L, Asikainen S (1993). Metronidazole in the treatment of localized juvenile periodontitis. J Clin Periodontol 20:166–171.

Saxer UP, Mühlemann HR (1975). Motivation und Aufklärung. SSO Schweiz Monatsschr Zahnheilkd 85:905–919.

Saxton CA (1973). Scanning electron microscope study of the formation of dental plaque. Caries Res 7:102–119.

Saxton CA (1975). The formation of human dental plaque: A study by scanning electron microscopy [thesis]. London: Univ of London.

Saxton CA (1976). The effects of dentifrices on the appearance of the tooth surface observed with the scanning electron microscope. J Periodontal Res 11:74–85.

Sbordone L, Ramaglia L, Gulletta E, Iacono V (1990). Recolonization of the subgingival microflora after scaling and root planing in human periodontitis. J Periodontol 61:579–584.

Scannapieco F, Stewart EM, Mylotte JM (1992). Colonization of dental plaque by respiratory pathogens in medical intensive care patients. Crit Care Med 20:740–745.

Scannapieco F, Mylotte J (1996). Relationships between periodontal disease and bacterial pneumonia. J Periodontol 67:1114–1122.

Scannapieco F (1998). Periodontal disease as a potential risk factor for systemic diseases [position paper].

Scannapieco FA, Genco RJ (1999). Association of periodontal infections with atherosclerotic and pulmonary diseases. J Periodontal Res 34:340–345.

Scannapieco FA, Wang B, Shiau HJ (2001). Oral bacteria and respiratory infection: Effects of respiratory pathogen adhesion and epithelial cell proinflammatory cytokine production. Ann Periodontol 6:78–86.

Schätzle M, Lang NP, Ånerud Å, Boysen H, Bürgen W, Löe H (2000). The influence of margins of restorations on the periodontal tissues over 26 years. J Clin Periodontol 27:57–64.

Schei O, Arnö A, Lövdal A, Waerhaug J (1959). Alveolar bone loss as a function of tobacco consumption. Acta Odontol Scand 17:3–10.

Scheie A (1989). Modes of action of currently known chemical antiplaque agents other than chlor-hexidine. J Dent Res 68(special issue):1609–1616.

Schenck K, Poppelsdorf D, Denis C, Tollefsen T (1993). Levels of salivary IgA antibodies reactive with bacteria from dental plaque are associated with susceptibility to experimental gingivitis. J Clin Periodontol 20:411–417.

Schenkein H, Genco RJ (1977). Gingival crevicular fluid and serum in periodontal disease. I. Quantitative study of immunoglobulins, complement components, and other plasma proteins. J Periodontol 48:772–777.

Schenkein H, Van Dyke T (1994). Early-onset periodontitis: Systemic aspects of etiology and pathogenesis. Periodontol 2000 6:7–25.

Schenkein H, Gunsolley J, Koertge T, et al (1995). Smoking and its effects on early-onset periodontitis. J Am Dent Assoc 126:1107–1113.

Schett G, Metzler B, Kleindienst R, et al (1997). Salivary anti-hsp65 antibodies as a diagnostic marker for gingivitis and a possible link to atherosclerosis. Int Arch Allergy Immunol 114:246–250.

Schlossman M, Knowler WC, Pettitt DJ, Genco RJ (1990). Type 2 diabetes mellitus and periodontal disease. J Am Dent Assoc 121:532–536.

Schneir M, Ramamurthy N, Golub L (1981). Diabetes reduces gingival collagen synthesis rather than enhancing its catabolism [abstract 1332]. J Dent Res 60(special issue):642.

Schroeder HE, Lindhe J (1980). Conditions and pathologic features of rapidly destructive, experimental periodontitis in dogs. J Periodontol 51:6–19.

References

Schürch E Jr, Minder C, Lang N, Geering A (1990). Comparison of clinical periodontal parameters with the Community Periodontal Index for Treatment Needs (CPITN) data. Schweiz Monatsschr Zahnmed 100:408–411.

Schürch E, Bürgin WB, Lang NP, et al (1991). The periodontal status of the population of 12 cantons in Switzerland [in German]. Schweiz Monatsschr Zahnmed 101:1393–1398.

Schwartz Z, Goultschin J, Dean D, Boyan B (1997). Mechanisms of alveolar bone destruction in periodontitis. Periodontol 2000 14: 158–172.

Scully C, Porter S, Mutlu S (1991). Changing, subject-based risk factors for destructive periodontitis. In: Johnson NW (ed). Risk Markers for Oral Diseases. Vol 3: Periodontal diseases. Cambridge, NY: Cambridge UP: 139–178..

Sefton AM, Maskell JP, Beighton D, et al (1996). Azithromycin in the treatment of periodontal disease. Effect on microbial flora. J Clin Periodontol 23:998–1003.

Seibold J, Uitto J, Dorward B, Prockop D (1985). Collagen synthesis and collagenase activity in dermal fibroblasts from patients with diabetes mellitus and digital sclerosis. J Lab Clin Med 105:664–667.

Selby C, Drost E, Brown D, Howie S, MacNee W (1992). Inhibition of neutrophil adherence and movement by acute cigarette smoke exposure. Exp Lung Res 18:813–827.

Selwitz R, Albander JM, Harris MI (1998). Periodontal disease in diagnosed diabetes: US population, 1988-94 [abstract 2139]. J Dent Res 77(special issue B).

Shah HN, Gharbia S (1992). Biochemical and chemical studies on strains designated Prevotella intermedia and proposal of a new pigmented species, Prevotella nigrescens sp nov. Int J Sys Bacteriol 42:542–546.

Shah HN (1993). Biology of the Species *Porphyromonas Gingivalis*. Boca Raton: CPC Press.

Shah HN, Gharbia S (1995). Oral and dental disease. The biochemical milleu of the host in the selection of anaerobic species in the oral cavity. Clin Infect Dis 20:291–300.

Shapira L, Frolov I, Halabi A, Ben-Nathan D (2000). Experimental stress suppresses recruitment of macrophages but enhanced their *P. gingivalis* LPS-stimulated secretion of nitric oxide. J Periodontol 71:476–481.

Shiloah J, Patters M, Dean J, Bland P, Toledo G (1997). The survival rate of *Actinobacillus actinomycetemcomitans, Porphyromonas gingivalis* and *Bacteroides forsythus*. Following 4 randomized treatment modalities. J Periodontol 68:720–728.

Silness J, Löe H (1964). Periodontal disease in pregnancy. II. Correlation between oral hygiene and periodontal condition. Acta Odontol Scand 22:121–135.

Silness J (1970). Periodontal conditions in patients treated with dental bridges. III. The relationship between the location of the crown margin and the periodontal condition. J Peridontal Res 5:225–229.

Simonson LG, Goodman C, Bial J, Morton H (1988). Quantitative relationship of *Treponema denticola* to severity of periodontal disease. Infect Immun 56:726–728.

Simonson LG, McMahon K, Childers D, Morton H (1992a). Bacterial synergy of *Treponema denticola* and *Porphyromonas gingivalis* in a multinational population. Oral Microbiol Immunol 7:111–112.

Simonson LG, Robinson P, Pranger R, Cohen M. Morton H (1992b). *Treponema denticola* and *Porphyromonas gingivalis* as prognostic markers following periodontal treatment. J Periodontol 63:270–273.

Sinusas K, Coroso JG, Sopher MD, Crabtree BF (1992). Smokeless tobacco use and oral pathoglogy in a professional baseball organization. J Fam Pract 34:713–718.

Sissons CH, Wong L, Cutress TW (1995). Patterns and rates of growth of microcosm dental plaque biofilms. Oral Microbiol Immunol 10:160–167.

Sjödin B, Crossner C, Unell L, Östlund P (1989). A retrospective radiographic study of alveolar bone loss in the primary dentition in patients with localized juvenile periodontitis. J Clin Periodontol 16: 124–127.

Sjödin B, Matsson L, Unell L, Egelberg J (1993). Marginal bone loss in the primary dentition of patients with juvenile periodontitis. J Clin Periodontol 20:32–36.

Slade GD, Spencer A, Gorkic E, Andrews G (1993). Oral health status and treatment needs of non-institutionalized persons aged 60+ in Adelaide, South Australia. Aust Dent J 38:373–380.

Slots J (1976). The predominant cultivable organisms in juvenile periodontitis. Scand J Dent Res 84:1–10.

Slots J (1977). Microflora in the healthy gingival sulcus in man. Scand J Dent Res 85:247–254.

Slots J, Reynolds H, Genco R (1980). *Actinobacillus actinomycetemcomitans* in human periodontal disease: A cross-sectional microbiological investigation. Infect Immun 29:1013–1020.

Slots J, Rosling B (1983). Suppression of the periodontopathic microflora in localized juvenile periodontitis by systemic tetracycline. J Clin Periodontol 10:465–486.

Slots J, Listgarten MA (1988). *Bacteroides gingivalis, Bacteroides intermedius* and *Actinobacillus actinomycetemcomitans* in human periodontal diseases. J Clin Periodontol 15:85–93.

Slots J, Rams TE, Listgarten MA (1988). Yeasts, enteric rods and pseudomonads in the subgingival flora of severe adult periodontitis. Oral Microbiol Immunol 3:47–52.

Slots J, Rams TE (1990). Antibiotics in periodontal therapy: Advantages and disadvantages. J Clin Periodontol 17:479–493.

Slots J, Feik D, Rams T (1990). Prevalence and antimicrobial susceptibility of *Enterobacteriaceae, Pseudomonadaceae* and *Acinetobacter* in human periodontitis. Oral Microbiol Immunol 5:149–154.

Slots J (1999). *Actinobacillus actinomycetemcomitans* and *Porphyromonas gingivalis* in periodontal disease. Periodontol 2000 20:1–362.

Socransky SS (1977). Microbiology of periodontal disease. Present status and future considerations. J Periodontol 48:497–504.

Socransky SS, Haffajee AD, Goodson JM, Lindhe J (1984). New concepts of destructive periodontal disease. J Clin Periodontol 11:21–32.

Socransky SS, Haffajee AD, Dzink J, Hillman J (1988a). Associations between microbial species in subgingival plaque samples. Oral Microbiol Immunol 3:1–7.

Socransky SS, Haffajee AD, Dzink JL (1988b). Relationship of subgingival microbial complexes to clinical features at the sampled sites. J Clin Periodontol 15:440–444.

Socransky SS, Haffajee AD (1990). Microbiological risk factors for destructive periodontal diseases. In: Beck JD, Bader JD. Risk Assessment in Dentistry [Proceedings of a conference, 2-3 Jun 1989, Chapel Hill]. Chapel Hill: University of North Carolina Dept of Dental Ecology: 79–90.

Socransky SS, Haffajee AD (1991). Microbial mechanisms in the pathogenesis of destructive periodontal diseases: a critical assessment. J Periodontal Res 26:195–212.

Socransky SS, Haffajee AD (1992). The bacterial etiology of destructive periodontal disease: Current concepts. J Periodontol 63:322–331.

Socransky SS, Smith C, Martin L, Paster BJ, Dewhirst FE, Levin A (1994). "Checkerboard" DNA-DNA hybridization. Biotechniques 17:788–792.

Socransky SS, Haffajee AF (1997). Microbiology of periodontal disease. In: Lindhe J, Karring T, Lang NP (eds). Clinical Periodontology and Implant Dentistry. Copenhagen: Munksgaard: 138–188.

Socransky SS, Haffajee AD, Smith C, Duff GW (2000). Microbiological parameters associated with IL-1 gene polymorphisms in periodontitis patients. J Clin Periodontol 27:810–818.

Söder B, Jun L, Söder P, Wikner S (1995). Clinical characteristics of destructive periodontitis in a risk group of Swedish urban adults. Swed Dent J 19:9–15.

Söder B (1998a). Neutrophil elastase activity, levels of prostaglandin E_2 and matrix metalloproteinase-8 in refractory periodontitis sites in smokers and non-smokers [in manuscript].

Söder B (1998b). Studies on plaque distribution and gingival crevicular fluid after non-surgical treatment in smokers and non-smokers with periodontal diseases [thesis]. Huddinge, Sweden: Karolinska Institute.

Söder B, Nedlich U, Jin L (1999). Longitudinal effect of non-surgical treatment and systemic metronidazole for 1 week in smokers and non-smokers with refractory periodontitis: A 5-year study. J Periodontol 70:761–771.

Söderholm G (1979). Effect of a dental care program on dental health conditions. A study of employees of a Swedish shipyard [thesis]. Malmö, Sweden: Univ of Lund.

Solomon HA, Priore R, Bross I (1968). Cigarette smoking and periodontal disease. J Am Dent Assoc 77:1081–1084.

Sorsa T, Vitto VJ, Suomalainen K, Vauhkonen M, Lindy S (1988). Comparison of interstitial collagenases from human gingiva, sulcular fluid and polymorphonuclear leukocytes. J Periodontal Res 23:386–393.

Soskolne W (1998). Epidemiological and clinical aspects of periodontal diseases in diabetics. Ann Periodontol 3:3–12.

Soskolne W, Klinger A (2001). the relationship between periodontal diseases and diabetes: An overview. Ann Periodontol 6:91–98.

Spinks GC, Carson RE, Everett B, Hancock, Pellen GB Jr (1985). A SEM study of overhang removal methods. J Periodontol 57:632–636.

Sreenivasan P, Meyer D, Fives-Taylor P (1993). Requirements for invasion of epithelial cells by *Actinobacillus actinomycetemcomitans*. Infect Immun 61:1239–1245.

Stambough RV, Dragoo M, Smith DM, Carasali L (1981). The limits of subgingival scaling. Int J Periodontics Restorative Dent 1:31–41.

Steidley KE, Thompson SH, McQuade MJ, Strong SL, Scheidt MJ, Van Dyke TE (1992). A comparison of T4:T8 lymphocyte ratio in the periodontal lesion of healthy and HIV-positive patients. J Periodontol 63:753–756.

References

Sternberg E, Chrousos G, Wilder R, Gold P (1992). The stress response and the regulation of inflammatory disease. Ann Intern Med 117:854–866.

Stewart R, Hollister D, Rimoin D (1977). A new variant of Ehlers-Danlos syndrome: An autosomal dominant disorder of fragile skin, abnormal scarring and generalized periodontitis. Birth Defects Orig Artic Ser13:85–93.

Stoltenberg JL, Osborn J, Pihlström B, et al (1993). Association between cigarette smoking, bacterial pathogens and periodontal status. J Periodontol 64:1225–1230.

Stoner J (1972). An investigation into the accuracy of measurements made on radiographs of the alveolar crests of dried mandibles. J Periodontol 43:699–701.

Straub A, Salvi G, Lang N (1998). Supragingival plaque formation in the human dentition. In: Lang NP, Attström R, Löe H. Proceedings of the European Workshop on Mechanical Plaque Control. Berlin: Quintessence: 72–84.

Strömberg N (1996). Salivens fingeravtryck avslöjar risk för tandlossning. Tandlakartidningen 88:138–141.

Suomi JD, Greene JC, Vermillion JR, Doyle J, Chang JJ, Leatherwood EC (1971). The effect of controlled oral hygiene procedures on the progression of periodontal disease in adults: Results after third and final year. J Periodontol 42:152–160.

Susser M (1991). What is a cause and how do we know one? A grammar for pragmatic epidemiology. Am J Epidemiol 133:635–648.

Suzuki JB, Collison BC, Falkler WA, Nauman RK (1984). Immunologic profile of juvenile periodontitis. II. Neutrophil chemotaxis, phagocytosis and spore germination. J Periodontol 55:461–467.

Syrjänen J, Peltola J, Valtonen V, Livanainen M, Kaste M, Huttunen J (1989). Dental infections in association with cerebral infarction in young and middle-aged men. J Intern Med 225:179–184.

Szopa TM, Titchener PA, Portwood ND, Taylor KW (1993). Diabetes mellitus due to viruses—Some recent developments. Diabetologia 36:687–695.

Tal H (1984). Relationship between interproximal distance of roots and the prevalence of intrabony pockets. J Periodontol 55:604–607.

Tal H, Panno JM, Vaidyanathan TK (1985). Scanning electron microscope evaluation of wear of dental curettes during standardized root planing. J Periodontol 56:532–537.

Tal H, Soldinger M, Dreiangel A, Pitaru S (1989). Periodontal response to long-term abuse of the gingival attachment by supracrestal amalgam restorations. J Clin Periodontol 16:654–669.

Tangada S, Califano J, Nakashima K, et al (1997). The effect of smoking on serum IgG2 reactive with Actinobacillus actinomycetemcomitans in early-onset periodontitis patients. J Periodontol 68:842–850.

Tanner A, Haffer C, Bratthall G, Visconti R, Socransky S (1979). A study of the bacteria associated with advancing periodontitis in man. J Clin Periodontol 6:278–307.

Tanner A, Socransky S, Goodson J (1984). Microbiota of periodontal pockets losing crestal alveolar bone. J Periodontal Res 19:279–291.

Tanner A, Dzink J, Ebersole J, Socransky S (1987). Wolonella recta, Campylobacter concisus, Bacteroides gracilis, and Eikenella corrodens from periodontal lesions. J Periodontal Res 22:237–330.

Tanner A, Bouldin H (1989). The microbiota of early periodontitis lesions in adults. J Clin Periodontol 16:467–471.

Tanner A, Maiden M, Paster B, Dewhirst F (1994). The impact of 16S ribosomal RNA-based phylogeny on the taxonomy of oral bacteria. Periodontol 2000 5:26–51.

Tanner A, Maiden M, Kent R, Macuch P, Murray L (1998). Microbiota of health, gingivitis and initial periodontitis. J Clin Periodontol 25:85–98.

Tatakis DN (1993). Interleukin-1 and bone metabolism: A review. J Periodontol 64:416–431.

Taubman M, Haffajee A, Socransky S, Smith D, Ebersole J (1992). Longitudinal monitoring of humoral antibody in subjects with destructive periodontal diseases. J Periodontal Res 27:511–521.

Taylor G, Burt B, Becker M, Genco R, Shlossman M (1998). Glycemic control and alveolar bone loss progression in type 2 diabetes. Ann Periodontol 3:30–39.

Taylor G (2001). Bidirectional interrelationships between diabetes and periodontal diseases: An epidemiologic perspective. Ann Periodontol 6:99–112.

Tempel T, Kimball H, Kakehashi S, Amen C (1972). Host factors in periodontal manifestations of Chediak-Higashi syndrome. J Periodontal Res 7(suppl 10):26–27.

Tenovuo J, Lagerlöf F. Saliva; Thylstrup A, Fejerskov O (1994). Textbook of Clinical Cariology. Copenhagen: Munksgaard: 17–43.

Ter Steeg P, Van der Hoeven J, de Jong M, van Munster P, Jansen M (1987). Enrichment of subgingival microflora leading to accumulation of Bacteroides species, peptostreptococci and fusobacteria. Antonie van Leeuwenhoek 53:261–272.

Ter Steeg P, Van der Hoeven J, de Jong M, van Munster P, Jansen M (1988). Modeling the gingival pocket by enrichment of subgingival microflora in human serum in chemostats. Microb Ecol Health Dis 1:73–84.

Tervonen T, Knuuttila M, Pohjamo L, Nurkkala H (1991). Immediate response to nonsurgical periodontal treatment in subjects with diabetes mellitus. J Clin Periodontol 18:65–68.

Tervonen T, Karjalainen K (1997). Periodontal disease related to diabetic status. J Clin Periodontol 24:505–510.

Tervonen T, Karjalainen K, Knuuttila M, Huumonen S (2000). Alveolar bone loss in type-1 diabetic subjects. J Clin Periodontol 27:567–571.

Tew JG, Zhang J-B, Quinn S, et al (1996). Antibody of the IgG2 subclass, *Actinobacillus actinomycetemcomitans* and early-onset periodontitis. J Periodontol 67(suppl 1):317–322.

Theilade E, Theilade J (1976). Role of plaque in the etiology of periodontal disease and caries. Oral Sci Rev 9:23.

Theilade E, Fejerskov O, Horsted M (1976). A transmission electron microscopic study of 7-day old bacterial plaque in human tooth fissures. Arch Oral Biol 21:587–598.

Theilade J, Attström R (1985). Distribution and ultrastructure of subgingival plaque in beagle dogs with gingival inflammation. J Periodontal Res 20:131–145.

Theilade E (1986). The non-specific theory in microbial etiology of inflammatory periodontal diseases. J Clin Periodontol 13:905–911.

Thorstensson H, Falk H, Hugoson A, Olsson J (1989). Some salivary factors in insulin-dependent diabetics. Acta Odontol Scand 47:175–183.

Thorstensson H (1995). Periodontal disease in adult insulin-dependent diabetics [thesis]. Gothenburg, Sweden: Univ of Gothenburg.

Thorstensson H, Dahlén G, Hugosson A (1995). Some suspected periodontopathogens and serum antibody response in adult long-duration insulin-dependent diabetics. J Clin Periodontol 22:449–458.

Thorstensson H, Kuylenstierna J, Hugosson A (1996). Medical status and complications in relation to periodontal disease experience in insulin-dependent diabetics. J Clin Periodontol 23:194–202.

Tinanoff N, Tanzer J, Kornman K, Maderazo E (1986). Treatment of the periodontal component of Papillon-Lefevre syndrome. J Clin Periodontol 13:6–10.

Tomar SL, Asma S (2000). Smoking-attributable periodontitis in the US: Findings from NHANES III. J Periodontol 71:743–751.

Tonetti MS (1994). Etiology and pathogenesis. In: Lang N, Karring T (eds). Proceedings of the 1st European Workshop on Periodontics, 1993. London: Quintessence: 54–89.

Tonetti MS, Pino-Prato G, Cortellini P (1995). Effect of cigarette smoking on periodontal healing following GTR in infrabony defects. A preliminary retrospective study. J Clin Periodontol 22:229–234.

Tonetti MS, Mombelli A (1997). Early onset periodontitis. In: Karring T, Lang N (eds). Clinical Periodontology and Implant Dentistry. Copenhagen: Munksgaard: 226–257.

Tonetti MS (1998). Cigarette smoking and periodontal diseases: Etiology and management of disease. Ann Periodontol 3:88–101.

Tonetti MS, Mombelli A (1999). Early onset periodontitis. Ann Periodontol 4:39–52.

Turesky S, Gilmore N, Glickman I (1970). Reduced plaque formation by the chloromethyl analogue of vitamine C. J Periodontol 41:41–43.

US Department of Health and Human Services (1982). The health consequences of smoking: Cancer. A report of the surgeon-general [DHHS Publication (CDC) 82-50179]. Washington, DC: USDHHS, Public Health Service, Centers for Disease Control Office on Smoking and Health.

US Public Health Service (1965). National Center for Health Statistics. Periodontal disease in adults, United States 1960-1962 [PHS Publication 1000, series 11, 12]. Washington DC: Government Printing Office.

US Public Health Service (1979). Basic data on dental examination findings of persons 1-74 years, United States 1971-1974 [DHEW Publication (PHS) 79-1662, series 11 No. 214]. Besthesda, MD: National Center for Health Statistics.

US Public Health Service (1987). Oral Health of US Adults; National findings 1987 [NIH Publication 87-2868]. Bethesda, MD: National Institute of Dental Research.

Vale JD, Caffesse RG (1979). Removal of amalgam overhangs. A profilometric and scanning electron microscopic evaluation. J Periodontol 50:245–249.

Valtonen VV (1991). Infection as a risk factor for infarction and atherosclerosis. Ann Med 23:539–543.

Van der Hoeven JS, Camp P (1991). Synergistic degradation of mucin by *Streptococcus oralis* and *Streptococcus sanguis* in mixed chemostat cultures. J Dent Res 70:1041–1044.

Van der Velden U (1991). The onset age of periodontal destruction. J Clin Periodontol 18:380–383.

Van Dyke TE, Horoszewicz HU, Genco RJ (1982). The polymorphonuclear leukocyte (PMNL) locomotor defect in juvenile periodontitis. J Periodontol 53:682–687.

Van Dyke TE, Levine M, Tabak L, Genco R (1983). Juvenile periodontitis as a model for neutrophil function: Reduced binding of complement chemotactic fragment, C5a. J Dent Res 62:870–872.

References

Van Dyke TE, Taubman MA, Ebersole JL, et al (1984). The Papillon-Lefevre syndrome: Neutrophil dysfunction with severe periodontal disease. Clin Immunol Immunopathol 31:419–429.

Van Dyke TE, Schweinebraten M, Cianociola LJ, Offenbacher S, Genco RJ (1985). Neutrophil chemotaxis in families with localized juvenile periodontitis. J Periodontal Res 20:503–514.

Van Dyke TE, Zinney W, Winkel K, Taufiq A, Offenbacher S, Arnold RR (1986). Neutrophil function in localized juvenile periodontitis. Phagocytosis, superoxide production and specific granule release. J Periodontol 57:703–708.

Van Dyke TE, Offenbacher S, Kalmar (1988). Neutrophil defects and host parasite interactions in the pathogenesis of localized juvenile periodontitis. Adv Dent Res 2:354–358.

Van Dyke TE, Hoop GA (1990). Neutrophil function and oral disease. Crit Rev Oral Biol Med 1:117–133.

Vanooteghem R, Hutchens LH, Garrett S, Kieger R, Egelberg J (1987). Bleeding on probing and probing depth as indicators of the response to plaque control and root debridement. J Clin Periodontol 14:226–230.

Vanooteghem R, Hutchens LH, Bowers G, et al (1990). Subjective criteria and probing attachment loss to evaluate the effects of plaque control and root debridement. J Clin Periodontol 17:580–587.

Van Steenbergen T, Petit MD, Scholte LE, van der Velden U, de Graaff J (1993). Transmission of *Porphyromonas gingivalis* between spouses. J Clin Periodontol 20:340–345.

Van Winkelhoff AJ, van der Velden U, Winkel E, de Graaff J (1986). Black-pigmented *Bacteroides* and motile organisms on oral mucosal surfaces in individuals with and without periodontal breakdown. J Periodontal Res 21:434–439.

Van Winkelhoff AJ, van der Velden U, Clement M, de Graaff J (1988a). Intra-oral distribution of black-pigmented *Bacteroides* species in periodontitis patients. Oral Microbiol Immunol 3:83–85.

Van Winkelhoff AJ, van der Velden U, de Graaff J (1988b). Microbial sucession in recolonizing deep periodontal pockets after a single course of supra- and subgingival debridement. J Clin Periodontol 15:116–122.

Van Winkelhoff A, van der Velden U, de Graaff J (1988c). Microbial succession in recolonizing deep periodontal pockets after a single course of supra- and subgingival debridement. J Clin Periodontol 15:116–122.

Van Winkelhoff AJ, Tijhof CJ, de Graaff J (1992). Microbiological and clinical results of metronidazole plus amoxicillin therapy in *Actinobacillus actinomycetemcomitans*-associated periodontitis. J Periodontol 63:52–57.

Villela B, Cogen RB, Bartolucci AA, Birkedal-Hansen H (1987). Collagenolytic activity in crevicular fluid from patients with chronic adult periodontitis and gingivitis, and from healthy control subjects. J Peridontal Res 22:381–389.

Vincent M (1899). Recherches bactériologiques sur l´angine a bacilles fusiformes. Ann Inst Pasteur 8:609–620.

Von Troil-Lindén B, Torkko H, Alaluusua S, Wolf J, Jousimies-Somer H, Asikainen S (1995). Periodontal findings in spouses. A clinical, radiographic and microbiological study. J Clin Periodontol 22:93–99.

Vrahopoulos T, Barber P, Liakoni H, Newman H (1988). Ultrastructure of the periodontal lesion in a case of Papillon-Lefevre syndrome. J Clin Periodontol 15:17–26.

Wactawski-Wende J (2001). Periodontal diseases and osteoporosis: Associations and mechanisms. Ann Periodontol 6:197–208.

Waerhaug J (1960). Histologic considerations which govern where the margins of restorations should be located in relation to the gingiva. Dent Clin North Am 4:161–176.

Waerhaug J (1975). Presence or absence of plaque on subgingival restorations. Scand J Dent Res 83:193–201.

Waerhaug J (1976). Subgingival plaque and loss of attachment in periodontosis as observed in autopsy material. J Periodontol 47:636–642.

Waerhaug J (1977). Subgingival plaque and loss of attachment in periodontosis as evaluated on extracted teeth. J Periodontol 48:125–130.

Waerhaug J (1978). Healing of dento-epithelial junction following subgingival plaque control. II. As observed on extracted teeth. J Periodontol 49:119–134.

Waerhaug J (1979). The infrabony pocket and its relationship to trauma from occlusion and subgingival plaque. J Periodontol 50:355–365.

Waerhaug J (1980). The furcation problem. Etiology, pathogenesis, diagnosis, therapy and prognosis. J Clin Periodontol 7:73–95.

Wakai K, Kawamura T, Umemura O, et al (1999). Association of medical status and physical fitness with periodontal disease. J Clin Periodontol 26:664–672.

Waldrop TC, Anderson DC, Hallmon WW, Schmalstieg FC, Jacobs RL (1987). Periodontal manifestations of the heritable Mac-1, LAF-1 defiency syndrome. Clinical histopathologic and molecular characteristics. J Periodontol 58:400–416.

Wang HL, Yuan K, Burgett R, Shyr Y, Syed S (1994). Adherence of oral microorganisms to guided tissue membranes: An in vitro study. J Periodontol 65:211–218.

Wennström A, Wennström J, Lindhe J (1986). Healing following surgical and nonsurgical treatment of juvenile periodontitis. A 5-year longitudinal study. J Clin Periodontol 13:869–882.

Wennström J, Serino G, Lindhe J, Eneroth L, Tollskog G (1993). Periodontal conditions of adults regular dental care attendants. A 12-year longitudinal study. J Clin Periodontol 20:714–722.

Wenzel A, Sewerin I (1991). Sources of noise in digital subtraction radiography. Oral Surg Oral Med Oral Pathol 71:503–508.

Weringer E, Arquilla E (1981). Wound healing in normal and diabetic chinese hamsters. Diabetologia 21:394–401.

Westfelt E, Nyman S, Lindhe J, Socransky S (1983). Significance of frequency of professional tooth cleaning for healing following periodontal surgery. J Clin Periodontol 10:148–156.

Westfelt E, Rylander H, Blohme G, Jonasson P, Lindhe J (1996). The effect of periodontal therapy in diabetics. Results after 5 years. J Clin Periodontol 23:92–100.

Whitney C, Ant J, Moncla B, Johnson B, Page R, Engel D (1992). Serum immunoglobulin G antibody to P gingivalis in rapidly progressive periodontitis: Titre, avidity and subclass distribution. Infect Immun 60:2194–2200.

Wiktorsson AM (1995). Dental caries and dental fluorosis among adults in two Swedish communities with optimal and low water fluoride concentrations [thesis]. Stockholm, Sweden: Karolinska Institute.

Williams RC, Paquette D (1997). Advances in periodontal diagnosis. In: Lindhe J, Karring T, Lang N (eds). Clinical Periodontology and Implant Dentistry. Copenhagen: Munksgaard.

Wilson M, Gibson M, Strahan D, Harvey W (1992). A preliminary evaluation of the use of a redox agent in the treatment of chronic periodontitis. J Periodontal Res 27:522–527.

Wilson AG, di Giovine FS, Duff GW (1995). Genetics of tumor necrosis factor alpha in autoimmune, infectious and neoplastic diseases. J Inflammation 45:1–12.

Wilton JM (1986). Crevicular neutrophils: Protective or damaging? In: Lehner T, Cimasoni G (eds). The Borderland Between Caries and Periodontal Disease III. Geneva: Editions Medecine et Hygiene: 71–85.

Wilton JM, Griffiths GS, Curtis MA, et al (1988). Detection of high-risk groups and individuals for periodontal diseases. Systemic predisposition and markers of general health. J Clin Periodontol 15:339–446.

Wilton JM (1991). Unchanging, subject-based risk factors for destructive periodontitis: Race, sex, genetic, congenital and childhood systemic diseases. In: Johnson NW (ed). Risk Markers for Oral Diseases. Vol 3: Periodontal diseases. Cambridge, NY: Cambridge UP: 109.

Wilton JM, Hurst T, Austin A (1992). IgG subclass antibodies to Porphyromonas gingivalis in patients with destructive periodontal disease. A case-control study. J Clin Periodontol 19:646–651.

Winkler JR, Murray P, Greenspan D, Greenspan J (1986). Periodontal disease of male homosexuals as related to AIDS virus infection. In: Gluckman J, Vilmer E (eds). Proceedings of the 2nd International Conference on AIDS, June 1986, Paris, France. Amsterdam: Elsevier.

Winkler JR, Grassi M, Murray P (1988). Clinical description and etiology of HIV-associated periodontal diseases. In: Robertson P, Greenspan J (eds). Perspectives on Oral Manifestation of AIDS. Littleton, MA: PSG Publishing: 49–70.

Wolfe MD, Carlos JP (1987). Periodontal disease in adolescents: Epidemiologic findings in Navajo Indians. Community Dent Oral Epidemiol 15:33–40.

Wolff LF, Anderson L, Sandberg GP, Aeppli D (1991). A fluorescence immunoassay for detecting periodontal bacterial pathogens in plaque. J Clin Microbiol 29:1645–1651.

Wolff L, Dahlén G, Aeppli D (1994). Bacteria as risk markers for periodontitis. J Periodontol 65(suppl): 498–510.

Wolff L, Koller N, Smith Q, Mathur A, Aeppli D (1997). Subgingival temperature: Relation to gingival crevicular fluid enzymes, cytokines and subgingival plaque micro-organisms. J Clin Periodontol 24:900–906.

World Health Organization (1985). WHO Expert Committee on Diabetes Mellitus: Third Report, No. 727, World Health Organization Technical Report Series. Geneva: WHO.

World Health Organization (1993). DMFT levels at 12 years 1993. WHO/OHU/DMFT 12. Geneva: WHO.

World Health Organization (1994). WHO Oral Health Country Profile Programme 1994. Geneva: WHO.

World Health Organization (1997). Global Oral Data Bank 1997. Geneva: WHO.

World Health Organization (1999). The World Health Report 1999. Geneva: WHO.

Wouters FR, Salonen L, Frithiof L, Helldén L (1993). Significance of some variables on interproximal alveolar bone height based on cross-sectional epidemiologic data. J Clin Periodontol 20:199–206.

References

Wu T, Trevisan M, Genco RJ, Dorn JP, Falkner KL, Sempos CT (2000a). Periodontal disease and risk of cerebrovascular disease. Arch Intern Med 160: 2749–2755.

Wu T, Trevisan M, Genco RJ, Falkner KL, Dorn JP, Sempos CT (2000b). Examination of the relation between periodontal health status and cardiovascular risk factors: Serum total and high density lipoproproten cholesterol, C-reactive protein and plasma fibrinogen. Am J Epidemiol 151:273–282.

Ximénez-Fyvie LA, Haffajee AD, Socransky SS (2000). Comparison of the microbiota of supra- and subgingival plaque in health and periodontitis. J Clin Periodontol 27:648–657.

Xu Q, Wick G (1996). The role of heat shock proteins in protection and pathophysiology of the arterial wall. Mol Med Today 2:372–379.

Yalda B, Offenbacher S, Collins J (1994). Diabetes as a modifier of periodontal expression. Periodontol 2000 6:37–49.

Yang M, Namgung Y, Marks R, Magnusson I, Clark W (1993). Change detection on longitudinal data in periodontal research. J Periodontal Res 28:152–160.

Yang S, Sun C, Gillanders E, et al (1996). Genome scan for susceptibility loci to the complex disorder early onset periodontitis [abstract]. Am J Hum Genet 59:1386.

Yoneyama T, Okamoto H, Lindhe J, Socransky SS, Haffajee (1988). Probing depth, attachment loss and gingival recession. J Clin Periodontol 15:581–591.

Yoon JW (1991). Role of viruses in the pathogenesis of IDDM. Ann Med 23:437–445.

Young RA, Elliot TJ (1989). Stress proteins, infection, and immune surveillance. Cell 59:5–8.

Yuan A, Yang PC, Lee L, Chang DB, Kuo SH, Luh KT (1992). *Actinobacillus actinomycetemcomitans* with chest wall involvement and rib destruction. Chest 101:1450–1452.

Yuan A, Luh KT, Yang PC (1994). *Actinobacillus actinomycetemcomitans* pneumonia with possible septic embolization (comments). Chest 105:645–646.

Zambon JJ, Christersson L, Slots J (1983a). *Actinobacillus actinomycetemcomitans* in human periodontal disease. Prevalence in patient groups and distribution of biotypes and serotypes within families. J Periodontol 54:707–711.

Zambon JJ, Slots J, Genco R (1983b). Serology of oral *Actinobacillus actinomycetemcomitans* and serotype distribution in human periodontal disease. Infect Immun 41:19–27.

Zambon JJ, Reynolds H, Chen P, Genco R (1985). Rapid identification of periodontal pathogens in subgingival dental plaque. Comparison of indirect immunofluorescence microscopy with bacterial culture for detection of *Bacteroides gingivalis*. J Periodontol 56:32–40.

Zambon JJ, Reynolds H, Fisher J, Schlossman M, Dunford R, Genco R (1988). Microbiological and immunological studies of adult periodontitis in patients with noninsulin-dependent diabetes mellitus. J Periodontol 59:23–31.

Zambon JJ, Reynolds H, Genco R (1990). Studies of the subgingival microflora in patients with acquired immunodeficiency syndrome. J Periodontol 61: 699–704.

Zambon JJ, Haraszthy V (1995). The laboratory diagnosis of periodontal infections. Periodontol 2000 7:69–82.

Zambon JJ (1996). Periodontal diseases: Microbial factors. Ann Periodontol 1:879–925.

Zambon JJ, Grossi S, Machtei E, et al (1996a). Cigarette smoking increases the risk for subgingival infection with periodontal pathogens. J Periodontol 67(suppl 10):1050–1054.

Zambon JJ, Haraszthy V, Hariharan G, Lally E, Demuth D (1996b). The microbiology of early-onset periodontitis: Association of highly toxic *Actinobacillus actinomycetemcomitans* strains with localized juvenile periodontitis. J Periodontol 67:282–290.

Zappa U, Smith B, Simona C, Graf H, Case D, Kim W (1991). Root substance removal by scaling and root planing. J Periodontol 62:750–754.

LIST OF ABBREVIATIONS

ABE—acute bacterial endocarditis
ABL—alveolar bone loss
AGE—advanced glycation end product
AIDS—acquired immunodeficiency syndrome
AMI—acute myocardial infarction
ANUG—acute necrotizing ulcerative gingivitis
AST—aspartate aminotransferase

BANA—benzoly-DL-arginine-2-naphthylamide
βG—β-glucuronidase
BMP—bone morphogenetic protein

CAL—clinical attachment loss
CCHD—chronic coronary heart disease
CEJ—cementoenamel junction
CHD—coronary heart disease
CHX—chlorhexidine
CI-S—Simplified Calculus Index
CNUG—chronic necrotizing ulcerative gingivitis
CPITN—Community Periodontal Index of Treatment Needs
CVD—cardiovascular disease

DI-S—Simplified Debris Index
DMFS—decayed, missing, or filled surfaces
DMFT—decayed, missing, or filled teeth

ECAM—endothelial cell adhesion molecule

EDTA—ethylenediaminetetraacetic acid
ELISA—enzyme-linked immunosorbent assay
EMD—enamel matrix derivative
EMRIRF—external modifying risk indicators, risk factors, and prognostic risk factors
ESI—Extent and Severity Index

FDI—Fédération Dentaire Internationale
fMLP—N-formyl-methionyl-leucyl-phenylalanine

GAD—glutamic acid decarboxylase
GAP—generalized aggressive periodontitis
GBI—Gingival Bleeding Index
GCF—gingival crevicular fluid
GDM—gestational diabetes mellitus
GI—Gingival Index
GODB–Global Oral Data Bank
GTR—guided tissue regeneration

Hag A—hemagglutinin gene A
HAL—horizontal attachment loss
HCMV—human cytomegalovirus
HSP—heat shock protein
HIV—human immunodeficiency virus

IAL—incidental attachment loss
ICAM—intercellular adhesion molecule
IE—infective endocarditis

IgA—immunoglobulin A
IgE—immunoglobulin E
IgG—immunoglobulin G
IgM—immunoglobulin M
IGT—impaired glucose tolerance
IL—interleukin
IMRIRF—internal modifying risk indicators, risk factors, and prognostic risk factors
INF—interferon

LAD—leukocyte adhesion deficiency
LADA—latent autoimmune diabetes in the adult
LAP—localized aggressive periodontitis
LF—lactoferrin
LPS—lipopolysaccharide
LZ—lysozyme

MCP—monocyte chemoattractant protein
MHC—major histocompatibility complex
MIP—macrophage inflammatory protein
MMP—matrix metalloproteinase
MRDM—malnutrition-related diabetes mellitus

NE—neutrophil elastase
NEEDS—New England Elders Dental Study
NS—necrotizing stomatitis
NSAID—nonsteroidal anti-inflammatory drug
NUG—necrotizing ulcerative gingivitis
NUP—necrotizing ulcerative periodontitis

OECD—Organization for Economic Development
OHI—Oral Hygiene Index
OHI-S—Simplified Oral Hygiene Index
OR—odds ratio

PAAP—platelet aggregation–associated protein
PAL—probing attachment loss
PBI—Papillary Bleeding Index

PDHS—Public Dental Health Service
PFRI—Plaque Formation Rate Index
PGE$_2$—prostaglandin E$_2$
PI—Plaque Index
PLBW—preterm, low–birth weight
PMNL—polymorphonuclear leukocyte
PMTC—professional mechanical toothcleaning
PPT—periodontal pocket temperature
PRF—prognostic risk factor
PROS—pathogen-related oral spirochete
PRP—proline-rich glycoprotein
PST—Periodontal Susceptibility Test
PTNS—Periodontal Treatment Needs System

RANTES—regulated-on-activation normal T cell, expressed and secreted
RF—risk factor
RI—risk indicator
RLTSI—Roughness Loss of Tooth Substance Index
RM—risk marker
RP—risk predictor

SBE—subacute bacterial endocarditis
SEC—socioeconomic condition
SEM—scanning electron micrograph
SES—socioeconomic status
sRAGE—soluble receptor for advanced glycation end product

TGF—transforming growth factor
TIMP—tissue inhibitor of metalloproteinases
TNF—tumor necrosis factor

VAL—vertical attachment loss
VCAM—vascular cell adhesion molecule
VWF—von Willebrand factor

WHO—World Health Organization

INDEX

Page references followed by "f" denote figures; those followed by "t" denote tables; those followed by "b" denote boxes

A